Child and Adolescent Psychiatry The Essentials

Second Edition

Keith Cheng, MD
Adjunct Associate Professor
Department of Psychiatry
Oregon Health & Science University
Chief Medical Officer
Trillium Family Services
Portland, Oregon

Kathleen M. Myers, MD, MPH, MS, FAACAP
Associate Professor
University of Washington
School of Medicine
Director, Telemental Health Service
Seattle Children's Hospital
Seattle, Washington

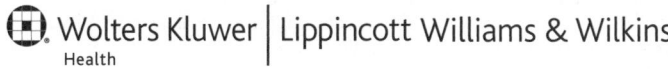
Wolters Kluwer | Lippincott Williams & Wilkins
Health
Philadelphia • Baltimore • New York • London
Buenos Aires • Hong Kong • Sydney • Tokyo

Acquisitions Editor: Charles Mitchell
Product Manager: Tom Gibbons
Vendor Manager: Bridgett Dougherty
Senior Manufacturing Manager: Benjamin Rivera
Marketing Manager: Brian Freiland
Design Coordinator: Teresa Mallon
Production Service: MPS Limited, A Macmillan Company

Second Edition

Printed in China

Library of Congress Cataloging-in-Publication Data

Child and adolescent psychiatry: the essentials/[edited by] Keith Cheng, Kathleen M. Myers.—2nd ed.
   p. ; cm.
  Includes bibliographical references and index.
  Summary: "Child and Adolescent Psychiatry: The Essentials, Second Edition presents comprehensive yet practical information about psychiatric problems in children and adolescents that can be used in a wide variety of clinical settings. Written by both psychiatrists and primary care providers, this concise and readable text is divided into four sections on evaluation, specific disorders, special issues, and treatment. Clinical case studies reinforce the major points in each chapter and tables present at-a-glance information on psychotropic drugs for various disorders. This edition has fifty percent new contributing authors, more information on evaluating polypharmaceutic approaches, and new chapters on fetal alcohol syndrome, nutritional psychiatry, and evidence-based psychotherapies"—Provided by publisher.
  ISBN-13: 978-1-60547-443-4 (alk. paper)
  ISBN-10: 1-60547-443-6 (alk. paper)
  1. Child psychiatry. 2. Adolescent psychiatry. I. Cheng, Keith. II. Myers, Kathleen M.
  [DNLM: 1. Mental Disorders—therapy. 2. Adolescent. 3. Child. WS 350 C53504 2011]
  RJ499.C48235 2011
  618.92'89—dc22

                  2010023516

10 9 8 7 6 5 4 3 2 1

Dr. Myers would like to acknowledge her family members,
Len, Mary, Lenny, Karen, Jeffery, and Jacqueline

Dr. Cheng would like to dedicate the second edition
in memory of his parents, George and Arlene.

CONTENTS

CONTRIBUTORS

My Banh, PhD
Postdoctoral Fellow
Department of Psychiatry and Behavioral
  Sciences
University of Washington School of Medicine
Psychiatry and Behavioral Medicine
Seattle Children's Hospital
Seattle, Washington

Rebecca A. Baum, MD
Clinical Assistant Professor of Pediatrics
The Ohio State University
Nationwide Children's Hospital
Columbus, Ohio

Gail A. Bernstein, MD
Endowed Professor in Child and Adolescent
  Anxiety Disorders
Division of Child and Adolescent Psychiatry
University of Minnesota Medical School
Minneapolis, Minnesota

David Breiger, PhD
Clinical Associate Professor
Department of Psychiatry and Behavioral
  Sciences
University of Washington School of Medicine
Department of Child Psychiatry and Behavioral
  Medicine
Seattle Children's Hospital
Seattle, Washington

Oscar G. Bukstein, MD, MPH
Professor of Psychiatry
Department of Psychiatry
Western Psychiatric Institute and Clinic
University of Pittsburgh School of Medicine
Pittsburgh, Pennsylvania

Rosemary Calderon, PhD
Associate Professor
Division of Child and Adolescent Psychiatry
Department of Psychiatry and Behavioral Sciences
University of Washington School of Medicine
Clinical Director
Eating Disorders Program
Department of Child Psychiatry and Behavioral
  Medicine
Seattle Children's Hospital
Seattle, Washington

Keith Cheng, MD
Adjunct Associate Professor
Department of Psychiatry
Oregon Health & Science University
Medical Director
Trillium Family Services
Portland, Oregon

Ann Childers, MD
Staff Psychiatrist
Clackamas County Mental Health
Oregon City, Oregon

Brent Collett, PhD
Assistant Professor
Department of Psychiatry and Behavioral
  Sciences
University of Washington School of Medicine
Attending Psychologist
Department of Child Psychiatry and Behavioral
  Medicine
Seattle Children's Hospital
Seattle, Washington

Joan M. Daughton, MD
Assistant Professor
Department of Psychiatry
University of Nebraska Medical Center
Omaha, Nebraska

Cynthia Flynn, PhD
Acting Assistant Professor
Department of Psychiatry and Behavioral
 Sciences
University of Washington School of Medicine
Staff Psychologist
Department of Child Psychiatry and Behavioral
 Medicine
Seattle Children's Hospital
Seattle, Washington

William P. French, MD
Acting Assistant Professor
Department of Psychiatry and Behavioral
 Sciences
University of Washington School of Medicine
Staff Psychiatrist
Department of Child Psychiatry and Behavioral
 Medicine
Seattle Children's Hospital
Seattle, Washington

Mary Margaret Gleason, MD, FAAP
Assistant Professor
Tulane University School of Medicine
New Orleans, Louisiana

Chia Granda, MD
Fellow, Triple Board Program
Brown University
Providence, Rhode Island

Gretchen R. Gudmundsen, PhD
Acting Assistant Professor
Department of Psychiatry and Behavioral
 Sciences
University of Washington School of Medicine
Attending Psychologist
Department of Child Psychiatry and Behavioral
 Medicine
Seattle Children's Hospital
Seattle, Washington

Toi Blakley Harris, MD
Assistant Professor
Menninger Department of Psychiatry and
 Behavioral Sciences
Baylor University
Houston, Texas

Robert J. Hilt, MD
Assistant Professor
Department of Psychiatry and Behavioral
 Sciences
University of Washington School of Medicine
Director, Emergency Psychiatric Services
Department of Child Psychiatry and Behavioral
 Medicine
Seattle Children's Hospital
Seattle, Washington

Stefanie A. Hlastala, PhD
Assistant Professor
Department of Psychiatry and Behavioral
 Sciences
University of Washington School of Medicine
Attending Psychologist
Department of Child Psychiatry and Behavioral
 Medicine
Seattle Children's Hospital
Seattle, Washington

Jenise Jensen, PhD
Children's Neurodevelopmental Services, Inc.
Salt Lake City, Utah

Ajit N. Jetmalani, MD
Director of Child Psychiatry Training
Joseph Professorship in Child and Adolescent
 Psychiatry Education
Division of Child and Adolescent
Oregon Health & Sciences University
Portland, Oregon

Kyle P. Johnson, MD
Associate Professor
Co-Medical Director of the Oregon Health &
 Science University Sleep Disorders Program
Departments of Psychiatry and Pediatrics
Oregon Health & Science University
Portland, Oregon

Kelly J. Kelleher, MD, MPH
ADS/Chlapaty Endowed Chair for Innovation
in Pediatric Practice
Professor of Pediatrics, Public Health, and
Psychiatry
Departments of Pediatrics and Psychiatry
Colleges of Medicine and Public Health
Ohio State University
Vice President for Community Health and
Community Health Services Research
The Center for Innovation in Pediatric Practice
The Research Institute at Nationwide Children's
Hospital
Columbus, Ohio

Bryan H. King, MD
Professor and Vice Chair
Department of Psychiatry and Behavioral
Sciences
University of Washington School of Medicine
Director
Department of Child Psychiatry and Behavioral
Medicine
Seattle Children's Hospital
Seattle, Washington

Stephanie King, PhD
Intervention Specialist/School Psychologist
Northern Suburban Special Education District
Northshore Academy Integrated Program
Highland Park, Illinois

Ian Kodish, MD, PhD
Acting Assistant Professor
Department of Psychiatry and Behavioral
Sciences
University of Washington School of Medicine
Attending Psychiatrist
Department of Child Psychiatry and Behavioral
Medicine
Seattle Children's Hospital
Seattle, Washington

Alison Leary, PhD
Child Clinical Psychologist
Evidence-Based Treatment Centers of Seattle
Seattle, Washington

Andrea K. Maikovich-Fong, PhD
Psychology Resident
University of Pennsylvania
Philadelphia, Pennsylvania
Department of Child Psychiatry and Behavioral
Medicine
Seattle Children's Hospital
Seattle, Washington

Elizabeth McCauley, PhD, ABPP
Professor
Division of Psychiatry and Behavioral Medicine
Seattle Children's Hospital
Department of Psychiatry and Behavioral
Sciences
University of Washington School of Medicine
Psychiatry and Behavioral Medicine
Seattle Children's Hospital
Seattle, Washington

Jon M. McClellan, MD
Professor
Department of Psychiatry and Behavioral
Sciences
University of Washington School of Medicine
Medical Director
Child Study and Treatment Center
Steilacoom, Washington

Kathleen M. Myers, MD, MPH, MS, FAACAP
Associate Professor
University of Washington School of Medicine
Director
TeleMental Health Service
Department of Child Psychiatry and Behavioral
Medicine
Seattle Children's Hospital
Seattle, Washington

Heather Carmichael Olson, PhD
Senior Lecturer
Department of Psychiatry and Behavioral
Sciences
University of Washington School of Medicine
Families Moving Forward FASD Intervention
Research Program
Seattle Children's Hospital Research Institute
Seattle, Washington

Francheska Perepletchikova, PhD
Yale University School of Medicine
New Haven, Connecticut

Norm Reed, PhD
Consulting Psychologist
Oregon Youth Authority
Salem, Oregon
Trillium Family Services
Portland, Oregon

Carol Rockhill, MD, PhD, MPH
Acting Assistant Professor
Division of Psychiatry and Behavioral Medicine
Seattle Children's Hospital
Department of Psychiatry and Behavioral Sciences
University of Washington School of Medicine
Psychiatry and Behavioral Medicine
Seattle Children's Hospital
Seattle, Washington

John Sargent, MD
Professor of Psychiatry and Pediatrics
Tufts Medical Center
Boston, Massachusetts

Kelly Schloredt, PhD
Clinical Assistant Professor
Department of Psychiatry and Behavioral Sciences
University of Washington School of Medicine
Clinical Director
Inpatient Psychiatric Unit
Department of Child Psychiatry and Behavioral
 Medicine
Seattle Children's Hospital
Seattle, Washington

Cindy Smith, MD, MPH
Medical Director
Children's Farm Home
Corvallis, Oregon

Jamie Snyder, MD
Assistant Professor
Creighton University
Training Director
Child and Adolescent Psychiatry, Post-Pediatric
 Portal Program
Omaha, Nebraska

Dorothy E. Stubbe, MD
Associate Professor
Program Director
Yale Child Study Center
Department of Child and Adolescent Psychiatry
Yale University School of Medicine
New Haven, Connecticut

Elizabeth Super, MD
Assistant Professor
Department of Pediatrics
Oregon Health & Science University
Portland, Oregon

Karen Toth, PhD
Assistant Professor
Department of Psychiatry and Behavioral
 Sciences
University of Washington School of Medicine
Staff Psychologist
Department of Child Psychiatry and Behavioral
 Medicine
Seattle Children's Hospital
Seattle, Washington

Jenny Tsai, MD
Child Psychiatrist
Parry Center
Trillium Child and Family Services
Portland, Oregon

Andrea M. Victor, PhD
Assistant Professor
Division of Child and Adolescent Psychiatry
University of Minnesota Medical School
Minneapolis, Minnesota

Nancy C. Winters, MD
Department of Psychiatry, Division of Public
 Psychiatry
Oregon Health & Science University
Portland, Oregon

Child and adolescent psychiatry continues to be a severely underserved medical specialty. The shortage of child and adolescent psychiatrists disproportionately affects certain populations. In particular, children of ethnic minorities and those living in rural communities and inner cities experience shortages that are now considered to have reached a crisis level. There are approximately 7500 child psychiatrists practicing in a country with more than 74 million children. Child and adolescent psychiatry is the only medical specialty that comprehensively trains physicians to treat youth with complex mental disorders. Yet only approximately 300 child and adolescent psychiatrists graduate annually from training programs. Thus, there is little hope that this disparity in access to specialty mental health services will be remedied through child and adolescent psychiatry alone.

Primary care clinicians continue to provide the majority of psychiatric treatment for pediatric populations. Pediatricians estimate that 20% of their patients have behavioral and emotional disorders in need of psychiatric treatment. There has been an increasing emphasis from families, insurers, professional organizations, and other stakeholders for children's mental disorders to be treated in primary care. Indeed, the American Academy of Pediatrics has developed guidelines to improve the delivery of evidence-based care to children with common psychiatric disorders, such as attention-deficit hyperactivity disorder (ADHD) and depression.

Noting these changes in the direction of mental health care of children since the first edition was published in 2005, this second edition emphasizes timely research findings in the evaluation and treatment of childhood psychiatric disorders that will help to guide the medical and nonmedical professionals treating children with mental health problems.

Recent studies have given new emphasis on the primary role of pharmacologic treatments for various childhood disorders, including ADHD, depressive disorders, and anxiety disorders. The use of antidepressants continues to be controversial. The Food and Drug Administration (FDA) still maintains a black box warning regarding the risk of suicidality in youth prescribed antidepressants, but some research over the past 5 years has concluded that curtailing prescriptions of antidepressants actually has led to an increased rate of youth suicide. In these 5 years since the first edition, research with youth suffering from schizophrenia, bipolar disorder, and autism have led to the FDA approval of three second-generation antipsychotics for use in pediatric populations. Research in psychotherapy has also increased the evidence base for selected psychotherapies for depression, anxiety, and disruptive disorders. Trauma-focused cognitive–behavioral therapy (CBT) has been shown in several randomized trials to be effective in the treatment of trauma-related symptoms. Exposure and response prevention has been shown effective in the treatment of obsessive–compulsive disorder (OCD).

Perhaps the most interesting findings during the past 5 years are for mood and anxiety disorders. The combination of psychotropic medication and psychotherapy is superior to medication or psychotherapy alone. The Treatment of Adolescent Depression Study (TADS) has shown that combination treatment is significantly superior to antidepressants alone or CBT alone in the treatment of depression and that psychotherapy protects against suicidality in those youth also treated with antidepressants. The Child/Adolescent Anxiety Multimodal Study (CAMS) also showed that combination therapy is superior to treatment with either medication or psychotherapy alone. These developments point to the need for clinicians to be aware that collaboration among clinicians with specific areas of expertise is necessary to provide a comprehensive treatment for youth who suffer from serious psychiatric illness.

Thus, the major audiences for this textbook are pediatricians, family physicians, and nurse practitioners who increasingly encounter children with diverse mental health needs in their practices. General psychiatrists who are often recruited to treat childhood mental disorders particularly in rural areas, and trainees interested in children's mental health, are also a target audience. These medical professionals should find valuable information on diagnosis and treatment to guide their practices. The emphasis is on basic information that will guide clinical practice. We avoid emphasis on esoteric information that, while interesting and cutting edge, can cloud clinical practice. Other mental health clinicians such as psychiatric social workers, special education teachers, and psychologists should appreciate learning of the status of child and adolescent psychiatry and what transpires in clinical treatment.

The second edition of *Child and Adolescent Psychiatry: The Essentials* continues to strive to meet the needs of clinicians wanting a concise but detailed source for practical information to guide treatment planning for youth with psychiatric illness. The second edition has retained many chapters and authors from the first edition. We have retained chapters on all of the disorders covered in the first edition and added a chapter on elimination disorders as this is a disorder often encountered in primary care. In Section III (Special Issues), we now add a chapter on the treatment of mental health problems in the general health setting, such as primary care. Two chapters address young children, early childhood mental health, and fetal alcohol spectrum disorders. Finally, given the increasing emphasis on nutrition for our nation's youth as well as a growing interest in complementary, alternative, and integrative medicine, we have included a chapter on nutritional aspects of psychiatric disorders. The "Treatment" section has been consolidated into three chapters. The psychopharmacology and systems of care chapters have been retained. A new chapter on evidence-based psychotherapies provides medical specialists and nonpsychiatric mental health professionals updated information on the evidence base supporting various psychotherapies for youth.

Finally, this second edition also includes updated bibliographies, tables, case vignettes, and suggested readings. Many clinicians are now using the Internet as a reference for clinical information. To keep up with this trend, the second edition now includes suggested useful websites for each chapter. Review questions for each chapter provide a quick check on material learned. These questions should help those using the textbook as a review before board examination or residency or fellowship in-service examinations.

The first edition has served a broad readership from child psychiatry trainees to pediatricians. Some training programs have used the first edition for organizing readings for seminars. Behavioral health training programs for pediatricians have also used the first edition as the major textbook for their courses. Child psychiatrists have used the first edition to assist them in preparing for board examinations. We hope the second edition continues to serve the needs of primary care clinicians as well as psychiatrists, through the overall goal of providing existing information in child and adolescent psychiatry in a succinct and organized volume so we can all improve the lives of our young patients who are among the most needy and underserved youths.

Since the publication of the first edition of *Child and Adolescent Psychiatry: The Essentials,* the amount of new research regarding the assessment and treatment of pediatric psychiatric disorders has continued to increase dramatically. Our goal in the second edition has been to incorporate this new information in our quest to keep our readers up to date. More importantly, there has been an emphasis on making this volume useful for primary care clinicians. This is in concert with the national drive to integrate psychiatric and primary clinicians in the provision of mental health treatment to children and adolescents. In order to address the shortage of child psychiatrists, both psychiatric and primary care clinicians must work together to meet this challenge. Therefore, the education of all clinicians treating youth with mental health problems continues to be the primary goal for the second edition. We hope that all those who use this volume will find their ability greatly enhanced in treating youth with psychiatric disorders.

Keith Cheng
Kathleen Myers

CHAPTER 1

Nancy C. Winters, MD,
and Jenny Tsai, MD

Psychiatric Assessment of Children and Adolescents

Introduction

The primary goal of psychiatric assessment of a child or an adolescent is to determine whether psychopathology is present and, if so, to establish a differential diagnosis, articulate a tentative diagnostic formulation, and develop a treatment plan in collaboration with the child or adolescent, and family. In order to reach this goal, much clinical and historic information needs to be gathered. We describe here a comprehensive psychiatric assessment. There are, however, situations in which specialized or focused assessments occur (e.g., forensic evaluation or risk assessment), and we will briefly review some such situations. Since time for assessment may be limited by external constraints such as funding or resources, a cogent method of assessment and treatment planning is pertinent. The aim of this chapter is to bring nonchild psychiatrists an understanding of the goals of psychiatric evaluation as well as a picture of what happens during psychiatric assessment. In this chapter, we refer to both children and adolescents as "children," except when discussing specific developmental variations. The term "parents" is used for the child's caregivers, who may include biologic, adoptive, or foster parents, or other family caregivers.

History Gathering

As summarized in Table 1-1, a comprehensive psychiatric assessment should include the following elements: (a) important identifying information, for example, child's age, sex, and grade in school; (b) the referral source and reason for referral; (c) sources of information; (d) history of the current problem(s); (e) past psychiatric history; (f) medical and developmental history including intrauterine experiences, and past and current medications; (g) educational history; (h) family social and psychiatric history; (i) social history including substance and tobacco use, sexual behavior, peer relationships, and legal history; (j) history of trauma and/or stressors; (k) mental status evaluation; (l) clinical formulation and *Diagnostic and Statistical Manual of Mental Disorders*, Fourth Edition (DSM-IV-TR) multiaxial diagnosis; (m) a problem list; and (n) treatment plan keyed to the problem list.

TABLE 1-1	Essentials of Psychiatric Assessment
• Identifying information (age, sex, grade in school, etc.) • Sources of information • Referral source • Chief complaint or reason for referral (note that chief complaint may differ between parent and child) • History of present situation • Past psychiatric (mental health) history • Current medications (and psychotropic medication history) • Medical/developmental history • Educational history (including special education services) • Family history (both psychiatric and social aspects)	• Cultural context (migration history, ethnic identification, religious affiliation) • Trauma history • Social history (peer relationships, activities, sexual behavior) • Use of electronic media, including Internet, cellular phone, video games, and movies • Substance and tobacco use • Legal history • Mental status examination • Clinical formulation (including strengths and prognosis) • *DSM-IV* diagnosis • Problem list • Treatment plan, including patient and family's goals for treatment

Special Considerations in Evaluating Children

There are important differences between the psychiatric assessment of children and that of adults. The most pertinent issue is that an evaluation of a child is generally initiated by the child's parents or other adults involved in the child's care (as in the case of a school referral). An exception may be the older adolescent who independently seeks treatment. Children may thus be anxious or even shamed in the initial contacts, and it is thus important to establish a positive and safe climate for them.

The rapid pace of children's development, especially in early childhood, requires familiarity with the different competencies, vulnerabilities, and tasks of each stage of development. Different methods of collecting data and interviewing the child apply at different ages. For example, the infant or toddler is generally assessed with the parent, with special attention to the dyadic interactions, whereas adolescents are best able to furnish relevant clinical information when interviewed alone. There are also differences in the way children at different ages are able to report their symptoms. The younger child tends to have less ability to self-observe and may not have the vocabulary to describe feeling states. Also, symptoms developed early, such as obsessions or compulsions, may be experienced by the child as part of himself or herself and not be recognized as problems.

Because children are more dependent on their adult caretakers, an adequate assessment requires a comprehensive understanding of important environmental characteristics and family relationships, as well as the child's response to them. Factors such as poverty, family violence, and parental substance abuse or mental health problems all increase the risk of a child developing a psychiatric disorder, and may also impair the family's ability to adequately respond to the child's problem.

Development of a differential diagnosis also differs when evaluating children. First, those disorders not specific to childhood, such as depression or obsessive–compulsive disorder, may show developmental variations. For example, depressed children may present as more irritable than sad, and compulsions in children may be experienced as acceptable, or egosyntonic. Additionally, a psychiatric disorder in evolution may have a different, possibly less "differentiated" earlier presentation. For example, young children with early oppositional behavior may later develop mood or anxiety disorders, and schizophrenia may be preceded by social abnormalities and neuropsychological deficits. Thus, the clinician must inform the parents that there can be some uncertainty about the eventual diagnosis. In practice, child psychiatric assessment is generally an ongoing process that occurs over time. The reality, however, is that children with serious mental health problems who experience significant functional impairment cannot wait for intervention because of negative impact on their development as well as caretaker burnout and community safety. Also there is growing evidence that early treatment can improve the outcome of child psychiatric disorders. Therefore, even in conditions of uncertainty, a preliminary diagnosis and treatment plan are important, as well as a plan for further data collection based on an initial hypothesis. To arrive at a diagnosis, many pieces of information must be brought together. The child psychiatrist is in the unique position of integrating the medical, psychological, social, and developmental aspects of the child, while other clinicians may address specific components.

Sources of Information

The assessment of the child requires that information be obtained not only from the child but also from the family, school, primary physician, and past mental health providers. Obtaining information from multiple sources allows the clinician to better gauge whether the problem is global (occurring across all settings) or circumscribed to a certain environment. For children involved in the juvenile justice, child welfare, special education, or developmental disabilities systems, review of information from the agency records or caseworker is essential. Past and current medical records are helpful in discerning any medical issues that may contribute to behavioral or mood problems.

Clarifying the purpose and goal of the referral at the very outset is essential. Although the child's behavioral and mood problems may be the obvious reason for referral, other more covert intentions may be present. For example, a pending juvenile court decision may be the motivating factor for an adolescent to seek "treatment," rather than his or her condition itself propelling the desire for treatment. Parental custody conflicts and threats of school expulsion may be other motivating factors that promote the initial visit to a clinician's office. These other intentions have implications regarding diagnosis and treatment recommendations, in addition to prognosis. For example, parental custody conflicts may influence a parent to overreport or underreport the child's symptoms. At times, the referral may have been requested by adults other than the parents, for example, by the school or court, in which case parental permission usually is needed unless the child is a ward of the state, in which case consent of the caseworker is needed.

One informative question to ask at the beginning of an assessment is "why now?" Often, there is an acute stress incident that finally makes the parents realize their child needs professional help. Whether the parent recognizes the child's need for help soon after problems develop or after the child has become very disturbed provides information about the closeness of the parent–child relationship and how well the family functions in promoting the health of family members. Often, fear of stigma delays seeking help for mental health conditions, and understanding the parents' or child's apprehensiveness facilitates forming a more collaborative relationship. This may be especially important when there are cultural, ethnic, religious, or even social class differences between the patient and the clinician, and these differences may contribute to delays in seeking treatment.

The Clinical Interview

The structure of assessment interviews depends on the individual case. It may be appropriate to have one or two initial interviews with the parents alone, especially when the patient is a younger child. This allows the parents to share a complete history of the problem without concern about what the child may hear. It also allows the parents to communicate about their response to the child and their own personal issues or concerns that may impact the child's mental health. That is not to say this is the only approach. One advantage of an initial conjoint interview with the child and parents is the opportunity to observe family interactions, such as the family's manner of communicating with and about the child, whether the family exhibits aggression or affection, concern or derision toward one another, who sets the rules, and whether the parents argue in front of the child. How the parent communicates with the child also provides information as to his or her understanding of the child's developmental capacity and the parent's attunement to the child's state of mind. During the conjoint interview, one can also appreciate the stress a child's difficulties place on a parent, even with otherwise normal parenting skills.

With adolescents, however, it is usually preferable to include the adolescent in interviews with the parents, as not doing so may risk the teenager's feeling that the clinician is colluding with the parents, with the result that a therapeutic alliance may be much more difficult to establish. An older adolescent may prefer to attend the first appointment alone. In either case, the child or adolescent should be prepared for the evaluation. At times, when parents think their child may refuse to come for a psychiatric evaluation, they may deceive the child by saying he or she will be taken to a medical doctor or a special school. The clinician then has the extra challenge to overcome the child's sense of betrayal by the parent and to manage the child's displaced anger and annoyance. It is also helpful to advise the parent to communicate the purpose of the evaluation in a manner that is supportive and nonblaming of the child, such as "we are going to see a kind doctor who will help you with your worries."

Once the family comes in, the primary task is to build a therapeutic alliance with the family and child. This means setting up an ambience of respect, warmth, and trustworthiness. Some means of doing this include having good eye contact, allowing ample time for all participants to describe their concerns, and speaking in a respectful, concerned way. Some adults and children may be intimidated by visiting a clinician. Asking the child simple questions such as his or her name or birthday, and the names of his or her siblings may help put the child at ease. Asking the child to spell his or her name or write down his or her birthday and other family members' birthdays on a piece of paper may lend valuable information regarding the child's cognitive abilities. With regard to teens, discussing hobbies, interests, and job responsibilities can create a sense of ease and convey that the clinician is interested in what they have to say.

Once a sense of mutual regard is established, the next stage of the interview involves exploring the reason for bringing the child in for evaluation, that is, the chief complaint. The goal is to ascertain the child's current difficulties and the impact of his or her symptoms on parents and the family. If there are several complaints, it is important to understand how disturbing each one is from the child's and the parents' points of view, and which ones they would like to address first in treatment. As the assessment progresses, it is not uncommon for the prioritization of concerns to change. Elaborating on the chief complaint entails careful data gathering of the frequency and severity of the problem, as well as the where, when, and how of the situation. A functional analysis of behavioral disturbance is helpful. Any elucidated triggering or alleviating factors should be explored. Does the behavior occur only at school, at home, or at both places? Is it in relation to only specific people, or does the child's behavior occur globally? What impact has this had on the child and family? How long has this behavior or symptom been occurring?

In addition to exploring current issues, it is crucial to learn about past psychiatric history, medical history, medications, family psychiatric history, social history, school functioning, legal involvement, and a review of systems. Each of these realms may provide a clue and/or have an influence on the present complaint. For example, if it is found in the substance abuse history that a teenager has abused illicit drugs in the past, it is possible that the parent's complaints that he or she is displaying agitated behaviors might be related to drug use. Similarly, in a child presenting with depressive symptoms, a review of the past medical history and medications may yield clues regarding the etiology. If a parent has a particular psychiatric disorder, he or she may be requesting an evaluation to see whether the child might be similarly affected. Such a situation requires balancing sensitivity to the parent's concerns with conducting an objective assessment of the child as a separate individual. Social history should also include a review of the child's extracurricular activities and peer relationships, especially whether the child is being bullied at school. Also, clarifying the nature and extent of the child's use of electronic media, including the Internet, video/computer games, text messaging, and movies, may be related to the presenting complaint, as in the case of a teenager who met with a stranger she met on the Internet, or the child at risk for aggression whose behavior is exacerbated by violent content in movies or video games, or the socially isolated teenager who spends excessive time playing Internet games. The importance of investigating the child's use of electronic media is highlighted by several recent investigations that have found a role in psychiatric disturbances, sexual victimization, and suicide. As reviewed by Huesmann, exposure to violence in electronic media is associated with increased aggression, especially in youth already at risk for psychiatric disorder. Other work has shown cyberspace-related victimization and promotion of suicide among young people. Even simple television viewing as toddlers appears related to the development of attention-deficit hyperactivity disorder (ADHD). Family members' use of electronic media is also important to explore, as parental preoccupation with online relationships may be disturbing to children. Similar to parental tobacco, drug, and alcohol use, excessive use of electronic media in adults may influence these behaviors in children.

It is worth noting that each individual family member may have a different perspective about the child's problem. This is relevant in the case of the child's parents, who, whether living together or divorced, are likely to perceive the child differently. Each point of view is likely to contain some kernel of truth. The parents may disagree in a way that compromises their ability to function together as parents and thereby contributes to the presenting problem. Such differences may relate to the parents' family-of-origin issues, differences in parenting styles, current psychiatric conditions, or stressors. How a parent describes the child's difficulties is also informative about the parent–child relationship. For example, a parent who describes the child's behavior in pejorative terms may be angry at home and may need additional help to support the child.

An analysis of the child's environment is an integral part of the assessment. The child's functioning is highly influenced by his or her ecologic context, which includes the "microsystem" of his or her family, school, and immediate neighborhood and the "macrosystem" of his or her larger community and culture. Exploring contributing factors within the home, school, community, and larger culture can yield clues for effective interventions. Culture is an integral aspect of family life, and this area should be included in the child's psychiatric assessment. Important aspects of the cultural interview include the family's ethnic identification, their relationship with a cultural community, the family's migration history, the structure of the extended family including languages spoken and roles of each family member, religious affiliations, child-rearing practices that may be related to culture, and the family's attitudes about illness and health care, including use of traditional healing. Of particular relevance to the presenting problem may be the child's attempts to live within both his or her family's traditional values and his or her new American culture. As described by Abad and Sheldon, differences in the degree of acculturation between immigrant parents and their children may cause family turmoil. Such issues should be explicitly raised with the child and family so that they realize these are appropriate issues to discuss and that the clinician is interested in their circumstances. The essentials of obtaining a psychiatric history are summarized in Table 1-2.

Developmental Issues
One main goal during the history gathering and mental status examination is to gauge the child's developmental stage in order to recommend appropriate interventions. This entails the evaluator's understanding variations of normal and abnormal child development, including

TABLE 1-2	Essentials of History Taking
• Clarify the chief complaint(s) and the goals for treatment • Clarify who is requesting the assessment and for what purpose • Determine the contexts in which problems occur • Incorporate information from school or child care, the other parent, health care or other mental health provider, and any other involved agencies, for example, juvenile justice and child welfare	• Interview the child or adolescent alone, as well as the family • Use open-ended questions; with young children, observing and describing play is more helpful • Ask about sexuality, substance use, and self-harm behaviors or impulses • Integrate information from parent(s) and child, especially in disruptive behavior disorders • Observe and consider parent–child and family dynamics • Consider discrepancies between different adults' perceptions of the child, and discrepancies between adults' and child's perceptions

the expected range of behaviors at different ages and the typical manifestations of sundry forms of disturbances in each developmental phase. The evaluator ideally would be skilled in verbal and nonverbal techniques for assessing the child. In general, children are not silver-tongued historians who narrate their travails in a straightforward verbal fashion, although there are exceptions. Hence, in order to elicit information that may be helpful in evaluating the child's current mental status and developmental level, the evaluator should be familiar with a variety of techniques that may facilitate information sharing on the child's part. Relevant aspects of the developmental assessment are summarized in Table 1-3.

Younger children, particularly preschool and early-school-aged children, are more able to communicate their thoughts, fears, and perceptions of themselves and others through play. Techniques for engaging the child in evaluative play include following the child's lead, using humor, exploring the child's interests, encouraging imaginative play, and matching the affect the child expresses during the interview. For younger children, it is usually advisable to start out making observations about the child's play. Small children can easily become frustrated with too many questions, and refuse to interact further. Other ways of engaging young children include reflecting the child's ideas and vocabulary, and using projective questions, for example, "If you had three wishes, what would they be?" "What animal would you choose to be if you could be one?" "Who would you take with you if you went on a trip to Mars?"

One common nonverbal projective technique is children's drawings. The results of free drawing can yield insights into the child's present state and developmental level. An unstructured drawing allows the child to demonstrate his or her interests and preoccupations. Children who have experienced trauma will frequently show the trauma event in their drawing when asked to draw whatever they wish. What the child chooses to include or leave out in the drawing is also informative. For example, a child leaving his or her father out of the family drawing may indicate the father's lack of presence in the child's life. Where the child positions himself or herself in a family drawing also may suggest to whom the child feels closest. There are also several structured drawings with psychometric properties that may be used to ascertain the child's developmental level or internal processes. These include the Draw-a-Person, Kinetic Family Drawing, and House-Tree-Person Drawing. The child's sharing of his or her drawings also gives the clinician an experience of the child's interpersonal relatedness. If the child shows a good capacity for drawing mechanical objects, but people are absent or minimally represented in his or her drawings, this may signal difficulties in the interpersonal sphere and lead one to consider a pervasive developmental disorder diagnosis as opposed to a motor coordination disorder.

TABLE 1-3   Developmental Aspects of the Child Interview

Preschool
- Use observational and play interaction as opposed to verbal assessment.
- Assess motor functioning, language skills, and social relatedness.
- Assess parent–child interaction.
- Allow more time for evaluation in order to provide child the opportunity to demonstrate skills that cannot be conveyed verbally at this age.

School age
- Consider the wide normal variation in the ability to verbalize.
- Integrate verbal techniques and play, encouraging imaginative themes.
- Use board games to facilitate verbal interaction, especially regarding rules.
- Obtain children's perspective as they are capable of reporting both internalizing and externalizing symptoms, but integrate with parents' report, especially for internalizing symptoms.
- Provide anchors for symptom onset and evolution as children have difficulty comprehending the chronology or time frame for symptom development.
- Consider the role of peers as they take on increasing importance at this stage of development.

Adolescence
- Incorporate abstract concepts and time frames, for example, the adolescent's perspective on significance of symptoms, comparing current symptoms with usual baseline.
- Increase reliance on adolescents' perspective as they are able to give accurate history of symptoms, particularly internalizing symptoms.
- Ask about adolescents' type of peer group that will reveal their self-perception.
- Assess the adolescent's ability to show empathy for others, which should be evident at this age, including for parents.

Toys can also facilitate the interaction with small children. A large number of toys are not needed; examples are shown in Table 1-4. Ideally, the office would have toys that can allow a wide range of self-expression, fantasy, and role-play of child-relevant themes. Such toys include a set of play telephones; a family set of dolls; a dollhouse; action figures to allow for possible themes of dependency, avoidance, or aggression to be expressed; and materials such as modeling clay, which the child may shape into whatever he or she has on his or her mind. Having a few board games may be helpful for latency-aged children, who may enjoy competition with the interviewer. This provides an opportunity to assess the child's appreciation of the use of rules and ability to interact reciprocally and fairly.

In general, it is best to have toys available that are tailored to the child's developmental stage and issues, for example, toys that promote imaginative play; are not noisy, overly complex, or overstimulating; and, especially for the younger child, are simple to manipulate and safe. It is

---

TABLE 1-4   Essentials for Evaluation through Play

- Dollhouse with family of dolls (including mother, father, and children), furniture, and toilet
- Set of play telephones
- Doctor's kit
- Set of blocks or Legos for building
- Paper, pencils, and crayons for drawing and writing; clay or Play-Doh
- Puppets
- Animal and human figures, motor vehicles for action-oriented play
- Board games (e.g., Checkers and Candyland)

helpful to keep toys in a cabinet so the child is not distracted by a roomful of toys and can select what he or she wants. In an increasingly ethnically diverse population, it is helpful to have a variety of dolls of different ethnic appearances. This allows children of various cultures and ethnicities to easily express their family-of-origin issues as well as patterns of identification within the community. Observation of the child drawing or playing not only yields important information regarding the child's inner fantasy world and perceptions, but also provides preliminary data regarding the child's relatedness, motor coordination, cognitive abilities, impulsivity, distractibility, ability to concentrate, and compulsivity. For example, a child unable to make eye contact would bring into consideration not only a pervasive developmental disorder but also attachment disorder, social anxiety, psychosis, or depression. The child's choices in play can also help with differential diagnosis. For example, a child who repetitively acts out traumatic themes such as a serious house fire or physical abuse is showing symptoms of re-experiencing suggestive of posttraumatic stress disorder.

When interviewing teens, it is important to offer some degree of confidentiality to allow them to openly discuss issues such as sexuality, substance use, use of electronic media, illegal activity, or impulses to harm themselves. However, they should also be told that their parents need to be informed about potential danger to them. It is best in that situation to help the teen to share the information with his or her parent. It is always important to spend some time in the assessment process interviewing the child or the adolescent alone. Not only does this allow for direct assessment of his or her mental and emotional state, but it also gives him or her the opportunity to share thoughts and concerns that he or she may be unable or unwilling to share with his or her parents. Essential aspects of interviewing adolescents are summarized in Table 1-5.

Confidentiality Issues

Several aspects of confidentiality should be kept in mind during the evaluation. In the course of obtaining ancillary information, disclosing that a child is being evaluated psychiatrically requires consent by the child's legal guardian. Additional requirements as specified by the Health Insurance Portability and Accountability Act (HIPAA) concerning release of medical information, patients' review of records, and contacting patients also need to be observed. The clinician should also be aware of additional state laws relating to confidentiality and consent,

TABLE 1-5   Essentials of Interviewing Adolescents
• Include the adolescent in the initial interview with his or her parents to allay concerns about collusion with the parents.
• Interview the adolescent alone, providing him or her ample opportunity to share his or her point of view, interests, and concerns, without judgment.
• Inform the adolescent that what he or she shares will be confidential, with the exception of anything representing harm to him or her or to others. Let him or her know that should this information need to be shared with his or her parents, he or she will be informed and, if possible, present.
• Pursue tactful questioning, if the adolescent denies problems, to collaboratively understand why his or her parents are concerned.
• Demonstrate an ability to empathize with the adolescent and show a willingness to see things from his or her point of view.
• Provide positive feedback to reinforce the adolescent's strengths and adaptive behaviors within his or her cultural context.
• Address right away the problems the adolescent is experiencing. Problem solve with the adolescent, supporting his or her ability to generate solutions within his or her own life constraints, rather than giving advice.

particularly in relation to adolescents' right with respect to releasing records to their parents. Confidentiality requirements do not absolve a clinician from the legal requirement to report suspected child abuse or neglect, although some states may have an exception for clinicians conducting psychotherapy.

The Mental Status Examination

During the mental status examination, the clinician assesses many aspects of the child; some of the following will already have been observed during history gathering.

The child's physical appearance and behavior: What is his or her general state of health? Is the child well nourished? Is the child small, average, or large for age? Are there dysmorphic features, bruises, or cuts? If the child appears to be small and poorly nourished, or has dysmorphic features such as unusual eye spacing or ear shape, he or she will need a more comprehensive medical evaluation, including genetic testing. How is the child's grooming? Does the young child seem to be well cared for? What is the child's mode of dress (especially relevant to an adolescent), and is it appropriate to the child's gender, circumstances, and current fashion? Does the child look happy or sad in general, or anxious or angry?

Motor function: Is the child hyperactive, or does he or she have psychomotor retardation? Are there any abnormal movements such as tics, dystonias, or chorea? Are there motor asymmetries? How is the child's gait? Can the child do simple age-appropriate tasks such as hopping or drawing a circle? Subtle indices of neurologic functioning include pencil grasp, penmanship, smoothness of rapid alternating movements, and toe walking. This is a very useful part of the mental status exam as motor coordination difficulties are underidentified, and can lead to learning problems, low self-esteem, and withdrawal from physical activities with peers.

Affect and mood: What is the range of affects displayed (full or constricted), and are they appropriate to the situation? What does the child say about his or her mood? Is this consistent with the child's affect? Young children may need prompts such as drawings of faces with different expressions to describe their emotions. A persistently sad affect in a preadolescent child who does not show enthusiasm even when offered a variety of interesting toys to play with is very suggestive of mood disturbance, even if the child is unable to express in words that he or she is sad.

Speech and language: How well is the child able to use language to communicate? Is his or her vocabulary and overall use of language developmentally appropriate? How is his or her verbal fluency? Does he or she have articulation problems? Is the speech frenetic or pressured? Is the prosody normal? Does the child use nonverbal communication effectively? How does the child respond to "why" questions; for example, can the child express and embellish his or her ideas beyond answering "yes" or "no"? Is he or she able to converse reciprocally? A child or an adolescent with apparently normal or even advanced language abilities who speaks at length but shows no awareness of the clinician's response or level of interest may have Asperger disorder.

Thought process and content: Is the thought process organized, logical, and goal directed? Is the child's thinking idiosyncratic or delusional? Does the child have hallucinations? Does the child have suicidal thoughts/plans? Does the child engage in other self-injurious behavior, and what is the intent of the behavior? Does he or she have aggressive or homicidal thoughts or plans? Does the child display any fears or worries? Are there specific themes to his or her play, such as repeated traumatic themes? How does the child describe himself or herself in play or words (and what does this suggest about his or her self-image)? What is the child's vision of his or her future? Who are the important people in the child's life? What are his or her attitudes toward family, school, and peers? Young children may use storytelling as a way of communicating their preoccupations.

For example, a child who tells a story about a lost puppy may be feeling abandoned after the birth of a sibling.

Social relatedness: Does the child make eye contact? What is the parent–child interaction like? Is he or she able to separate from his or her parents? When with the interviewer, what is the level of the child's engagement, relatedness, and ability to interact reciprocally? How does he or she use verbal and nonverbal communication? Does the child appear to derive pleasure from the interaction? Does the child show expected curiosity and interest in the playroom, and does he or she have an appropriate understanding of physical boundaries? A child who runs to a clinician he or she has never met and asks for a hug should alert the clinician to consider diagnoses of reactive attachment disorder, sexual abuse, pervasive developmental disorder, or impulsivity related to ADHD.

Intellectual functioning: While considering where the child should be developmentally, intellectual functioning should be roughly gauged based on the following: vocabulary and language complexity, general fund of knowledge, level of play, complexity of drawings, and orientation to time, person, and place. A variety of standardized instruments also may be used for the younger child, such as the Goodenough–Harris Draw-a-Person test. Examination of the older child or adolescent's intellectual functioning can include more typical verbal approaches such as immediate recall of numbers, long-term recall of events, age-appropriate fund of knowledge, reading ability, and abstract thinking.

Judgment and insight: Judgment and insight vary with age and developmental level. Hypothetical questions that are keyed to the child's ability may be asked, for example, for a younger child, "What do you do when it's cold outside?," or for an adolescent, "What would you do if you were at a party and the friend who drove you was drinking alcohol?". Regarding insight, as adolescents do not initiate the evaluation, they may appear to have poor insight into the presenting problem. They may, however, have the capacity to develop insight over time or recognize how others perceive their behavior. Young children may be able to tell you they are sad or mad, or may be aware that they get in trouble for certain behaviors.

Rating Scales/Assessment Instruments

Over the years, many adjunctive tools such as rating scales have been developed to assess psychiatric symptoms in children. The interested reader is referred to Chapter 3 of this book. Rating scales range from systematized questionnaires that assess psychiatric symptoms in general to those that probe in depth a specific area of difficulty. Advantages to using rating scales include their assisting the clinician in the systematic evaluation of the child, including detecting problems that are clinically significant but are not part of presenting problem. Some youth may reveal concerns in writing that they do not verbalize. Rating scales also play an important part in evidence-based interventions by providing an easy numeric score for monitoring response to treatment. For example, an ADHD rating scale can be used to assess the child's response to stimulant treatment. Also, children's self-report questionnaires such as the Children's Depression Inventory (CDI) can be used by busy primary care practitioners to decide whether to treat or refer to a specialist, for example, if the child endorses suicidality or the score indicates severe depression. Disadvantages of using rating scales include the time needed to complete them, the feeling of being "check-listed," and clinicians' tendency to overrely on rating scales for diagnosis.

One must also be aware of the limits of what the scores of a rating scale might add to the overall clinical assessment. For example, one mental health worker had inquired of a psychiatrist why a patient was hospitalized when his or her Beck Depression Inventory (BDI) score was only a "3." As it turned out, the answer was that the patient had endorsed on the BDI that he or she wanted to kill himself or herself, and on further clinical interview, this patient had

TABLE 1-6	Medical Factors with Possible Psychiatric Presentation

- *Medications/drug-induced*: corticosteroids, benzodiazepines, amphetamines, anticholinergics, hallucinogens, antihypertensives
- *Endocrinologic*: Cushing disease, adrenal insufficiency, diabetes, hypothyroidism, hyperthyroidism, hypopituitarism, androgenization
- *Infectious/immunologic*: infectious mononucleosis, HIV, tuberculosis, neoplasms, lupus erythematosis, chronic fatigue syndrome, PANDAS (pediatric autoimmune neuropsychiatric disorders associated with streptococcal infection)
- *Neurologic*: epilepsy, migraine headache, central nervous system tumor, traumatic brain injury (recent or old), anoxia, demyelinating processes
- *Genetic*: Wilson disease, Prader–Willi syndrome, Klinefelter's syndrome, fragile X syndrome, velocardiofacial syndrome
- *Other*: uremia, hypoglycemia, electrolyte abnormalities, paraneoplastic syndrome

endorsed enough intention that the psychiatrist felt that he or she warranted hospitalization, especially when taking into account factors that were not in the scale, such as the patient's psychiatric history, substance use history, and current social support.

This being said, however, rating scales have numerous advantages that can contribute to efficient data gathering and improved clinical assessment. For example, the Conner's ADHD Rating Scale and the Child Behavior Checklist are straightforward questionnaires that can easily be given to the child's parents in the waiting room while the child is being assessed. These scales also have versions that can be completed by the child or adolescent and the child's teacher. Rating scales with demonstrated reliability and validity for the presenting clinical concern will be most useful. Also important are the scale's sensitivity and specificity; whether the scale is suitable for the population, setting, and the training of the rater; and the scale's sensitivity to change during treatment. Ultimately, diagnosis and assessment are based on clinical judgment, with rating scales used as adjuncts to a competent history and examination.

At times, the clinician may refer the child for other specialized evaluations. Such evaluations would include formal psychological testing, including psychometric and projective evaluation and/or neuropsychological testing. These evaluations would be especially pertinent if the diagnosis continues to be unclear and the clinician needs further clarification of the child's cognitive abilities, personality and temperament, thought disturbances, and added information about symptoms. Medical consultation also would be appropriate when there are questions concerning the child's physical conditions and medications that may be influencing the child's psychiatric presentation. Such conditions can especially include conditions of a neurologic, metabolic, endocrinologic, or genetic nature, as summarized in Table 1-6.

Clinical Formulation and Diagnosis

In this stage of the assessment, the clinician must formulate the most likely explanation of why the problem is occurring. This involves synthesizing the data that have been gathered and identifying the contributing factors that have brought the patient to assessment. A comprehensive clinical formulation includes a summary of predisposing, precipitating, perpetuating, and protective factors contributing to the current problem. Each of these factors may be described along the following dimensions: (a) biologic/constitutional (including prenatal, birth, and early temperament), (b) psychological/personality/temperament, (c) family/interpersonal, and (d) socioenvironmental. For example, in a 10-year-old boy presenting with disruptive behavior, predisposing factors (i.e., vulnerabilities) can range from genetic loading for ADHD (constitutional factor) to a disrupted early attachment relationship (family/interpersonal factor). Precipitating factors (i.e., stressors) may include an acute medical illness (biologic factor) or loss of family housing (socioenvironmental factor). Perpetuating factors may include low self-esteem (psychological factor) or parental substance abuse (family factor). Protective factors (i.e., strengths) may include intelligence (constitutional factor) or a positive relationship with a warm, caring adult outside the family (family/interpersonal factor). Consideration of risk factors such as poverty, abuse, low birth weight, difficult temperament, trauma exposure, and genetic factors is helpful in considering vulnerability to mental health disorders. Winters and colleagues have discussed how to construct a formulation and provide examples of multifactorial case formulations. The overall focus of the formulation is to understand what brings the child or youth to this point in life. In developing a formulation, it is helpful to consider the following:

- Why is the problem surfacing now?
- Has the child been experienced any changes, losses, or other stressors?
- What is the interplay between constitution, personality, and environment?
- How are the parent(s)' and child's vulnerabilities interacting?
- How does the child's view compare with the parents' view of the problem?
- How have the child and family adapted to the problem? Might this explain some of the symptoms?
- How is the child's development being affected by the primary problem?
- What are the child's and family's strengths that can support positive change?
- What social structures or natural supports are available to further support the family's strengths?

It should be remembered that just because a factor is present does not mean that it explains the problem. For example, a traumatic event may be less relevant to a child's disruptive behavior than mental retardation. Thus, the factors believed to be most relevant to the presenting problems should be emphasized. With this caveat, the following components should be included in a comprehensive clinical formulation:

- Brief case summary (several sentences, including demographic information, chief complaint, presenting problems, major signs and symptoms, and course of illness)
- Biologic characterization (genetic, medical, and constitutional)
- Precipitating stressors
- Psychological characterization (personality, intrapsychic issues, defense mechanisms, and cognitive style)
- Family and interpersonal factors
- Sociocultural factors (environment and larger ecologic context)
- Integrative statement: how the above-mentioned factors interact to lead to the current situation and the child's current level of functioning

This multifactorial synthesis need not comprise a major treatise. The purpose of the clinical formulation is not to rehash the specific data but to make succinct, integrative statements that lead to understanding how the child got to this point in his or her life and to the subsequent differential diagnosis. It is useful to think of stating the formulation much as one clinician would do when referring a patient to a colleague. A brief formulation provides a useful opportunity to think about and understand the child. It is a springboard for generating a broad differential diagnosis, allowing the clinician to determine whether there is sufficient evidence of a diagnosable syndrome, as well as prognostic factors that may contribute to worsening or improving the condition. One should not forget to include in the differential diagnosis any relevant parent–child conditions, organic factors, and personality features, and to address both internalizing and externalizing symptoms (which are often comorbid). It is essential that the full *DSM-IV* multiaxial diagnostic system be applied, as this system includes factors that may be contributing to the clinical picture as a whole and provides an overall assessment of how the child is functioning in the face of these psychiatric difficulties.

In many cases there are multiple factors to consider and/or comorbid conditions that complicate the diagnostic profile. A definitive diagnosis may not be appropriate initially. When the diagnostic picture is still unclear, it may be necessary to extend the evaluation period. The clinician should explain to the child and parents that ongoing assessment during treatment may be appropriate.

Special Situations

A number of special situations may lead to a request for psychiatric evaluation. Common among these are evaluations directly requested by another agency such as the school, juvenile justice, or child welfare agency. In these cases, it is important to clarify the specific reason for the referral and whether the custodial parent has given permission for the evaluation. Confidentiality issues differ in these specialized situations in that the parents and child need to understand that the evaluation report will be sent to the requesting agency. The specific question dictates the areas to be addressed in the evaluation. For example, a school may request evaluation of whether a child who has made a violent threat can safely return to school. Although this may appear to be a circumscribed question, a thorough evaluation must be done to assess the nature of the child's threat and risk of acting on the threat. The clinician should inquire about the event in some detail, including precipitating factors and chronic stressors in the environment in which the threat occurred, such as chronic bullying. A comprehensive evaluation is then conducted. In the written report, the clinician's recommendations should emphasize the most helpful and cautious approach that is in the best interest of the child. Recommendations offered should take into account the realities of the child's home life, as well as parental concerns and sensitivities.

Other assessments may focus on a particular clinical question such as evaluation of suicidal risk to determine need for hospitalization. In this case, issues pertaining to safety must be emphasized. These include the presence of psychiatric disorder and severity of symptoms, history of suicide attempts, nature of the suicidal ideation and lethality of intent, access to means, personality variables (e.g., impulsivity), capacity for problem-solving, presence of social stressors, current substance abuse, availability of meaningful psychological support, and ability of the family to monitor the child at home.

When asked to conduct a psychiatric evaluation in the midst of custody disputes, it is important to discern whether the evaluation is for legal purposes or for the purpose of helping the child with an emotional or behavioral problem. If the evaluation may be used in legal proceedings, Schetky and Benedek recommend that it should be done according to specific guidelines for forensic evaluation and not done by a treating clinician. In a forensic evaluation, the clinician must inform the child and family of the purpose of the evaluation and that the contents of the interview will not be reflected in the report. Evaluations of physical or sexual abuse generally require additional medical and specialized forensic methods as described by the American Academy of Child and Adolescent Psychiatry. In preliminary assessments to decide whether to refer to a specialist, only open-ended, nonleading questions should be asked, for example, "Have you been touched in a way that made you uncomfortable?" rather than "Tell me what Mr. X did to you." In situations of suspected abuse, asking detailed questions about the abuse may prejudice a subsequent examination that may be used in legal proceedings.

Communicating Findings and Recommendations

Effectively communicating the clinician's findings to the parents and child is an essential part of the psychiatric assessment. Depending on the nature of the problem and the developmental level of the child, communicating the findings and recommendations may take place either with the child and family together or separately. Communicating information that is sensitive, such as discussing concerns that the child is mentally retarded or autistic, requires considerable tact, as well as education of the parents. Presenting diagnostic impressions of major mental illness such as schizophrenia or bipolar disorder, that may be disconcerting or controversial requires time, sensitivity, and opportunity for questions, even for denial. It is important to emphasize the child's strengths, in addition to providing suggestions on what can assist with the child's difficulties. In situations when diagnostic clarity remains uncertain, this should be communicated to the family. This discussion should take place in a collaborative manner, allowing the child and parents to articulate areas of disagreement with the clinician, which may change the formulation.

On the basis of the clinical formulation and diagnosis, the clinician's goal is to formulate a developmentally suitable approach to the treatment of the child's difficulties that considers the child's and family's preferences. Selection of appropriate treatment is based on multiple factors, including diagnosis and symptom severity, acute and ongoing risk of harm, capacity of the family to support treatment and provide a safe environment, capacity of the child to use interactive treatment approaches, and availability of treatment options in the community. A biopsychosocial treatment plan should also include adjunctive interventions such as special education services for children with learning disorders, or social skills training for children with problems in peer relationships.

Conclusions

The comprehensive psychiatric assessment of a child is a challenging task. Because of the variable capacity of the child to describe his or her symptoms, the interaction of the child's vulnerabilities and symptoms with his or her environment, and the evolving and often unclear nature of childhood psychiatric disorders, child psychiatric assessment generally requires a longer time than assessment of adults. Thus, primary care physicians and general psychiatrists may want to collaborate with a child and adolescent psychiatrist or child psychologist to help clarify complex diagnostic and treatment issues.

Ultimately, a comprehensive psychiatric assessment is well worth the time and resources involved. It holds the key to clarifying the causes of emotional and behavioral disturbances and can open doors to future improvements. A comprehensive treatment plan based on an accurate clinical formulation and diagnosis can greatly improve a child's functioning, making a difference in the lives of the child and family.

BIBLIOGRAPHY

Abad NS, Sheldon KM. Parental autonomy support and ethnic culture identification among second generation immigrants. *J Fam Psychol.* 2008;22:652–657.

Alao AO, Soderberg M, Pohl EL, et al. Cybersuicide: review of the role of the internet on suicide. *Cyberpsychol Behav.* 2006;9:489–493.

American Academy of Child and Adolescent Psychiatry. Practice parameters for the psychiatric assessment of children and adolescents. *J Am Acad Child Adolesc Psychiatry.* 1997;36(suppl 10):4S–20S.

American Academy of Child and Adolescent Psychiatry. Practice parameters for the forensic evaluation of children and adolescents who may have been physically or sexually abused. *J Am Acad Child Adolesc Psychiatry.* 1997;36(suppl 10):37S–56S.

Barker P. Assessing children and their families. In: *Basic Child Psychiatry.* Oxford, England: Blackwell Science, Ltd; 1995:60.

Christakis DA, Zimmerman FJ, DiGiuseppe DL, et al. Early television exposure and subsequent attentional problems in children. *Pediatrics*. 2004;113:708–713.

Huesmann LR. The impact of electronic media violence: scientific theory and research. *J Adolesc Health*. 2007;41(6 suppl 1):S6–13.

Myers KM, Winters NC. Ten-year review of rating scales, I: overview of scale functioning, psychometric properties, and selection. *J Am Acad Child Adolesc Psychiatry*. 2002;41:114–122.

Pynoos RS, Eth S. Witness to violence: the child interview. *J Am Acad Child Psychiatry*. 1986;25:306–319.

Schetky DH, Benedek EP, eds. *Principles and Practice of Child and Adolescent Forensic Psychiatry*. Washington DC: American Psychiatric Press; 2002.

Wolak J, Ybarra ML, Mitchell K, et al. Current research knowledge about adolescent victimization via the internet. *Adolescent Med State Art Rev*. 2007;18:325–341.

Winters N, Hanson G, Stoyanova V. The case formulation in child and adolescent psychiatry. *Child Adolesc Psychiatric Clin N Am*. 2007;16:111–132.

SUGGESTED READINGS

Bostic JQ, King RA. Clinical assessment of children and adolescents: content and structure. In: Martin A, Volkmar FR, eds. *Lewis's Child and Adolescent Psychiatry: A Comprehensive Textbook, Fourth Edition*. Philadelphia, PA: Wolters Kluwer/Lippincott Williams & Wilkins; 2007:323–343. (Contains list of suggested parent interview questions to elicit history.)

Cepeda C. *The Psychiatric Interview of Children and Adolescents*. Washington DC: American Psychiatric Press; 2000.

Koplewicz H. *It's Nobody's Fault: New Hope and Help for Difficult Children and Their Parents*. New York, NY: Random House, Inc; 1996.

SUGGESTED WEBSITES

On this website, see in particular "Facts for Families and Other Resources": http://www.aacap.org.

American Academy of Pediatrics: Policy statement—the future of pediatrics: mental health competencies for pediatric primary care. Available at: http://aappolicy.aappublications.org/cgi/reprint/pediatrics;124/1/410.pdf. Accessed May 6, 2010.

National Institute for Health Care Management (NIMHCM): Strategies to support the integration of mental health into pediatric primary care. August 2009. Available at: http://nihcm.org/pdf/PediatricMH-FINAL.pdf. Accessed May 6, 2010. (Contains list of screening and assessment tools.)

National Institutes of Mental Health: Child and adolescent mental health website. Available at: http://www.nimh.nih.gov/health/topics/child-and-adolescent-mental-health/index.shtml. Accessed March 25, 2010. (Contains materials on all major psychiatric disorders and psychiatric medications.)

REVIEW QUESTIONS

1. Which of the following elements should be included in a comprehensive psychiatric assessment?
   a. Identifying information
   b. Reason for the referral
   c. Medical and developmental history
   d. Educational history
   e. All of the above

2. What is a key difference between psychiatric assessment of children and adults?
   a. A mental status exam can be done only with adults
   b. Children should be interviewed conjointly with parents
   c. Diagnosis cannot be made reliably in children
   d. The evaluation of a child is generally initiated by the child's parents or other adults involved in his or her care

3. Which strategy can be problematic in evaluating adolescents?
   a. Meeting with the parents first to better understand their concerns
   b. Including the adolescent in the first interview
   c. Offering them some degree of confidentiality
   d. Discussing the adolescent's interests

4. Which of the following is the most useful play material for evaluating a young child?
   a. Board games
   b. Computer games
   c. Dollhouse and family
   d. Children's books

5. The clinical mental status examination includes all but which of the following:
   a. Appearance and behavior
   b. Intellectual functioning
   c. Judgment and insight
   d. Social relatedness
   e. Educational history

6. Which statement best describes the clinical formulation?
   a. A five-axis DSM diagnosis
   b. A succinct synthesis of how the clinician understands the child's problem
   c. A comprehensive document restating all major findings of the evaluation

7. Reasons for inquiring about the child's or adolescent's use of electronic media include:
   a. Its association with increased risk for ADHD in young children
   b. Its association with increased violence
   c. Risks posed for victimization
   d. Influence on suicidal behavior
   e. All of the above

Answers: 1-e, 2-d, 3-a, 4-c, 5-e, 6-b, 7-e

Psychological Assessment

Introduction

Diagnosis and treatment planning are complicated activities that attempt to determine a course of treatment affecting an individual's affect, thinking, behavior, and social systems. Often treatment planning decisions are made based on assessments that rely on gaining information through unstructured interview and informal observations obtained over a very short period of time. Treatment plans based on these one-dimensional assessments often ignore the complex context of a client's problems by not collecting information from multiple environmental settings using multiple methods of measurement. Managed health care organizations are often hesitant to allow physicians to refer clients for more in-depth assessment pushing instead a strategy focused on simple, single method ratings with quick turnaround and superficial survey of symptoms. As a result, clinicians may overlook important areas of functioning and miss the context of the client's complaints. Further difficulty occurs when using the single method, usually an interview, with children, youth, and their parents as they can be poor historians, or biased informants adding error to information collection and leading to invalid conclusions. For example, the client may have an agenda when presenting for an interview, such as obtaining medication, proving there are no problems, or affixing blame on certain individuals or circumstances. A further source of error can be the context of the interview often leading to denial or exaggeration of presenting problems. For example, if youths believe that they will have to take medication for the rest of their life, which is not to their liking, they may admit to no symptoms during the interview. Drastic diagnostic errors may occur when relying on single method assessment leading to inappropriate or inadequate treatment. This, in turn, can lead to further clinical problems and complications. In Perry's review of the assessment literature reported in 1992, diagnosis by one clinician using a single method of assessment (semi-structured interview) can yield a 70% error in personality diagnoses when compared to a more complex integrated assessment using multiple methods of gathering information.

When Is Assessment Useful?

Psychological assessment offers a tool to improve the accuracy and reliability of diagnosis and treatment planning. Although time consuming and adding to immediate expense, in the long run, there can be savings due to fewer false starts and inappropriate treatment interventions. Not everyone needs in-depth psychological assessment. In fact, it would be too costly to provide this for every client. Yates and Taub suggested in 2003 that a clinician needs to weigh the cost/benefit for an in-depth assessment before making a referral. Psychological assessment consultations are useful when clients have complex, multiple problems; the diagnosis is unclear; the client is unresponsive to treatment attempts; the client is dissatisfied with previous mental health treatment; it is difficult to engage the client; secondary gains or symptoms are suspected;

TABLE 2-1	Common Indications for Psychological Assessment

- Difficult to engage patients/families
- Historians are biased or unreliable
- Suspicions of secondary gain
- Presence of complex and/or multiple presenting problems (diagnostic clarity)
- Poor responsiveness to multiple treatment interventions
- Questions about risk of harm to self or others
- Faced with litigious family/youth situations
- Questions about lingering effects of trauma

liability risk appears to be high; and clients are seeking certain medications or medical treatments that are of questionable utility to presenting problems. Examples of common indications for psychological assessment are summarized in Table 2-1.

Testing Versus Assessment

It is important to distinguish between psychological testing and psychological assessment. A psychological test has been defined as a systematic procedure for measuring a sample of behavior. Systematic procedure refers to the fact that the test was constructed to be administered in the same standard manner thereby minimizing sources of measurement error related to situational variables, clinician error, and clinician–client interaction error. Thus, testing is the process of administering a particular test to obtain a specific score on a relatively narrow dimension of behavior. Well-constructed tests allow for developmental and normative descriptions. For example, once the score is obtained on an attention-deficit hyperactivity disorder (ADHD) or depression rating scale, the score can be compared to a large group of individual scores previously collected and studied. The score can then inform the clinician whether it is high, average, or low for the age group represented by the client and even give critical "cutoff" scores suggesting significant presence of whatever the test measures. It allows for empirically quantified information with standardized administration, information about reliability, a validity of the construct measured, and an overall more precise measurement of client dimensions than is typically obtained with interviews. However, tests are usually a single method of measure such as self-report measures, observer ratings, and performance tasks that yield single method bias and may only measure a single construct. Again, using the simple ADHD or depression symptom checklists as examples, the rater is faced with a list of symptoms or behaviors that make up a single diagnostic construct. The rater assigns a level of disorder or quantity score to each symptom or behavior about himself or herself or someone else. The rater may actually have little knowledge of the client, only view him or her in limited settings such as in physical education class or at youth group outings, or have a biased preconceived view that influences such observations. Self-raters may have little self-awareness, be seeking certain treatments, exhibit intense denial or resistance, or have exaggerated symptoms in the narrow situational context of the single test. Thus, self-raters may give biased responses to the rating scale, possibly based on limited knowledge or distorted by personal views. Since it is a single method rating, it is difficult to examine the accuracy of the report. This can easily lead to a misdiagnosis and inadequate or inappropriate treatment interventions. Obtaining a single sample of behavior, thought, or affect through one measurement method can easily lead to making judgments that are highly inaccurate. In addition, these simple tests often do not measure a sufficient domain of behaviors to differentiate among various diagnostic subtleties. For example, when inattention is rated high on an ADHD rating scale might that not also represent the attention problems seen with some depressed children or children with anxiety disorders? Since there were no items for rating mood behaviors, it is difficult to tease out what the inattention means.

Psychological assessment, on the other hand, comprises focusing on a number of scores obtained through multiple methods and combining the data in the context of historical information, referral information, interview data, and behavior observations in order to generate a cohesive and comprehensive understanding of the client. Thus, multiple test scores, or a battery of tests, are examined in the context of current situational circumstances, developmental history, and family social system factors. The high score obtained on a self-report ADHD scale is now compared to the low scores obtained from teachers, the high anxiety scores on a performance test, the history of average school performance, the recent episode of sexual abuse by a peer at school, and the information that a parent has recently dropped out of treatment for methamphetamine abuse. The experienced psychologist can take these multiple sources of information or samples of functioning and derive a more accurate description of the client's diagnosis and develop a more accurate treatment plan.

In general, the use of a battery of tests that obtains information through multiple methods including self-report, information derived from performance tests, observer information, and information derived from behavioral or functional assessment strategies is more reliable and accurate than reliance on a single clinician using a single method (i.e., an interview). These psychological assessments, however, cannot be completed by a minimally trained clinician and requires an extensive knowledge of psychopathology, personality, psychological measurement, research methods, assessment methods, and skill to integrate information with complex history, situational context, and developmental information.

The *Standards for Educational and Psychological Testing* in the 1999 edition suggests test publishers use competency-based qualification guidelines in determining who can purchase and administer various tests. This is to assure the ethical test use and appropriate interpretation of test results. Tests are usually assigned to one of several qualification levels. Psychological Assessment Resources, Inc. uses the following qualification guidelines. Qualification level A indicates no special qualifications are required. Qualification level B indicates a degree from an accredited 4-year college in psychology or related field plus satisfactory completion of coursework in testing. Qualification C indicates all qualifications for Level B plus an advanced professional degree that provides appropriate training in the administration and interpretation of psychological tests or a license or certification from an agency that requires training and experience in ethical and competent use of psychological tests. Finally, there is Qualification level S that requires a degree or license to practice in a health care profession or occupation including the following: medicine, neurology, nursing, occupational therapy, and other allied health care professions, physicians' assistants, psychiatry, social work, speech and language pathology, plus appropriate training and experience in the ethical administration, scoring, and interpretation of clinical behavior assessment instruments. The first time a clinician purchases from a supplier, he/she is asked to supply supporting credentials.

Common Tests Used with Children and Youth

There are numerous testing techniques utilized in the assessment of children and youth. These numerous tests can be divided into categories based on domains measured, the approach or method of measurement (e.g., individual, group, questionnaire, observation, and so on), or types of testing based on content. For example, Van Ornum et al. in their 2008 test suggest categorizing tests using a seven approaches model while the *Standards for Educational and Psychological Testing* in the 1999 text utilizes a categorization of tests based on domains measured. The classification of tests utilized here generally follows a model focusing on the psychological domain measured, but under the domain of personality there is a subcategorization based on the method of measurement. The various tests illustrated here that are the most likely utilized in a good assessment include: achievement, behavioral problems, adaptive behavior, intelligence, personality—self-report, personality—projective, neuropsychological, and parenting/family.

The purpose of achievement testing is to measure an individual's development, strengths and weaknesses in various areas of learning such as written expression, reading, spelling, math, nonverbal reasoning, language skills, expressive and receptive vocabulary, and so on. Often a child has behavioral problems in school or with peers due to learning and processing problems. These tests will help in identifying learning disabilities and deficits in learning various academic content areas requiring special focus.

The purpose of behavioral problem ratings is to get a concrete description of behavioral functioning across various living environments or settings such as school, home, day care, restaurants, and so on. Scales with a broad sampling of behavioral items are more useful than narrow samples. Also, scales that elicit ratings from various individuals in the client's life (such as teacher, parent, friend, sibling, or self) are more useful than single rater forms. Ratings on various items are often combined into different scales such as aggression, level of isolation, externalizing behavior, internalizing behavior, and so on. These are most useful in helping to determine which behaviors are most excessive, the environments in which the behavior is most excessive, and whether the behavior is excessive for age.

Adaptive behavior techniques usually consist of other rating or semi-structured interview formats aimed at measuring a patient's adaptive behavior or functional skills. These are skills considered important for personal responsibility, self-care, daily living, social functioning, and/or independent living. This type of measurement is required in assessing for developmental disabilities.

Intelligence testing measures the performance of a number of different tasks. These tasks represent certain abilities including the ability to learn or understand from experience, the ability to retain knowledge, reasoning ability, the ability to respond to new situations, and ability to direct behavior. These abilities are measured through the performance of verbal tasks and nonverbal tasks. These measures are often used in school settings to help determine placement, handicapping conditions, or appropriate modalities of treatment. For example, a child with low verbal skills would not do well in a high verbal reasoning type of therapy.

Personality tests measure the way in which a person may habitually or typically respond emotionally, cognitively, and behaviorally in various situations. This type of test often measures various manifest symptoms but also coping mechanisms, defenses, affect, perception of reality, thinking processes, ego functioning, conflicts, drives, motivators, level of distress, and so on. This category is broken into two types or methods of measurement, self-report and projective. Self-report usually entails having the client respond to a number of statements and indicating whether they are true or false. Projective tests involve the presentation of an ambiguous stimulus to a client in order to measure how his or her personality influences the way in which he/she perceives, organizes, and interprets his or her environment and experiences. These tests are often used to assist in differential diagnosis, treatment planning, and risk assessment.

Neuropsychological testing is concerned with the measurement of brain–behavior relations. In general, neuropsychological testing measures the human adaptive function dependent on the organic integrity of the brain. Consequently, there is a need to systematically measure most major adaptive behavior functions. Thus, neuropsychological assessment examines areas of learning, information processing, planning, sensory-motor functioning, perceptions, memory, executive functioning, attention, and personality changes. Neuropsychological testing is most useful when damage to the brain is suspected to be interfering with performance and adaptive functioning.

Parent/family types of tests are used to describe parent–child relationships, describe family functioning, identify stressful areas of parent–child interactions, identify strength of child rearing alliance between parents, or identify parenting skills. This is most useful in helping identify contextual issues affecting a child/youth's symptom presentation.

Examples of tests commonly used by psychologists for the assessment of childhood or adolescent disorders are listed in Table 2-2 by type of test, appropriate age ranges to take the test, and where the test can be purchased.

TABLE 2-2	Commonly Used Tests for the Assessment of Children and Youths		
Test Category	**Test Name**	**Test Age Range**	**Supplier**
Intelligence	Stanford–Binet	2–23 years	a
	Wechsler Preschool and Primary Scale of Intelligence	2.6–7.3 years	b
	Wechsler Intelligence Scale for Children–IV (WISC-IV)	6–16.11 years	b
	Wechsler Abbreviated Scale of Intelligence (WASI)	6–89 years	b
	Kaufman Assessment Battery for Children (K-ABC)	2.5–12.5 years	c,h
	Test of Nonverbal Intelligence	6– 85 years	c,h
Achievement	Kaufman Test of Educational Achievement (KTEA)	4.6–90 years	d,g
	Wechsler Individual Achievement Test II (WIAT)	4–85 years	b
	Wide Range Achievement Test	5–85 years	b,c,f,h
Adaptive	Adaptive Behavior Scale	3–21 years	c
	Adaptive Behavior Assessment System-II	0–89 years	b,c,f,h
	Vineland Adaptive Behavior Scales	3 to 21.11 years	d,g
Behavior problems	Achenbach System of Empirically Based Assessment (CBCL; TRF; YSR)	1.5–59 years	c,e
	Autism Diagnostic Observation Schedule	Toddlers to adults	h
	Behavior Assessment System for Children (BASC)	2.6 to 18.11 years	d,g
	Conners Rating Scales—3rd edition	6–18 years	c,f,h
Personality—self-report	Jesness Inventory–Revised (JI–R)	8 years and older	f
	Million Adolescent Clinical Inventory	13–19 years	g
	Minnesota Multiphasic Personality Inventory (MMPI)	14 years and older	g
	Personality Inventory for Child	5–19 years	h
	Personality Inventory for Youth	9–19 years	b,c,h
	Trauma Symptom Checklist for Children	8–16 years	b,c
Personality—projective	Rorschach	5 years and older	b,c,g,f,h
	Tell Me A Story	5–18 years	h
	Thematic Apperception Test	4 years and older	b,c,g
Neuropsychological tests	Conners Continuous Performance Test	6 years and older	b,c,h
	Delis–Kaplan Executive Function System	8–89 years	b
	NEPSY—Developmental Neuropsychological Assessment	3–12 years	b,c
	Rey–Osterrieth Complex Figure Test	5–94 years	c
	Tests of Memory and Learning	5–59 years	h
	Wide Range Assessment of Memory and Learning (WRAML)	5–90 years	b,c
	Wisconsin Card Sorting Test	6.5–89 years	c

(continued)

TABLE 2-2	Commonly Used Tests for the Assessment of Children and Youths *(continued)*		
Test Category	**Test Name**	**Test Age Range**	**Supplier**
Parenting/family	Family Assessment Measure	10 years to adults	c
	Parenting Stress Index	Parents of children 0–12 years	b,c
	Parenting Satisfaction Scale	Parents of elementary children	b
	Parent–Child Relationship Inventory	Parents of children	h
	Parenting Relationship Quest.	Parents of children/youth	g

Suppliers:
a) Riverside Publishing Company (http://www.riverpub.com);
b) PsychCorp (a subsidiary of Pearson products) (http://www.PsychCorp.com);
c) Psychological Assessment Resources (http://www.parinc.com);
d) AGS Publishing (http://www.agsnet.com);
e) ASEBA Research Center (http://www.ASEBA.org);
f) Multi Health Systems (http://www.mhs.com);
g) Pearson Assessments (http://www.pearsonassessments.com);
h) Western Psychological Services (http://www.wpspublish.com).

When to Refer

Psychological assessment can be used for a number of purposes. Referrals can be made for issues pertaining to description of current functioning, confirmation or refutation of clinical impressions, differential diagnosis, identification of treatment needs and appropriate treatment interventions, predictions of outcome, monitoring treatment over time, and risk management.

When making referrals for psychological assessment, it is important to be specific about the goal of the assessment. Often, specific tests are requested without reference to the goal of the assessment. A preferable method of referral makes clear the questions being asked by referring clinician, family, patient, or agency so as to allow the psychologist to pick the appropriate methods to gather information given the situational and personal characteristics of the child. Thus, questions such as "Is the child suffering from depression or is there some other difficulty present?"; "What seems to be the meaning of the child's poor attention or restlessness?"; "What is behind the child's aggression?"; "Is there some way to effectively treat his or her aggression?"; and "Does the child exhibit any suicidal or homicidal risk?" are preferable referral questions. Examples of such referral questions are included in Table 2-3.

Once the referral is made, the clinician will select the battery of tests most useful to utilize to answer the questions. The psychologist will attempt to develop a battery that uses multiple source or samples of information gathered with multiple methods. A common battery for children or youth will include historical information, baseline observations gathered over multiple sites (i.e., home and school), with multiple raters (i.e., parents, teachers, or self), interview data, self-report data, projective testing, and intelligence/achievement measures. When selecting a battery, the client's characteristics such as age, ethnicity, ability to read, language disabilities, and physical disabilities are taken into consideration. Issues such as prior testing history, time constraints, and who will have access to the results (i.e., estranged parents, juvenile court, insurance companies, and so on) are also taken into consideration when choosing the battery.

TABLE 2-3	Examples of Referral Questions for Psychological Assessment

- Does this child qualify for a handicapping condition and special education services?
- Does this child qualify for services for mental retardation or developmental disabilities?
- Does this child's attention problem suggest attention-deficit hyperactivity disorder, bipolar disorder, or an anxiety disorder?
- Does this child's impulsivity and attention problems relate to a brain injury?
- Is this child's behavior problems related to trauma?
- Is this child a dangerous sex offender?
- Should this child be placed in 24-hour care for the safety of others?
- Does this child's complaint of hearing voices in the absence of other psychotic symptoms represent the
- development of a thought disorder?
- Is this child's aggression and irritability related to depression or conduct problems?
- Is this child a homicide or suicide risk?

Psychological Reports

Results from a psychological assessment are often reported out in the form of a report rather than only reporting specific test scores. These reports along with the actual testing data are considered confidential and the psychologist is ethically bound to maintain the confidentiality. Confidentiality rules vary according to individual state's regulations and should be similar to those followed for any medical record document.

Reports can vary greatly depending on the psychologist's training and the referral question. Psychological assessment reports usually include presenting problems, relevant background information, interview information with child/youth and parents, testing results, a formulation or summary of data collected, and recommendations or answers to the referral questions. The psychologist will go over these results and conclusions with the child (if age-appropriate), youth, and parents. Turnaround time of the report depends on many factors including the availability of the client, difficulty in testing the client, difficulty of the referral questions, and workload of the clinician. However, a 1- to 2-week turnaround for more extensive assessment protocols is a guideline to utilize. Forensic assessments are often more time consuming and require more data gathering time making it a longer turnaround time. Common components of a psychological assessment report are summarized in Table 2-4.

TABLE 2-4	Common Components of the Psychological Assessment Report for Children and Adolescents

- Specific referral question
- List of specific data gathering techniques
- Relevant background history
- Interview with significant adults in child/youth's life (parents, teachers, other family)
- Interview with child/youth
- Behavioral rating scales collected from multiple environments and multiple observers
- Testing—varied depending on question but usually covers multiple domains
- Summary of data or formulation of results
- Diagnostic impression if requested
- Recommendations or addressing of specific referral questions

Conclusions

Psychological assessment provides a valuable adjunct to optimize the evaluation and treatment planning of youths with mental health and developmental problems. A variety of clinical problems can be addressed ranging from the broad evaluation of symptoms and behaviors, to in-depth assessment of a specific symptom, to elucidation of broad constructs such as intelligence and personality. Psychological assessment offers such evaluation in a comprehensive, yet efficient testing battery. While psychological assessment is often thought to increase the cost of mental health evaluation and treatment, it may instead ensure that the most appropriate treatment is implemented in the timeliest manner. Clinicians seeking to integrate psychological assessment into their evaluation and treatment will profit from collaborating with a few psychologists whose work they can get to know well. In that manner, referring clinicians can best hone their referral questions and the psychologists can best hone their feedback so that the referral process ensures the best clinical service for young patients.

CASE VIGNETTES

VIGNETTE 1: 8 YEAR OLD GIRL WITH DIFFERENTIAL DIAGNOSES OF ADHD VS BIPOLAR DISORDER

A pediatrician was presented at an appointment with an 8-year-old girl with a question from parents about whether their child would need stimulant drugs, as the school believes she has ADHD. A typical assessment battery for ADHD would include an interview with parents and child focusing on early development and family history; behavior ratings such as the Conners Rating Scales or the Child Behavior Checklist (CBCL); tests of cognitive ability and academic achievement aimed at ruling out possible learning disabilities; and, in some cases, neuropsychological tests such as the Continuous Performance Test. The pediatrician was presented only with ADHD rating scores completed in the school setting and at home. This particular test yielded a score on inattentiveness, hyperactivity, and an overall ADHD score. Both parents and a teacher had completed the rating scale and all suggested high scores significant of ADHD. Other testing or interviewing was not completed. The pediatrician attempted to gather more background information to aid in formulating a differential diagnosis. In gathering this information, the pediatrician noted the biological mother had a great aunt with a history of depression and possible bipolar disorder; the child had no history of overactivity or poor attention in the classroom or home prior to this last 6 months and the child was recently discovered to be playing doctor with a neighborhood boy 1 year her junior. Rather than prescribing a stimulant, the pediatrician thought that the diagnostic picture was unclear and so made a referral to a child psychologist with the goal of making a differential diagnosis and treatment suggestions.

The psychologist, in examining the referral, noted a thorough ADHD assessment had not been completed by the school and the apparent symptoms could be observed with the child suffering from bipolar disorder, posttraumatic stress disorder, ADHD, or even an anxiety disorder caused by recent family upheaval. Thus, the testing battery chosen needed to be able to sort out these various symptoms and etiologies. The battery chosen included the CBCL and Teacher's Report Form, the Trauma Symptom Checklist for Children; Personality Inventory for Youth (which is filled out by the child), Rorschach Test, the Wechsler Individual Achievement Test Screener, and the Wechsler Intelligence Scale for Children-IV. The latter was utilized as it has been noted that children with intellectual delays sometimes have difficulty focusing in a classroom setting or in the home. Upon presenting the standardized testing to the young girl, the psychologist noted she had difficulty concentrating, was restless, and answered impulsively. In addition, she was aggressive and boisterous with siblings and mother during the family interview and she complained of problems with sleep.

The intelligence testing yielded scores in the average range for her age and suggested that despite her impulsive style, she was able to express her intelligence adequately. Achievement testing measured by the WIAT-Screener suggested she functioned at her intelligence level in school thereby ruling out a possible learning disability. Behavioral ratings, which were compared to others her age, yielded high scores on the aggression, inattentive, and depression scales as rated by parents and teachers. This is a pattern often seen with children who may be exhibiting early symptoms of juvenile mania. The girl's responses on the Personality Inventory for Youth yielded significantly high scores on the Psychological Discomfort scale, particularly the depression and sleep disturbance subscales, and the Impulsivity/Distractibility scale, particularly the brashness and distractibility/overactivity subscales. The Trauma Symptom Checklist for Children indicated no significant problems in any of the areas such as sexual concerns, dissociation, defensive avoidance, or anxiety but did have elevations on the depression subtest. In addition, her responding was considered to be consistent and did not exhibit a pattern of malingering or deceptiveness. Finally, the Rorschach Test indicated severe problems with mood and a tendency toward depression or hypomania, aggression, and disorganized thinking in emotionally charged situations. There was an indication of a pattern similar to those found suffering from juvenile mania or bipolar disorder. There was also indication, given her age, that she may have been having difficulty with processing information in emotionally charged, ambivalent situations. Altogether, the various test results yielded a picture of a child who suffers from a juvenile bipolar disorder. The treatment approach would be very different from that assumed by a diagnosis of ADHD.

In the field of child and youth mental health, use of behavioral ratings to measure treatment effectiveness has become increasingly more prevalent. In their standards of practice, the American Academy of Child and Adolescent Psychiatry recommends the integration of behavioral ratings from multiple settings with interview and observational data if ADHD is suspected and to use a series of behavioral rating measures to evaluate the success of medication treatment over time. Use of depression or anxiety rating scales is also encouraged for use with children or youths to measure treatment effectiveness with medication treatment. Referrals for behavioral ratings aimed at measuring the effect of a treatment protocol are also common. Thus, data are gathered using standard single construct behavior rating scales to gather baseline information about symptoms before medication treatment is started and at various points along the way to help determine whether the treatment is working. In these situations, it is not necessary to be concerned about developmental norms or multiple diagnostic constructs as the diagnosis is already made and one is only measuring against an individual's baseline measurement. In such cases, psychological testing can help reduce potential legal liability for health care professionals by providing a "baseline" reference point or outside opinion should a client claim a provider was negligent, committed malpractice, or is damaged by the treatment provided. In this vignette, however, the pediatrician was being asked to make a diagnosis based on limited construct behavioral ratings and could easily have gone down the wrong treatment path.

VIGNETTE 2: 7 YEAR OLD CHILD WITH DIFFERENTIAL DIAGNOSES OF LEARNING DISORDER VS DEVELOPMENTAL DELAY

A typical referral in school involves trying to understand why a child is unable to perform age-appropriate school work or tasks. In this example, a 7-year-old child is referred as due to inability to perform tasks in the first-grade classroom and immature behavior with peers and family. The psychologist will focus on the child's abilities as compared to peers and developmental history.

A typical battery would include a detailed developmental and family history from parents, a child interview, an intelligence test, an achievement test, and a test of adaptive functioning. In particular, the WISC-IV, the Wide Range Achievement Test 3 (WRAT), and the Vineland Adaptive Behavior Scales were used. The child obtained a Full Scale IQ of 60 on the WISC-IV, an overall Adaptive Behavior Score of 55 on the Vineland and standard scores of 51 in reading, 52 in spelling, and 53 in arithmetic on the WRAT3.

The Full Scale IQ score on the WISC-IV is an overall measure of one's ability on various tasks as compared to one's age group. If a child is considered to be of average intellect, or about the same as peers, then the IQ score would fall in the range of 90 to 110. Most children's scores fall between 70 and 130 (approximately 95 %). Those children whose scores fall below 70 are considered to be mentally deficient and are considered to be functioning at or below the 2.5 percentile when compared to others their age. Some children, however, score low on the intelligence test but then score in the average range for adaptive functioning. One would not expect this for a child who is mentally deficient, but may see this pattern with a child who has not been exposed to formal learning experiences but has excelled at learning to care for himself or herself at home and in the community. Thus, the child's abilities may not be developed well, but are not considered mentally deficient or mentally retarded. The referred child, however, scores below 70 on both IQ and adaptive functioning suggesting significant deficits on both more formally learned skills and daily care/social skills. This indicates the child does exhibit a mild mental retardation and would qualify for special education planning.

VIGNETTE 3: 13 YEAR OLD GIRL WITH DIFFERENTIAL DIAGNOSES OF MOOD DISORDER VS PSYCHOSIS

In this example, there is a 13-year-old girl who was first seen for problems associated with depression but was not responding well to standard treatment. The girl was referred for psychological assessment to aid with diagnosis and treatment planning. At the time of the referral she was residing in a psychiatric state hospital unit and was exhibiting symptoms of withdrawal, lethargy, sleep problems, complaints of anxiety in school and difficulty in concentrating. She would have periodic aggressive outbursts where she hurt younger children. These symptoms were exhibited in a family context of a divorced family system in which she had been exposed to neglect, parental substance abuse, and abandonment by her father and limited contact with her mother. She had been in foster home placement and had prior placement in the hospital. There were historical complaints that she may have heard voices on occasion and sometimes appeared confused. The psychologist chose a testing battery including intelligence testing (WISC-IV), the CBCL completed by hospital staff, as parents were unavailable; the Youth Self-Report, which is a version of the Child Behavior Check List completed by the client; the Personality Inventory for Youth; and the Rorschach Test. The presenting problem suggests possible difficulty with depression, anxiety, and/or ADHD. In getting the results it was noted the teenager tended to respond slowly to the standardized testing. Her responses to the Similarities subtest on the WISC-IV, which measures verbal abstract reasoning, suggest very loose associations or overly concrete associations. She obtained a score in the low average range of intelligence both in the Verbal and Performance portions of the intelligence testing. The CBCL completed by both swing and day staff indicated high scores on the thought problem scale, depression scale, attention-deficit scale, and anxiety scale. Her own behavioral report indicated problems with depression and anxiety. In particular, she reported symptoms suggestive of being fearful, being somewhat hypervigilant and lacking in self-worth. The Personality Inventory for Youth indicated high scores on the clinical scales of reality distortion (feelings of alienation, hallucinations, and delusions subscales), psychological discomfort (depression subscale), social withdrawal (isolation subscale), and social skill deficit (limited peer status). Finally, the Rorschach

Test indicated problems with reality testing and logical reasoning. It suggested a pattern significantly similar to those who suffer from a psychotic disorder. Depression was not as evident on this particular procedure. Instead, the results from the projective testing seemed to support the concept of a slow developing incipient psychosis.

What was perceived initially as an affective disorder leading to an ineffective treatment plan was reassessed using psychological assessment. The treatment plan was changed based on the testing results and focused more on the thinking, poor social interactions, and poor emotional controls that are associated with a psychotic disorder. The teenager was started on an antipsychotic medication and showed very good improvement over a short period of time leading to her being able to be released from the hospital. As can be seen, the battery approach can often tease out the complicated symptoms and place them in the proper context when data are gathered over multiple methods.

BIBLIOGRAPHY

American Academy of Child and Adolescent Psychiatry. Practice parameters for the assessment and treatment of children, adolescents, and adults with attention-deficit/hyperactivity disorder. *J Am Acad Child Adolesc Psychiatry*. 1997;36:1312.

American Educational Research Association, American Psychological Association, National Council on Measurement in Education. *Standards for Educational and Psychological Testing*. Washington, DC: American Educational Research Association; 1999.

Franzer MD, Berg RA. *Screening Children for Brain Impairment*. 2nd ed. New York: Springer; 1998.

Groth-Marnat G. *Handbook of Psychological Assessment*. 4th ed. New York: Wiley; 2003.

Meyer GJ, Finn SE, Eyde LD, et al. *Benefits and Costs of Psychological Assessment in Healthcare Delivery: Report of the Board of Professional Affairs Psychological Assessment Work Group, Part I*. Washington, DC: American Psychological Association; 1998.

Perry JC. Problems and considerations in the valid assessment of personality disorders. *Am J Psychiatry*. 1992;149:1645–1653.

Reynolds CR, Kamphaus RW. *Handbook of Psychological and Educational Assessment of Children*. 2nd ed. Vols 1 and 2. New York: Guilford; 2003.

Van Ornum W, Dunlap LL, Shore MF. *Psychological Testing Across the Life Span*. New Jersey: Pearson Education; 2008.

Yates BT, Taub J. Assessing the costs, benefits, cost-effectiveness, and cost-benefit of psychological assessment: We should, we can, and here's how. *Psycholog Assess*. 2003;15:478–495.

SUGGESTED READINGS

Title: Assessment of Children: Behavioral, Social, and Clinical Foundations (5th edition)
Authors: Jerome M Sattler and Robert D Hoge
Publisher: Jerome M Sattler, Publisher, Inc., 2006
(A comprehensive guide to psychological assessment of children)
Title: Essentials of Neuropsychological Assessment
Authors: Nancy Hebben and William Milberg
Publisher: John Wiley and Sons, 2002.
(A comprehensive guide to basic tests and practical issues related to neuropsychological assessment)
Title: Essentials of School Neuropsychological Assessment
Authors: Daniel C. Miller
Publisher: John Wiley and Sons, 2007
(Provides a current overview of neuropsychological assessment in schools)
Title: Psychological Testing Across the Life Span
Authors: William Van Ornum, Linda L. Dunlap, and Milton F Shore
Publisher: Pearson Education, Inc., 2008
(An excellent guide to all aspects of psychological testing and how it integrates with developmental and abnormal psychology)
Title: Straight Talk about Psychological Testing for Kids
Authors: Ellen Braaten and Gretchen Felopuols
Publisher: The Guilford Press, 2004
(An excellent, pragmatic guide for parents and allied health professionals about the process of psychological testing)

Title: The Clinical Assessment of Children and Adolescents: A Practitioner's Guide
Authors: Steven R. Smith and Leonard Handler (Editors)
Publisher: Routledge, 2006
(Practical guide to psychological assessment techniques providing guidance for referral, test selection, and application. Includes case material)

REVIEW QUESTIONS

1. Psychological assessment:
   a. Can improve the accuracy and reliability of diagnostic formulation
   b. Be offered to every new client
   c. Is especially useful in cases of suspected malingering
   d. Both a and c

2. Psychological testing:
   a. Is the process of administering a particular test to obtain a specific score on a relatively narrow dimension of behavior
   b. Is comprised of focusing on a number of scores obtained through multiple methods and combining the data in the context of historical information, interview data, and behavior observations
   c. Is never used to determine a diagnosis
   d. Is made up of a battery of tests

3. Child psychiatrists are qualified to purchase and administer psychological tests:
   a. Only if they have taken three testing classes in a qualified clinical psychology training program
   b. Only if they are supervised by a clinical or neuropsychologist
   c. With a license to practice in a health care profession and appropriate training and experience in the ethical administration, scoring, and interpretation of clinical behavior assessment instruments
   d. None of the above

4. The appropriate tests to assess learning disabilities include:
   a. Rorschach
   b. IQ test
   c. CBCL
   d. Achievement tests
   e. Both b and d

5. Reasons to obtain information from multiple raters include:
   a. Different raters have different perspectives depending on their experience with the child
   b. Some tests are more reliable with more input from multiple raters
   c. Multiple raters address the contextual aspects of a child's behavior
   d. Tests vary from person to person
   e. Both a and c

Answers: 1-d, 2-a, 3-c, 4-e, 5-e

CHAPTER **3**

Andrea K. Maikovich-Fong, PhD,
Alison Leary, PhD, Brent Collett, PhD,
and Kathleen Myers, MD, MPH

Rating Scales

Rating scales are instruments that provide rapid assessment of behaviors or psychological dimensions, and that yield numerical scores with relatively straightforward scoring and interpretative guidelines. They can be used without extensive training in both research and clinical applications. As psychiatric disorders do not yet have identified genes, serum tests, or functional imaging profiles, rating scales have assumed an important role in identifying criterion symptoms for making a diagnosis, establishing the severity of a disorder, and tracking symptoms over time. This chapter introduces several rating scales pertaining to childhood disorders that are frequently treated in general psychiatric practice but that are also readily applicable to other clinical settings. From the large number of available scales, those presented in this chapter were selected on the basis of their frequency of use in clinical practice and the adequacy of their psychometric properties. Whenever possible, emphasis is on scales that are available in the public domain. Information on obtaining these scales is included at the end of the chapter. To avoid redundancy, the individual scales are not also cited in the bibliography, although relevant other citations are included.

Functioning of Rating Scales

Advantages and Disadvantages of Rating Scales

Myers and Winters have reviewed the role and functioning of rating scales in child and adolescent mental health research and clinical practice. An abbreviated overview is provided in Table 3-1. One of the most common ways in which people describe a child's difficulties is via *comparisons*. For example, parents might express concerns that their younger daughter is more aggressive than their older daughter was at that age, teachers might report that a child's moods are more labile than those of his classmates, and a teenager might worry that she has a harder time focusing at school than her friends do. One of the overarching advantages of rating scales is that they allow for multiple such comparisons in structured, scientific ways. First, ratings scales can be used to compare youth to other youth. For example, a youth's score on a self-report scale is often derived by comparing his or her answers to those of some comparison group—ideally a large, representative sample of same-aged, same-gendered peers. On the Child Behavior Checklist (CBCL) (described later in text), a teenaged female will have a "clinically significant" internalizing score if her self-reported symptoms of internalizing problems are significantly above those of same-aged females from a nationally representative sample. If a caregiver or teacher is the informant, then this adult's answers are compared to the answers from a sample of parents or teachers of same-aged youth in order to derive scores. Second, rating scales can be used to compare a youth's functioning to his or her own functioning at previous points in time. For example, if a child experiences a major stressor, such as invasive treatment for cancer or the loss of a parent, comparisons between pre- and poststressor scores can assist with understanding how the event affected the youth's functioning from

TABLE 3-1	Essentials of Rating Scales in Data Collection

Rating scales cannot be used alone to make a diagnosis; they are adjunctive tools used to complement a diagnostic evaluation.

Rating scales have several valuable roles in clinical practice, including diagnostic corroboration, establishing severity of a disorder or symptom, screening for a disorder or symptom, identifying treatment goals, and monitoring treatment response.

Rating scales' *utility* is highest when the scale is brief and easy to complete, and has a single total score, or several subscale scores, that can be easily derived and interpreted.

Rating scales must be *suitable*; that is, they must be geared to the youth's developmental abilities. Therefore, scales developed with adults cannot be administered to youth without examining their functioning in this age group.

Rating scales for youth are best used with multiple informants in order to consider ecological, or contextual, aspects of a youth's disorder. Typical informants include the youth, parents/guardians, teachers, coaches, other relevant adults, and sometimes peers.

The younger the child, the worse the agreement, or concordance, between the youth's own report and that of a relevant adult, demonstrating both developmental issues and personal perspective. Such disconcordance does not invalidate results.

Relevant adults show only poor to moderate agreement, or concordance, in their reports of a youth's behavior, demonstrating both contextual aspects of a youth's behavior and each individual's personal perspective. This does not invalidate either individual's report.

For self-report scales, reliability and validity are lower at younger ages and for youths with externalizing behaviors, rather than with internalizing symptoms.

multiple people's perspectives. Rating scale scores taken at different points in time can also help establish a trajectory for a child's functioning and show, for example, whether the youth is experiencing increasing or decreasing symptoms. Increasing symptoms, even if not yet at the "clinically significant" level, may suggest that the child is at risk for later problems and that early intervention is warranted. When used to establish trajectories, rating scales can provide a cost-efficient means of documenting evidence-based treatment effects. Third, rating scales can be useful in comparing a youth's functioning across different settings. Youth often function differently at home and at school, for example, so comparing a teacher's perspective to that of a primary caregiver can be critical to understanding the pattern and nature of a youth's difficulties. The *Diagnostic and Statistical Manual, Fourth Edition* (*DSM-IV*) requires evidence of impaired functioning in multiple settings in order to raise symptom clusters to the level of diagnosis. Therefore, multiple perspectives help to establish the contextual variation and context of the youth's symptoms and support formal diagnoses.

Rating scales can also be useful because they allow for a systematic investigation of a youth's perspective on his or her own functioning. Studies suggest that adults, including caregivers, are not always aware of the extent and exact nature of a child's symptoms, particularly "internalizing" symptoms such as depression or anxiety. Youth may also be more willing to disclose distress on a written rating scale than in a face-to-face interview. This may be particularly true among certain groups of youth, such as sexually abused males.

There are also several disadvantages to using rating scales. Most of these stem from false assumptions about rating scales or a poor understanding of their role in an overall assessment. For example, problems arise when physicians, psychiatrists, and other evaluators assume that an elevated score on a measure automatically equates to a diagnosis. The data collected with rating scales should be considered only in conjunction with other evaluation procedures and clinical judgment. Similarly, the text printouts generated by computer scoring systems should be treated with caution. When selecting a scale, it is important to evaluate its developmental suitability, particularly when working with special populations (e.g., those with developmental delays or very young children). A scale is not necessarily suited for all children, even if they fall into the age range for which the scale was designed. If, for example, a developmentally delayed 8-year-old is given a self-report measure designed for 8-year-olds, he or she may not understand the task at hand and misinterpret items and/or circle answer choices randomly, yielding an invalid score.

Unfortunately, many popular scales do not have sufficient data to determine how well the scale discriminates clinical groups, how reliable scores are, and how suitable the scale may be for a particular youth or clinical population. For example, if a scale has been developed with a school-based sample, it may not function as well with a clinic-based sample. This is a particular problem when it comes to using scales with minority and immigrant youth, as many of the most popular scales were validated on samples of Caucasian children. Simply translating a scale into another language does not ensure that the meaning of a score will equate across cultures.

Rating scales rely on the reports of youth and those individuals in their environment who know them well, and are subsequently only as useful as the informants are honest and perceptive. Individual and situational factors can affect a youth's score on rating scales. Youth who seek social acceptance may underreport symptoms ("denial" or "lying"), whereas those who feel overwhelmed or who are seeking access to diagnosis-based services may overreport symptoms ("faking" or "malingering"). Similarly, on observer-rated scales, adult respondents may convey their own distress and frustration with the youth by exaggerating symptoms, or may minimize their child's problems in an effort to protect him or her. Caregivers who are involved in custody disputes, or who are being monitored by child protective services, may have other reasons for inflating or deflating their child's scores, and caution should be used when interpreting scores from scales completed by parents under circumstances such as these.

Finally, it is important to be aware that there is typically low agreement among adults who rate a youth in different settings, such as teachers and parents, and only moderate agreement among adults in the same environment, such as mothers and fathers. Such disparities reflect both subjective differences in reporters' perceptions and objective variations in youths' behavior across settings. Not surprisingly, correlations between youths' self-reports and adults' reports are low. These disparities highlight the need to gather information from multiple informants across settings.

Psychometric Properties of Rating Scales

Rating scales are a means of measuring a construct, and all measurement is subject to error. Examining the psychometric properties of a measure is one way to examine this error in order to determine whether a measure is appropriate for use. Several psychometric properties are relevant to rating scales. This chapter briefly introduces these properties. More information is available in the resources listed in the "Suggested Readings" section at the end of this chapter.

Reliability refers to the consistency with which a scale's items measure the same construct the same way, every time. There are several types of reliability to consider. Internal reliability, or internal consistency, represents the degree to which individual items are consistent with each other. Items that are not internally consistent detract from the scale. Test–retest reliability, or stability, assesses whether a scale is stable over time. If the construct measured has not changed, then repeated measurements should be similar. This might be more difficult to determine for a "state" construct that is expected to wax and wane, such as suicidality, than for a "trait" construct, such as hyperactivity. Interrater reliability represents the agreement, or concordance, between different informants. As noted above, even well-regarded scales may have relatively low interrater reliability.

Validity indicates whether the scale accurately assesses what it was designed to assess. There are several types of validity. Content validity assesses whether the scale's items represent the construct being measured. Criterion-related validity refers to whether there is a relationship between the rating scale and other types of criteria or outcomes, such as other rating scales, verbal report, clinical data, etc. There are two subtypes: predictive validity assesses whether the scale correlates with an event that will occur in the future (such as whether a high score on a suicidality scale predicts later suicide attempts); concurrent validity assesses whether the scale correlates with an event assessed at the same time the scale is administered (such as whether a self-report anxiety scale correlates with clinicians' ratings of children's anxiety). Often, it is of interest to determine whether a scale effectively differentiates a group of youth who have been diagnosed with a condition using some "gold standard" evaluation from those without the diagnosis. This is a type of criterion validity, sometimes termed discriminant validity. Finally, convergent validity refers to whether the measure relates to, or correlates with, other measures that are designed to assess the same construct, whereas divergent validity refers to whether the measure does *not* correlate with measures that are supposed to measure some other construct. For example, ideally scores on a new measure of teen depression would more highly correlate with scores on other established measures of teen depression (demonstrating convergent validity) than with measures of teen anxiety (demonstrating divergent validity).

Psychometric properties and other characteristics of rating scales should be matched to the intended application. For example, screening requires high sensitivity (i.e., a low number of "false negatives") and a relatively brief instrument to reduce respondent burden. Monitoring requires good stability and a response format that is sensitive to response variation. Finally, the cutoff score that would indicate a clinically significant score varies in part due to factors like a youth's developmental status, culture, and clinical status, but such information is often not available. Thus, as mentioned earlier in text, caution is needed when using scales that were developed with groups that differ from the youth in question. Even when a scale has strong psychometric properties, it is often appropriate to use more than one scale to tap various aspects of a problem.

Broadband Rating Scales

Broadband scales assess youths' functioning across broad dimensions of behavior and symptoms, and are not designed to focus on one specific domain. They have high utility for initial evaluation and serve as guides for identifying problem areas that might warrant further evaluation. Broad coverage is important as a youth referred for one concern often has other problems needing attention which are not mentioned during an initial evaluation. Despite their utility, these scales suffer some limitations. To minimize respondent burden without sacrificing coverage of a broad range of problems, these scales often contain few items per subscale. Further, because broadband scales are often lengthy and cover multiple domains, they are not as useful for some applications, such as treatment monitoring. In short, these scales are best used to identify problems needing further evaluation with interview, observation, or narrowband scales.

The **Child Behavior Checklist** is a commercially available scale from the Achenbach System of Empirically Based Assessment (ASEBA). These scales have been the "gold standard" among broadband rating scales for over two decades. They include multiple versions for different reporters and age groups, including the CBCL 1½–5 and Caregiver-Teacher Report Form (C-TRF) for preschoolers, the parent report (CBCL) and Teacher Report Form (TRF) for youth 6 to 18 years old, and the Youth Self-Report (YSR) for youth 11 years and older. Although details vary by version, there are approximately 140 items that take 15 to 30 minutes to complete. These scales were updated in 2001 with new normative data and modifications to item content and subscale structure. In 2007, the authors updated the CBCL 6–18, TRF, and

YSR computer scoring profiles to offer norms relevant to several different cultures, which is helpful to avoid misinterpreting culture-based behavior.

The CBCL, TRF, and YSR include subscale scores for several specific problem areas, as well as composite scores for internalizing, externalizing, and total problems. The items can also be scored using factors that approximate the diagnostic criteria of the *DSM-IV*. There are also items to assess youths' adaptive functioning in the home, community, and school. The structure of the CBCL 1½–5 and C-TRF is comparable, with a few differences in subscales for this developmental stage, and the inclusion of a screen for communication deficits. Ivanova and colleagues have provided strong evidence that the basic eight-syndrome structure of the CBCL is upheld in 30 international societies across continents.

One aspect of the CBCL warrants comment. The CBCL subscale labels are sometimes misleading and should not be taken at face value. For example, the Aggressive Behavior subscale contains items about oppositional and defiant behaviors with only a few items actually describing physical aggression. Scores on the Thought Problems subscale can be affected by various cognitive problems, and elevated scores are not equivalent to a thought disorder. It is therefore important to review a respondent's responses to ascertain what he or she is really reporting. It is also important to inquire further about unusual responses to ensure understanding, particularly with younger children or lower-functioning caregivers. Overall, the CBCL has high utility due to its rapid coverage of a wide range of problems in various settings, the assessment of adaptive functioning, cross-cultural normative data, and its extensive use in the research literature. Computer scoring increases ease of use.

The **Early Childhood Inventory-4** (ECI-4), **Child Symptom Inventory-4** (CSI-4), **Adolescent Symptom Inventory-4** (ASI-4), and **Youth's Inventory-4** (YI-4) by Gadow and Sprafkin comprise another commercially available series of broadband scales for children aged 3 to 18 years. They have the advantage of being based on *DSM-IV* diagnostic criteria for the most common disorders of childhood and adolescence, as well as less common disorders such as schizophrenia, reactive attachment disorder, and somatization disorder. Parent and teacher forms exist for all ages, and a self-report form exists for youth aged 12 to 18 years (YI-4). Thus, the scales provide easy comparison of symptoms endorsed over time and across informants. There are approximately 100 items per scale that take 15 to 20 minutes to complete.

Two scoring procedures are available. The Symptom Severity procedure simply sums the items endorsed, which can then be compared to normative data. Kamphaus and Frick have cautioned, however, that the moderate size and diversity of the scales' normative sample limit the utility of this dimensional scoring approach. The Symptom Count procedure is more commonly used and allows clinicians to identify whether the child or adolescent is exhibiting the sufficient number of clinical symptoms (i.e., rated as occurring "often" or "very often") necessary to consider a *DSM-IV* diagnosis. However, the scales do not consider age of onset of symptoms or functional impairment, both of which are needed to make a formal diagnosis.

Many clinicians and investigators prefer this series of scales, as item responses can help to focus the diagnostic interview on the most likely problematic categories and related comorbidities. Another strength is the inclusion of disorders that are severe but rarely covered in other broadband scales. Thus, these scales may be helpful with children who present with more severe symptomatology. The psychometric properties of the scales vary by age, informant, and disorder, but substantial data guide users toward the most effective uses of these scales.

Narrowband Rating Scales: Externalizing Symptoms

Collett and colleagues have discussed the use of externalizing scales in child and adolescent psychiatry. Externalizing symptoms are observable by others, and include behaviors such as hyperactivity, aggression, and oppositionality. Youth displaying these behaviors are typically referred for services because of the challenges they pose to others. Given that youth tend to underestimate their externalizing symptoms, adults are generally considered to be the optimal respondents. Ratings are generally obtained from multiple adults in order to ascertain varied perspectives and to assess the ecological aspects of youths' behaviors (i.e., if aggression occurs both at home and at school). Many of these scales were developed for school-aged boys, and suitability is less clear for younger and older youth, and for girls.

Multiple available scales purport to measure attention-deficit hyperactivity disorder (ADHD), the most common, and best studied, externalizing disorder.

The **Conners' Rating Scale-Revised** (CRS-R), and its recently updated version—the Conners' Rating Scale-3 (CRS-3)—are commercially available ADHD-rating scales that have been the prototypical ADHD scale for two decades. The 2008 CRS-3 includes normative data, an assessment of executive functioning, a measure of impairment, and a validity scale. The coverage of executive functioning is especially useful given the overlap between ADHD and executive dysfunction. The CRS-R and the CRS-3 cover core ADHD subtypes in addition to comorbid problems, such as oppositional-defiant disorder (ODD) and conduct disorder (CD). They can be used with children aged 3 through 17 years (parent and teacher forms) and 12 through 17 years (self-report form). There are short and long form options for each informant that vary from 39 to 115 items and take 5 to 20 minutes to complete. The CRS-R and CRS-3 are strong choices for comprehensive assessment given the multiple indices, normative base, and strong psychometrics. The high sensitivity, particularly for the parent report version, makes these scales a good choice for screening. There is also an abbreviated version that has been useful in monitoring medication treatment. Relative disadvantages include the scales' somewhat poorer functioning of the comorbidity indices, and poor discrimination between ADHD, ODD, and CD. The CRS-3 does not yet have a body of literature supporting its use.

The **Swanson, Nolan, and Pelham-IV Questionnaire (SNAP-IV)** is an ADHD-rating scale that is available in the public domain. The SNAP was the first of several scales to utilize DSM symptoms of ADHD in a rating scale format that can be completed by both parents and teachers. The scale was the primary outcome measure in the Multisite Multimodal Treatment Study of Children with ADHD (MTA). The short version of the SNAP-IV includes the core *DSM-IV*-derived ADHD subscales of inattention, hyperactivity/impulsivity, as well as ODD, along with summary questions in each domain. The longer version (90 items, which take 20 minutes to complete) includes these core subscales along with items selected from other scales measuring ADHD and associated features. Finally, the SNAP-IV contains 40 items that have been extracted from *DSM-IV*-based criteria for several other disorders, such as internalizing symptoms, and motor disturbances. Thus, this scale incorporates multiple dimensions into a single scale. Clinicians and investigators often adapt selected indices or subscales from the SNAP-IV to their specific applications. Scoring information for the SNAP-IV is conveniently provided free on a website.

Representative normative data are not available, and cutoff scores are based on a study of 5- to 11-year-olds from low socioeconomic status and predominantly Hispanic heritage. Recent studies by Bussing and colleagues in 2008 identified two ADHD factors, an ODD factor and acceptable reliability, as well as race differences in teacher reports, which merit further examination. Internal consistency appears good to excellent.

Advantages include the SNAP-IV's basis in the *DSM-IV* and its coverage of other problems to gain a brief assessment of comorbidity. Several of the additional SNAP-IV indices (e.g., the SKAMP) have been useful to assess functioning. Its free, online availability and scoring make it readily available. However, the collapsed age and gender data preclude optimal interpretation of an individual's scores. There is no adolescent data or self-report version.

The **Eyberg Child Behavior Inventory** and the **Sutter–Eyberg Student Behavior Inventory-Revised** (ECBI and SESBI-R) are commercially available, well-established scales assessing externalizing behaviors corresponding to diagnoses of ADHD, ODD, and CD. The ECBI is completed by parents and the SESBI-R by teachers. Both versions use the same format with item overlap. The ECBI contains 36 items and the SESBI-R 38 items, and both take 5 to 10 minutes to complete. Respondents rate each item on two dimensions: an intensity scale (I) assesses behavior frequency, and a problem scale (P) assesses reporters' perceptions of whether the behavior is problematic. This format is clinically useful, as respondents may rate behaviors as problematic even if they occur at a normative rate, thus indicating a low threshold and/or inappropriate expectations. Conversely, a respondent may rate problem behaviors as frequent but not problematic, reflecting a high threshold. In 2008, Butler and colleagues found support for the ECBI discrepancy hypothesis; that is, discrepancy in elevated scores on the I and P scales is associated with problematic parenting, such as intolerance of misbehavior or permissive parenting.

The ECBI and SESBI-R have been extensively used to discriminate clinical samples of disruptive youth and to assess the efficacy of interventions, such as Hutchings and colleagues's 2006 study of the relation of parenting programs for high-risk preschoolers to crime rates. Although norms are available for youth up to 16 years of age, these scales are most suitable for younger children, not for older children with major CDs. These measures are widely used across ethnic and racial groups in the United States. There are no major disadvantages.

Rating Scales Assessing Internalizing Symptoms

Myers and Winters have reviewed rating scales that assess youths' internalizing symptoms, specifically depression and anxiety. These symptoms are manifestations of psychological distress that may not be readily observable by others, such as anxiety and depression, and it is important to assess these symptoms via youth self-report; ideally, relevant adults complete parallel parent-report and/or teacher-report forms. Youth generally endorse more symptoms than these adults appreciate, and interrater reliability is often low. Clinician-rated scales integrate youths' and adults' responses and may provide greater accuracy in treatment studies. Given that youths' feelings of depression, anxiety, or suicidality wax and wane, it is difficult to know whether observed change over time is due to a real clinical change or random error in the scale unless test–retest reliability has been established. Finally, many internalizing symptom scales detect symptoms of other internalizing disorders; for example, depression-rating scales generally detect anxiety and suicidality, making scales with good discriminative and divergent validity especially valuable.

Rating Scales Assessing Mood Symptoms

Depression-rating scales have many challenges. Many measure distress rather than depression. Also, it can be difficult to discriminate clinically depressed youth from their nondepressed peers, as depressive symptoms are common in both clinical and community samples.

The **Beck Depression Inventory-II** (BDI-II) is a commercially available scale developed for adults that has become the most popular depression-rating scale for adolescents over 13 years. It has been used in multiple diverse applications. The BDI-II contains 21 items that take 10 minutes to complete. This measure assesses the same aspects of depression in adolescents that it does in adults: cognitive, behavioral, affective, and somatic. The BDI-II discriminates outpatient depressed teens from those with anxiety and CDs. This scale is also useful for monitoring treatment process. The BDI-II has been translated into several languages and used with various ethnic populations, but caution is warranted as cutoff scores vary with culture and are not always available. One of the scale's weaknesses is that it lacks an adult-report form to provide a contextual perspective.

The **Children's Depression Inventory** (CDI) is a commercially available scale that was developed by Kovacs as a downward extension of the BDI. It can be used with youth 7 to 17 years old. It is the most frequently studied and utilized measure of juvenile depression. Its 27 items take 15 minutes to complete. Scoring yields five subscales: negative mood, interpersonal problems, ineffectiveness, anhedonia, and negative self-esteem. The CDI functions well psychometrically and has good predictive validity. It has been translated into several languages and has been used extensively across cultures. However, sensitivity, specificity, and discriminative validity are suboptimal and the CDI appears to measure distress, rather than depression. Nonetheless, the CDI enjoys a broad literature supporting its use.

The **Children's Depression Rating Scale-Revised** (CDRS-R) is a commercial, clinician-rated scale patterned by Poznanski and Mokros on the Hamilton Depression Rating Scale. It can be used with youth aged 6 years and older. It consists of 17 items that take 15 to 20 minutes to administer. The CDRS-R is unique in that it integrates information from both the child and the parent, incorporates behaviors observed during the interview, and includes several items not specific to depression. Thus, the measure's construct of depression differs somewhat from *DSM-IV.* Jain and colleagues have recently found solid psychometric properties for the CDRS-R. There is some evidence of discriminative validity, and impressive interrater reliability supports the alleged benefit of clinician-rated scales over lay scales. The short form facilitates screening and repeated assessment. Wagner and colleagues have found it to be sensitive to treatment. Use of the CDRS-R in combination with self-reports and global ratings offers comprehensive, yet efficient, assessment.

The **Moods and Feelings Questionnaire** (MFQ) is a scale in the public domain developed by Angold and colleagues to screen for depression in youth aged 8 to 18 years. It is available as a child-self-report and a parent-report form. The 33 items of the long form (MFQ) take 15 minutes to complete and the 13 items of the short form (SMFQ) take 5 minutes to complete. The MFQ covers symptoms of major depressive disorder and dysthymia as specified by the *Diagnostic and Statistical Manual, Third Edition, Revised* (*DSM-III-R*), but includes other symptoms of clinical significance as well. This construct of depression approximates *DSM-IV* criteria sufficiently to remain relevant. Several studies, including that by Daviss and colleagues in 2006, demonstrate solid psychometric properties, including high internal consistency for all forms, strong test–retest reliability, and good concordance with depressive diagnoses derived from standardized diagnostic interviews. Furthermore, the MFQ discriminates between pediatric and psychiatric patients and depressed and nondepressed youth with good sensitivity and specificity. The MFQ has two major advantages. First, it is based on a clear diagnostic construct of depression, which distinguishes it from other depression-rating scales. Second, the MFQ can be readily downloaded from the author's website free of charge.

The **Mania Rating Scale** (MRS) is an older, brief scale available in the public domain to assess mania. It was developed for completion by the clinician after he or she collects data from the patient and relevant other individuals, typically on inpatient units. It consists of 11 items that take around 15 minutes to administer. The MRS has been increasingly used with youth diagnosed with bipolar disorder (BPD), but the lack of consensus regarding the diagnostic criteria for juvenile BPD impedes interpretation of these studies. In 2004, Youngstrom and colleagues developed a parent-report version that shows good concordance with the clinician-administered MRS. The MRS has shown some ability to discriminate BPD from ADHD, other disruptive behaviors, and depression. Several investigators including Wagner and colleagues have found that the MRS is sensitive to treatment with mood stabilizers. Overall, however, the MRS has not been adequately examined to establish its utility for clinical applications with youth, despite its increasingly wide usage.

Rating Scales Assessing Suicidality and Hopelessness

Winters and colleagues have reviewed scales relevant to suicidality. The term *suicidality* encompasses suicidal ideation, suicide attempts, and completed suicide. Suicidal ideation and attempts are relatively common, but completed suicide is not. It is therefore difficult to attain strong predictive validity with these scales, and the goal is for scales with high sensitivity to identify youth in need of further assessment. Hopelessness strongly predicts suicidality, and scales measuring hopelessness are often used instead of suicide-rating scales.

The **Suicidal Ideation Questionnaire** (SIQ) by Reynolds consists of two very popular, commercially available scales that are widely used to assess suicidality, one for high school students and one for middle school students. Each contains 15 to 30 items that take 10 to 15 minutes to complete. These scales are most commonly used as part of suicide prevention efforts in schools, although they are appropriate to clinical settings as well. Both scales measure the intensity and frequency of suicidal ideation during the past month. Standardization was conducted with large normative samples, a major strength of the measure. Psychometric properties are quite good over various samples and across cultures. Large differences in scores between suicide attempters and other youth, combined with good sensitivity and specificity, suggest discriminative validity. These scales have been used to elucidate the relationship of suicidality to hopelessness, depression, and loss.

The **Columbia Suicide Screen** (Teen Screen) was developed by Shaffer and colleagues in 2004 as part of a program to assess high school students' functioning and need for services, particularly in the primary care setting. The Teen Screen is an 11-item screen for suicidality that is embedded within a larger 32-item questionnaire. The entire questionnaire takes about 10 minutes to complete. It was developed with a large sample of high school students of mixed race and ethnicity in New York City. There has been some concern about the specificity of this scale; that is, it identifies false positives due to youth endorsing general mood or substance use items. This feature may not be such a disadvantage if the scale is used for screening and there is an opportunity to follow up youth with a personal interview. A main advantage of this scale is its availability in the public domain on the author's website that contains much other useful information and a newsletter particularly geared to primary care and community providers.

The **Beck Hopelessness Scale** (BHS) is one of the commercially available Beck series of scales developed for adults, but widely used with adolescents as young as 12 years old. It contains 20 items that take 5 to 10 minutes to complete. Hopelessness is correlated with depression, but more powerfully predicts suicidal ideation and eventual suicide. The proposed subscales of the BHS have not been consistently validated with adolescents, and total scores are generally used. The BHS strongly discriminates suicidal adolescents from nonsuicidal ones, and predicts serious suicide attempts. It has good utility for screening and longitudinal assessment. Its utility for monitoring treatment is less clear due to lack of stability data. McMillan and colleagues recently conducted a meta-analysis that indicated that while the standard cutoff point identifies a group of youth at high risk for potential suicide, the actual magnitude of risk may not be as high as typically thought. This study also found that the cutoff point does identify youth at risk for self-harm, but has a low specificity rate (i.e., yields a large number of false positives).

The **Hopelessness Scale for Children** (HSC) was developed by Kazdin and colleagues as a downward modification of the BHS. It is available in the public domain. It functions best with children aged 6 to 13 years. Hopelessness in children relates to a negative attributional style fostered through aversive developmental conditions, and correlates with depression and suicidality, but not with anxiety. High scores on the HSC, along with high scores on measures of depression, should alert clinicians to serious risk for self-harm. The HSC has discriminated suicidal children from nonsuicidal ones. The HSC should function well in screening applications, and Voeltz has shown some sensitivity to treatment. It has a long history of use with diverse psychiatric and medical samples and enjoys an extensive literature supporting its use with suicidal as well as nonsuicidal youth. Its brevity (it consists of 17 items that can be completed in 5 to 10 minutes with a yes/no format) makes it easily completed by children.

Rating Scales Assessing Anxiety Symptoms

Myers and Winters have reviewed anxiety-rating scales for youth. They note that newer scales have been developed with youth rather than being modified from adult scales, making them more developmentally relevant.

The **Multidimensional Anxiety Scale for Children** (MASC) is a popular, commercially available scale developed by March with diverse clinical and community samples 8 to 19 years old. The MASC has four subscales, three of which can be subdivided: physical symptoms (tense/restless and somatic/autonomic), social anxiety (humiliation/rejection and performance fears), harm avoidance (perfectionism and anxious coping), and separation anxiety. It has 39 items that take 10 to 20 minutes to complete. Two factors map onto the *DSM-IV* diagnoses of social phobia and separation anxiety disorder, while the total score maps onto generalized anxiety disorder. The MASC offers several advantages. Its construct of anxiety diverges from depression, it includes an Inconsistency Index that identifies invalid profiles, and it is sensitive to treatment. The MASC has strong psychometric properties. Baldwin and Dadds have recently reported similarly good functioning of both parent and child versions in cross-cultural samples. This scale has become the favored anxiety-rating scale for research and clinical work. However, in 2008, van Gastel and Ferdinand did not find support for the MASC as a valid screening instrument for *DSM-IV* disorders, so additional research may be warranted.

The **Screen for Child Anxiety–Related Emotional Disorders** (SCARED) was developed by Birmaher and colleagues with youth presenting to a mood and anxiety disorders clinic. It is available in the public domain. Its five factors conform to *DSM-IV* criteria for generalized anxiety disorder, separation anxiety disorder, social phobia, panic, and school phobia. It has 41 items that take 10 to 20 minutes to complete. This scale shows divergence from disruptive behaviors and, more impressively, from depression. Cohen and colleagues found that it is sensitive to treatment effects. The SCARED has been used cross-culturally, particularly in the Netherlands. Its broad coverage, basis on *DSM-IV* criteria, and cost-free availability make it appealing especially for clinical work. It can be used with children 6 years and older (parent report) or 8 years and older (self-report).

The **Social Phobia and Anxiety Inventory for Children** (SPAI-C) is a commercially available scale that measures the specific anxiety construct of social anxiety in youth between the ages of 8 and 14 (26 items, 15 to 20 minutes to complete). Beidel and colleagues found three subscales: assertiveness, traditional social encounters, and public performance. Inderbitzen-Nolan and colleagues have found robust sensitivity, specificity, and construct validity. The SPAI-C is impressive in its ability to discriminate among anxiety disorders. However, its sensitivity to treatment needs clarification, as variable results have been reported in treatment studies. A parent-report version is available that has demonstrated good internal consistency (SPAI-P) in a recent study by Higa and colleagues. The special focus of this scale has found many uses with school and clinical samples. Sanna and colleagues have noted that different clinical cutoffs may be appropriate for various translated versions of this scale, due to cultural differences in the expression of social phobia.

Rating Scales Assessing Trauma Symptoms

Ohan and colleagues have summarized scales assessing trauma and its associated symptoms. Psychological trauma symptoms, often referred to as posttraumatic stress symptoms (PTSS), are a subcategory of anxiety symptoms that are sometimes exhibited by children who have experienced a traumatic event. Because interest in measuring posttraumatic stress disorder (PTSD) and its ramifications in children is relatively recent, many of the available scales have not been fully examined. Therefore, recommendations made now may change as new data are published. Nevertheless, with caution, the following scales can provide useful information.

The **Impact of Events Scale** (IES) and the revised IES (IES-R) were designed to assess the psychological impact of a specific trauma or stressor on adults. They are available in the public domain. As these scales were developed before the inclusion of PTSD in the *DSM* nomenclature, they do not reflect *DSM-IV* criteria. These scales have been used as self-report measures with youth as young as 8 years old, but generally without adequate developmental modifications. Factor analysis with trauma-exposed adolescents has produced the original two main factors, avoidance and intrusions, as well as a third factor, numbing. Solid factor structures and psychometric properties have been established with adults, and preliminary data are available with youth including moderate sensitivity and specificity for a PTSD diagnosis. The IES's major advantages are its translation into various languages, applications with adolescents in various cultures, and demonstration that reactions to trauma are consistent across cultures. The major disadvantages relate to the lack of optimal developmental modifications and the lack of psychometric properties for childhood samples. The factor structure is also not clear. Overall, the IES is best used to screen for youth in need of full PTSD evaluation and to understand the breadth of symptoms that may develop in response to trauma. It has found a role in pediatric psychology, such as cancer patients and their families. A relatively new 13-item version (5 to 10 minutes to complete) called the **Children's Revised Impact of Events Scale** (CRIES) has been used by Smith with children who experienced war in Bosnia. Giannopoulou and colleagues have found initial support for a three-factor structure: arousal, intrusion, and avoidance. However, additional research is needed before the CRIES can be routinely used in practice.

The **Children's PTSD-Reaction Index** (CPTS-RI) is the best known and most widely used scale assessing the sequelae of trauma. It was developed by Pynoos and colleagues as a clinician-administered scale that can also be used as a self-report scale with youth over the age of 8 years. It is available in the public domain and is a widely used measure of PTSD symptoms for children and adolescents. The items are based on an adult measure of PTSD derived from the *DSM-III-R*. Factor analysis has revealed three factors: reexperiencing/numbing, fear/anxiety, and concentration/sleep. This structure partially overlaps with the three *DSM-IV* factors of reexperiencing, arousal, and avoidance. Interrater reliability appears very good, and test–retest reliability is excellent. Validity is suggested by extensive evidence that children who had greater exposure to traumatic events have higher CPTS-RI scores. Sensitivity and specificity for diagnosis of PTSD are moderate to good.

The CPTS-RI has extensive research supporting its suitability for children of varying ages, cultures, and traumatic experiences, and has been translated into multiple languages. In 2006, Thienkrua and colleagues used the CPTS-RI to evaluate tsunami-affected youth in southern Thailand, and in 2009, Pat-Horenczyk and colleagues used it to assess youth involved in the Israeli–Palestinian conflict. It is one of the best studied and most frequently used scales for evaluating traumatized youths. Normative data are not available.

The **Trauma Symptom Checklist for Children** (TSCC) was developed by Briere as a self-report scale for youth aged 8 to 16 years to assess distress and related symptoms after an acute or chronic trauma. It does not assess the *DSM-IV* construct of PTSD. It is commercially available. The TSCC has six clinically derived subscales: anxiety, depression, anger, posttraumatic stress, dissociation, and sexual concerns. It contains 54 items that take 20 to 25 minutes to complete. The TSCC-Alternate Form (44 items) does not contain sexual trauma symptoms. There are two validity indices to detect underresponding (underresponse, i.e., denial) and overresponding (hyperresponse, i.e., faking or "crying for help"). The dissociation scale of the TSCC contains two components identified through factor analysis: fantasy and overt dissociation. Similarly, the sexual concerns scale contains sexual preoccupation and sexual distress components.

The internal consistencies of the subscales are good, with the exception of the sexual concerns and hyperresponse subscales, which are moderate. Elliott and Briere have reported support for concurrent, convergent, divergent, and discriminant validity. Lanktree and Briere found that the TSCC is sensitive to psychotherapy for sexually abused children. Unlike many other trauma scales, the TSCC has a large normative base of ethnically and economically diverse children who do not have a history of trauma. The **Trauma Symptom Checklist for Young Children**

(TSCYC) was developed by Briere in 2005 as a parallel caregiver report for children aged 3 to 12 years. The TSCYC has 90 items (15 to 25 minutes to complete) that yield eight clinical sub-scales—anxiety, depression, anger/aggression, posttraumatic stress-intrusion, posttraumatic stress-avoidance, posttraumatic stress-arousal, dissociation, and sexual concerns—as well as a summary posttraumatic stress scale (posttraumatic stress-total). In 2001, Briere and colleagues reported initial evidence for good reliability and validity of the TSCYC.

The **Child PTSD Symptom Scale** (CPSS) by Foa and colleagues addresses the need for a self-report scale specific to the *DSM-IV* concept of PTSD for youths aged 8 to 15 years. It is available in the public domain. The items directly assess *DSM-IV*-defined PTSD symptoms with a format and wording that are suitable for children and adolescents. It contains 24 items that take 15 minutes to complete. The three CPSS subscales were not derived by factor analy-sis but are based on the *DSM-IV*: reexperiencing, avoidance, and arousal. The CPSS also in-cludes seven items measuring youths' functional impairment as a result of PTSD.

Foa and colleagues investigated the psychometric properties with children who survived a serious earthquake. They found that the subscales are highly correlated and may not measure meaningfully separate constructs. Internal reliability was moderate to very good. Test–retest reli-ability was good. There is also support for convergent and divergent validity. The brevity, ease of administration and scoring, efficiency, and no-cost availability of the CPSS afford excellent util-ity for clinical and research use. Scores can be examined dimensionally in order to judge severity, as well as categorically to examine overlap with the *DSM-IV* guidelines. However, the CPSS does not have a normative base and needs to be examined with larger and more diverse samples to better understand its functioning and define potential applications in young populations. Furthermore, although the authors suggest cutoffs for concordance with *DSM-IV*-based PTSD, sensitivity and specificity have not been investigated. In 2008, Kohrt and colleagues used the CPSS to assess the mental health of Nepalese child soldiers.

Rating Scales Assessing Autism Spectrum Disorders

There has been an increased emphasis on early diagnosis and treatment of pervasive develop-mental disorders, or as noted here, autism spectrum disorders (ASD), given the demonstrated efficacy of early interventions. While the diagnosis of ASD is best determined by a multidisci-plinary, multimethod assessment, a number of scales can help in gathering relevant informa-tion about the child's behavior. These screening scales are most appropriately used as aids for identifying children who require more extensive diagnostic evaluation.

The **Social Communication Questionnaire** (SCQ) was originally developed by Rutter and colleagues as the Autism Screening Questionnaire. It is based on the Autism Diagnostic Interview, and items correspond to *DSM-IV* criteria for the diagnosis of autism. It is a com-mercially available parent-report scale used specifically to screen children for deficits in social skills or communication. Its 40 items take approximately 10 minutes to complete. The SCQ is simple to complete and to score. While it has demonstrated high specificity and sensitivity in identifying children with ASD, it may be less sensitive for children with "high functioning autism" who are more verbal or who have highly developed cognitive abilities. It can be used with children 4 years of age and older. Bolte and colleagues reported initial evidence of cross-cultural validity.

The **Modified Checklist for Autism in Toddlers** (M-CHAT) is a screening instrument available in the public domain for the assessment of behaviors consistent with ASD in children 18 months to 2 years old. Robins and colleagues designed the M-CHAT as a two-step process including (1) a parent questionnaire (23 items taking approximately 5 to 10 minutes to com-plete) and (2) a clinical interview of the parent. The interview is structured to provide follow-up questions to clarify items that were "failed" (i.e., consistent with ASD) on the parent question-naire. Use of the parent-rating form alone without follow-up interview has not been validated.

Ventola and colleagues recently reported high levels of sensitivity and specificity in identifying children with ASD. These features make the M-CHAT desirable for use in primary care and other settings where a brief screening measure is needed.

The **Autism Behavior Checklist** (ABC), developed by Krug and colleagues, is a screening checklist in the public domain for assessing ASD that is completed by the parent or a teacher familiar with the child. It has 57 questions that take 10 to 20 minutes to complete. It is one component of the Autism Screening Instrument for Education Planning (ASIEP), a more comprehensive system of ASD assessment, but it has frequently been used alone for screening purposes. The scale includes a number of behaviors that are frequently seen in children with ASD, and the informant is asked to identify whether or not the child exhibits that behavior. The ABC was originally researched for use with school-aged children but has effectively been used with children as young as 1.5 years. As supported by Eaves and colleagues, the greatest strength of the ABC is its demonstrated ability to discriminate children with ASD from those who exhibit other disorders that are often confused with ASD, such as mental retardation.

Rating Scales Assessing Functional Impairment and Adaptive Functioning

Winters and colleagues have reviewed scales that assess adaptive functioning in youth. These scales differ from those reviewed earlier in the text in that they are not keyed to specific psychiatric symptoms, but rather tap deficits in functioning or adaptation. Impairment may result from the psychiatric illness or may have a shared etiology with the illness. Global scales assign a summary score to describe the youth's overall functioning. The simplicity of a single score allows for easy comparison of impairment across diagnoses and time. However, because they do not distinguish which domains of functioning are most impaired, they may not optimally inform treatment planning. Multidimensional scales are therefore often more helpful.

The **Children's Global Assessment Scale** (CGAS) is a unidimensional, widely used clinician-rated scale adapted from the adult version, the Global Assessment of Functioning (GAF) Scale. It is available in the public domain. During the diagnostic interview, the rater gathers a broad range of data regarding the youth's functioning in relation to history, symptomatology, and behavior across settings. This information is summarized into an overall score ranging from 1 to 100. The psychometric properties of the CGAS are sound. It has been used extensively in research and clinical work, domestically and internationally, to characterize psychosocial functioning in clinical samples, including medically ill youth. The CGAS has been used as an outcome variable to complement measures of syndromal improvement in both psychosocial and pharmacological studies, such as the 2006 Treatment of Adolescent Depression Study described by Vitiello and colleagues. In 2007, Wagner and colleagues modified the CGAS for children with pervasive developmental disorders (DD-CGAS). While the psychometric properties of the DD-CGAS appear sound, its utility in clinical and research samples has yet to be determined.

The **Columbia Impairment Scale** (CIS) is another global impairment scale in the public domain. Bird developed the CIS for administration by a lay interviewer as it is "respondent based;" that is, the interviewer does not make a clinical judgment, but relies on the patient's responses to the items. The downside is that this approach requires time from staff. The CIS contains 13 items scored on a five-point Likert-type scale that can be completed in 5 to 10 minutes. It is available in both parent-report (CIS-P) and child/adolescent-report (CIS-C) versions. It covers functioning in interpersonal relations, schoolwork or job, use of leisure time, and psychopathology, although it is usually used as an overall global rating with a single score. It is available in both English and Spanish.

The CIS has good stability, but its sensitivity to change has not been established. However, both parent and child versions of the CIS discriminate clinical samples of youth, making it useful for detecting differences between different groups of youth. Also, the CIS performs better than checklists in detecting youth in need of mental health treatment, making it a good screening tool. The ability to look at the four domains of functioning may offer advantages over the CGAS. Overall, the CIS has good utility for applications that call for a brief measure that requires little training and allows comparison of parents' and youth's perceptions of a youth's functioning.

The **Vineland Adaptive Behavior Scales-Second Edition** (VABS-II) is a commercially available series of scales that comprise the prototypical measure of adaptive functioning. Sparrow and colleagues developed the VABS-II as a semi-structured interview with caregivers for individuals from birth through adulthood. Multiple forms are available. The survey form is most frequently used. Although lengthy (varies from taking 20 to 90 minutes to complete), it is a comprehensive scale whose items cover developmental skills in five clinically and empirically derived domains: communication, daily living skills, socialization, motor skills, and an optional maladaptive behavior domain. Rather than administering all items, estimated starting points are provided by age, and basal and ceiling rules are used to ensure that a youth's abilities are adequately represented. The expanded form adds further content to assist with the development of education and treatment programs. Parent and teacher rating forms are available.

The VABS-II has a good normative base, and its supplemental norms for selected developmental groups are a strength. Reliability and validity are robust. The VABS has a strong history of use in many diverse applications. It has been used with very young developmentally impaired infants and preschoolers, and with children diagnosed with ASD and other developmental disorders. It is often used to establish functional deficits in order to qualify children for school services and for disability insurance. In 2009, Goldberg and colleagues found psychometric support for a version designed for non-Western populations, for example, Vietnamese preschoolers.

The **Adaptive Behavior Assessment System-Second Edition** (ABAS-II) by Harrison and Oakland is another popular, commercially available measure of adaptive functioning that provides information based on age-related norms. The ABAS-II uses caregivers' reports of children's behaviors and abilities to assess adaptive functioning in individuals from birth through 89 years. The number of items varies by age, but it consists of approximately 240 items that take 30 to 45 minutes to complete. The structure of the ABAS-II is based on recommendations of the American Association on Intellectual and Developmental Disabilities and confirmed with factor analysis: conceptual, social, practical, and a general adaptive composite score. There are 10 individual skill area scores that are correlated, but not so highly as to be redundant. The ABAS-II appears to be psychometrically sound with high internal consistency and concurrent validity, assessed in relation to the VABS, as reported by Rust and Wallace. Overall, the ABAS-II offers a comprehensive assessment of children's adaptive functioning in various domains using a simple and relatively short measure. It is increasingly used to establish disability status to obtain services and funding for children with cognitive limitations. Given its ease of use and the utility of its information, the ABAS-II will likely be increasingly used in research and clinical settings.

Conclusions

Rating scales have a core role as adjunctive tools in the assessment and treatment of youth suffering with psychiatric disorders. They complement a diagnostic evaluation and cannot be used alone to make a diagnosis or to inform specific treatment recommendations.

Rating scales must be geared to the youth's developmental abilities, not just to his or her chronological age. They are best used with multiple informants to provide context and ecological validity to a youth's symptoms. The low to moderate concordance among informants does not invalidate a scale's utility. For rating scales assessing externalizing behaviors adult report is often most helpful, while internalizing symptoms are best assessed with a youth's self-report.

The increasing focus on the effects of experiencing a traumatic event on children's functioning has led to the development and increased use of available trauma-specific scales. These scales detect symptoms not well addressed by other internalizing rating scales. Rating scales for ASD can be helpful in identifying youth who require more extensive diagnostic evaluation. Rating scales assessing functional impairment or adaptive functioning measure a construct that differs from, but overlaps with, symptomatology. Perhaps, the major contribution of rating scales has been their role in establishing evidence-based assessment and treatment of children and adolescents suffering with psychiatric disorders.

CLINICAL VIGNETTES

VIGNETTE 1: CHILD WITH MIXED EXTERNALIZING AND INTERNALIZING BEHAVIORS

RS is a 10-year-old boy whose parents had him repeat kindergarten due to his teacher's report of "immaturity" regarding self-control and socialization. In first grade he seemed to be settling down, but still struggled academically and socially. His parents spent a lot of time helping him complete his schoolwork, and set up social activities for him. But when his fourth-grade teacher expressed concerns about his falling behind academically, his parents brought him in for evaluation. They note that he has always been a good boy but rather disorganized, "spacey," and restless. He also does not do well with new events or transitions, and worries a lot about bad things that might happen, especially when beginning new activities. He also has a lot of aches and pains. When a third child was born to the family, RS's parents could no longer spend so much extra time helping him with homework and social activities, and he fell further behind. His teacher and parents decided to ask his doctor about ADHD and to consider medication.

After an initial evaluation, the doctor asked the teacher to complete the TRF and the mother to complete the CBCL. Both scales showed elevations on the *DSM-IV*-Oriented Scale for ADHD. Additionally, the teacher's TRF showed an elevated Internalizing Index and a *DSM-IV*-Oriented Scale suggesting anxiety. Like 30% of children diagnosed with ADHD, RS seemed to have a comorbid anxiety disorder. To better sort this out, the doctor had the teacher and mother complete the SNAP ADHD rating scales, both of which were highly consistent with a diagnosis of ADHD. RS also completed the MASC. On this measure, he endorsed high levels of anxiety consistent with generalized anxiety disorder. His mother was quite surprised to learn of her son's level of anxiety. The doctor initially treated the ADHD symptoms with a stimulant medication and monitored RS's ADHD symptoms with monthly ratings on the follow-up form of the SNAP rating scales. RS did better but developed several tics that were stigmatizing, and his anxiety worsened per the follow-up form of the MASC. The doctor then switched him to atomoxetine (Strattera), and the mother started a course of parent-behavior training. RS's ADHD symptoms improved as evident on subsequent administrations of the SNAP, the tics stopped, and his anxiety abated considerably over the ensuing year.

VIGNETTE 2: ADOLESCENT WITH INTERNALIZING SYMPTOMS

AG is a 16-year-old female who does not have a history of mental health difficulties. She has always performed well in school, has a relatively large social network, and is described as a "happy person" by her parents. However, 10 weeks ago she witnessed the accidental drowning death of her younger brother in their family's pool. Since then, her grades have plummeted, she has withdrawn from her friends, and she appears moody, anxious, and irritable to her family. She is also complaining of a "jumpy heart," and of regular stomachaches. Her mother reported that she has a very difficult time waking AG up for school in the mornings. Her parents expressed concern that AG has "fallen into a deep depression" and requested medication for her.

When interviewed, AG endorsed feeling worried and unhappy, although she denied suicidality. She was unable to maintain eye contact, and looked down at the floor as she spoke. She reported having trouble focusing at school due to "images that won't go away," and said that she often has the feeling that she is back by the pool, helplessly watching her brother. She endorsed feeling tired all the time.

It seemed clear that AG was affected by the trauma of witnessing her brother's death, but the degree to which she was experiencing anxiety, depression, or PTSS was less clear. To better understand her internalizing symptoms, several self-report scales were administered. The BDI-II was moderately elevated, indicating subclinical levels of depression and distress. AG had written comments next to most of the items she endorsed, such as "because of my brother's death" or "only because my brother died." AG also completed the MASC. She showed a severely elevated score on the subscale of physical symptoms, which was consistent with her self-report. Nothing else was elevated. While completing this measure, AG commented that filling out the questionnaire reminded her of some other physical feelings she has that she forgot to share during the interview. Finally, AG completed the TSCC. She had significant elevations on the subscales of anxiety, depression, and posttraumatic stress. Again, completing the questionnaire caused AG to remember symptoms that she had forgotten to share or did not think were important, such as the fact that she often cannot sleep due to severe nightmares. The TSCC suggested PTSD, and AG was subsequently referred to a psychologist who did further evaluation and confirmed the diagnosis. AG participated in a course of trauma-focused cognitive–behavioral therapy, and her parents were referred for their own treatment related to the loss of their son. AG responded well to therapy and did not require medications, and is now functioning at her baseline level.

BIBLIOGRAPHY

American Psychiatric Association. *Diagnostic and Statistical Manual of Mental Disorders, Third Edition-Revised (DSM-IIIR)*. Washington, DC: American Psychiatric Association; 1987.

American Psychiatric Association. *Diagnostic and Statistical Manual of Mental Disorders, Fourth Edition (DSM-IV)*. Washington, DC: American Psychiatric Association Press; 1994.

Angold A, Erkanli A, Silberg J, et al. Depression scale scores in 8–17 year-olds: Effects of age and gender. *Journal of Child Psychology & Psychiatry & Applied Disciplines*. 2002;43:1052–1063.

Baldwin JS, Dadds ME. Reliability and validity of parent and child versions of the multidimensional anxiety scale for children in community samples. *J Am Acad Child Adolesc Psychiatry*. 2007;46:252–260.

Bolte S, Holtmann M, Poustka F. The social communication questionnaire (SCQ) as a screener for autism spectrum disorders: additional evidence and cross-cultural validity. *J Am Acad Child Adolesc Psychiatry*. 2008;47:719–720.

Briere J, Johnson K, Bissada A, et al. The trauma symptom checklist for young children (TSCYC): reliability and association with abuse exposure in a multi-site study. *Child Abuse Negl*. 2001;25:1001–1014.

Birmaher B, Khetarpal S, Brent D et al. The Screen for Child Anxiety Related Emotional Disorders (SCARED): Scale construction and psychometric characteristics. *J Am Acad Child Adolesc Psychiatry*. 1997;36:545–553.

Bussing R, Fernandez M, Harwood M, et al. Parent and teacher SNAP-IV ratings of attention deficit hyperactivity disorder symptoms: psychometric properties and normative ratings from a school district sample. *Assessment*. 2008;15:317–328.

Butler AM, Brestan EV, Eyberg SM. Examination of the Eyberg child behavior inventory discrepancy hypothesis. *Child Fam Behav Ther*. 2008;30:257–262.

Cohen JA, Mannarino AP, Staron VR. A pilot study of modified cognitive-behavioral therapy for childhood traumatic grief (CBT-CTG). *J Am Acad Child Adolesc Psychiatry*. 2008;45:1465–1473.

Collett BR, Ohan JL, Myers KM. Ten-year review of rating scales. V: scales assessing attention deficit hyperactivity disorder. *J Am Acad Child Adolesc Psychiatry*. 2003;42:1015–1037.

Collett BR, Ohan JL, Myers KM. Ten-year review of rating scales. VI: scales assessing externalizing behaviors. *J Am Acad Child Adolesc Psychiatry*. 2003;42:1143–1170.

Daviss WB, Birmaher B, Melhem NA, et al. Criterion validity of the mood and feelings questionnaire for depressive episodes in clinic and non-clinic subjects. *J Child Psychol Psychiatry*. 2006;47:927–934.

Eaves RC, Campbell HA, Chambers D. Criterion-related and construct validity of the pervasive developmental disorders rating scale and the autism behavior checklist. *Psychol Sch*. 2000;37:311–321.

Elliott DM, Briere JN. Forensic sexual abuse evaluations of older children: disclosures and symptomatology. *Behav Sci Law*. 1994;12:261–277.

Foa EB, Johnson KM, Feeny NC, et al. The child PTSD symptom scale: a preliminary examination of its psychometric properties. *J Clin Child Psychol*. 2001;30:376–384.

Giannopoulou I, Smith P, Ecker C, et al. Factor structure of the children's revised impact of event scale (CRIES) with children exposed to earthquake. *Pers Individ Dif*. 2006;40:1027–1037.

Goldberg MR, Dill CA, Shin JY, et al. Reliability and validity of the Vietnamese *Vineland adaptive behavior scales* with preschool-age children. *Res Dev Disabil*. 2009;30:592–602.

Gracious BL, Youngstrom EA, Findling RL, et al. Discriminative validity of a parent version of the young mania rating scale. *J Am Acad Child Adolesc Psychiatry*. 2002;41:1350–1359.

Higa CK, Fernandez SN, Nakamura BJ, et al. Parental assessment of childhood social phobia: psychometric properties of the social phobia and anxiety inventory for children–parent report. *J Clin Child Adolesc Psychol*. 2006;35:590–597.

Hutchings J, Bywater T, Davies C, et al. Do crime rates predict the outcome of parenting programmes for parents of "high-risk" preschool children? *Educ Child Psychol*. 2006;23:15–24.

Inderbitzen-Nolan H, Davies CA, McKeon ND. Investigating the construct validity of the SPAI-C: comparing the sensitivity and specificity of the SPAI-C and the SAS-A. *J Anxiety Disord*. 2004;18:547–560.

Ivanova MY, Achenbach TM, Dumenci L, et al. Testing the 8-syndrome structure of the child behavior checklist in 30 societies. *J Clin Child Adoles Psych*. 2007;36:405–417.

Jain S, Carmody TJ, Trivedi MH, et al. A psychometric evaluation of the CDRS and MADRS in assessing depressive symptoms in children. *J Am Acad Child Adolesc Psychiatry*. 2007;46:1204–1212.

Kamphaus RW, Frick PJ. *Child and adolescent personality and behavior-2nd Edition*. New York: Springer Science and Business Media; 2005.

Kohrt BA, Jordans MJD, Tol WA, et al. Comparison of mental health between former child soldiers and children never conscripted by armed groups in Nepal. *JAMA*. 2008;300:691–702.

Lanktree CB, Briere JN. Outcome of therapy for sexually abused children: a repeated measures study. *Child Abuse Negl*. 1995;19:1145–1155.

McMillan D, Gilbody S, Beresford E, et al. Can we predict suicide and non-fatal self-harm with the *Beck hopelessness scale?* A meta-analysis. *Psychol Med*. 2007;37:769–778.

Myers K, Winters NC. Ten-year review of rating scales. I: overview of scale functioning, psychometric properties, and selection. *J Am Acad Child Adolesc Psychiatry*. 2002;41:114–122.

Myers K, Winters NC. Ten-year review of rating scales. II: scales for internalizing disorders. *J Am Acad Child Adolesc Psychiatry*. 2002;41:634–659.

Ohan J, Myers K, Collett B. Ten-year review of rating scales. IV: scales assessing trauma and its effects. *J Am Acad Child Adolesc Psychiatry*. 2002;41:1401–1422.

Pai ALH, Lewandowski A, Youngstrom E, et al. A meta-analytic review of the influence of pediatric cancer on parent and family functioning. *J Fam Psychol*. 2007;21:407–415.

Pat-Horenczyk R, Qasrawi R, Lesack R, et al. Posttraumatic symptoms, functional impairment, and coping among adolescents on both sides of the Israeli–Palestinian conflict: a cross-cultural approach. *Appl Psychol-Int Rev*. 2009;58:688–708.

Robins DL, Fein D, Barton ML, et al. The modified checklist for autism in toddlers: an initial study investigating the early detection of autism and pervasive developmental disorders. *J Autism Dev Disord*. 2001;31:131–144.

Rust JO, Wallace MA. Review of the adaptive behavior assessment system-2nd edition. *J Psychoeduc Assess*. 2004;22:367–373.

Sanna K, Pollock-Wurman R, Ebeling H, et al. Psychometric evaluation of social phobia and anxiety inventory for children (SPAI-C) and social anxiety scale for children-revised (SASC-R). *Eur Child Adolesc Psychiatry*. 2009;18:116–124.

Shaffer D, Scott M, Wilcox H, et al. The Columbia Suicide Screen: validity and reliabililty of a screen for youth suicide and depression. *J Am Acad Child Adolesc Psychiatry*, 2004;43:71–79.

Smith P, Perrin S, Yule W, et al. War exposure among children from Bosnia–Hercegovina: psychological adjustment in a community sample. *J Trauma Stress*. 2002;15:147–156.

Swanson JM, Kraemer HC, Hinshaw SP, et al. Clinical relevance of the primary findings of the MTA: success rates based on severity of ADHD and ODD symptoms at the end of treatment. *J Am Acad Child Adolesc Psychiatry*. 2001;40:168–179.

Thienkrua W, Cardozo BL, Chakkraband MLS, et al. Symptoms of posttraumatic stress disorder and depression among children in tsunami-affected areas in southern Thailand. *JAMA*. 2006;296:549–559.

van Gastel W, Ferdinand R. Screening capacity of the multidimensional anxiety scale for children for DSM-IV anxiety disorders. *Depress Anxiety*. 2008;25:1046–1052.

Ventola P, Kleinman J, Pandey J, et al. Differentiating between autism spectrum disorders and other developmental disabilities in children who failed a screening instrument for ASD. *J Autism Dev Disord*. 2007;37:425–436.

Vitiello B, Rohde P, Silva S, et al. Functioning and quality of life in the treatment for adolescents with depression study (TADS). *J Am Acad Child Adolesc Psychiatry*. 2006;45:1419–1426.

Voelz ZR, Haeffel GJ, Joiner TE Jr., et al. Reducing hopelessness: the interaction of enhancing and depressogenic attributional styles for positive and negative life events among youth psychiatric inpatients. *Behav Res Ther*. 2003;41:1183–1198.

Wagner A, Lecavalier L, Arnold LE, et al. Developmental disabilities modification of the children's global assessment scale. *Biol Psychiatry*. 2007;61:504–511.

Wagner KD, Jonas J, Findling RL, et al. A double-blind, randomized, placebo-controlled trial of escitalopram in the treatment of pediatric depression. *J Am Acad Child Adolesc Psychiatry*. 2006;45:280–288.

Wagner KD, Kowatch RA, Emslie GJ, et al. A double-blind, randomized, placebo-controlled trial of oxcarbazepine in the treatment of bipolar disorder in children and adolescents. *Am J Psychiatry*. 2006;163:1179–1186.

Winters NC, Collett BR, Myers KM. Ten-year review of rating scales, VII: scales assessing functional impairment. *J Am Acad Child Adolesc Psychiatry*. 2005;44:309–338.

Winters NC, Myers K, Proud L. Ten-year review of rating scales, III: scales for suicidality, cognitive style, and self-esteem. *J Am Acad Child Adolesc Psychiatry*. 2002;41:1050–1181.

Youngstrom EA, Findling RL, Calabrese JR. Effects of adolescent manic symptoms on agreement between youth, parent, and teacher ratings of behavior problems. *J Affect Disord*. 2004;82(suppl 1):S5–S16.

SUGGESTED READINGS

J Clin Child Adolesc Psychol. 2005;34(3):362–596. Available at: http://www.informaworld.com/smpp/title~content= t775648094~db=all/title~db=all~content=g783754988.

This article is a special section devoted to evidence-based = assessment, including scales for establishing evidence-based practice.

Verhulst FC, van der Ende J. *Assessment Scales in Child and Adolescent Psychiatry*. UK: Informa Healthcare; 2006.

This volume in the *Assessment Scales in Psychiatry Series* provides a nice description of multiple scales for youth and provides copies of the reviewed scales.

Sattler J, Hoge R. *Assessment of Children: Behavioral, Social, and Clinical Foundations*. San Diego: Author; 2005.

This excellent resource includes descriptions of how reliability and validity relate to assessment. It also discusses other relevant dimensions of assessment tools, such as the quality and appropriateness of the standardization sample, and important assessment concepts related to interpreting rating scale scores, such as standard scores, standard deviations and variance, statistical significance, and T and z scores.

SUGGESTED WEBSITES

Massachusetts General Hospital: http://www2.massgeneral.org/schoolpsychiatry/screeningtools_table_print.asp

This website, managed by Massachusetts General Hospital, provides a comprehensive list of screening tools and rating scales that can be used to help measure a youth's mental health functioning after interventions at home or at school. Many of the measures described in this chapter are included on the website, in addition to several others.

OBTAINING THE SCALES (IN ORDER OF PRESENTATION IN TEXT)

Child Behavior Checklist (CBCL)/Teacher Report Form (TRF)/Youth Self-Report (YSR) and Child Behavior Checklist 1½–5 Years Old (CBCL 1½–5)/Caregiver–Teacher Report Form (C-TRF)

Achenbach TM, Rescorla LA. *Manual for the ASEBA School-Age Forms & Profiles; Manual for the ASEBA Preschool Forms & Profiles; Multicultural Supplement to the Manual for ASEBA School-Age Forms & Profiles*. Burlington, VT: University of Vermont, Research Center for Children, Youth, and Families; 2000, 2001, 2007. Available from Achenbach System of Empirically Based Assessment (ASEBA), Room 6436, 1 South Prospect Street, Burlington, VT 05401-3456, 1-802-656-8313 or 1-802-656-2608; Available at: www.aseba.org (accessed March 2010).

Child Symptom Inventories
Gadow KD, Sprafkin J. *Early Childhood Inventory 4: Norms Manual; Early Childhood Inventory 4: Screening Manual; Childhood Symptom Inventory –4: Screening and Norms Manual; Youth's Inventory 4; Adolescent Symptom Inventory 4: Norms Manual*. Stony Brook: Checkmate Plus; 1997–2000, 2002. Available from Western Psychological Services, 12031 Wilshire Boulevard, Los Angeles, CA 90025-1251, 1-800-648-8857; Available at: http://portal.wpspublish.com (accessed March 2010).

Conners' Rating Scales-Revised (CRS-R)
Conners C. *Conners' Rating Scales-Revised Technical Manual; Conners 3 Manual*. 2002, 2008. Available from Multi-Health Systems, 908 Niagra Falls Boulevard, North Tonawanda, NY 14120-2060, 1-800-456-3003; Available at: www.mhs.com (accessed March 2010).

Swanson, Nolan, and Pelham-IV Questionaire (SNAP-IV)
Swanson J, Schuck S, Mann M, et al. *Categorical and Dimensional Definitions and Evaluations of Symptoms of ADHD: The SNAP and SWAN Ratings Scales (Draft)*; 2001. Available at: http://www.adhd.net (accessed March 2010).

Eyberg Child Behavior Inventory (ECBI) and Sutter–Eyberg Student Behavior Inventory-Revised (SESBI-R)
Eyberg SM, Pincus D. *Eyberg Child Behavior Inventory and Sutter-Eyberg Student Behavior Inventory-Revised Professional Manual*. 1999. Available from Psychological Assessment Resources, Inc., 16204 North Florida Avenue, Lutz, FL 33549, 1-813-968-3003, 1-800-331-8378; Available at: www.parinc.com (accessed March 2010).

The Beck Depression Inventory-II (BDI-II)
Beck A, Steer RA. *Beck Depression Inventory (BDI) Manual*. 2nd ed; 1996. Available from Psychological Corporation, 555 Academic Court, San Antonio, TX 78204-2498, 1-800 211-8378; Available at: www.psychcorp.com (accessed March 2010).

Children's Depression Inventory (CDI)
Kovacs M. *Children's Depression Inventory Manual*. 1992. Available from Multi-Health Systems, 908 Niagra Falls Boulevard, North Tonawanda, NY 14120-2060, 1-800-456-3003; Available at: www.mhs.com (accessed March 2010).

Moods and Feelings Questionnaire (MFQ)
Available at the authors' website: http://devepi.duhs.duke.edu/mfq.html (accessed March 2010).
Also available in: Verhulst FC, van der Ende J. *Assessment Scales in Child and Adolescent Psychiatry*. UK: Informa Healthcare; 2006:92.

Children's Depression Rating Scale-Revised (CDRS-R)
Poznanski EO, Mokros HB. *Children's Depression Rating Scale-Revised (CDRS-R)*. 1999. Available from Western Psychological Services, 12031 Wilshire Boulevard, Los Angeles, CA 90025-1251, 1-800-648-8857; Available at: http://portal.wpspublish.com (accessed March 2010).

Young Mania Rating Scale (Y-MRS)
Young RC, Biggs JT, Ziegler VE, et al. A rating scale for mania: reliability, validity and sensitivity. *Br J Psychiatry*. 1978;133:429–435.
Also available in: Young RC, Biggs JT, Ziegler VE, et al. Young mania rating scale (YMRS): Mood Disorders Measures. In: American Psychiatric Association, eds. *Handbook of Psychiatric Measures*. 2nd ed. Washington, DC: American Psychiatric Association; 2008:540–542 (printout from CD ROM).

Suicidal Ideation Questionnaire (SIQ)
Reynolds CR. *Suicidal Ideation Questionnaire (SIQ): Professional Manual*. 1987. Available from Psychological Assessment Resources, Inc., 16204 North Florida Avenue, Lutz, FL 33549, 1-813-968-3003; Available at: www.parinc.com (accessed March 2010).

The Columbia Suicide Screen (aka the Teen Screen)
All available online at their websites, as follows: http://www.teenscreen.org
There is also a free newsletter available at:
http://www.teenscreen.org/images/_mediacenter/pdfs/CheckupSummerIssuesept.pdf (accessed March 2010).

The Beck Hopelessness Scale (BHS)
Beck A. *Beck Hopelessness Scale (BHS) Manual*. 1988. Available from Psychological Corporation, 555 Academic Court, San Antonio, TX 78204-2498, 1-800-211-8378; Available at: www.psychcorp.com (accessed March 2010); email: beckinst@gim.net.

The Hopelessness Scale for Children
Kazdin AE. *The Hopelessness Scale for Children (HSC)*, 2009. Available from the author: Alan Kazdin, PhD, Yale University; 1-203-432-9993; email: Alan.Kazdin@yale.edu.

Multidimensional Anxiety Scale for Children (MASC)
March JS. *Manual for the Multidimensional Anxiety Scale for Children (MASC)*. 1997. Available from Multi-Health Systems, 908 Niagra Falls Boulevard, North Tonawanda, NY 14120-2060, 1-800-456-3003; Available at: www.mhs.com (accessed March 2010).

Screen for Child Anxiety–Related Emotional Disorders (SCARED)
Available at the author's website at: http://www.wpic.pitt.edu/research/ OR E-mail: birmaherb@msx.upmc.edu.
Also in: Verhulst FC, van der Ende J, eds. *Assessment Scales in Child and Adolescent Psychiatry*. Part of the Assessment Scales in Psychiatry Series. Burns A, series ed. UK: Informa Healthcare; 2006:62–63.

Social Phobia and Anxiety Inventory for Children (SPAI-C)

Beidel DC, Turner SM, Morris TL. *Social Phobia and Anxiety Inventory for Children (SPAIC-C).* Available from Multi-Health Systems, 908 Niagra Falls Boulevard, North Tonawanda, NY 14120-2060, 1-800-456-3003; Available at: www.mhs.com (accessed March 2010).

The Impact of Events Scale-Revised (IES-R)

Weiss D, Marmar CR. *The Impact of Events Scale-Revised.* In: Wilson J, Keane TM, eds. *Assessing Psychological Trauma and PTSD.* New York: The Guilford Press; 1997:399–411. Also available from Daniel Weiss, PhD, Department of Psychiatry, University of California at San Francisco (UCSF), Box F-0984, San Francisco CA 94143; 2002; email: daniel.weiss@ucsf.edu.

The Child Posttraumatic Stress-Reaction Index (CPTS-RI)

Pynoos RS. *The Child Post Traumatic Stress-Reaction Index (CPTS-RI).* 2002. Available from Robert Pynoos, MD, Trauma Psychiatry Service, UCLA, 300 UCLA Medical Plaza, Los Angeles, CA 90024-6968; Tel: (310) 2068973; Fax: (310) 2064310; email: rpynoos@npih.medsch.ucla.edu.

The Clinician-Administered PTSD Scale, Child and Adolescent Version(CAPS-C)

The scale is available from the national center for PTSD, while river junction, VT: www.ptsd.va.gov/professional/pages/assessments/caps-ca.asp

Trauma Symptom Checklist for Children (TSCC) and Trauma Symptom Checklist for Young Children (TSCYC)

Briere J. *Trauma Symptom Checklist for Children (TSCC), Professional Manual.* 1996.

Briere J. *Trauma Symptom Checklist for Young Children: Professional Manual.* 2005. Available from Psychological Assessment Resources, Inc., 16204 North Florida Avenue, Lutz, FL 33549, 1-800-899-8378; Available at: http://www3.parinc.com (accessed March 2010).

Child PTSD Symptom Scale (CPSS)

Foa EB, Johnson KM, Feeny NC, et al. *The Child PTSD Symptom Scale.* 2002. Available from author: Edna Foa, PhD, Center for the Treatment and Study of Anxiety, University of Pennsylvania School of Medicine, Department of Psychiatry, 3535 Market Street, Sixth Floor, Philadelphia, PA 19104; Tel: (215) 746-3327; email: foa@mail.med.upenn.edu.

Social Communication Questionnaire (SCQ)

Rutter M, Bailey A, Lord C, et al. *Social Communication Questionnaire.* 2002. Available from Western Psychological Services, 12031 Wilshire Boulevard, Los Angeles, CA 90025-1251, 1-800-648-8857; Available at: http://portal.wpspublish.com (accessed March 2010).

Modified Checklist for Autism in Toddlers (M-CHAT)

Robins DL, Fein D, Barton ML, et al. *Modified Checklist for Autism in Toddlers.* 2001. Available at: http://www2.gsu.edu/~psydlr/Diana_L._Robins,_Ph.D..html (accessed March 2010).

Autism Screening Instrument for Educational Planning, ASIEP

Krug DA, Arick JR, Almond PJ. *Portland: Pro-Ed Incorporated;* 1980.

Autism Behavior Checklist (ABC)

Verhulst FC, van der Ende J, eds. *Assessment Scale in Child and Adolescent Psychiatry. Part of the Assessment Scales in Psychiatry Series.* Burns A, series ed. UK, Informa Healthcare; 2006:120. Autism Behavior Checklist.

The Children's Global Assessment Scale (CGAS)

Shaffer D, Gould MS, Bird H, Fisher P. Children's global assessment scale (CGAS): child and adolescent measures of functional status. In: American Psychiatric Association, eds. *Handbook of Psychiatric Measures.* 2nd ed. Washington, DC: American Psychiatric Association; 2008:363–365 (printout from CD ROM).

Verhulst FC, van der Ende J, eds. *Assessment Scales in Child and Adolescent Psychiatry.* UK: Informa Healthcare; 2006:205–206.

Also available from the author: David Shaffer MD, New York State Psychiatric Institute (Unit 78). 1051 Riverside Dr., New York, NY 10032; email: shafferd@childpsych.columbia.edu.

The Columbia Impairment Scale (CIS)

Verhulst FC, van der Ende J, eds. *Assessment Scales in Child and Adolescent Psychiatry.* UK: Informa Healthcare; 2006:207–208.

Bird HR. Columbia impairment scale (CIS): child and adolescent measures of functional status. In: American Psychiatric Association, eds. *Handbook of Psychiatric Measures;* Washington, DC: American Psychiatric Association; 2000:367–369 (printout from CD ROM).

Also available from the author: Hector R, Bird MD, Division of Child Psychiatry, New York State Psychiatric Institute, Unit 78, 1051 Riverside Dr., New York, NY 10032; Tel: (212) 5435191; Fax: (212) 5435730; email: birdh@childpsych.columbia.edu (accessed March 2010).

Vineland Adaptive Behavior Scales: Interview Edition Survey Form Manual

Sparrow SS, Balla DA, Cicchetti DV. *Interview Edition Survey Form Manual: Vineland Adaptive Behavior Scales.* Circle Pines, MN: American Guidance Service, AGS Publishing; 2005. Available from 4201 Woodland Road, Circle Pines, MN 55014-1796; Tel: (800) 328 2560; Fax: (651) 287-7220, (800) 471 8457; email: www.customerservice@agsnet.com (accessed March 2010).

Adaptive Behavior Assessment System-Second Edition (ABAS-II)

Harrison PL, Oakland T. *Adaptive Behavior Assessment System–2nd Edition Manual (ABAS-II)*. 2003. Available from Western Psychological Services, 12031 Wilshire Boulevard, Los Angeles, CA 90025-1251, 1-800-648-8857; Available at: http://portal.wpspublish.com (accessed March 2010).

REVIEW QUESTIONS BASED ON VIGNETTE 1

1. The CBCL and TRF, which you administered initially to the mother and the teacher, respectively, provided information about multiple different problem areas. These scales are examples of:
   a. Narrowband scales
   b. Diagnostic scales
   c. Broadband scales
   d. Impairment scales

2. The reasons the child's doctor administered the SNAP rating scales and the MASC when the CBCL and TRF already indicated ADHD and anxiety included:
   a. The low concordance of the CBCL and TRF invalidates the scales' results
   b. The narrowband SNAP rating scale and the MASC are used to make the diagnosis of ADHD and an anxiety disorder
   c. The narrowband SNAP rating scale and the MASC aid in making the diagnosis, help to establish severity of the disorder, and set a baseline for following symptom course during treatment
   d. The teacher and mother showed low concordance on the internalizing scale of the TRF and CBCL, respectively

3. Which of the following statements are true regarding youth and adults who complete rating scales?
   a. Caregivers and other adults familiar with the child are the preferable reporters for scales assessing externalizing problems
   b. Important adults may underestimate youth's internalizing symptoms on depression and anxiety rating scales
   c. Scales are administered to various adult observers in order to assess the youth's symptoms contextually
   d. Even adults who know the youth well may show low concordance on a scale assessing the youth's behavior
   e. All of the above

4. The doctor administered the SNAP rating scales and the MASC repeatedly over time. Such scales must have which of the following so that the doctor can rely on the scores each time?
   a. Strong face validity
   b. High test–retest reliability
   c. At least good discriminant validity
   d. Strong interrater reliability
   e. b and d

Answers: 1-c, 2-c, 3-e, 4-b

REVIEW QUESTIONS BASED ON VIGNETTE 2

1. You used several ratings scales in AG's case in order to help differentiate between anxiety, depression, and posttraumatic stress symptoms. This approach was useful only because the scales you selected have demonstrated evidence of:
   a. Convergent validity
   b. Divergent validity
   c. Discriminant validity
   d. Criterion-related validity

2. About a year after you referred AG for psychological treatment for trauma, she returned complaining of increased moodiness, difficulties at school, and heightened anger. She did not experience additional trauma. You decide to give her the Youth Self-Report, and also give the appropriate versions to her parents (CBCL) and teacher (TRF). As compared to the measures you administered to her a year ago, the measures you are now administering are referred to as:
   a. Broadband versus narrowband
   b. Narrowband versus broadband
   c. Criterion-based versus convergent-based
   d. None of the above; they are not in different categories

3. You chose to administer measures to multiple informants the second time you saw AG. Which of the following is *not* true about multiple informants and rating scales?
   a. Getting data from multiple informants is a good way to learn about the contextual influences of a youth's symptoms
   b. Typical informants include the youth, caregivers, teachers, and even coaches
   c. Youth and their caregivers often show low concordance on rating scales
   d. Adults often show high rates of concordance on rating scales
   e. All of the above are true

4. Select the answer(s) that is/are true of self-report rating scales.
   a. Reliability is lower for younger-aged youth
   b. Validity is higher for younger-aged youth
   c. Reliability is lower for kids with internalizing rather than with externalizing symptoms
   d. Validity is lower for youth with externalizing rather than with internalizing symptoms

Answers: 1-b, 2-a, 3-d, 4-a

CHAPTER

4

Dorothy E. Stubbe, MD

Attention-Deficit/Hyperactivity Disorder

Introduction

Attention-deficit/hyperactivity disorder (ADHD) is the single most commonly diagnosed psychiatric disorder of childhood, with an estimated prevalence rate of 4% to 12% of youths in the United States. ADHD is characterized by developmentally inappropriate levels of hyperactivity, inattention, impulsivity, and other deficits of executive function. ADHD is often comorbid with other psychiatric disorders, both externalizing and internalizing, as well as bipolar disorder and learning disabilities. These children frequently experience peer rejection and engage in a broad array of impulsive and disruptive behaviors with subsequent consequences on self-esteem and adaptive coping. This disorder is a major public health problem with enormous negative impact on the child, the family, schools, and society. Billions of dollars are spent annually for school services, mental health services, and increased use of the juvenile justice system for children and adolescents suffering from ADHD. In contrast with historical notions, children do not typically "outgrow" ADHD. Morbidity and disability often persist into adult life.

Background

The conceptualization and diagnostic terminology related to ADHD have changed over the years. Historically, three views of the disorder have dominated: (1) behavioral (e.g., hyperactivity), (2) etiologic (e.g., minimal brain dysfunction), and (3) cognitive (e.g., attention deficit disorder). These changes in conceptualization have led to alterations in diagnostic criteria, research design, prevalence rates, and interventions.

Although initially described in 1902 as "morbid defects of moral control," the thinking about ADHD as an organic disorder occurred around the time of World War I following the influenza pandemic which left many survivors with high levels of overactivity, impulsivity, and behavioral difficulties. The title "minimal brain dysfunction" was accepted in the 1950s. The next iteration in diagnosis occurred in 1968 with the second edition of the *Diagnostic and Statistical Manual of Mental Disorders*, 2nd Edition (DSM-II) and the corresponding International Classification of Diseases, 9th Revision (ICD-9) as "hyperkinetic syndrome of childhood." This disorder remains in the ICD-10 (used clinically in Europe and for billing coding in the United States) and includes children with pervasive overactivity and inattention, but excludes children with co-occurring conduct difficulties. The DSM criteria used in the United States include children with co-occurring conduct difficulties, thus consisting of a larger population of children.

A conceptual shift occurred in the late 1970s in which the disorder was coined "attention-deficit disorder," and the core deficiency was postulated to be a failure to regulate attention, arousal, and inhibitory control. The present conceptualization in the fourth edition of the DSM (DSM-IV) published in 1994 consists of three subtypes: predominant symptoms of inattention (ADHD-IA), predominant symptoms of hyperactivity with impulsivity (ADHD-HI), and the combination of the two (ADHD-Combined).

Clinical Features and Differential Diagnosis

ADHD is clinically diagnosed by functional deficits in attention and/or hyperactivity and impulsivity and is most noticeable in the classroom setting. By epidemiological estimates, a classroom with 25 students would be expected to have between 1 and 3 students suffering from functionally impairing ADHD. If there are three ADHD children, the following scenario may be expected: Ms. Jones, the teacher, is discussing the states in New England in the third-grade class. The children have their books open to a map of New England. She asks a question, and Paul's hand shoots up, he leaps up from his seat in enthusiasm, in the process tipping the desk and causing his pencil and book to fall to the ground. When called on, he looks perplexed and is not able to answer the question. Sam, who is sitting in the back of the class, laughs at Paul and shouts out, "Clutz!" The teacher, in exasperation, calls on Tasha, who is gazing out the window, her book opened to the wrong page. "What was the question?" Tasha asks, coming out of her dreamy state.

As this brief vignette illustrates, children with ADHD may struggle in multiple ways within a classroom. Elementary students most frequently present with ADHD-Combined, which includes functionally interfering symptoms of both inattention and hyperactivity with impulsivity. In the vignette, one might postulate that both Paul and Sam are suffering from this disorder. Tasha, on the other hand, demonstrates symptoms more consistent with ADHD-IA.

Inattention may be thought of as a combination of difficulties with selective attention (difficulties attending to the task at hand), and difficulties with sustained attention and problem solving (distractibility and difficulties considering options). Children with ADHD-IA are often diagnosed at an older age as behavioral difficulties tend to be infrequent and these children are not noted by teachers as disruptive. However, severe underachievement in academic functioning may bring these children to educators' attention. Parents may be frustrated as distractibility leads to difficulty with organization, and "taking forever" to get ready for school.

ADHD must be differentiated from age-appropriate overactivity and other disorders. For preschool children, this may be difficult. ADHD is most notable in group situations for children who are attending a preschool or a daycare program. These youngsters are usually overly active, but also struggle with "circle-time," and have a great difficulty sharing, playing cooperatively, and inhibiting impulses. Early diagnosis is helpful in addressing safety, monitoring, teaching parents techniques to help their children, and teaching the children methods to control impulses.

The differential diagnosis for ADHD is extensive. Many medications or other substances may cause overactivity or activation, such as the commonly used bronchodilators to treat asthma. Additionally, other medical disorders such as hearing or vision impairment, seizure disorder, genetic abnormalities, thyroid disorders, and sleep disorders may present with ADHD-type symptoms. Traumatized children and those who have experienced severe psychosocial adversity may be anxious and inattentive. Depressed youths may complain of problems concentrating. Bipolar disorder, manic phase, may mimic the hyperactivity and impulsivity of ADHD. Additionally, any of these disorders and learning difficulties may be comorbid with ADHD, further complicating the clinical diagnosis.

TABLE 4-1	Diagnostic Symptoms of Attention-Deficit/Hyperactivity Disorder

1. Onset before 7 years old of symptoms of inattention and/or hyperactivity and impulsivity.
2. Symptoms should have occurred for at least 6 months and are not explained by developmental level.
3. Acronym for symptoms of inattention: Careless mistakes; Attention difficulty; Listening Problem; Loses things; Fails to finish what he/she starts; Organizational skills lacking; Reluctant to do tasks that require sustained mental effort; Forgetful in Routine activities; Easily Distracted (CALL FOR FRED). If prominent hyperactivity and impulsivity are not present, the disorder is termed attention-deficit hyperactivity disorder, predominantly inattentive type.
4. Acronym for symptoms of hyperactivity and impulsivity: Runs or is restless; Unable to wait his or her turn; Not able to play quietly; Slow—oh no, on the go!; Fidgets with hands or feet; Answers are blurted out; Staying seated is difficult; Talks excessively; Tends to interrupt (RUNS FASTT). If prominent inattention is not present, the disorder is diagnosed as attention-deficit/hyperactivity disorder, predominantly hyperactive–impulsive type.
5. Prominent symptoms of inattention *with* hyperactivity and impulsivity are diagnosed as attention-deficit/hyperactivity disorder, combined type.
6. Symptoms must be impairing to daily functioning in more than one setting, such as social, academic or employment settings.
7. Symptoms should not be better explained by another disorder.

The onset of ADHD impairment must be in early childhood, at least before the age of 7 years, even if it was not diagnosed until later in life. There must be functional impairment in a variety of life settings (home, school, work, etc.). ADHD should not be diagnosed if it presents only concomitantly with a pervasive developmental disorder or a psychotic disorder. Table 4-1 gives diagnostic features and Table 4-2 a comprehensive differential diagnosis for ADHD.

Comorbidity

Individuals with ADHD are at increased risk of suffering from other psychiatric disorders. It is important to diagnose comorbid disorders, as the ADHD child with a comorbid condition may have a different clinical presentation, life course, and response to treatment. The most common disorders comorbid with ADHD are other disruptive behavior disorders and learning disorders, although anxiety disorders and mood disorders (bipolar disorders and major depressive disorders) frequently cooccur. Neurological soft signs (e.g., coordination difficulties and immature reflexes) are also common. Tourette syndrome and other tic disorders frequently present with concomitant ADHD.

It is estimated that 50% of children with ADHD meet criteria for either oppositional defiant disorder (ODD) or conduct disorder (CD). ADHD comorbid with conduct difficulties confers an increase in impairment and risk. In one study, ADHD boys without delinquency were no different from controls on neuropsychological measures, whereas the ADHD delinquents were impaired in the areas of verbal skill, visual motor integration, and visuospatial skills. Additionally, children with ADHD and CD have a much stronger family history of antisocial behavior. Interestingly, there is some evidence that a positive response of ADHD symptoms to stimulant medication may also lead to a decrease in antisocial behaviors.

Learning disabilities are common in children suffering from ADHD—an estimated 20% to 50% suffer from reading, spelling, or arithmetic learning disorders. Both ADHD and reading disorders have strong genetic components but seem to be inherited independently. Children with learning disability alone do not respond to stimulant medications, but children with comorbid ADHD and reading disability show an increase in reading achievement scores when there inattentiveness is successfully controlled with medication.

TABLE 4-2	Differential Diagnosis for Attention-Deficit/ Hyperactivity Disorder

Psychiatric Disorders
- Oppositional defiant disorder
- Conduct disorder
- Mood disorders (depression and bipolar disorder)
- Anxiety disorders
- Tic disorders
- Substance use disorders
- Pervasive developmental disorder
- Learning disorders
- Posttraumatic stress disorder
- Mental retardation or borderline intellectual functioning

Psychosocial Conditions
- Abuse and/or neglect
- Poor nutrition
- Neighborhood violence
- Chaotic family situation
- Being bullied at school

Medical Disorders
- Partial deafness
- Poor eyesight
- Seizure disorder
- Fetal alcohol syndrome
- Genetic abnormalities (such as fragile X)
- Sedating or activating medications
- Substance abuse
- Thyroid abnormality
- Heavy metal poisoning

Approximately 25% to 30% of children diagnosed with ADHD will meet criteria for an anxiety disorder compared to 5% to 15% of the general population. Children with ADHD and comorbid anxiety report anxiety symptoms that their parents may not have appreciated, as internalizing symptoms may be less overtly noticeable to others especially in the presence of disruptive hyperactive and impulsive behaviors. ADHD-anxious children also tend to report more social difficulties. Factors associated with comorbid ADHD and anxiety include problems during the pregnancy, developmental delays, and stressful life events. Genetic studies suggest that anxiety and ADHD are inherited independently of each other. Major depressive disorder is another internalizing disorder that is diagnosed in some ADHD children, although the prevalence is unknown. Its course is independent of ADHD symptoms.

The prevalence of comorbid bipolar disorder is an area of much controversy. First, the clinician must differentiate the two disorders and then determine whether they are comorbid. Children with comorbid mania demonstrate more grandiosity, elated or irritable mood, racing thoughts, and hypersexuality than children suffering from ADHD alone. These children tend to respond better to mood stabilizers, with or without stimulants, than stimulant medications alone. This issue is complicated and suspicion of bipolar disorder warrants referral to child psychiatry.

Epidemiology

The changing diagnostic criteria over time, different diagnostic schemes used worldwide, and the complex task of integrating diagnostic information from multiple sources complicate epidemiological studies of ADHD. However, based on DSM-IV criteria, prevalence rates seem to be consistent globally, suggesting that ADHD affects 4% to 12% of children worldwide. The male-to-female ratio is about 3:1 in community samples, but as high as 9:1 in the mental health clinical population, most likely due to the higher proportion of disruptive behaviors in ADHD boys which promotes referral for treatment. For the inattentive type of ADHD, the ratio of boys to girls is about equal. Boys tend to demonstrate more hyperactive, impulsive, and other disruptive behaviors, while girls present with more inattention and comorbid anxiety and depression. According the to the American Academy of Child and Adolescent Psychiatry (AACAP), a higher prevalence of ADHD is found in individuals with younger age, lower socioeconomic status, and male gender.

Preschool children are increasingly diagnosed with ADHD. Prevalence has been estimated at 2% to 5% in primary care settings. In a 2008 study by Ghuman and colleagues, up to 59% of preschool children presenting to child guidance clinics met criteria for ADHD, indicating how distressing these symptoms can be even at very young ages. The hyperactive–impulsive type of ADHD is most commonly diagnosed. In general, symptoms related to hyperactivity decline as the child matures. In school-aged children, ADHD-Combined is most commonly diagnosed, while ADHD-IA is increasingly diagnosed in middle school and high school. It is estimated that clinically significant symptoms of ADHD persist into adulthood for about 60% of individuals.

Etiology, Risk, and Resilience Factors

Neurochemistry

Available research suggests that ADHD is a complex disorder resulting from the combined effects of several genes in interactions with the environment. Stahl describes ADHD as primarily a disorder of prefrontal cortex functioning, along with associated interconnections, projections, and circuits to selected parts of the brain regulating attention and motor functioning. Chemically, signals mediated by the neurotransmitters norepinephrine (NE) and dopamine (DA) are thought to be weak in the prefrontal cortex. This is consistent with the idea that the arousal system is deficient and that tonic NE and DA firing rates are too low. Selective attention is hypothesized to be mediated primarily by the anterior cingulate cortex (ACC). Disruptions or inefficient processing by the ACC is related to ADHD or other disorders with impaired ability to attend. Impairments in executive functioning have been postulated by Brown and others to comprise a primary deficit in ADHD. Developmental difficulties with activation, focus, sustained effort, planning and organization, emotion regulation, working memory and behavior regulation are all subsumed under the construct of impairments in executive functioning. Neuropsychological tests have consistently identified deficits in the executive functions of individuals diagnosed with ADHD. Executive functions are thought to involve neural networks that encompass the dorsolateral prefrontal cortex (DLPFC), with connections to the thalamus and basal ganglia. Hyperactive symptoms in ADHD are linked to the prefrontal motor cortex, while impulsive symptoms are thought to be related to the orbital frontal cortex. Barkley postulates that the primary deficit in ADHD-Combined is behavioral disinhibition, which underlies deficits in working memory, self-regulation of affect, motivation, arousal, the capacity for reasoning and reflection, and goal-directed behavior. The cortico–striatal–thalamic–cortical (CSTC) loops are hypothesized to regulate the complex aspects of attention and activity. Inefficiencies anywhere along this loop may cause symptoms of ADHD, and individual patients may vary in symptoms, severity, and type depending upon the unique pattern of neurocircuitry disruption.

NE and DA are intricately involved in modulating prefrontal cortical functioning and are a major focus of treatment. Stimulants approved to treat ADHD include various preparations of methylphenidate and amphetamine, and both are considered to boost NE and DA signals in a number of different ways. It is evident that moderate amounts of these neurotransmitters are essential to prefrontal cortical functioning, and deficits, particularly in the prefrontal cortex, lead to attentional deficiencies. By contrast, very high levels of NE and DA (as found in extreme stress) may impair optimal functioning. Indeed, substance abuse and anxiety disorders are correlated with excess neurotransmission of DA and NE in the prefrontal cortex.

Early neurodevelopmental problems such as obstetrical complications, prematurity, other genetic abnormalities (such as fragile X disorder and others), and exposure in utero to alcohol, cocaine, or other toxins may predispose to ADHD. It is postulated that fetal insults, particularly during the second trimester during the height of neural development, may cause subtle functional abnormalities to the frontal cortex and other brain structures, resulting in the disorder. Soft neurological signs and subtle deficits on electroencephalograms (EEG) findings are also noted in populations of individuals with ADHD compared with controls.

Early findings are also provocative regarding the neuronal–environmental interactions. Specifically, the efficiency of brain functioning may be molded in the perinatal period via neuronal pruning, which is enhanced by appropriate levels of stimulation and nurturance. Efficient CSTC tracks depend upon early activation of these circuits, as is facilitated in an optimally stimulating environment and as is inhibited in a chaotic or deprived environment. Therefore, severe psychosocial adversity in infancy may predispose to less efficient neuronal tracks and potentially to subtle neurodevelopmental disorders such as ADHD. Psychosocial correlates of ADHD include poverty, urban residence, family dysfunction, and parents with psychiatric disorders. These psychosocial risk factors suggest that there may be multiple pathways leading to the development of ADHD in vulnerable children. This information is important for public health prevention efforts and may guide early intervention efforts.

Neuroimaging

Imaging studies of ADHD have focused on the prefrontal cortex, basal ganglia, and cerebellum as these are areas that have been implicated in the pathways that mediate ADHD or are rich in DA. Although results have been mixed, there is evidence of structural and functional differences in the brains of children and adults with ADHD. Volumetric measures have detected smaller right-sided prefrontal regions overall in boys with ADHD. These reductions have been correlated with performance on tasks that require response inhibition, and are consistent with a postulated etiologic role for prefrontal deficits. Girls with ADHD have been found to have smaller left and total caudate volumes. A consistent finding in ADHD has been reduced volume of the posterior–inferior cerebellar vermis, a region that exhibits a high degree of DA receptor reactivity.

Neuroimaging is an important tool to assist in understanding the neurophysiological correlates of ADHD. Functional neuroimaging with positron emission tomography (PET) and single photon emission computerized tomography (SPECT) with adults diagnosed with ADHD has demonstrated decreased frontal cerebral metabolism. Decreased perfusion in the striatum and prefrontal cortex has also been reported. Although functional magnetic resonance imaging (fMRI) has not been conclusive, early results also suggest subtle deficits in frontal lobe and basal ganglia activity. Such results support the notion that catecholamine dysregulation is central to the pathophysiology of ADHD and not just to its treatment. Most interestingly, McNab and colleagues found that when patients conducted mental exercises to train their working memory, an increase in the number of central DA receptors was detected on PET scanning. Despite these intriguing findings, currently there is no clinical role for neuroimaging in diagnosis, determining treatment, or predicting treatment response.

Genetics

It is helpful to conceptualize ADHD as a disorder in which genes may "bias" an individual's brain circuits toward inefficient information processing and the precipitation of ADHD under adverse environmental circumstances. Data from family, twin, and adoption studies, as well as segregation analyses, show very high heritability coefficients, strongly supporting a genetic etiology for ADHD. Preliminary molecular genetic studies have implicated candidate genes associated with the DA system, including D2 and D4 receptors and the DA transporter. There is also preliminary evidence that genes involved in alpha-2A adrenergic receptors, serotonin receptors, and other proteins may be important. Given the importance of these catecholamines for the modulation of attentional circuits, it is not surprising that alterations in these systems would disrupt attention. Despite these intriguing findings, large genome-wide linkage studies conducted by Castellano and Swanson intended to identify chromosomal regions shared within families with ADHD have been inconsistent. Thus, much work is still needed to clarify the roles of genes and the gene–environment interaction in the etiology of ADHD.

Clinical Course

Although many of the symptoms of ADHD may remit, it has become clear that ADHD is frequently a chronic disorder, which leads to a negative impact on functioning throughout the life cycle. Studies following children with ADHD into adolescence have fairly consistently shown that ADHD children, as compared with controls, exhibit impaired academic functioning, perform more poorly on cognitive tasks, and are characterized by lower self-esteem and poorer social functioning. About three quarters of these children continue to show symptoms of ADHD into adolescence, and serious conduct problems are common.

In general, preschool children demonstrate the highest rates of hyperactivity and impulsivity. Although it is normative for preschool children to interrupt others and have high energy levels, the ability to pay attention and inhibit motor activity can generally differentiate children with functional disability from ADHD and the normal exuberance of preschool children. Children with early-onset severe symptoms, including preschool expulsion, peer rejection, and aggression, may predict a more serious prognosis. Preschool children with ADHD are also at higher risk for corporal punishment, or abuse. These children are challenging to parents, and parents who lack support and effective coping skills may resort to physical discipline.

ADHD-Combined is the most common type of ADHD diagnosed among school-aged children and generally adversely affects their social and academic development. These children have fewer friends and are more often the recipient of disciplinary measures. In general, the hyperactivity tends to wane with maturity, although feelings of restlessness are often reported. Adolescents with ADHD may have less hyperactivity, but they are more prone to school underachievement, substance abuse, and high-risk behaviors. Impulsivity declines after adolescence. The most persistent symptom cluster involves inattention, distractibility, lack of organization, and poor perseverance.

Follow-up studies into adulthood suggest that up to 33% of ADHD teens versus 1% to 9% of controls drop out of high school. ADHD youths complete less education (by 2 to 3 years) and fewer obtain a graduate degree. Likewise, ADHD youths demonstrate lower occupational rankings at the age of 25 years, a higher rate of divorce, increased motor vehicle accidents, poor money management, and a higher rate of unwed pregnancy. Youths with ADHD are also at increased risk for developing antisocial personality disorder and substance-use disorders in adulthood. An estimated 60% of adults continue to suffer from impairing symptoms of ADHD.

Of note, there are a number of very high achievers with ADHD. Talented athletes (such as Michael Phelps, Olympics swimmer, and multiple gold medalist), businesspeople, and other highly accomplished and creative individuals who have been diagnosed with ADHD have found successful methods of harnessing their energy and exuberance. Higher cognitive functioning, athletic talents, and a supportive environment improve outcomes. Assisting children, adolescents, and adults to develop their strengths and talents, in addition to treating the disability, may be the most successful method of optimizing prognosis.

Assessment

ADHD is a clinical diagnosis. There is no diagnostic test for ADHD. The diagnosis is established by clinical judgment based on a comprehensive assessment, which involves multiple domains, informants, methods, and settings. The AACAP Practice Parameter for ADHD describes five components of the ADHD assessment including history, school data, rating scales, medical evaluation, and tests.

An accurate and complete assessment of a child for ADHD involves a careful history that includes the child's prenatal and developmental history, current symptoms, psychosocial functioning, medical history, and family psychiatric and medical history (with a focus on family history of cardiac arrhythmias or disease). The diagnosis of ADHD generally cannot be made simply by observing the child in the office. The structured setting, individualized attention, and novelty may mask the ADHD, at least at the first appointment. Whenever possible, symptom history should be gathered from multiple sources, including the parents or primary caretakers, teachers, the primary care physician, and the child. The younger the child, the poorer will be the concordance between the child and his or her parents', or other adults', reports. Low concordance does not negate the diagnosis, but reflects the ecological aspects of ADHD, that is, contextual factors affect the child's behavior across settings, as well as differences in observers' experiences of the child and their attributions to the child's behavior.

It is crucial to gather data from a child's school to compare with information gathered from parents or guardians. Data to be obtained should include any psychoeducational testing, grades, teacher comments, grades, and standardized achievement tests. Informal clinical observations of classroom behavior can provide useful data regarding a child's level of disruptive or inattentive behavior. These data can be quite helpful in making the diagnosis of ADHD, especially when information from parents and teachers are equivocal.

Parent and teacher rating scales can provide valuable information in an efficient manner. Commonly used instruments are described in chapter 3. While rating scales should not be used to make the diagnosis of ADHD, they are useful in providing a baseline of current severity and then for measuring treatment progress, including assisting in titrating medication to therapeutic doses.

Information from a medical history and physical examination within the past 12 months should be reviewed. Vision and hearing deficits should be ruled out, as well as over-the-counter, illicit, or prescription drug use. If indicated, tests such as an EEG, thyroid panels, ferritin, and lead levels may be helpful to rule our medical causes of ADHD symptoms. The history should guide decision making regarding further testing and evaluations.

Psychological tests are useful to assess specific deficits but are not routinely obtained as part of an ADHD evaluation. Such testing should be obtained as indicated from the individual child's presentation and needs. Similar to rating scales, computerized tests of attention are considered useful for baseline documentation and measuring treatment progress. Table 4-3 gives a summary of the diagnostic assessment for ADHD in children and adolescents.

Treatment

ADHD is a complex disorder affecting every area of functioning and thereby requires a comprehensive treatment program. Psychosocial interventions, medication treatment, and ensuring an appropriate educational plan are all part of the effective treatment for ADHD.

TABLE 4-3	Evaluation Essentials for Attention-Deficit Hyperactivity Disorder

Clinical diagnosis based on careful history and clinical evaluation
- Prenatal and developmental history
- Current symptoms and longitudinal timeline of symptom development
- Assessment of associated symptoms to determine any comorbidities
- Psychosocial history
- Educational history
- Medical history
- Family history (psychiatric and medical—especially cardiac)
- Multiple historical informants (parents, teachers, child, primary care physician)

Physical and neurological examination
- Neurological evaluation, as needed
- Electrocardiogram (ECG)-based cardiovascular and family history
- Vital signs, height, and weight
- Blood work for thyroid, lead, and other screening laboratory assessments

Individual assessment of the child
- Social connectedness, attention, comorbidities, and strengths and assets
- Hyperactivity (may be masked in one-on-one setting)
- Mental status examination and other diagnostic questions
- Child's view of personal strengths and difficulties

Psychoeducational assessment, as needed
- Cognitive and/or neuropsychological and psychoeducational testing
- Computerized continuous performance task (CPT)
- Baseline and follow-up rating scales (e.g., Vanderbilt ADHD Rating Scales, and Conners Rating Scales) prior to medication treatment and as follow-up of effectiveness

The diagnosis and treatment of ADHD during preschool is becoming more common. The Preschool ADHD Treatment Study (PATS) by Greenhill and colleagues has shown the importance of early intervention services, including behavioral management and parent training. For those who do not respond to behavioral interventions, medication can be effective. However, preschool children have higher rates of adverse effects, especially sleep and appetite difficulties, than older patients. Emotional lability is also more common.

The Multimodal Treatment Study of ADHD (MTA) was sponsored by the National Institute of Mental Health (NIMH) to compare the effectiveness of four treatment groups with specific interest in addressing the long standing debate of whether medication or behavioral treatment is more helpful to children diagnosed with ADHD. A total of 579 children were enrolled into four treatment groups: medication alone, behavioral therapy alone, medication and behavioral therapy combined, and treatment as usual with the community physician. Treatment continued for 14 months. Methylphenidate was used in the medication and combined treatment arms, using an algorithm to titrate medication to an individually optimal dose based on teacher and family feedback. The psychosocial intervention included regular parent training and teacher consultation on classroom behavior along with an 8-week, all-day summer treatment program that utilized contingency management and social skills training. Children in the community care condition also received medication, adjusted per the physician's discretion.

The study found that for the core symptoms of ADHD, medication management and combined treatment were equally effective. Medication management alone was also superior to behavioral treatment alone and treatment in the community. Of particular interest, doses utilized in the medication and combined treatment arms of the study were higher than the doses used by the community physicians. For non-ADHD aspects of functioning, the combined treatment was superior to the other groups in the treatment of oppositional and aggressive symptoms, internalizing symptoms, teacher-rated social skills, parent–child relations, and reading achievements. These results suggest that the single best treatment for the most children is stimulant medication and that children with comorbid disorders can further benefit from the addition of parent training and behavioral interventions.

The MTA sample has been followed up at multiple points over time. As soon as the study ended, children began to deviate from their assigned treatment condition. Many discontinued medication altogether while others received community care. Most children exhibited impairment in adolescence. Outcomes for the four study groups started to converge by the third year, and there was no difference among the original four treatment groups. The most recent follow-up at 8 years showed that the 14-month treatment for ADHD in childhood did not predict later functioning. Children with behavioral and sociodemographic advantages, and those who displayed the best response to any of the MTA treatments, have had the best long-term prognosis. Early ADHD symptom trajectory tended to be prognostic.

The interpretation of these results is complicated. The decreased functioning is not surprising given that medication use decreased by 62% after the controlled trial ended; psychosocial interventions were not as intensive; and community physicians were on their own in treating these youths. Most youths do not have complete remission of symptoms even with state-of-the-art treatment, and so families seek other interventions. Overall, a year long course of treatment does not "rectify" an underlying deficit, and the deficit continues into adolescence and needs ongoing treatment to optimize outcomes. In fact, as original work by Mannuzza and colleagues showed and as more recent work by Lara and colleagues for the World Health Organization confirmed, ADHD persists into adulthood in an average of 50% of individuals diagnosed in childhood (range of 32 to 84% across countries). The take-home message is that ADHD is a chronic, serious disorder requiring evidence-based treatment approaches that target specific impairments, and such treatments must be maintained and individualized from childhood, adolescence, and often into adult life.

Psychosocial Treatments

Pelham and colleagues have recently reviewed evidence-based psychosocial interventions for children with ADHD. They note that behavioral parent training and behavioral classroom management are well supported, and that there is also a role for intensive peer-focused behavioral interventions implemented in recreational settings. Chronis and colleagues have updated the behavioral parent training paradigm. This training focuses on issues such as helping the parents to give effective commands so that the child can be successful in following through with an activity, differentially attending to positive over negative behaviors, and helping the child to contain impulsive responses or calm himself in the face of arousal. Other authors note the importance of psychoeducation in developing an ongoing alliance among the therapist, the child and the family, and in ensuring treatment adherence. Close collaboration among treatment providers and school personnel is equally important. Families and clinicians often elect to initiate treatment with these nonmedication interventions and most children treated pharmacologically also need such interventions concurrently with medication.

School is where ADHD symptoms may be most disabling, with the inherent demands to sit quietly, pay attention, and work cooperatively. School interventions include ensuring that learning needs are appropriately assessed and addressed. Additionally, contact with teachers regarding treatment is required. It is crucial that the teacher understands the disorder provides an environment that optimizes the child's learning. Preferential seating (seating within the class to optimize paying attention and minimize distractions), a behavioral management plan that highlights positive reinforcement for desired work habits and behavior, social skills groups, and other interventions may help the child gain school success. More intensive interventions (a small self-contained classroom, special educational services, or a more intensive therapeutic educational plan) may be required for children who are more impaired by the disorder and/or comorbidities. Active collaboration among treatment providers, school personnel, and the child's caregivers improves outcomes.

Medication Treatment

The impact of the MTA study has been significant. Most experts, organizations, and consensus panels such as the Texas Children's Medication Algorithm Project (TCMAP) now recommend stimulant medication as the first-line treatment and propose behavioral interventions as second-line, or complementary to medication, interventions. Medication treatment is the single most effective treatment for core ADHD symptoms, at least over the short term. Less clear is how medication performs over the long term. There is a large body of literature documenting the efficacy of stimulants on core features of ADHD as well as their substantial effects on cognition, social function, and aggression. The stimulants are the best studied medications in child and adolescent psychiatry, and have demonstrated safety and efficacy in over 200 controlled trials. Despite concerns of many families about the abuse and addiction potential of the stimulants, this has not been the case. In fact, there is evidence that youths under treatment are at decreased risk for substance abuse, legal difficulties, and other sequelae of poor impulse control. Finally, concerns that stimulant medication might be responsible for the smaller structures in the central nervous system described for ADHD children have not been supported.

At times, medication "holidays" may be indicated during nonschool days. Although this practice may be helpful for children who experience side effects in appetite, growth, and sleep, many other children require the medication consistently, even when not in school, to maintain appropriate social behavior and to contain impulsive behaviors that pose a safety risk. Essential tips for the treatment of ADHD are listed in Table 4.4.

Psychotropics Used in the Treatment of ADHD

The stimulant medications are considered the first-line treatment for the core symptoms of ADHD. Atomoxetine is an antidepressant that has been approved by the Food and Drug Administration as a long-acting, noncontrolled medication for the treatment of ADHD. However, atomoxetine does not have the same benefits as stimulants for core ADHD symptoms. The stimulants are generally very well tolerated but not without potential adverse effects. Common side effects include appetite suppression, sleep disturbances, and minor, clinically irrelevant, increases in pulse and blood pressure. Stimulants may precipitate or exacerbate tics. At times, stimulant medications may cause more serious side effects, such as dsyphoria, irritability, lability, or even hallucinations, particularly in younger children. Recent research indicates that children treated long term with stimulants may show some mild growth suppression at 18 years of age.

The cardiovascular safety of stimulant medications has been a topic of controversy intermittently for 20 years. In particular, there have been concerns about an increased potential for sudden death. Recently, the American Heart Association (AHA) and the American Academy of Pediatrics (AAP) issued a joint statement noting that medications that treat ADHD have not been shown to cause heart conditions or sudden cardiac death, although the potential for cardiotoxicity may warrant special monitoring in some children, especially those with cardiac defects or family histories of cardiac disease. The AAP and AHA recommendations for cardiac

TABLE 4-4	Essentials of Treatment for Attention-deficit Hyperactivity Disorder

- Engagement and psychoeducation of the child, caregivers, and teacher about the diagnosis and treatment options are the cornerstones of treatment.
- Pretreatment and intermittent posttreatment rating scales (e.g., Conners Rating Scales and Vanderbilt ADHD Rating Scales) should be used to monitor treatment effectiveness.
- Pharmacologic treatment is the single most effective treatment for most of the children diagnosed with ADHD with or without comorbid disorders. Individual dose titration to the optimal effective dose with fewest side effects is recommended.
- Parent management training should be included in any treatment plan, particularly skill-building training for parents in how to engage and discipline a disruptive child.
- Behavioral plans that reinforce appropriate and adaptive behaviors are most effective when consistent between home and school.
- Individual psychotherapy may be useful for skill building, psychoeducation, and treatment of comorbid disorders (e.g., supportive psychotherapy, cognitive–behavioral therapy for depression or anxiety, anger management skill building to control aggression, etc.).
- Comorbid disorders should be treated with psychosocial interventions and medications, as indicated.
- A section 504 accommodation plan or individualized education plan (IEP) is indicated for children whose ADHD interferes with education.
- Children who are so impaired that they are not able to function in a less restrictive setting may require a self-contained classroom designed for children with ADHD.
- Monthly follow-up of medications with modifications required to optimize response is needed.
- Medication holidays should be individualized to the child's unique situation and utilized only if the child's social functioning and safety would not be compromised.
- In the case of poor response, reassessment of the diagnosis or comorbidities is indicated; consultation may be helpful.

assessment are given in Table 4.5. This controversy is likely to continue as a recent study by Gould and colleagues has again raised concern about an increased risk for sudden death in children treated with stimulants.

The TCMAP developed by Pliszka and colleagues provides treatment algorithms for ADHD with and without comorbidities. Relevant comorbidities include anxiety, depression, tics, and aggression. These algorithms reflect consensus guidelines in the absence of randomized clinical trials for the treatment of ADHD with comorbidities. In general, stimulants (methylphenidate or amphetamine preparations) are first-line medication treatments, with a second stimulant tried if the first one is ineffective or is not well-tolerated (Table 4.6). With the selection of the appropriate stimulant and dosing, over 75% of children with ADHD will improve considerably. Atomoxetine is considered the second-line treatment for ADHD

TABLE 4-5	AAP and AHA Recommendations for Cardiac Assessment during Treatment with Stimulant Medication

- Carefully assess children for underlying cardiac conditions if medication treatment is indicated.
- Obtain a patient and family health history and conduct a physical examination focused on cardiovascular risk factors.
- Obtain an electrocardiogram (ECG) based on physician's clinical judgment (not mandatory).
- Treatment of a patient for ADHD should not be withheld because an ECG is not done.
- Monitor heart rate and blood pressure for children with heart conditions.

without comorbidities, and may be considered first-line for children with comorbid anxiety, although not all investigators prioritize atomoxetine. Bupropion, tricyclic antidepressants, and alpha-2 agonists are considered third-line in the medication algorithm. Stimulants should be titrated slowly in children with comorbid tic disorders, and the addition of an alpha agonist (guanfacine or clonidine), atypical or typical antipsychotic may be used for severe tics. The concomitant use of selective serotonin reuptake inhibitors (SSRIs) is considered for children with comorbid major depression. Several studies have described the safety and efficacy of combined SSRI and stimulant pharmacotherapy. However, all of the antidepressants contain a "Black Box" warning for increased risk of suicidal behavior, which needs to be considered. For children with functionally disabling ADHD and aggression that remains unaltered after the use of stimulant medication, the addition of an atypical antipsychotic followed by lithium or divalproex sodium are suggested.

General principles of pharmacotherapy should be followed in the treatment of children and adolescents with ADHD. These include beginning with one medication and slowly titrating dosage up to optimal effectiveness with minimal side effects. At times, changing the dosing schedule may help to decrease side effects such as appetite suppression or sleep disturbance. Routine monitoring of blood pressure, pulse, height, and weight is indicated.

Conclusions

ADHD is the single most frequently diagnosed and most thoroughly researched psychiatric illness of childhood. However, there continues to be major challenges to the assessment and treatment of children with ADHD. The high prevalence of comorbid diagnoses complicates both evaluation and treatment. ADHD remains a diagnosis made on the basis of history, mental status, and corollary data. Despite years of study and thousands of publications regarding the etiology and treatment of ADHD, there are no brain scans, psychological tests, or laboratory studies that reliably render a valid diagnosis of ADHD. Current research indicates that stimulants are the primary treatment of ADHD in school-aged children, but controversy persists regarding their risks for cardiac complications and growth. Nonmedical interventions focus on parent training for preadolescent children complemented by interventions in the classroom to promote learning. Medications have also been utilized safely in preschool children, although this is another area of controversy, as longer-term effects on neurological processes are not known. Thus, psychosocial interventions emphasizing behavioral and skill-building treatments, parent training, and educational interventions should be the first approach for these younger children.

TABLE 4-6	Medication Algorithm for Treating Attention-Deficit/Hyperactivity Disorder

First Line
- Methylphenidate or amphetamine preparations
- Second stimulant medication, in other stimulant class

Second Line
- Atomoxetine; it may be the first-line treatment in children with clinically relevant anxiety

Third Line
- Bupropion
- Tricyclic antidepressant (nortriptyline, imipramine, amitriptyline, desipramine)
- Alpha agonist (guanfacine or clonidine)

If above medications are ineffective, reassess for misdiagnosis or significant comorbidities; consider clinical consultation.

While children with ADHD present many challenges, effective treatments are available. As ADHD is a disorder that manifests in multiple settings and persists into adulthood for most individuals, multidisciplinary, multimodal interventions are indicated and are most effective if they are consistent and implemented at school and at home. Good outcomes are very rewarding for parents, families, and the children suffering from this disorder, as well as for their treatment providers. Hopefully, as our understanding of ADHD increases, new treatments will be targeted to individual children's needs.

CASE VIGNETTES

VIGNETTE 1: SCHOOL-AGED GIRL WITH ANXIETY COMORBID WITH ADHD AND ODD

Tania is a 10-year-old fifth-grade girl who is referred to a child and adolescent psychiatrist for treatment by her parents on the recommendation of her teachers due to difficulties with anxiety and oppositionality. She has a history of separation anxiety in preschool and kindergarten. Although she is a sweet girl who is not openly disrespectful, her teachers and parents are frustrated by her refusal to do schoolwork and chores. She is getting Ds and Fs in several of her academic classes due to failure to complete assignments. She avoids written schoolwork, and tends to be oppositional or ignore prompts. In fact, the teacher notes that Tania doesn't listen, is "dreamy" (perhaps worrying?), and is not available for learning. The child and adolescent psychiatrist takes a full history and discovers that Tania had low normal developmental milestones. She has always been dependent upon her mother for emotional support and for activities of daily living. Her mother complains that Tania's room is a disorganized mess, and that it is "like pulling teeth" to get Tania ready for school in the morning. It is as if she is in "slow motion". She often forgets instructions and is easily distracted. She avoids homework and her writing is slow and labored. Psychological testing is requested and reveals average cognitive functioning, no specific learning disability, but with low average to borderline processing speed and notable executive functioning deficits. An ADHD scale is positive for inattentive symptoms, but not hyperactivity or impulsivity. Anxiety level is higher than most of the children, but there are no acute worries. Sleep and appetite are normal. ADHD of inattentive type is diagnosed, with concern about comorbid anxiety disorder. A low dose of stimulant medication (methylphenidate 5 mg) is initiated and increased slowly. Within a few weeks, Tania is getting her classwork completed for the first time in her life. Her grades improve and oppositionality and work avoidance decrease. She is switched to a long-acting preparation, as Tania does not want to take medication at school (Concerta 18 mg is increased to 36 mg over the course of the school year). Upon psychiatrist's recommendation, Tania's seat is placed closer to the teacher; the teacher and Tania set up a nonintrusive manner to prompt Tania to pay attention; Tania receives extra time for tests; she takes tests in a quiet area; and she has a checklist to organize her materials and a homework log that is reviewed with a teacher prior to dismissal. Tania has some difficulties falling asleep at night (remedied with a standard bedtime routine and occasional melatonin), but no exacerbation of anxiety.

VIGNETTE 2: PRESCHOOL BOY WITH ADHD AND A CHRONIC MOTOR TIC

John is a 4-year-old boy who is in preschool. He has had a difficult time in school and at home due to his high levels of activity, inattention, and impulsivity. John interrupts conversations, cannot sit at the dinner table, and disrupts his preschool classroom on a daily basis due to talking out, inability to sit in circle, pushing children to be first in line, constant touching of other children, and unsafe behaviors, such as jumping off the swing. The other children have started to avoid him, due to his difficulties waiting his turn, following rules, and his anger outbursts when he loses at a game. He is frequently sent to the "quiet chair" for oppositional and disruptive behaviors. His teacher is "wearing out" spending so much of the day dealing with John. Developmental screening suggests that John is average in all areas. The Behavioral Assessment Scale for Children (BASC) is significant for symptoms of ADHD and behavioral difficulties. John has a normal physical exam except for mild blinking tics. He weighs 18 kg. He has a very difficult time slowing down in the evening to get to sleep. Family history is significant for an aunt with obsessive–compulsive disorder and his father had mild motor tics and similar symptoms to John when he was young.

John was diagnosed with motor tic disorder and ADHD-Combined type. Parent management training and a behavioral plan for the school were implemented. John's overall behavior began to improve, but his impulsive unsafe behavior and aggression persisted. John was at risk of being dismissed from the preschool when he threw a rock at another child after he lost a game. He was unable to complete work without one-on-one assistance. He broke his arm when he impulsively jumped off a stone fence on a dare. He pushed another child off the swing when he was unable to wait his turn. It was determined that medication treatment was indicated. A trial of stimulant medication was initiated (methylphenidate started at 2.5 mg once daily and increased up to 5 mg twice daily) to address his impairing ADHD symptoms. His motor tics exacerbated on the medication. Appetite decreased, but he otherwise tolerated the medication well. Due to concerns of tic exacerbation, John was started on a trial of guanfacine, which was increased to 1.5 mg daily (0.5 mg in the morning and 1.0 mg in the evening). John's tics decreased in frequency and severity over 2 months of treatment, and his sleep habits improve substantially. School behavior problems were markedly improved and tics were mild. John was able to sit in circle; his impulsive and unsafe behaviors were notably diminished; and he was able to complete most assignments without individualized assistance. On the recommendation of his psychiatrist, the preschool provided John with special services, which included preferential seating (near the teacher), a behavioral plan that provided rewards for appropriate behavior, social skills assistance (lunch with a teacher and one other child to practice social skills), and a school–home log of behavior, and John started extracurricular activities to assist him in burning his extra energy, learning to be a good sport at games, and developing athletic skills (e.g., playing with a preschool soccer team). By the time John was to start kindergarten, he was completing more of his worksheets, having less anger outbursts, and getting along better with his peers. His teacher noted that John was able to participate appropriately in the class most of the time; he did not substantially disrupt the classroom; he had several friends; and he was less oppositional and seemed happier and less reactive.

BIBLIOGRAPHY

American Academy of Child and Adolescent Psychiatry. Practice Parameter for the assessment and treatment of children and adolescents with attention-deficit/hyperactivity disorder. *J Am Acad Child Adolesc Psychiatry.* 2007;46:894–921.

American Heart Association. American Academy of Pediatrics/American Heart Association clarification of statement on cardiovascular evaluation and monitoring of children and adolescents with heart disease receiving medications for ADHD. *AAP News.* 2008;29:1–2.

American Psychiatric Association. *The Diagnostic and Statistical Manual of Mental Disorder.* 2nd ed. Washington DC: American Psychiatric Press; 1968.

American Psychiatric Association. *The Diagnostic and Statistical Manual of Mental Disorders.* 4th ed. Washington DC: American Psychiatric Press; 1994.

Arnsten AFT, Castellanos FX. Neurobiology of attention regulation and its disorders. In: Martin A, Scahill L, Charney DS, Leckman JF, eds. *Pediatric Psychopharmacology: Principles and Practice*. New York, NY: Oxford University Press; 2003:99–109.

Barkley R. *Attention Deficit Hyperactivity Disorder: A Handbook for Diagnosis and Treatment*. 3rd ed. New York, NY: Guilford; 2005.

Brown TE. *Attention Deficit Disorder: The Unfocused Mind in Children and Adults*. New Haven, CT: Yale University Press; 2005.

Castellanos FX, Swanson J. Biological underpinnings of ADHD. In: Sandberg S, ed. *Hyperactivity and Attention Disorders of Childhood: Cambridge Monographs in Child and Adolescent Psychiatry*. Cambridge, UK: Cambridge University Press; 2002.

Conners CK. *Conners ADHD DSM-IV Scale for Parents and Teachers: Technical Manual*. North Tonowanda, NY: Multi Health Systems; 2007.

Chronis AM, Chacko A, Fabiano GA, et al. Enhancements to the behavioral parent training paradigm for families of children with ADHD: review and future directions. *Clin Child Fam Psychol Rev*. 2004;7(1):1–27.

DuPaul GJ, McGoey KE, Eckert TL, et al. Preschool children with attention-deficit/ hyperactivity disorder: impairment in behavioral, social, and school functioning. *J Am Acad Child Adolesc Psychiatry*. 2001;40:508–515.

Faraone SV, Biederman J. The neurobiology of attention deficit hyperactivity disorder. In: Charney DS, Nestler EJ, and Bunney BS, eds. *Neurobiology of Mental Illness*. New York, NY: Oxford University Press; 1999:788–801.

Lara C, Fayyad J, de Graaf R, et al. Childhood predictors of adult attention-deficit/hyperactivity disorder: results from the World Health Organization World Mental Health Survey Initiative. *Biol Psychiatry*. 2009;65(1):46–54.

Ghuman JK, Arnold LE, Anthony BJ. Psychopharmacological and other treatments in preschool children with attention-deficit/hyperactivity disorder: current evidence and practice. *J Child Adolesc Psychopharmacol*. 2008;18(5):413–447.

Gould MS, Walsh BT, Munfakh JL, et al. Sudden death and use of stimulant medication in youths. *Am J Psychiatry*. 2009;166:992–1001.

Greenhill L, Kollins S, Abikoff H, et al. Efficacy and safety of immediate-release methylphenidate treatment for preschoolers with ADHD. *J Am Acad Child Adolesc Psychiatry*. 2006;45:1314–1224.

Kuehn BM. Stimulant use linked to sudden death in children without heart problems. *JAMA*. 2009;302:613–614.

Mannuzza S, Klein RG, Bessler A, et al. Adult psychiatric status of hyperactive boys grown up. *Am J Psychiatry*. 1998;155:493–498.

McNab F, Varrone A, Farde L. Changes in cortical dopamine D1 receptor binding associated with cognitive training. *Science*. 2009;4:86–90.

MTA Cooperative Group. A 14-month randomized clinical trial of treatment strategies for attention deficit/ hyperactivity disorder. *Arch Gen Psychiatry*. 1999;56:1073–1086.

MTA Cooperative Group. The MTA at 8 years: prospective follow-up of children treated for combined-type ADHD in a multisite study. *J Am Acad Child Adolesc Psychiatry*. 2009;48:484–500.

Murray DW, Arnold E, Swanson J, et al. A clinical review of outcomes of the multimodal treatment study of children with attention-deficit/hyperactivity disorder (MTA). *Current Psychiatry Reports*. 2008;10:424–431.

National Institutes of Health. National Institutes of Health Consensus Development Conference Statement: diagnosis and treatment of attention-deficit hyperactivity disorder (ADHD). *J Am Acad Child Adolesc Psychiatry*. 2000;39:182–193.

Olfson M, Gameroff MJ, Marcus SC, et al. National trends in the treatment of ADHD. *Am J Psychiatry*. 2003;160: 1071–1077.

Pelham WE , Fabiano GA. Evidence-based psychosocial treatments for attention-deficit/hyperactivity disorder. *J Clin Child Adolesc Psychol*. 2008;37(1):184–214.

Pliszka SR, Crismon ML, Hughes CW, et al. The Texas children's medication algorithm project: revision of the algorithm for pharmacotherapy of attention-deficit/hyperactivity disorder. *J Am Acad Child Adolesc Psychiatry*. 2006;45:642–657.

Stahl SM. *Stahl's Essential Psychopharmacology: Neuroscientific Basis and Practical Applications*. 3rd ed. New York, NY: Cambridge University Press; 2008.

Stubbe DE. Attention-deficit/hyperactivity disorder. *Child and Adolescent Psychiatric Clin N Am*. 2000;9:469–479.

Swanson J, Arnold LE, Kraemer H, et. al. Evidence, interpretation, and qualification from multiple reports of long-term outcomes in the multimodal treatment study of children with ADHD (MTA). Part I: executive summary. *J Atten Disord*. 2008;12:4–14.

Swanson J, Arnold LE, Kraemer H, et. al. Evidence, interpretation, and qualification from multiple reports of long-term outcomes in the multimodal treatment study of children with ADHD (MTA). Part II: supporting details. *J Atten Disord*. 2008;12:15–43.

Szatmari P. The epidemiology of attention-deficit hyperactivity disorders. In: Weiss G, ed. *Attention-Deficit/ Hyperactivity Disorder*. Philadelphia, PA: WB Saunders; 1992:361–371.

Taylor E. Development of clinical services for attention-deficit/hyperactivity disorder. *Arch Gen Psychiatry.* 1999;56:1097–1099.

Vetter VL, Elia J, Erickson C, et al. Cardiovascular monitoring of children and adolescents with heart disease receiving medications for attention-deficit/hyperactivity disorder: a scientific statement from the American Heart Association Council on Cardiovascular Disease in the Young Congenital Cardiac Defects Committee and the Council on Cardiovascular Nursing. *Circulation.* 2009;117:2407–2423.

World Health Organization. *International Statistical Classification of Diseases and Related Health Problems.* Geneva: WHO; 1979.

World Health Organization. *International Statistical Classification of Diseases and Related Health Problems.* Geneva: WHO; 1994.

Zito JM, Safer DJ, dosReis S, et al. Trends in the prescribing of psychotropic medications to preschoolers. *JAMA.* 2000;283:1025–1030.

SUGGESTED READINGS

Taking Charge of ADHD: The Complete, Authoritative Guide for Parents, 3rd ed.
Author: Russell A. Barkley, PhD
Publisher: Guilford Publications, Inc., 2005

Delivered from Distraction: Getting the Most Out of Life with Attention Deficit Disorder
Authors: Edward M. Hallowell, John J. Ratey
Publisher: Random House Publishing, 2005

You Mean I'm Not Lazy, Stupid or Crazy?!
Authors: Kate Kelly and Peggy Ramundo
Publisher: Simon & Schuster Adult Publishing Group, 2006

ADHD: A Complete and Authoritative Guide
Authors: American Academy of Pediatrics, Sherill Tippins (Editor), Michael I. Reiff (Editor)
Publisher: American Academy of Pediatrics Press: Washington DC, 2004

Attention-Deficit Hyperactivity Disorder: A Handbook for Diagnosis and Treatment
Author: Russell A. Barkley
Publisher: Guilford Publications, Inc., 2005

Teenagers with ADD: A Parent's Guide
Author: Chris A. Zeigler Dendy
Publisher: Woodbine House, 1995

ADHD in the Schools, Second Edition : Assessment and Intervention Strategies
Authors: George J. DuPaul, Gary Stoner
Publisher: Guilford Publications, Inc., 2005

Attention-Deficit Hyperactivity Disorder : A Clinical Workbook
Authors: Russell A. Barkley, Kevin R. Murphy
Publisher: Guilford Publications, Inc., 2005

SUGGESTED WEBSITES

ADHD: A Guide for Families. Available at: http://www.aacap.org/cs/adhd_a_guide_for_families/resources_for_families_adhd_a_guide_for_families.

Children and Adults with Attention-Deficit/Hyperactivity Disorder (CHADD). Available at: http://www.chadd.org.

National Attention Deficit Disorder Association (ADDA). Available at: http://www.add.org.

Texas Department of State Health Services Children's Medication Algorithm Project. Available at: http://www.dshs.state.tx.us/mhprograms/adhdpage.shtm.

REVIEW QUESTIONS

1. In community samples, attention-deficit/hyperactivity disorder, inattentive type is
   a. Three times as common in boys as in girls
   b. Three times as common in girls as in boys
   c. About equal between girls and boys
   d. Unknown

2. In community samples, attention-deficit/hyperactivity disorder, hyperactive–impulsive type is
   a. Three times as common in boys as in girls
   b. Thee times as common in girls as in boys
   c. About equal between girls and boys
   d. Unknown

3. Referral for treatment is *least* common with which subtype of ADHD?
   a. ADHD, combined type
   b. ADHD, hyperactive–impulsive type
   c. ADHD, inattentive type
   d. All of the above

4. The most common comorbid psychiatric disorder diagnosed in youths with ADHD is
   a. Anxiety disorder
   b. Learning disorder
   c. Mood disorder
   d. Oppositional defiant disorder or conduct disorder

5. Evidence suggests that the most effective treatment for inattention in ADHD is
   a. Behavioral modification therapy
   b. Stimulant medication
   c. Alpha agonist medication
   d. Antidepressant medication

6. Which of the following treatments of ADHD is contraindicated in children and adolescents with tic disorders?
   a. Methylphenidate (Ritalin)
   b. Bupropion (Wellbutrin)
   c. Guanfacine
   d. None of the above

7. Children with Tourette syndrome and ADHD are at greater risk for
   a. Conduct disorder
   b. Anxiety disorder
   c. Mood disorder
   d. All of the above

8. When treating children and adolescents who have tics with psychostimulant medication for ADHD, it is most appropriate to
   a. Give a fairly large "loading dose" medication trial to see if the tics worsen before starting a more prolonged medication trial
   b. Start at about half of the usual dose and increase dosages more slowly
   c. Avoid using stimulant medication at all costs in individuals with tics
   d. Be sure the tics are eradicated with an antipsychotic or alpha agonist (clonidine or guanfacine) medication prior to initiating a stimulant medication trial

9. Children with ADHD tend to respond most positively to behavioral plans with
   a. Clear negative consequences (punishment) for inappropriate behavior
   b. Clear positive consequences (positive reinforcement) for appropriate behavior

    c. Time alone for misbehavior
    d. None of the above

10. The most common side effect of stimulant medication is
    a. Arrhythmia
    b. New onset of tics
    c. Decreased appetite
    d. Growth retardation

Answers: 1-c, 2-a, 3-c, 4-d, 5-b, 6-d, 7-d, 8-b, 9-b, 10-c

5

Francheska Perepletchikova, PhD

Oppositional Defiant Disorder and Conduct Disorder

Introduction

Oppositional defiant disorder (ODD) and conduct disorder (CD) encompass a range of dysfunctional behaviors that emerge over the course of childhood. Both ODD and CD include hostile and defiant behavior toward authority, such as disobedience, temper tantrums, argumentativeness, and refusal to comply with requests. However, individuals with ODD do not exhibit the more severe and persistent behavior patterns of CD, such as aggression toward others, destruction of property, theft, and deceit. Although this chapter covers both ODD and CD, greater attention is accorded to the latter disorder. Much more is known about the onset, clinical course, and long-term outcomes of CD. Also, CD has more deleterious consequences for the individual, the family, and the society at large.

Disruptive behaviors encompass a variety of acts that reflect social rule violations and actions against others. Many of these behaviors such as argumentativeness, temper tantrums, resentfulness, lying, fighting, and bullying others are relatively common among children over the course of normal development. Formal ODD and CD diagnoses are reserved for instances in which disruptive behaviors lead to impairment in everyday functioning, as reflected in unmanageability at home and at school or disorderly acts that affect others.

Contemporary diagnosis, as reflected in the 1994 *Diagnostic and Statistical Manual of Mental Disorders, Fourth Edition* (*DSM-IV*), has recognized an increased number of disorders among children and adolescents. Antisocial, disruptive, obstreperous, oppositional, unmanageable, and delinquent child behavior has been acknowledged throughout history even though their identification as psychiatric disorders is quite recent. The behaviors have been attributed to possession by the devil, criminality, and only quite recently mental illness. Extreme measures often have been allowed. For example, early in the history of the United States, Massachusetts had a law that such children could be killed if their parents so approved. The fact that conduct problems represent dysfunction that warrants intervention has not been questioned. The challenge and advances within the past 25 years have been to delineate the disorders of conduct and to identify ways for their treatment or prevention.

Clinical Features

As Rowe and colleagues have shown, ODD and CD are closely related. Several somewhat different models of the nature of this relationship have been proposed. Because all features of ODD are evident in CD, ODD is usually viewed as its precursor. CD is also seen as a more severe form of the same underlying disorder. Furthermore, ODD is sometimes viewed as a subtype of CD. Finally, because these disorders are closely similar in etiology, the distinction between CD and ODD itself has been questioned. In short, the precise nature of the relationship between these disorders is still a matter of debate and empirical attention.

TABLE 5-1	Major Diagnostic Symptoms of Oppositional Defiant Disorder

1. Often loses temper
2. Often argues with adults
3. Often actively defies or refuses to comply with adult's requests or rules
4. Often deliberately annoys people
5. Often blames others for his or her mistakes or misbehavior
6. Is often touchy or easily annoyed by others
7. Is often angry or resentful
8. Is often spiteful or vindictive

Diagnostic Criteria for Oppositional Defiant Disorder

DSM-IV delineates ODD as a recurrent pattern of negativistic, hostile, and defiant behavior. Table 5-1 lists the main symptoms. A diagnosis of ODD is provided if (1) the individual shows at least four symptoms (2) within the past 6 months. To meet the criteria, the behavior must occur more frequently than is typically observed in individuals of compatible age and developmental level, and must be associated with impaired functioning.

Diagnostic Criteria for Conduct Disorder

Current diagnosis using the *DSM-IV* delineates CD as the violation of basic rights of others and age-appropriate societal norms as the essential features. Table 5-2 lists the main symptoms. A diagnosis of CD is provided if (1) the individual shows at least three symptoms (2) within the past 12 months (3) with at least one of the symptoms evident in the last 6 months. To meet the criteria, the behaviors must be repetitive and persistent and be associated with impaired functioning.

Many ways of subtyping have been proposed. Historically, the greatest evidence has accumulated for aggressive and nonaggressive subtypes. These are characterized by youth who engage primarily in fighting as opposed to stealing. Some youth are of a mixed type, show

TABLE 5-2	Major Symptoms of Conduct Disorder

1. Bullying or threatening others
2. Fighting
3. Using a weapon that can cause serious physical harm to others
4. Being physically cruel to people
5. Being physically cruel to animals
6. Stealing and confronting a victim (e.g., mugging, purse snatching, extortion, and armed robbery)
7. Forcing someone into sexual activity
8. Fire setting
9. Destroying others' property
10. Breaking into someone else's house, building, or car
11. Frequent lying or "conning" others
12. Stealing without confronting a victim
13. Staying out late at night despite parental prohibitions
14. Running away from home
15. Being truant from school

symptoms of both, and have a particularly untoward prognosis. In current research, another way of delineating subtypes has focused on age of onset. Two types are distinguished that vary in the nature of conduct problems: developmental course and prognosis, and gender ratio.

Childhood-onset CD is characterized by aggressive behavior. Symptoms usually emerge early in childhood. Individuals with this subtype are usually male, are aggressive, have disturbed peer relationships, have more persistent CD, and are more likely to develop adult antisocial personality disorder than are those with adolescent-onset CD. These individuals usually have had ODD during early childhood, and have symptoms that meet full criteria for CD before puberty.

Adolescent-onset CD is defined by the absence of CD symptoms prior to age 10. Individuals with this type usually have more normative peer relationships, and are less likely than those with childhood-onset type to display aggressive behaviors, have persistent CD, and develop antisocial personality disorder. Moreover, the adolescent-onset type is more evenly distributed among males and females. Symptoms are more likely to reflect vandalism and illegal behaviors than aggressive acts.

There has been support for the subtypes, but a great deal more work is needed to identify whether there are key characteristics that can be identified to refine this grouping further. Also, age of onset as childhood versus adolescence is not very sensitive to large differences seen clinically. For example, among prepubertal children (all considered childhood-onset types), onset, symptom pattern and severity, family history, and long-term course can vary widely.

Limitations in Contemporary Diagnosis of ODD and CD

There are several limitations to the *DSM-IV* diagnostic criteria of ODD and CD. First, the criteria for diagnosis of ODD and CD are somewhat arbitrary. For example, there is no firm empirical basis for selecting the minimal number of symptoms or a time period as part of the criteria. Variation in the number or time period on either side of the cutoff points does not appear to be clinically or prognostically meaningful. Furthermore, diagnosis of ODD relies on the subjective estimation of whether the behavior occurs more frequently than if typically observed in normal development. Such decisions are arbitrary because no specific criterion is present or based on evidence that would consider sex, cultural, and ethnic differences. Second, the diagnostic criteria do not include a core set of symptoms. This allows for a vast heterogeneity of symptom pattern within the diagnosis. Indeed, the requirement of at least 3 of 15 criteria yields an astonishing 32,647 ways in which the CD diagnosis may be met. Third, features of ODD and CD are observable in other disorders, which raise concerns about the meaningfulness of the current categorical delineation of disruptive behavior problems. Fourth, diagnosis of CD seems to be age biased. The diagnostic symptoms are the same or applied in the same way across ages. However, some behaviors, such as stealing, running away, and fire setting, may be less evident in younger ages. There is a need for a more flexible system with symptoms varying depending on age. Finally, *DSM-IV* criteria do not account for sex differences. Diagnostic symptoms of CD focus on aggressive and violent actions that are more likely in boys. Females, on the other hand, are more likely to engage in less obvious acts, such as stealing or lying. Such bias may account for the higher prevalence of CD among boys.

Differential Diagnoses and Comorbid Disorders

Oppositional Defiant Disorder

ODD is comorbid with attention-deficit hyperactivity disorder (ADHD), anxiety disorders, and depressive disorders, as detailed by Angold and Costello. The comorbid condition of ODD and ADHD is associated with greater family conflict, teen management difficulties, rebelliousness, antisocial acts, and earlier substance abuse. Furthermore, symptoms of ODD are sometimes evident in individuals with mental retardation. A diagnosis of ODD is given only if the oppositional behavior is markedly greater than is commonly observed among individuals of comparable age, gender, and severity of cognitive problems.

Features of ODD can be evident in other disorders, such as mood disorder, psychotic disorders, and disorders of language comprehension. Differential diagnosis is based on the associated behavioral patterns and accompanying symptoms. Both ODD and CD include hostile and defiant behavior toward authority, such as disobedience, argumentativeness, temper tantrums, and refusal to comply with requests. However, individuals with ODD do not exhibit more severe and persistent behavior patterns such as aggression toward others and destruction of property. When a behavior pattern meets both diagnoses, the diagnosis of CD takes precedence. Oppositional behavior is a common feature of mood and psychotic disorders and should not be diagnosed separately if symptoms occur exclusively during the course of these disorders. ODD should also be distinguished from a failure to follow directions that result from impaired language comprehension, such as in hearing loss and mixed receptive–expressive language disorder.

Conduct Disorder

CD has a high rate of comorbidity over the course of childhood and adolescence, especially with ADHD, depression, anxiety, and substance abuse, as described by Angold and Costello. The combination of ADHD and CD is especially common, with estimates from 45% to 70% of children with one of these disorders also meeting criteria for the other. Children with both diagnoses show high levels of conduct problems, peer rejection, school problems, and conflictual interactions with parents. Comorbid anxiety disorder has been linked to lower levels of aggression and violence (at least in younger children), but higher rates of shyness and social withdrawal. Comorbid among adolescents, depression is strongly associated with suicide, especially when coupled with substance use disorders.

Features of CD are also evident in other disorders, including adjustment disorders, mania, child or adolescent antisocial behavior, antisocial personality disorder, and pervasive developmental disorders (PDD). Differential diagnoses can be discerned from the onset and course of each disorder, associated behavioral patterns, and accompanying symptoms. A manic episode can occur in children and adolescents with conduct problems. The episodic course and accompanying core symptoms of mood elevation distinguish a manic episode from CD. Adjustment disorders with disturbance of conduct are differentiated from CD by an associated psychosocial stressor preceding the conduct problems. Isolated behavior problems that do not meet criteria for CD or adjustment disorder can be coded as child or adolescent antisocial behavior. Antisocial personality disorder is diagnosed when the individual is at least 18 years old, meets criteria for CD before the age of 15 years, and continues antisocial behavior. For individuals over age 18, a diagnosis of CD is given only if the criteria for antisocial personality disorder are not met. Aggression is also a common reason for referral of children with PDD, and CD or ODD can be comorbid with PDD. The severity of CD or ODD symptoms is lower in younger children with PDD than in children with non-PDD disorders. This can be attributed to the withdrawal from social interactions, characteristic of children with Asperger disorder or autism. However, aggressive behaviors in older children and adolescents with PDD represent a greater clinical problem.

Epidemiology

The prevalence of a disorder refers to the percentage of cases in the population at a given point in time. Among school-aged community samples, the prevalence of ODD and CD combined is approximately 2% to 16%. This estimate is conservative in representing the scope of the problem because research suggests that meeting the diagnostic criteria cutoff is not meaningful in relation to ODD and CD course. Children who approach, but do not quite meet, the diagnostic criteria are also likely to have significant impairment in everyday lives and poor long-term prognoses, especially in the case of CD.

ODD is more prevalent in boys than in girls, especially before puberty. Such differences can be explained by more consistent parental expectations and reinforcement of girls, and more unresponsive and rejecting parenting of boys. Parents also tend to tolerate more excessive behaviors from boys. Furthermore, girls may have more difficulty in expressing anger and are more inclined to refrain from behaviors that would negatively affect relationships, such as oppositionality that evokes frustration and annoyance.

Boys also show approximately three to four times higher rates of CD than do girls. The sex difference may also be explained by the above-mentioned factors and by differences in predispositions toward responding in aggressive ways and the base rates in the different symptoms that comprise CD. Age variations reveal interesting patterns in prevalence rates. Rates of CD tend to be higher for adolescents (approximately 7% for youths aged 12 to 16) than for children (approximately 4% for children aged 4 to 11 years). Childhood-onset and adolescent-onset of CD are often considered to represent distinguishable patterns in light of the symptom patterns, sex distribution, and long-term course, as highlighted later in text.

The prevalence does not convey the scope of the problem from a clinical or social perspective. Symptoms of CD represent clinically important criteria for referring one third to one half of youth for inpatient and outpatient treatment. Moreover, CD has been identified as the most costly mental health problem, at least in the United States. This is due in large part to the findings that children referred for treatment are likely to become involved in several service systems (e.g., mental health, juvenile justice, and special education), and this may continue throughout childhood and well into adulthood.

Etiology and Pathogenesis

Risk Factors

There is no single defining set of symptoms that constitute ODD or CD. Children who meet the diagnosis for either of these disorders may not share any symptoms, in light of the heterogeneity of the current diagnostic criteria. Consequently, on a priori grounds, it is unlikely that there would be a simple etiology. The diagnosis may require finer distinctions in terms of subgroups, time of onset, and clinical course before advances will be made. A great deal is known about the onset of CD, which has been studied much more thoroughly than ODD.

Rather than etiology, research focuses on multiple risk factors that contribute to the onset. This shift is in recognition that there are multiple factors that contribute to CD and multiple paths. *Risk factors* refer to characteristics, events, or processes that increase the likelihood (risk) for the onset of a problem or dysfunction. Risk factors, as antecedents to the dysfunction, may provide clues as to the development and progression of CD, possible mechanisms and processes through which the dysfunctions come about, and foci for possible intervention. Several factors that predispose children and adolescents to behavior problems are highlighted in Table 5-3.

Protective Factors

Even under very adverse conditions with multiple risk factors present, many individuals will not experience adverse outcomes. Protective factors refer to characteristics, events, or processes that decrease the impact of a risk factor and likelihood of an adverse outcome. Protective factors are identified by studying individuals known to be at risk (who show several risk factors) and by delineating subgroups of those who do, versus those who do not, later develop CD. Among a high-risk sample, children are less likely to develop CD if they are first born, are perceived by their mothers as affectionate, show high self-esteem and locus of control, and have alternative caretakers in the family (in addition to the parents) and a supportive same-sex model who played an important role in their development. Other factors that reduce or attenuate risk include above-average intelligence, competence in various skill areas, getting along with peers, and having friends.

TABLE 5-3	Factors That Place Youths at Risk for the Onset of Oppositional Defiant Disorder and Conduct Disorder

Child factors

- *Child temperament.* A more difficult child temperament (on a dimension of "easy-to-difficult"), as characterized by more negative mood, lower levels of approach toward new stimuli, and less adaptability to change.
- *Neuropsychological deficits and difficulties.* Deficits in diverse functions related to language (e.g., verbal learning, verbal fluency, and verbal IQ), memory, motor coordination, integration of auditory and visual cues, and "executive" functions of the brain (e.g., abstract reasoning, concept formation, planning, and control of attention).
- *Subclinical levels of CD.* Early signs of mild (subclinical) levels of unmanageability and aggression, especially with early age of onset, multiple types of antisocial behaviors, and multiple situations in which they are evident (e.g., at home, in school, and in the community).
- *Academic and intellectual performance.* Academic deficiencies and lower intellectual functioning

Parent and family factors

- *Prenatal and perinatal complications.* Pregnancy- and birth-related complications including maternal infection, prematurity, low birth weight, impaired respiration, and minor birth injury.
- *Psychopathology and criminal behavior in the family.* Criminal behavior, antisocial personality disorder, and alcoholism of the parent.
- *Poor parental practices.* Coercive parent–child communications, inconsistent disciplining, harsh or corporal punishment, and permissive or overcontrolling parenting.
- *Monitoring of the child.* Poor supervision, lack of monitoring of whereabouts, and few rules about where youth can go and when they can return.
- *Quality of the family relationships.* Less parental acceptance of their children; less warmth, affection, and emotional support; and less attachment.
- *Marital discord.* Unhappy marital relationships, interpersonal conflict, and parental aggression.
- *Family size.* Larger family size, that is, more children in the family.
- *Sibling with antisocial behavior.* Presence of a sibling, especially an older brother, with antisocial behavior.
- *Socioeconomic disadvantage.* Poverty, overcrowding, unemployment, receipt of social assistance (welfare), and poor housing.

School-related factors

- *Characteristics of the setting.* Attending schools where there is little emphasis on academic work, little teacher time spent on lessons, infrequent teacher use of praise and appreciation for schoolwork, little emphasis on individual responsibility of the students, poor working conditions for pupils (e.g., furniture in poor repair), unavailability of the teacher to deal with children's problems, and low teacher expectancies.

Note: The list of risk factors highlights major influences. Identified factors are generally stronger predictors of CD than of ODD. The number of factors and the relations of specific factors to risk are more complex than the summary statements noted here.

See Burke JD, Loeber R, Birmaher B. Oppositional defiant disorder and conduct disorder: a review of the past 10 years, part II. *J Am Acad Child Adolesc Psychiatry.* 2002;41:1275–1293; Hendren RL. Disruptive behavior disorders in childhood and adolescents. In: Oldham JM, Riba RM, eds. Review of Psychiatry, Washington, DC: American Psychiatric Press; 1999; Kazdin AE. *Conduct Disorder in Childhood and Adolescence.* 2nd ed. Thousand Oaks, CA: Sage; 1995.

The mechanisms through which risk and protective factors may exert their influence are not known. As an exception, parenting practices (e.g., harsh punishment and attending to aggressive child behavior) have been well studied. These practices directly contribute to aggressive and antisocial behavior. Moreover, Reid and colleagues have shown that altering these practices reduces aggressive and antisocial child behavior.

Antisocial behavior runs in families. Twin and adoption studies indicate a genetic influence on antisocial behavior and deviance in general. Advances in the molecular genetics will no doubt lead to breakthroughs that move closer to understanding mechanisms of action and subgroups of youths. For example, Caspi and colleagues found that children who are maltreated are especially likely to develop antisocial behavior if they have the genotype coding for low monoamine oxidase A activity. Further research relating genotype of vulnerability to subsequent risk factors will add considerably to identifying subgroups and pathways involved in CD.

Clinical Course

Typically, ODD becomes evident before age 8 years. In a significant proportion of cases, ODD is a developmental precursor of CD. Little is known, however, about the outcomes of children with ODD who do not develop antisocial and aggressive symptoms. As discussed earlier in text, CD can emerge in childhood or in adolescence. Adolescent-onset CD is more common and is more equally distributed among boys and girls. Childhood-onset CD is considered to be a more severe form as it usually leads to more severe outcomes. Longitudinal studies show that CD in childhood predicts aggressive and antisocial behavior up to 30 years later. Among CD youths identified in childhood, slightly less than 50% continue their CD into adulthood. If all comorbid diagnoses are considered, apart from CD, slightly over 80% are likely to show a psychiatric disorder as adults. Psychiatric disorder in adulthood is only one of many untoward prognostic features. As highlighted in Table 5-4, individuals with a history of CD evince a broad range of negative outcomes.

Assessment

ODD and CD are usually evaluated using multiple assessment modalities. These modalities have been described in detail by Kazdin as well as by Sommers-Flanagan and Sommers-Flanagan.

TABLE 5-4	Long-Term Prognosis of Youths Identified as Conduct Disordered: Major Characteristics Likely to be Evident in Adulthood
Major Characteristics	**Prognosis**
Psychiatric status	Greater psychiatric impairment including antisocial personality, alcohol and drug abuse, and isolated symptoms (e.g., anxiety and somatic complaints); also, greater history of psychiatric hospitalization
Criminal behavior	Higher rates of driving while intoxicated, criminal behavior, arrest records and conviction, and period of time spent in jail
Occupation adjustment	Less likely to be employed; shorter history of employment, lower status jobs, more frequent change of jobs, lower wages, and depend more frequently on financial assistance (welfare); served less frequently and performed less well in the armed services
Educational attainment	Higher rates of dropping out of school, lower attainment among those who remain in school
Marital status	Higher rates of divorce, remarriage, and separation
Social participation	Less contact with relatives, friends, and neighbors; little participation in organizations such as church
Physical health	Higher mortality rate, higher rate of hospitalization for physical problems

Note: These characteristics are based on comparisons of clinically referred children identified for CD relative to control clinical referrals or normal controls or from comparisons of delinquent and nondelinquent youths.

See Pepper DJ, Rubin KH. *The Development and Treatment of Childhood Aggression.* Hillsdale, NJ: Erlbaum; 1991; Peters RD, McMahon RJ, Quinsey VL. *Aggression and Violence Throughout the Life Span.* Newbury Park, CA: Sage; 1992.

TABLE 5-5	Essentials of Assessment of Oppositional Defiant Disorder and Conduct Disorder

1. Multimethod, multirater, and multisetting assessment approaches should be utilized in the evaluation of ODD and CD.
2. There are no specific assessment instruments that have been established to be individually diagnostic for ODD and CD.
3. There are no core symptoms associated with making the diagnosis of ODD and CD.
4. When a behavior pattern meets both diagnoses, the diagnosis of CD takes precedence.
5. Parental practices, parent–child interactions, parental psychopathology, and child's peer relationships should be assessed for treatment planning and delivery.
6. Educational assessment should be performed if school or learning problems are suspected.
7. Functional analysis of the behavior patterns, including baseline and follow-up ratings, should be performed to evaluate the effectiveness of treatment.

Each modality may be more or less relevant for the purposes of a particular assessment and may yield information not attainable by other forms of assessment. For example, raters can have limited knowledge about child's conduct problems. Conclusions about symptoms, severity of dysfunction, and changes over time will vary for different measures. Furthermore, youths with behavior problems tend to exhibit symptoms in some settings, but not others. Therefore, utilizing multimethod, multirater, and multisetting assessment approaches would provide a better picture of each psychopathology. Table 5-5 presents the essentials of assessment.

Self-Report Measures

Self-report measures are used in the assessment of childhood psychopathologies because they can elicit information not apparent to parents, obtainable from institutional records, or evident through direct observations. Children over 10 years old and adolescents readily report their disruptive behavior and can provide a valid account of their conduct. However, younger children rarely identify themselves as having a problem. The ability of children to report their psychological maladjustment is not as clear as that of adolescents or adults, at least in relation to conventional self-report measures. Although for these reasons self-report inventories are not usually used as primary measures among young children, they are still regarded as a valuable source of important information.

Several self-report measures are currently available to assess disruptive behavior problems. Selected examples of the measures that have been studied extensively include *Children's Action Tendency Scale* by Deluty; *Adolescent Antisocial Self-Report Behavior Checklist* by Kulik, Stein, and Sarbin; and *Self-Report Delinquency Scale* by Elliott, Dunford, and Huizinga. *Children's Action Tendency Scale*, intended for ages 6 to 15 years, is a 30-item questionnaire that asks a child to select what he or she would do in interpersonal situation. The format is forced-choice, and responses fall along three dimensions: aggressiveness, assertiveness, and submissiveness. *Adolescent Antisocial Self-Report Behavior Checklist* measures a broad range of behaviors, from mild misconduct to serious antisocial acts. It consists of 52 items rated on a five-point scale (from never to very often). Items load four factors: delinquency, drug use, parental defiance, and assaultiveness. *Self-Report Delinquency Scale* is intended for ages 11 to 21 years. This instrument asks about the occurrences of delinquent acts at home, at school, and in the community over the last year. The measure consists of 47 items rated on a four-point scale (from 1 = once to 4 = four or more times). The items encompass theft, property damage, illegal services (e.g., peddling drugs), public disorder, status offenses (e.g., running away), and index offenses (e.g., assaults).

Reports of Significant Others

Reports of significant others (e.g., parents, relatives, and teachers) are most frequently used as a measure of childhood psychopathology. Parents are in a unique position to provide accounts of a child's functioning and changes over time. Their reports correlate significantly with clinical judgments. Furthermore, such inventories are easy to administer and can cover a wide range of symptoms. However, reports of significant others have their own limitations. Parents sometimes are unaware of covert acts such as stealing and substance abuse. Also, parental evaluations can be influenced by parental stress and psychopathology.

The *Eyberg Child Behavior Inventory* is a frequently used and well-studied measure for oppositional and conduct problems completed by significant others. This measure is intended for ages 2 to 17 years. This 36-item inventory is designed to assess the frequency of a wide range of behavior problems that occur at home. A parent is asked to endorse whether each item is a problem (yes/no) and specify the frequency of occurrences on a seven-point scale (1 = never to 7 = always). The scores reflect the number of items endorsed as a problem and the intensity of problems.

Broadband scales that can be applied to conduct problems, but also across the full spectrum of symptoms, are commonly used. The most widely used measure is the *Child Behavior Checklist* by Achenbach. The measure has multiple versions completed by different raters (parent, teacher, and adolescent/child) and provides scores to evaluate externalizing and internalizing behaviors. The utility of this measure derives from widespread use and standardization among clinical and nonclinical samples. Also, broad and specific scales are available to assess aggression, delinquency, and attention-deficit disorder to provide fine-grained analyses of individual symptom domains.

Direct Observation

Observations directly sample behaviors and do not have to rely on recollections or general impressions. Also, observations can provide actual frequencies of selected behaviors. However, they have several drawbacks and limitations. Covert acts and infrequently occurring behaviors are not directly or readily observable. Also, the act of observation, if evident to the child or parent, can influence performance. Furthermore, direct observations may require extensive training to ensure accuracy and reliability, which makes them costly and time consuming.

An example of a relatively elaborate direct observational measure is the *Family Interaction Coding System* by Reid. This system is designed for ages 3 to 12 years. It records parent–child behaviors in home. The occurrences and nonoccurrences of 29 different behaviors are coded by observers within small intervals for 1 hour each day for a period of several days. Individual behaviors are usually summarized with a total aversive behavior score.

Institutional and Societal Records

Institutional records are frequently used to measure antisocial behavior because they represent an indicator of the impact of the problem on society, can reveal important social trends, facilitate decisions about allocation of resources, and can be utilized to evaluate interventions designed to reduce dysfunctional behavior problems. However, official records can greatly underestimate the occurrence of antisocial behavior, because most delinquent acts are not observed or recorded. Examples of institutional and societal records include school attendance, grades, graduation, suspensions, expulsions, contacts with police, arrests, and convictions.

Treatment

Many different treatments have been applied, including pharmacotherapy; psychotherapy; home, school, and community-based programs; residential and hospital treatment; and assorted social services. Relatively few treatments have been carefully evaluated in controlled

TABLE 5-6	Essentials of Treatment of ODD and CD

1. Pharmacologic treatment alone is not sufficient in the management of the majority of CD cases.
2. Evidence-based psychosocial treatments should be utilized.
3. Treatment planning should consider child's age, severity and range of problems, and family needs and commitment.
4. Comorbid diagnoses should be identified and treated.
5. Parental guidance is critical in the management of ODD and CD.
6. Parental psychopathology and stress should be considered.
7. All areas and setting in which a child exhibits behavior problems should be identified and addressed.

studies and shown to reduce ODD and CD problems and to improve functioning of the child in everyday life. Table 5-6 presents treatment essentials of ODD and CD, and key points are elaborated in the following sections.

Pharmacologic Treatment

Pharmacotherapy is rarely reported or studied for ODD, and there is no established database supporting their use. Medications for CD have been used primarily to alleviate aggression, reduce reactivity preceding aggressive behaviors, and moderate levels of emotional arousal as reported by multiple investigators (Table 5-7). Please see Chapter 22, on aggression, for more information on the use of medication in relation to types of aggression. Medication-based interventions are predicated on research findings that disruptive behavior problems are at least partially attributable to disturbances in neurobiologic mechanisms. Because few randomized controlled trials have been performed to establish the effectiveness of medications, ODD and CD have no standard pharmacologic treatment. All categories of psychotropic medications have been tried clinically to alleviate disruptive behavior problems, and so are briefly reviewed here.

Psychostimulants, such as amphetamine and methylphenidate, are thought to exert their primary neuropharmacologic effects by facilitating the release of neurotransmitters that positively correlate with levels of aggression. Stimulants have been demonstrated to reduce aggressive behaviors primarily in children with ADHD. There is some recent evidence, however, supporting their usefulness in reducing aggressive behaviors in ODD and CD children with and without ADHD. Stimulants are generally considered safe in the application to childhood disorders and are recommended as a good initial choice for the aggressive child with underlying ADHD. In considering the use of stimulants, consideration must be given to the recent concerns from the American Heart Association (AHA) and the American Academy of Pediatrics (AAP) regarding the potential risks of cardiotoxicity in children with cardiac disease, including whether an electrocardiogram (ECG) is indicated prior to initiating a stimulant and again during the course of treatment.

Mood stabilizers, such as lithium and selected anticonvulsants, have been used to modulate impulsivity, explosive temper, and mood liability. Antidepressants, such as the selective serotonin reuptake inhibitors (SSRIs) and the tricyclic antidepressants (TCAs), have also been used to reduce aggressive and impulsive symptoms particularly in the presence of mood symptoms. The high rate of comorbidity between disruptive behavior disorders and depression suggests the need for further examination of the utility of antidepressants for this population. However, their use must be considered with respect to a suggested association between the use of antidepressants and suicidality.

TABLE 5-7	Pharmacologic Agents Used in Treatment of Oppositional Defiant Disorder and Conduct Disorder		
Medication Class	**Medication**	**Clinical Effects/Indications**	**Side Effects**
Psychostimulants	Methylphenidate Amphetamine	Dose-dependent effect: diminish aggression, decrease motor activity level, reduce disinhibited behavior. May be indicated for youth with comorbid disruptive behavior disorders and ADHD	Potentially addictive, loss of appetite, insomnia, tachycardia, nervousness, abdominal pain, and weight loss; possible cardiotoxicity
Mood stabilizers and antiepileptics	Lithium Anticonvulsants Carbamazepine Sodium valproate Divalproex sodium	Reduce aggression, behavioral dyscontrol, and manic excitement. Often used for youth with explosive temper, mood lability, and disruptive behaviors	Fine tremor, polydipsia, polyuria, nausea, malaise, sedation, weight gain, anorexia, hair loss, gastrointestinal upset
Antidepressants	Trazodone Selective serotonin reuptake inhibitors	Reduce aggression and impulsivity. May be indicated for disruptive youth with mood dysregulation	Somnolence, headaches, drowsiness, nightmares, sleep disturbance, decreased appetite, bedwetting, hair loss; putative increased risk of suicidality
Antipsychotics	Chlorpromazine Haloperidol Risperidone Molindone Aripiprazole	Reduce level of central nervous system activation, reduce hostility and aggression	Tardive dyskinesia, extrapyramidal side effects, sedation, interference with learning, weight gain, metabolic syndrome, neuroleptic malignant syndrome
Adrenergic agents	Clonidine Guanfacine Propranolol	Reduce anger and aggression, decrease agitation and rage, increase frustration tolerance. May be indicated for comorbid disruptive behavior disorders and ADHD	Sedation, depressive symptoms, fatigue, headache, insomnia, orthostasis, dizziness

Adrenolytic drugs such as clonidine, guanfacine, and propranolol are often utilized in the treatment of disruptive behaviors as they help some children to mute aggression, reduce agitation and rage, and increase frustration tolerance, possibly by reducing adrenergic output.

Neuroleptics, or antipsychotic medications, including both the first-generation antipsychotics (FGA; e.g., chlorpromazine, haloperidol, and perphenazine) and the second-generation antipsychotics (SGA; risperidone, olanzapine, ziprasidone, aripiprazole, and quetiapine) are effective in reducing aggressive and violent behavior, hyperactivity, and social unresponsiveness. However, because of the potential risk of tardive dyskinesia with the FGA and metabolic syndrome with the SGA, these medications are recommended for youth with severely aggressive CD.

Psychotherapies

Kazdin has noted that over 550 therapies are in use for children and adolescents. A very small portion has been subjected to empirical tests. Interestingly, a few treatments have been well studied in relation to ODD and CD and qualify as evidence-based treatments in light of replications in controlled clinical trials. These interventions have a better evidence base than do pharmacologic interventions.

Parent management training refers to a treatment in which parents are trained to interact with the child in ways that promote prosocial behavior. The treatment focuses on the use of antecedents (e.g., prompts and setting events), reinforcement (e.g., praise and tokens), development of prosocial behavior, and other techniques to develop adaptive child behavior. Extensive research has shown that many parent–child interaction patterns in the home unwittingly foster and escalate child oppositional and aggressive behavior. Parent training teaches skills to the parent, develops interactions between parents and the child that promote positive parent and child behavior, and in the process, decreases disruptive behavior.

Cognitive problem-solving skills training is based on research showing that youths with aggressive and antisocial behavior often show distortions in various cognitive processes (e.g., how individuals perceive, code, interpret, and experience the world, as reflected in beliefs, attributions, and expectations). A variety of cognitive processes pertain to interactions with others, including the ability to generate solutions to interpersonal problems and consequences of action (e.g., what would happen after a particular behavior). Problem-solving skills therapy develops skills in approaching interpersonal situations and teaches ways to identify prosocial or adaptive solutions and alternative consequences of actions. Children practice the approach in treatment sessions and in other settings (home and school) outside of treatment.

Multisystemic therapy focuses on child behavior within the context of various systems (e.g., the family, peer group, and schools) that may contribute to the child's problem behavior or could be used to help alter that behavior. A focus on the family as a system is designed to build better communication, to reduce negative interactions, and to improve the ability of the parents to function. Factors that can affect these interactions and the child's problems, such as stress that the parent experiences, marital conflict, and association of the child with a deviant peer group, are also a focus of treatment. Many different techniques are applied to address these areas. Parent management training and problem-solving skills training, mentioned previously, often are incorporated into treatment. Several studies, especially with adjudicated adolescents, have attested to the efficacy and durability of the effects of multisystemic therapy.

The three treatments noted here are well studied. Others such as anger-management training and functional family therapy also have evidence on their behalf. Although there are now evidence-based treatments for ODD and CD, they are not widely available. In most clinical settings, general relationship therapy, play therapy, or psychodynamically oriented psychotherapy are more likely to be practiced with unclear benefits and outcomes.

Prevention

Early intervention programs with the family have been effective in reducing disruptive behaviors. These programs have been described by several investigators including McCord and Tremblay, and Mrazek and Haggerty. High-risk families are identified usually by factors such as low socioeconomic status, low educational attainment, and high stress living conditions. Intervention programs sometimes begin before the child is born to provide counseling related to maternal care, to provide support in the home to reduce stress, and to prepare the parents for child-rearing demands. After the infant is born, the program may continue for a few years to help support parents, to develop cognitive skills of the child, and to enroll the child in a preschool program. Adolescents who have received such programs as children show lower arrest rates, higher levels of educational attainment, and less substance use and abuse than other youths who did not receive early intervention.

During early and middle childhood, prevention programs are often conducted in the schools because there are opportunities to provide programs to youths in larger numbers, in the context of peers, and on a regular basis for extended periods. Programs often focus on developing positive skills and success experiences at home and at school. The reason for this focus is that bonding to deviant peers and poor family connections are risk factors for delinquency and substance abuse. Developing such success experiences in the schools among elementary school children has increased bonding to families and decreased rates of defiant and antisocial behavior and substance abuse. To date, evidence shows that preventive interventions can have significant impact on aggressive and antisocial behavior.

Conclusions

ODD and, to a much greater extent, CD in children and adolescents are significant clinical problems because of their prevalence and referral rates for services. CD is a large and costly social problem as it continues over the course of development and brings the child in contact with multiple special education, social, mental health, and juvenile justice services. The costs, monetary and social, extend to others. The symptoms often lead to disturbance or victimization of others in the form of oppositional or aggressive acts and, as the child enters into adulthood, abuse and domestic violence. Efforts to understand the underpinnings and paths leading to ODD and CD continue to advance. The heterogeneity of these disorders and the multiple risk factors involved challenge investigators and clinicians.

Treatment has advanced considerably in the past 20 years. A few medications look promising for key symptoms of CD. The strongest evidence is for stimulants and mood stabilizers. But there is no medication that has shown efficacy in randomized controlled trials, and thus the evidence base is lacking. The best evidence base is for psychotherapy, of which three interventions were mentioned in this chapter. Each of these evidence-based interventions has multiple replications in controlled trials and has shown to reduce symptoms of ODD or CD and to improve prosocial functioning. Advances are being made in prevention. Now that promising interventions are available, a key challenge is disseminating them to mental health professionals so they can be implemented as standard care.

For many individuals, severe antisocial behavior and associated dysfunction in multiple spheres represents a lifelong pattern. Because these disruptive disorders are often passed from parents to children, efforts to understand and intervene are critically important. Many questions remain about ODD and CD and their course. Even so, much of the available knowledge can have impact on the problem.

CLINICAL VIGNETTES

VIGNETTE 1: A 13-YEAR OLD BOY WITH CONDUCT DISORDER

A case vignette provides an example of someone who presents with CD to an outpatient service for children (ages 2–13), who are referred for oppositional, aggressive, and antisocial behavior. "I cannot take it anymore. It is so frustrating that sometimes I feel like running away from my own home," said David's mother during a clinical interview. David is a 13-year-old biracial male, who was referred to the outpatient clinic for physical and verbal aggression, noncompliance, destruction of property, running away, and disruptive behavior in school. His mother reports that he lies frequently and refuses to do homework and chores. David responds to requests with anger and, when frustrated, punches holes in doors. He was also recently charged with carrying a dangerous weapon, assault, and a risk of injury to a minor when he shot a girl with a BB gun. He is currently on probation due to these charges. Furthermore, he was involved in thefts outside of the home with confrontation of another person.

According to his mother, David has difficulty getting along with his siblings. He is particularly aggressive with his sister, who is 2 years younger. His mother indicated that David does not tolerate anything from his sister and takes every comment the wrong way. He also has problematic relationships with peers. At school, he argues and fights with children, and has been suspended several times for behavior problems. He is not liked by peers, which makes him angry, resentful, and aggressive. His mother states that children at school "pick on him and start with him," and he tends to react and fight back. In extracurricular activities, such as basketball, he loses his temper and is sometimes asked to leave the field. His mother also noted that none of David's friends or acquaintances serve as positive role models and that he spends too much time fooling around, getting into trouble, or just hanging out with delinquent peers.

David also shows academic difficulties. His intelligence is in the borderline range (full-scale IQ score of 77 on the Wechsler Intelligence Scale for Children-Revised). He is now two grades behind in school and also stayed back in the first and fifth grades. He was in special education in several grades, and tested out for sixth grade, in which he is currently placed. His teachers report that he is very disruptive in class, disrespects instructors, lacks motivation and attention, and is physically aggressive.

During assessment, David's mother indicated that she does not closely monitor his academic performance, rarely supervises his activities, and does not spend enough time with him after school or on weekends. Furthermore, she reported using physical, harsh verbal and prolonged punishment, such as verbal threats, frequent corporal punishment, criticizing in front of others, and taking away privileges for more than a week. She also indicated that her disciplining is inconsistent as she would often let go of the punishment or would ignore David's negative behavior one day and punish it the next day. Fortunately, David and his family live near a university psychology program that conducts multisystemic therapy (MST), and as part of a youth-at-risk petition that his mother filed, he and his family were enrolled in MST.

Several characteristics of David's family are noteworthy. He resides with his biologic mother and three siblings in a high-crime neighborhood. He is the oldest in the family and has two younger sisters and a baby brother. All children have different fathers. David's parents were never married; however, he has weekly contact with his father. His mother is currently separated from her last husband. She works part-time as a unit clerk in a hospital and receives public assistance. Her highest educational level is junior high school. As a child, David's mother was also in trouble with the law, ran away on several occasions, was a member of a gang, got into fights on a regular basis, and was arrested as a teenager. She also reported having a drug and alcohol problem as a teenager, but never sought treatment. She was also in therapy for mental health problems as a child.

Discussion

This case illustrates key symptoms of CD and also many of the contextual issues involved related to the child, parents, family, and living conditions. With both ODD and CD, research has advanced considerably by focusing on child symptom patterns, disorders, and related features within the child (e.g., comorbidity). What is often most striking about CD in particular is the fact that it is deeply embedded in contexts that extend well beyond features of the child's presenting symptoms. The risk factors for onset of CD illustrate many of the characteristics of families that continue to be present long after onset of the disorder. This makes delivery of treatment a special challenge. Advances in evidence-based treatments are remarkable. At the same time, delivering these treatments often requires attention to a host of parent and family dysfunctions that clinical trials of treatment rarely discuss.

VIGNETTE 2: A 10 YEAR OLD GIRL WITH OPPOSITIONAL DEFIANT DISORDER

Crystal is a 10-year-old girl from an upper middle class family and attends third grade at the local public elementary school. She is known to be a difficult child by her teachers and principal. She is stigmatized by her loud and violent tantrums when she does not get her way on the playground. In class, she frequently refuses to complete schoolwork. Crystal's achievement tests placed her at least one standard deviations above her peers. So her teacher advised her parents to not make homework a battle at home since she rarely complied with any assignments. There were concerns that Crystal's parents were too intrusive in the homework process. Born out of wedlock, Crystal was the only child living with both parents. She was considered spoiled by her parents, and they constantly complained about her "princess" demands. She was disliked at school and frequently tried getting her classmates in trouble by lying or provoking them by calling them names. She always lied about doing chores and was constantly being placed in "timeout" by her parents for being "bad." Relational problems plagued Crystal's parents for several years. Family history was positive bilineally for anxiety and hyperactivity.

An evaluation by a local therapist identified her parents' discord as the primary reason for Crystal's oppositional and defiant behaviors. A significant amount of time was spent on parenting-skills training and problem-solving skills in individual therapy. The frequency and intensity of tantrums decreased, but defiance persisted. In particular, school assignments were left incomplete or not even started. At home, chores were still left undone and bedtime struggles continued. Social isolation continued at school, and Crystal's teacher was concerned about how her classmates teased, or avoided, her due to her annoying and disruptive behaviors. After completion of parent management training and 6 months of individual skills coaching and continued defiance, psychological assessment was requested by Crystal's therapist. The psychologist found that Crystal had a very short attention span. With a full-scale IQ above 110, her school performance on tests was excellent, when she agreed to do the work. Crystal complained to the psychologist that schoolwork was stupid and boring, and that is why she never completed assignments. Crystal was found to be very impulsive, which correlated with her quick to anger responses to her peers and teachers. She thought that everyone hated her, and she preferred to attack first rather than be criticized. Furthermore, the psychological testing revealed anxiety symptoms of which neither her parents nor teachers were aware. Further family and individual therapy were recommended. Crystal's parents were "tired" of the months of therapy they had just completed and asked about other treatment modalities. She was referred to a child and adolescent psychiatrist.

Discussion

Crystal was at risk for both ADHD and anxiety disorders. She also had multiple risk factors for developing oppositional and disruptive behaviors. Her "rejecting" parents were punitive. Her social anxiety had led her to develop a pattern of being aggressive with peers to avoid being rejected. Her decreased attention span interfered with completion of assignments, and her impulsivity antagonized peers, especially on the playground. The psychiatrist noted that while evidence-based interventions of parent-skills training and social skills training have proven successful in oppositional and conduct-disordered youth, they are less likely to be successful when a child has multiple comorbid psychiatric illnesses. Thus, the psychiatrist recommended to the parents that they continue with family and individual psychotherapies, but also undertake a trial of atomoxetine to address the comorbid anxiety and ADHD symptoms, as supported by the Children's Medication Algorithm Project developed by the University of Texas. Crystal's symptoms improved with this multimodal treatment approach. The atomoxetine seemed to "take the edge off" of her reactivity, allowing her to better take advantage of the psychotherapies. She also started to take more interest in attempting to do her homework.

Acknowledgment

Completion of this chapter was facilitated by support from the William T. Grant Foundation (98-1872-98), the National Institute of Mental Health (MH59029), and the NRSA/NIMH Research Fellowship in Functional Disability Interventions.

BIBLIOGRAPHY

Achenbach TM, Rescorla LA. *Manual for the ASEBA School-Age Forms & Profiles*. Burlington: University of Vermont Research Center for Children, Youth, and Families; 2000.

Achenbach TM, Rescorla LA. *Manual for the ASEBA Preschool Forms & Profiles*. Burlington: University of Vermont Research Center for Children, Youth, and Families; 2001.

Achenbach TM, Rescorla LA. *Multicultural Supplement to the Manual for ASEBA School-Age Forms & Profiles*. Burlington: University of Vermont, Research Center for Children, Youth, and Families; 2007.

American Heart Association. American Academy of Pediatrics/American Heart Association clarification of statement on cardiovascular evaluation and monitoring of children and adolescents with heart disease receiving medications for ADHD. *AAP News*. 2008;29:1–2.

American Psychiatric Association. *Diagnostic and Statistical Manual of Mental Disorders, Fourth Edition*. Washington, DC: American Psychiatric Association; 1994.

Angold A, Costello EJ. Toward establishing an empirical basis for the diagnosis of oppositional defiant disorder. *J Am Acad Child Adolesc Psychiatry*. 1996;35:1205–1212.

Angold A, Costello EJ. The epidemiology of disorders of conduct: nosological issues and comorbidity. In: Hill J, Maughan B, eds. *Conduct Disorder in Childhood and Adolescence*. Cambridge, UK: Cambridge University Press; 2001.

Burke JD, Loeber R, Birmaher B. Oppositional defiant disorder and conduct disorder: a review of the past 10 years, part II. *J Am Acad Child Adolesc Psychiatry*. 2002;41:1275–1293.

Caspi A, McClay J, Moffitt TE, et al. Role of genotype in the cycle of violence in maltreated children. *Science*. 2002;297:851–854.

Deluty RH. Children's action tendency scale: a self-report measure of aggressiveness, assertiveness, and submissiveness in children. *J Consul Clin Psychol*. 1979;47:1061–1071.

Elliott DS, Dunford FW, Huizinga D. The identification and prediction of carrier offenders utilizing self-reported and official data. In: Burchard JD, Burchard SN, eds. *Preventing Delinquent Behavior*. Newbury Park, CA: Sage; 1987.

Eyberg SM, Robinson EA. Conduct problem behavior: standardization of a behavioral rating scale with adolescents. *J Clin Child Psychol*. 1983;12:347–354.

Gerardin P, Cohen D, Mazet P, et al. Drug treatment of conduct disorder in young people. *Eur Neuropsychopharmacol*. 2002;12:361–370.

Green WH. *Child and Adolescent Clinical Psychopharmacology*. 2nd ed. Baltimore: Williams & Wilkins; 1995.

Hammad TA, Laughren T, Racoosin J. Suicidality in pediatric patients treated with antidepressant drugs. *Arch Gen Psychiatry*. 2006;63(3):332–339.

Hendren RL. Disruptive behavior disorders in childhood and adolescents. In: Oldham JM, Riba RM, eds. *Review of Psychiatry*, Washington, DC: American Psychiatric Press; 1999.

Kazdin AE. *Conduct Disorder in Childhood and Adolescence*. 2nd ed. Thousand Oaks, CA: Sage; 1995.

Kazdin AE. *Psychotherapy for Children and Adolescents: Directions for Research and Practice*. New York: Oxford University Press; 2000.

Kazdin AE. *Parent Management Training: Treatment of Oppositional, Aggressive, and Antisocial Behavior in Children and Adolescents*. New York: Oxford University Press; 2005.

Kulik JA, Stein KB, Sarbin TR. Dimensions and patterns of adolescent antisocial behavior. *J Consul Clin Psychol.* 1968;32:375–382.

McCord J, Tremblay RE. *Preventing Antisocial Behavior.* New York: Guilford; 1992.

Mrazek PJ, Haggerty RJ. *Reducing Risks for Mental Disorders: Frontiers of Preventive Intervention Research.* Washington, DC: National Academy Press; 1994.

Pepper DJ, Rubin KH. *The Development and Treatment of Childhood Aggression.* Hillsdale, NJ: Erlbaum; 1991.

Perrin JM, Friedman RA, Knilans TK. The Black Box Working Group and the Section of Cardiology and Cardiac Surgery. *Pediatrics.* 2008;122:451–453.

Peters RD, McMahon RJ, Quinsey VL. *Aggression and Violence Throughout the Life Span.* Newbury Park, CA: Sage; 1992.

Pliszka SR, Crismon ML, Hughes CW, et al. The Texas Children's Medication Algorithm Project: Revision of the algorithm for pharmacotherapy of attention-deficit/hyperactivity disorder. *J Am Acad Child Adolesc Psychiatry.* 2006;45(6):642–657.

Reid JB (ed.). A social learning approach to family intervention. In: *Observation in Home Settings.* Eugene, OR: Castalia; 1978.

Reid JB, Patterson GR, Synder J. *Antisocial Behavior in Children and Adolescents: A Developmental Analysis and Model for Intervention.* Washington, DC: American Psychological Association; 2002.

Rowe R, Maughan B, Pickles A, et al. The relationship between DSM-IV oppositional defiant disorder and conduct disorder: finding from the Great Smoky Mountains Study. *J Child Psychol Psychiatry.* 2002;43:365–373.

Sommers-Flanagan J, Sommers-Flanagan R. Assessment and diagnosis of conduct disorder. *J Counsel Dev.* 1998;76:189–197.

Stoff DM, Breiling J, Maser JD. *Handbook of Antisocial Behavior.* New York: Wiley; 1997.

Vetter VL, Elia J, Erickson C, et al. Cardiovascular monitoring of children and adolescents with heart disease receiving medications for attention deficit/hyperactivity disorder: a scientific statement from the American Heart Association Council on Cardiovascular Disease in the Young Congenital Cardiac Defects Committee and the Council on Cardiovascular Nursing. *Circulation.* 2008;117:2407–2423.

Waslick B, Werry JS, Greenhill LL. Pharmacotherapy and toxicology of oppositional defiant disorder and conduct disorder. In: Quay HC, Hogan AE, eds. *Handbook of Disruptive Behavior Disorders.* New York: Plenum; 1999.

Werry JS, Aman MG. *A Practitioner's Guide to Psychoactive Drugs for Children and Adolescents.* 2nd ed. New York: Plenum; 1998.

SUGGESTED READINGS

Alan E. Kazdin
The Kazdin Method for Parenting the Defiant Child: With No Pills, No Therapy, No Contest of Wills
Boston: Houghton Mifflin Harcourt (2008)

Ross W. Greene
The Explosive Child: A New Approach for Understanding and Parenting Easily Frustrated, "Chronically Inflexible" Children (revised 4th ed.)
New York: HarperCollins (2009)

Robert J. McMahon and Rex L. Forehand
Helping the Noncompliant Child, Second Edition: Family-Based Treatment for Oppositional Behavior
New York: Guilford Press (2005)

Michael L. Bloomquist
Skills Training for Children with Behavior Problems, Revised Edition: A Parent and Practitioner Guidebook
New York: Guilford Press (2005)

SUGGESTED WEBSITES

The below-listed websites offer further information on ODD and CD in children and adolescents, treatment options, online parent support, and family resources, and provide links to additional websites that may be helpful for parents and clinicians.

http://www.conductdisorders.com
http://www.focusas.com/ConductDisorders.html
http://www.teenswithproblems.com/conduct_disorder.html
http://www.mentalhelp.net
http://www.aacap.org/cs/root/facts_for_families/conduct_disorder
http://childparenting.about.com/cs/disorders/a/conductdisorder.htm
http://www.myoutofcontrolteen.com/support.html
http://www.familymanagement.com/facts/english/odd.html

REVIEW QUESTIONS

1. Which of the following defines adolescent-onset conduct disorder?
   a. Aggressive behavior and problematic peer relationship at age 12
   b. Absence of conduct disorder symptoms by age 12
   c. Absence of conduct disorder symptoms by age 10
   d. Vandalism and illegal behaviors starting at age 10

2. Chris is 9 years old and exhibits multiple behavior problems. He frequently fails to follow his parent's directions, has anger outbursts and temper tantrums, argues with adults, interrupts others, fights with peers, destroys things when frustrated, and is easily distracted. Chris is most likely suffering from which of the following disorders?
   a. Conduct disorder
   b. Oppositional defiant disorder
   c. Attention-deficit hyperactivity disorder
   d. Disruptive behavior disorder NOS

3. Which of the following is *not* a risk factor for development of disruptive behavior disorders?
   a. Low IQ
   b. Prenatal complications
   c. Socioeconomic disadvantage
   d. Being first born

4. Which of the following is the most established psychopharmacologic intervention for treating conduct disorder?
   a. Psychostimulants
   b. Antidepressants
   c. Antipsychotics
   d. There is no standard pharmacologic treatment

5. Which of the following is *not* true?
   a. Boys show three to four times higher rates of CD than do girls
   b. Rates of conduct disorder is higher for children than for adolescents
   c. Childhood onset of conduct disorder is considered to be more severe form than adolescent onset
   d. A diagnosis of antisocial behavior can be given before an individual is 18 years old

6. Which of the following is true?
   a. When a behavior pattern meets both diagnoses, the diagnosis of conduct disorder takes precedence over the diagnosis of oppositional defiant disorder
   b. There are core symptoms associated with making the diagnosis of oppositional defiant disorder
   c. Play therapy is empirically supported for treatment of disruptive behavior disorders
   d. Early intervention programs with families have *not* been shown effective in reducing problematic behaviors

7. Which of the following is the most common symptom of disruptive behavior disorders targeted by medications?
   a. Impulsivity
   b. Hyperactivity

    c. Emotional arousal

    d. Aggression

8. Which of the following is a recommended initial choice for child with comorbid conduct disorder and ADHD?
   a. Atypical antipsychotic medication
   b. Psychostimulant
   c. Mood stabilizer
   d. Antidepressant

9. Which of the following is true for parent management training?
   a. Focuses on child's behavior within the context of various systems
   b. Targets marital problems as one of the risk factor for the development of disruptive behavior problems
   c. Teaches behavior modification techniques
   d. Teaches problem-solving skills

10. Multisystemic therapy teaches which of the following?
    a. Problem-solving skills
    b. Behavior modification techniques
    c. More effective communication strategies between family members
    d. All of the above

Answers: 1-c, 2-b, 3-d, 4-d, 5-b, 6-a, 7-d, 8-b, 9-c, 10-d

6

Oscar G. Bukstein, MD, MPH

Adolescent Substance-Use Disorders

Introduction

Substance use by adolescents remains an important public health problem due to the potential consequences of use, including accidents; the possible progression of use into the substance-use disorders (SUDs); and the persistence of SUDs into adulthood. Because of both health and mental health consequences of substance use, all health care professionals need to have a basic understanding of the risk for substance use and abuse by adolescents, the acquisition of use behaviors, and progression into SUDs within a developmental framework. As substance use is a common behavior for adolescents, primary health care professionals often must act as gatekeepers for adolescents, screening for SUDs and related problems, and refer adolescents for more comprehensive substance-use evaluation and treatment. To achieve optimal results, an understanding of assessment and screening and other assessment procedures as well as treatment should include the knowledge of evidence-based interventions which focus on specific substance-use behaviors, as well as risk factors that have a role in the onset and maintenance of SUDs.

Clinical Features

There is a range of substance-use behaviors and patterns of use from abstinence through to substance *use*, often without significant consequences or impairment, and on to substance-related diagnoses, *abuse* and *dependence*, as defined by the *Diagnostic and Statistical Manual, Fourth Edition* (*DSM-IV*). Substance use per se is not sufficient for a diagnosis of abuse or dependence, even in adolescents.

The diagnosis of *substance abuse* requires evidence of a maladaptive pattern of substance use with clinically significant levels of impairment or distress. Recurrent use by adolescents results in an inability to meet major role obligations, leading to impaired functioning in one or more major areas of their life and an increased likelihood of legal problems due to possession, risk-taking behavior, and exposure to hazardous situations. The diagnosis of *substance dependence* requires that the adolescent meet at least three criteria, including such symptoms as withdrawal, tolerance, and loss of control over use. For example, for alcohol-use disorders (AUDs), adolescents commonly exhibit tolerance (i.e., requiring increasing amounts of a substance to achieve the same effect) but less frequently show withdrawal or other symptoms of physiologic dependence. Many adolescents do manifest withdrawal symptoms with cannabis and opiate-use disorders. Preoccupation with use is often demonstrated by giving up previously important activities, increasing the time spent in activities related to substance use, and using more frequently or for longer amounts of time than planned. The adolescent may use these substances despite the continued existence or worsening of problems caused by substance use. Polysubstance use by adolescents appears to be the rule rather than the exception; therefore, adolescents often present with multiple SUD diagnoses. Adolescents' alcohol and drug symptom profiles often appear to vary along a severity dimension, rather than fitting into the *DSM-IV* categories of abuse and dependence categories.

Misuse and diversion are nonstandard terms that indicate behaviors may or may not result in an SUD diagnosis in adolescents. The term *misuse* can be defined as use for a purpose not consistent with medical guidelines including modifying dose, using to achieve euphoria, and/or using with other nonprescribed psychoactive substances. The term *diversion* is the transfer of medication from the individual for whom it was prescribed to one for whom it is not prescribed. While abuse and dependence are terms that connote psychopathology related to substance use, diversion and misuse are not. *Diversion and misuse* of prescription drugs are widespread, especially in high school and college students.

Epidemiology

The Prevalence of Substance-Use Disorders

The prevalence of SUDs increases with age through young adulthood when both SUDs and substance use peak. Data from the National Survey on Drug Use and Health indicate that very few youth (less than 3%) met criteria for any past-year SUD prior to age 14. SUDs increased steadily from age 14 (7%) to age 21 (25%), with peak prevalence occurring in the 20s. Among 12- to 17-year-olds, 9% met criteria for a past-year *DSM-IV* SUD abuse or dependence diagnosis, 6% had an alcohol-related diagnosis, and 4% had a cannabis diagnosis; 2% met criteria for use of both alcohol and at least one illicit substance. However, other studies show considerable variation of rates, especially when sampling different-aged adolescents. Recent national survey data indicate little to no difference in rates of past-year SUD prevalence by gender for alcohol or illicit drugs. Similar to ethnic differences in the prevalence of substance use, larger proportions of Caucasian and Hispanic youth aged 12 to 17 years met criteria for a past-year *DSM-IV* alcohol or drug diagnosis than African Americans (10%, 10%, and 6%, respectively), although American Indian adolescents had the highest proportion of alcohol or other drug diagnoses (20%).

The Prevalence of Substance Use

According to the National Survey on Drug Use and Health, the rates of current illicit drug use among youths aged 12 to 17 were 11.6% in 2002 and 9.9% in 2005. In 2005, 9.9% of youths aged 12 to 17 were current illicit drug users: 6.8% used marijuana, 3.3% used prescription-type drugs nonmedically, 1.2% used inhalants, 0.8% used hallucinogens, and 0.6% used cocaine. In 2008, adolescents in the United States continued to show a gradual decline in their use of certain drugs, especially stimulants including amphetamines, methamphetamine, crystal methamphetamine, cocaine, and crack, according to the Monitoring the Future (MTF) annual national survey of the US students in 8th, 10th, and 12th grades.

Rates of Intervention

Only a small percentage of adolescents with SUDs actually receive treatment. Among youths aged 12 to 17, there were 1.3 million (4.9%) who needed treatment for an illicit drug use problem in 2005. Of this group, only 142,000 received treatment at a specialty facility, that is, 11.3% of youths aged 12 to 17 who needed treatment, leaving 1.1 million youths who needed such treatment but did not receive it. Among 12- to 17-year-olds in publicly funded programs, most were referred by the criminal justice system, with smaller proportions referred by schools or family; rates of self-referral to treatment begin to increase in young adulthood.

TABLE 6-1	Essential Risk Factors for the Development of Substance-Use Disorders in Adolescents

Individual factors
Early disruptive behavior disorder, for example, ADHD
Early aggressive behavior, for example, conduct disorder
Poor academic performance, school failure
Positive beliefs and attitudes about substance use

Peer-related factors
Peer substance use
Peer beliefs and attitudes about substance use
Earlier involvement with peers and away from family

Familial factors
Parental substance use
Parental beliefs and attitudes about substance use
Parent tolerance of substance use
Lack of closeness or attachment between parent and child
Poor parental supervision and monitoring of child/adolescent

Sociocultural factors
Community or neighborhood characteristics
Low socioeconomic status
High population density
Physical deterioration
High crime
Media messages about substance use

Risk Factors

The early onset of substance use and a more rapid progression through the stages of substance use are among the risk factors for the development of SUDs. The literature on the development of substance use and SUDs in adolescents has identified a variety of individual, peer, family, and community risk factors, as summarized in Table 6-1. Within a developmental context, genetic predispositions to affective, cognitive, and behavioral problems are exacerbated by family and peer factors leading to early-onset substance use and pathologic use. Family factors identified as increasing SUD risk in children and adolescents include decreased affectional bonding, decreased parental supervision, and decreased adherence to religious beliefs. A harsher parental discipline style and affiliation with socially deviant peers have been shown in many studies to promote substance use.

Comorbidity

In both community surveys of adolescents with SUD and samples of adolescents in addictions treatment, the majority have a co-occurring non-substance-related mental disorder. More than half of adolescents in addictions treatment who have a co-occurring mental illness have three or more psychiatric disorders, which are summarized in Table 6-2. The most common disorders include conduct problems, attention-deficit/hyperactivity disorder (ADHD), mood disorders (e.g., depression), and trauma-related symptoms. Among treated adolescents, comorbid psychopathology generally predicted early return to substance use, particularly

TABLE 6-2	Comorbid Disorders

Disruptive behavior disorders
- Conduct disorder
- Oppositional defiant disorder
- Attention-deficit/hyperactivity disorder

Mood disorders
- Major depressive disorder: single episode vs. recurrent episodes
- Bipolar disorder
- Dysthymic disorder
- Cyclothymia

Anxiety disorders
- Social phobia
- Posttraumatic stress disorder
- Generalized anxiety disorder
- Panic disorder

Other disorders
- Schizophrenia
- Bulimia nervosa

conduct problems and major depression. Co-occurring psychopathology also generally predicted a more persistent course of substance involvement over 1-year follow-up.

Clinical Course

The clinical course of AUDs in community samples suggests some remission with maturation, as well as a more chronic course of adolescent-onset AUD for certain individuals. Although the majority of treated adolescents return to some substance use following treatment, they generally show reductions in substance use and problems over both short- and longer-term follow-up. Despite significant reductions in substance involvement and improvements in school performance, interpersonal relations, and other areas, treated adolescents continue to show greater problem severity across multiple domains compared to a community comparison sample, showing that adolescent-onset SUD, likely in combination with co-occurring psychopathology and other risk factors, interferes with the achievement of normative adolescent developmental tasks.

Assessment

There are two levels of assessment: screening and comprehensive assessment. Screening is a process in which adolescents are identified according to characteristics that indicate that they possibly have a problem with substance use. Screening does not inform the clinician of the severity of the adolescent's substance use or the presence of SUDs but rather identifies the *need* for a comprehensive assessment. It is not a substitute for an assessment. For primary health care professionals, screening is a critical task as these professionals are among the potential gatekeepers for adolescents with SUDs. The comprehensive assessment is a thorough process that includes inquiry of factors contributing to and maintaining substance abuse, the severity of the problems, and the variety of consequences associated with the adolescent's substance use.

TABLE 6-3	CRAFFT
C	Have you ever ridden in a car driven by someone (including self) high, drunk, or using drugs
R	Have you ever used drugs or alcohol to **Relax**?
A	Do you ever use **Alone**?
F	Do you ever **Forget** things that you did while using?
F	Do **Family or Friends** tell you to cut down?
T	Have you ever gotten into **Trouble** when using?

Screening

In order to screen large numbers of youth, clinicians and others such as school professionals, mental health professionals, and primary health care professionals often rely on the use of screening instruments. The two alternative approaches to screening involve (1) specific screening of substance use and related behaviors, focusing on this behavior alone, and (2) screening for SUD as part of a multidomain screen that includes mental health problems and high-risk behaviors. In a primary care setting, questions for all youth about substance use follow a general inquiry about health behaviors and should include questions about cigarette, alcohol, and other substance use. In settings such as child welfare, mental health, or juvenile justice, the high-risk status is sufficient to require screening of each adolescent. Primary health care staff (e.g., physicians and nurses) may use a brief series of questions to screen for substance-use problems. Although specific interview questions with established validity, such as the CRAFFT (see Table 6-3), are often sufficient, many clinicians or other relevant professionals use other specific screening instruments.

Professionals need to decide what screening threshold will trigger a comprehensive assessment. The CRAFFT has a threshold of two positive items. Other factors, such as past history of substance use, high-risk behaviors, and moderate to severe high-risk status, may prompt such a referral even in the absence of an adolescent report of regular use or consequences.

Comprehensive Assessment

The assessment process is used to identify those individuals who have an SUD and whether they meet criteria for a *DSM-IV* diagnosis. Substance-using behaviors, the pattern of use, and any consequences of use are also discussed. The results of the comprehensive assessment should also identify which adolescents require treatment, the level of treatment needed, and other problems that may need intervention. Many screening and comprehensive assessment instruments follow the Domain Model of assessment, shown in Table 6-4, that provides a review of the primary domains of adolescent functioning, including substance-use behaviors, psychiatric and behavioral problems, school and occupational functioning, family functioning, social competency and peer relations, and leisure and recreation.

The Interview

As primary health care professionals often have a long-standing relationship with the adolescent and his or her family, they are in an optimal position to track developmental risk factors that may lead to substance use and SUDs as well as identify these problems. Screening through the use of the CRAFFT allows for screening through a conversational format of a series of questions. Some primary care professionals may elect to proceed to a more comprehensive substance-use history, inquiring about age of onset, duration, frequency, and route of ingestion for each individual drug including alcohol, tobacco, illicit drugs, inhalants, over-the-counter medications,

TABLE 6-4	Essentials of Assessment

Use of Domain Model
- Substance use
- Psychiatric symptoms/disorders
- Family functioning
- School/vocational functioning
- School competency/peer relations
- Leisure/recreation
- Medical

Be nonjudgmental
Be aware of risk factors
Use urine toxicology for assessment and follow-up

and prescription drugs such as benzodiazepines, opiates, and stimulants. Additional questions should cover negative consequences as well as attempts and motivation to control use or quit. Questions detailing the context of use include the setting of use (time and place), whether the adolescent uses alone or with peers, and the attitudes of these peers about substance use. Variability in quantity and frequency of adolescent substance use is often great. The adolescent may report periods of abstinence as well as periods of rapid acceleration of use and heavy use of particular agents. A timeline drug chart or calendar is often useful to allow the adolescent to report quantity, frequency, and variability data across time with important dates, holidays, and other time cues as a guide. Additional substance-use-related information includes attitudes, expectancies of use, and motivation(s) or perceived benefits to use. Assessment of substance-use behavior may follow a functional analysis of use to determine usual antecedents to use and consequences of use. Such an analysis may allow a more specific targeting of relevant antecedents during treatment. Along with specific attitudes and beliefs about substance use, the interviewer may also inquire about the adolescent's values and attitudes in general.

Particularly in a medical setting, the other domains of adolescent functioning are also very important. In choosing the level of inquiry into psychopathology, the clinician is guided by the setting and the purpose of the assessment. Because of the considerable prevalence of SUD-psychiatric comorbidity, screening questions about depression, suicidality, aggression, psychosis, and treatment history may be important in determining when an adolescent should be referred for a more detailed, comprehensive psychiatric evaluation. The medical history and possible physical examination search for symptoms and illnesses that may be related to SUDs and behaviors, including trauma, pregnancies, human immunodeficiency virus (HIV), sexually transmitted diseases, infections or wounds, and possible liver diseases. School/vocational, peer and family domains would emphasize family and peer substance use and attitudes toward use, parental monitoring and supervision, family history of SUDs and psychiatric disorders, and the effect of substance use on academic and/or vocational functioning. Inquiry into recreational or prosocial activities such as sports, interests, and hobbies will provide the clinician with information about the adolescent's social repertoire and whether this will have to be targeted for change. Knowledge of risk factors in each domain is quite useful as the interview will often include an inventory of risk factors for SUDs.

Toxicology

Toxicologic tests of bodily fluids, usually urine but also saliva, and hair samples to detect the presence of specific substances should be part of the formal evaluation and the ongoing assessment of substance use. Guidelines published by the American Academy of Pediatrics indicate the importance of clinical suspicion of use as a basis for toxicologic screening and consideration of confidentiality and consent. The optimal use of urine screening requires proper collection techniques including monitoring of youth providing the sample, prevention of contamination, dilution or substitution, evaluation of positive results, and specific plan(s) of action should the specimen be positive or negative for the presence of substance(s). Because of the limited time a drug remains in the urine and possible adulteration, a negative urine test does not indicate that the youngster does not use drugs, while a positive specimen indicates only the presence of specific drug(s) and not the presence of an SUD or a specific pattern of use.

Confidentiality

Adolescents are more likely to provide truthful information if they believe that their information, at least the details, will not be shared. Prior to the adolescent interview, the health care professional should review exactly what information the clinician is obliged to share and with whom and under what considerations this would be done without the teen's permission, such as suicidal and/or homicidal ideation and behavior or physical/sexual abuse. Although the adolescent should provide consent before drug use is revealed and discussed with parents, the health care professional should encourage and support the adolescent's revealing to parents the extent of substance use and other problems. The health care professional may provide a general recommendation for treatment or impressions rather than a detailed report of specific behaviors.

The Validity of Adolescent Report

Especially in a health care setting, the majority of adolescents give temporally consistent reports of substance use, while specific populations, such as extremely antisocial youth, have much higher responses of "faking good" than clinical samples. The use of structured interviews or standardized questionnaires, either paper and pencil or computer administered, may also serve to support or validate the self-report. The adolescent may feel less threatened by a self-report questionnaire, many of which have questions to ascertain response bias. The use of toxicologic methods such as urine drug screens can validate self-report by testing for the use of a specific agent. Finally, the attitude and skill of the assessment interviewer is often the best promoter of the validity of self-report, with engagement with the adolescent predicting more valid responses.

Treatment

Reviews of studies of adolescent treatment outcome have concluded that treatment is better than no treatment. In the year following treatment, adolescents report decreased heavy drinking, marijuana and other illicit drug use, and criminal involvement as well as improved psychological adjustment and school performance. Longer duration of treatment is associated with several favorable outcomes. The in-treatment factors predictive of outcome are greater readiness to change, time in treatment, involvement of family, use of practical problem-solving, and provision of comprehensive services such as housing, academic assistance, and recreation. Posttreatment variables that are thought to be the most important determinants of outcome include association with nonusing peers and involvement in leisure time activities, work, and school. Variables reported to be most consistently related to successful outcome are treatment completion, low pretreatment use, and peer and parent social support and nonuse of substances.

The primary, explicit goal for the treatment of adolescents with SUDs is achieving and maintaining abstinence from substance use, while a realistic view recognizes both the chronicity

TABLE 6-5	Essentials for Treatment

- Motivation and engagement
- Family involvement to improve supervision, monitoring, and communication between parents and adolescent
- Improved problem-solving, social skills, and relapse prevention
- Comorbid psychiatric disorders through psychosocial and/or medication treatments
- Social ecology in terms of increasing prosocial behaviors, peer relationships, and academic functioning
- Adequate duration of treatment and follow-up care; self-support groups can be encouraged as adjuncts to the modalities above

of SUDs in some populations of adolescents and the self-limited nature of substance use and substance-use-related problems in others. Harm reduction may be an interim, implicit acceptable outcome, although "controlled use" of any nonprescribed substance should never be an explicit goal in the treatment of adolescents. Included in the concept of harm reduction is a reduction in the use and negative consequences of substances, a reduction in the severity and frequency of relapses, and improvement in one or more domains of the adolescent's functioning (e.g., academic performance or family functioning). While adolescents may not initially be motivated to stop substance use in treatment, the attainment of skills to deal with substance use may provide the adolescent with greater self-efficacy to not only reduce use but also ultimately move toward the future goal of abstinence. In addition, control of substance use should not be the only goal of treatment as a broad concept of rehabilitation involves targeting associated problems and domains of functioning for treatment. Integrated interventions that concurrently deal with coexisting psychiatric and behavioral problems, family functioning, peer and interpersonal relationships, and academic/vocational functioning not only will produce general improvements in psychosocial functioning, but also most likely will yield improved outcomes in the primary treatment goal of achieving and maintaining abstinence.

Based on the combination of empirical research and current clinical consensus, the clinician dealing with adolescents with SUDs should develop a treatment plan that uses modalities that target salient domains, shown in Table 6-5.

The primary care physician (PCP) has a potentially critical role in identification, referral, and even administration of brief interventions such as motivational interviewing. The ability to screen for substance use, SUDs, and associated behaviors and the knowledge of community resources, including SUD treatment providers, are critical for the PCP who deals with adolescents.

Pharmacologic Treatments

The majority of the research in pharmacotherapy of adolescents with SUD relates to the treatment of comorbid psychiatric disorders, such as depression and ADHD. Strategies in pharmacologic interventions for SUDs include detoxification, substitution therapies, aversion therapies, blocking therapies, and craving reduction therapy.

Detoxification strategies generally use agonists or medications that provide symptomatic relief (e.g., clonidine for opioid withdrawal and benzodiazepines for alcohol withdrawal). In the absence of adolescent data, it is reasonable to use pharmacotherapy protocols similar to those used for adults, when needed. Since adolescents may not use substances in the same amount, frequency, or duration as adults, they may be less likely to have withdrawal symptoms as compared to adults (e.g., alcohol).

Substitution therapies, which are used to prevent withdrawal, eliminate drug craving, and block the euphoric effects of illicit opiate use, use an agonist (e.g., nicotine replacement therapy [NRT] for nicotine dependence and methadone maintenance for opioid dependence), or a partial agonist (e.g., buprenorphine for opioid dependence) that acts on the same receptors that mediate the psychotropic effects of a substance.

Aversive interventions, such as disulfiram (Antabuse), blocking strategies (e.g., naltrexone for opiate dependence), and anticraving medications (naltrexone, acamprosate, topiramate, and ondansetron for alcohol; bupropion for nicotine; and buprenorphine for opioids) require medication adherence and are likely most effective among patients with high motivation. For these agents, efficacy is based on trials with adults and with the possible exception of bupro-prion and buprenorphine, there is very modest evidence supporting their use in adolescents. These agents should be prescribed to youth only after a thorough consideration of previous treatment attempts.

Nicotine dependence or cigarette smoking is commonly present in adolescents with SUDs and/or psychiatric disorders, but few are diagnosed with nicotine dependence and offered smoking cessation treatment. NRTs (with the transdermal patch, gum, inhaler, and lozenge), varenicline, and bupropion sustained release (SR) are currently approved by the FDA for smoking cessation in adults. NRT and bupropion SR are the agents most studied for adolescent smokers, with most studies of NRT using the transdermal nicotine patch (TNP). The efficacy of TNP has been modest among adolescents, with resulting abstinence rates ranging from 5% to 18%. Nicotine withdrawal symptoms may be a significant problem in situations where adolescents with nicotine dependence cannot smoke, such as psychiatric hospitals, and NRT may need to be provided to counter nicotine withdrawal symptoms, even to non-treatment-seeking adolescent smokers. Bupropion, approved for use in adult smoking cessation, has also shown promise in an open study in the treatment of adolescent smokers.

Buprenorphine is a partial agonist. It is difficult to overdose on buprenorphine, and its combination with naloxone (opiate antagonist) makes it difficult to abuse intravenously to obtain euphoric effects either with or without other opiates. In a recent double-blind, double-dummy trial of buprenorphine versus clonidine detoxification in a 28-day outpatient clinic with 36 adolescents with opiate dependence, buprenorphine had almost double the retention and half the number of positive urine tests for opiates compared to clonidine.

Recent emerging research and experience suggest that pharmacotherapy can be used safely and effectively in adolescents with SUDs and comorbid psychopathology. A double-blind placebo-controlled trial with cognitive–behavioral therapy (CBT) for SUDs plus fluoxetine or placebo for adolescents with major depressive disorder (MDD) and SUD showed greater improvement for the active medication for depressive symptoms, while there were no significant group differences for substance use. A double-blind, placebo-controlled trial of a stimulant medication (pemoline) demonstrated the efficacy of medication in improving ADHD symptoms in adolescents with comorbid ADHD and SUD, although there were no differences between groups on substance use. In a randomized controlled trial including adolescents with SUDs and comorbid bipolar disorder, lithium showed improvements over placebo on both mood and substance-use variables.

Some commonly used pharmacologic agents, such as psychostimulants and benzodiazepines, have inherent abuse potential. The risk of diversion or misuse of a therapeutic agent by the adolescent or his or her peer group or family members should prompt a thorough assessment of the risk of this outcome (e.g., history of abuse of the specific or other potentially abusable agents and family/parental history of substance abuse or antisocial behavior). Often, parental or adult supervision of medication administration can alleviate concerns about potential abuse. The clinician should also consider alternative agents to psychostimulants, such as atomoxetine or bupropion, which do not have abuse potential. The long-acting stimulant preparations may offer less potential for abuse or diversion due to their form of administration, reduced level of reinforcement due to more gradual and longer time to maximum plasma concentration, and the ability to more easily monitor and supervise once-a-day dosing. Many anxiety symptoms or disorders in adolescents can be treated successfully with psychosocial methods such as behavior therapy. If pharmacotherapy is required, the use of selective serotonin reuptake inhibitors, tricyclic antidepressants, or buspirone is preferred over the use of benzodiazepines.

Psychotherapeutic Treatments

Family therapy approaches have the most empirical support. Family interventions for substance-abuse treatment have common goals: providing psychoeducation about SUDs, which decreases familial resistance to treatment and increases motivation and engagement; assisting parents and family to initiate and maintain efforts to get the adolescent into appropriate treatment and achieve abstinence; assisting parents and family to establish or re-establish structure with consistent limit-setting and careful monitoring of the adolescent's activities and behavior; improving communication among family members; and getting other family members into treatment and/or support programs. Specific engagement procedures have been incorporated as part of many family-based interventions. Some of the specific evidence-based family therapies include multidimensional family therapy (MDFT) and multisystemic family therapy (MST). Based on a social ecology theory that suggests adolescent antisocial behavior is multidetermined and linked to variables of the individual and his or her family, peer group, school, and community, interventions are developed in conjunction with the family with the explicit goal of structuring the youth's environment to promote healthier, less risky behavior. MST services are usually intense and short term (average of 4 to 6 months) and are offered in the youth's natural environment, such as at home or in school. MST draws heavily on strategies and techniques found in cognitive–behavioral, behavioral, and family therapies.

Similarly, interventions with the adolescent alone such as CBT or CBT plus motivational enhancement therapy (MET) are also effective. Individual approaches such as CBT, both alone and with motivational enhancement, have shown to be efficacious. Community reinforcement approaches using contingency contracting and vouchers also appear to be promising. Modifications of motivational interviewing or enhancement techniques for adolescents have shown promise for both evaluation and treatment, based on limited treatment studies.

A controversial element of traditional treatment programs is the widespread use of group treatment. While there is evidence that group treatment can have negative effects on outcomes, other studies show positive effects for group modalities.

Twelve-step approaches, using Alcoholics Anonymous (AA) and Narcotics Anonymous (NA) as a basis for treatment, are perhaps the most common approaches for treatment in the United States. Naturalistic studies of adolescent SUD treatment find that attendance in aftercare treatment or self-support groups (e.g., AA or NA) is related to positive outcomes and higher rates of abstinence and other measures of improved outcome, when compared with those not participating in such groups following treatment.

In 12-step programs, adolescents work on specific steps toward recovery, attend self-support groups (AA or NA), and obtain the assistance of a sponsor (another person in recovery from substance-use problems). Developmentally appropriate, specific 12-step programs and self-support groups offer several benefits including a recovering (i.e., non-substance-using) peer group, available sponsors, and other types of support. Although 12-step programs may be effective for many adolescents, they have not been subjected to controlled clinical trials.

SUDs are often chronic disorders requiring ongoing intervention. While most of adolescent SUD treatment is accomplished on an ambulatory basis, resistance to lower levels of care (i.e., treatment failure), high levels of psychiatric comorbidity, and low social supports may necessitate residential treatment of varying duration. Participation in aftercare services following treatment in a program is related to improved outcomes. After the acute treatment for substance use, ongoing attention should be paid to comorbid psychopathology and other comprehensive needs of the adolescent and his family.

Conclusions

Substance use and SUDs in adolescents remain a critical problem due to the common use of psychoactive substances by youth, the consequences that result, and the persistence into adulthood. Clinicians seeking to understand the risk for substance use and abuse, the acquisition of use behaviors, and their development into SUDs should consider neurobiology, all aspects of development, and the adolescent and family. The treatment should focus on specific substance-use behaviors as well as risk factors that have a role in the onset and maintenance of SUDs.

Risk factors for the development of SUDs include individual, peer, and family factors, and are likely not specific for a particular substance but are common across substances. Comorbidity with other psychiatric disorders is the rule rather than the exception in adolescents with SUDs. Comorbid psychiatric disorders should be treated concurrently with SUDs. Evidence-based practices for SUDs include specific family therapies, CBT, and motivational interviewing/enhancement. Aftercare and involvement in prosocial activities with nondeviant peers are critical following an acute treatment episode.

CLINICAL VIGNETTES

VIGNETTE 1: OPIATE EVALUATION AND MANAGEMENT

Bill is a 16-year-old white single male who comes into your office for a physical examination required for a new job. He appears very tremulous and you notice needle tracks on his arms on physical examination. You are highly suspicious as he had a number of behavioral problems, including ADHD when he was young. When asked about substance use, he readily admits to recent intravenous heroin use, progressing form "snorting" it and using oral opiate analgesics. He admits to getting "dope sick" with prominent withdrawal symptoms on several previous occasions. He dropped out of school when he began to use on school days and missed a lot of school and fell hopelessly behind. He was arrested 6 weeks ago on burglary charges.

Comment: Bill's history and his presentation caused an increased level of suspicion for the physician. It is obvious that he has opioid dependence. The physician's challenge will be to evaluate the withdrawal symptoms, monitor detoxification, and refer for treatment. Given IV drug use, Bill should have testing for HIV and Hepatitis B and C.

VIGNETTE 2: COMORBID DEPRESSION

Melinda is a 17-year-old African American female whose mother tells you that she is concerned that Melinda is depressed as she is increasingly socially isolative and her formerly good grades have deteriorated. When asked about her mood, Melinda is initially quiet and minimizes problems. Later, she starts to spontaneously cry, admitting to depressed mood, anhedonia, poor sleep, decreased motivation, and hopelessness. When asked about substance use, she acknowledges marijuana use "occasionally."

Comment: Melinda's history will require screening for depression (already done), substance use (via CRAFFT), and suicidality, related to her increased risk by virtue of both depression and substance use. Based on the results of this screening, the physician will have to refer Melinda either to a substance use or psychiatric treatment center or to a program that offers integrated treatment for both SUD and mental health problems.

BIBLIOGRAPHY

American Academy of Child and Adolescent Psychiatry (AACAP). Practice parameters for the assessment and treatment of children and adolescents with substance use disorders. *J Am Acad Child Adolesc Psychiatry*. 2005;44:609–621.

American Psychiatric Association. *Diagnostic and Statistic Manual of Mental Disorders, Fourth Edition, Text Revision (DSM-IV-TR)*. Washington, DC: American Psychiatric Press; 2001.

Brown SA, D'Amico EJ, McCarthy DM, et al. Four-year outcomes from adolescent alcohol and drug treatment. *J Stud Alcohol*. 2001;62(suppl):381–388.

Casavant MJ. Urine drug screening in adolescents. *Pediatr Clin North Am*. 2002;49:317–327.

Chung T. Adolescent substance use, abuse, and dependence: prevalence, course, and outcomes. In: Kaminer Y, Bukstein OG, eds. *Adolescent Substance Abuse: Psychiatric Comorbidity and High Risk Behaviors*. New York: Haworth Press; 2007:29–52.

Chung T, Martin C. Classification and short-term course of DSM-IV cannabis, hallucinogen, cocaine, and opioid disorders in treated adolescents. *J Consult Clin Psychol*. 2005;73:995–1004.

Chung T, Martin CS, Grella C, et al. Course of alcohol problems in treated adolescents: symposium proceedings of 2002 Research Society on Alcoholism Meeting. *Alcohol Clin Exp Res*. 2002;27:253–261.

Dennis ML, Dawud-Noursi S, Muck RD, et al. The need for developing and evaluating adolescent treatment models. In: Stevens SJ, Morral AR, eds. *Adolescent Substance Abuse Treatment in the United States: Exemplary Models from a National Evaluation Study*. Binghamton, NY: Haworth Press; 2003:3–34.

Dennis N, Godley SH, Diamond G, et al. The Cannabis Youth Treatment (CYT) study: main findings from two randomized trials. *J Subst Abuse Treat*. 2004;27:197–213.

Dishion T, Poulin F, Burraston B. Peer group dynamics associated with iatrogenic effects in group interventions with high-risk young adolescents. In: Nangle DW, Erdley CA, eds. *The Role of Friendship in Psychological Adjustment. New Directions for Child and Adolescent Development, No. 91*. San Francisco: Jossey-Bass; 2001:79–92.

Geller B, Cooper TB, Sun K, et al. Double-blind and placebo-controlled study of lithium for adolescent bipolar disorders with secondary substance dependency. *J Am Acad Child Adolesc Psychiatry*. 1998;37:171–178.

Grant B, Dawson D. Age at onset of alcohol use and its associated DSM-IV alcohol abuse and dependence: results from the National Longitudinal Alcohol Epidemiologic Survey. *J Subst Abuse Treat*. 1997;9:103–110.

Grella C, Hser YI, Joshi V, et al. Drug treatment outcomes for adolescents with comorbid mental and substance use disorders. *J Nerv Ment Dis*. 2001;189:384–392.

Henggeler SW, Pickrel SG, Brondino MJ. Multisystemic treatment of substance abusing and dependent delinquents: outcomes, treatment fidelity, and transportability. *Ment Health Serv Res*. 1999;1:171–184.

Hogue A, Dauber S, Samuolis J, et al. Treatment techniques and outcomes in multidimensional family therapy for adolescent behavior problems. *J Fam Psychol*. 2006;20(4):535–543.

Hser YI, Grella CE, Hubbard RL, et al. An evaluation of drug treatments for adolescents in four U.S. cities. *Arch Gen Psychiatry*. 2001;58:689–695.

Knight JR, Sherritt L, Shrier LA, et al. Validity of the CRAFFT substance abuse screening test among adolescent clinic patients. *Arch Pediatr Adolesc Med*. 2002;156:607–614.

Kulig JW. Committee on substance abuse, American Academy of Pediatrics tobacco, alcohol, and other drugs: the role of the pediatrician in prevention, identification, and management of substance abuse. *Pediatrics*. 2005;115:816–821.

Marsch LA, Bickel WK, Badger GJ, et al. Comparison of pharmacological treatments for opioid-dependent adolescents. *Arch Gen Psychiatry*. 2005;62:1157–1164.

Moolchan ET, Robinson ML, Ernst M, et al. Safety and efficacy of the nicotine patch and gum for the treatment of adolescent tobacco addiction. *Pediatrics*. 2004;15:407–414.

Myers MG, Brown SA, Tate S, et al. Toward brief interventions for adolescents with substance abuse and comorbid psychiatric problems. In: Monti PM, Colby SM, O'Leary TA, eds. *Adolescents, Alcohol, and Substance Abuse: Reaching Teens through Brief Interventions*. New York, NY: Guilford Press; 2001:275–296.

Riggs PD, Hall SK, Mikulich-Gilbertson SK, et al. A randomized controlled trial of pemoline for attention-deficit/hyperactivity disorder in substance-abusing adolescents. *J Am Acad Child Adolesc Psychiatry*. 2004;43:420–429.

Riggs PD, Mikulich-Gilbertson SK, Davies RD, et al. A randomized controlled trial of fluoxetine and cognitive behavioral therapy in adolescents with major depression, behavior problems, and substance use disorders. *Arch Pediatr Adolesc Med.* 2008;161:1026–1034.

Substance Abuse Mental Health Services Administration (SAMHSA). *Results from the 2004 National Household Survey on Drug Use and Health: National Findings (NSDUH) Series H-28*, DHHS Publication No. SMA-05-4062. Rockville, MD: Office of Applied Studies; 2005.

Substance Abuse Mental Health Services Administration (SAMHSA). *Results from the 2005 National Household Survey on Drug Use and Health: National Findings (NSDUH).* Available at: http://www.oas.samhsa.gov/nsduh/2k5nsduh/2k5Results.htm#TOC (accessed July 15, 2007).

Tarter RE. Evaluation and treatment of adolescent substance abuse: a decision tree method. *Am J Drug Alcohol Abuse.* 1990;16:1–46.

University of Michigan. 2008 Monitoring the Future Survey. Available at: http://monitoringthefuture.org/pubs/monographs/overview2008.pdf (accessed April 20, 2009).

Upadhyaya HP, Deas D, Brady KT. A practical clinical approach to the treatment of nicotine dependence in adolescents. *J Am Acad Child Adolesc Psychiatry.* 2005;44:942–946.

Upadhyaya HP, Deas D, Brady KT, et al. Cigarette smoking and psychiatric comorbidity in children and adolescents. *J Am Acad Child Adolesc Psychiatry.* 2002;41:1294–1305.

Waxmonsky JG, Wilens TE. Pharmacotherapy of adolescent substance use disorders: a review of the literature. *J Child Adolesc Psychopharmacol.* 2005;15:810–825.

Wilens TW, Adler LA, Adams J, et al. Misuse and diversion of stimulants prescribed for ADHD: a systematic review of the literature. *J Am Acad Child Adolesc Psychiatry.* 2008;47:21–31.

Williams RJ, Chang SY. Addiction Centre Adolescent Research Group: a comprehensive and comparative review of adolescent substance abuse treatment outcome. *Clin Psychol: Sci Pract.* 2000;7:138–166.

Winters KC. Treating adolescents with substance use disorders: an overview of practice issues and treatment outcome. *Subst Abuse.* 1999;20:203–225.

Winters KC, Stinchfield RD, Henly GA, et al. Validity of adolescent self-report of alcohol and other drug involvement. *Int J Addict.* 1991;25:1379–1395.

Winters KC, Stinchfield RD, Opland E, et al. The effectiveness of the Minnesota Model approach in the treatment of adolescent drug abusers. *Addiction.* 2000;95:601–612.

World Health Organization. *Lexicon of Alcohol and Drug Terms.* Geneva, Switzerland: World Health Organization. Available at: http://www.who.int/substance_abuse/terminology/ICD10ClinicalDiagnosis.pdf.

SUGGESTED READINGS

Functional Family Therapy: An Evidence-based Clinical Model for Working with Troubled Adolescents and Their Families
Thomas Sexton
Routledge (July 2009)
Paperback 320 pages

Adolescent Substance Abuse: Research and Clinical Advances
Howard Liddle and Cynthia Rowe
Cambridge University Press (March 2006)
Hardback 528 pages

Adolescent Substance Abuse: Psychiatric Comorbidity and High Risk
Yifrah Kaminer and Oscar Bukstein
Routledge Press (December 2007)
Hardback 532 pages

Multisystemic Therapy and Neighborhood Partnerships: Reducing Adolescent Violence and Substance Abuse
Cynthia Swenson, Scott Henggeler, Ida Taylor, Oliver Addison, and Patricia Chamberlin
Guilford Press (February 2009)
Paperback 272 pages

SUGGESTED WEBSITES

Monitoring the Future (University of Michigan) Annual High School Survey:
    http://www.monitoringthefuture.org (accessed April 2010).
Substance Abuse & Mental Health Services Administration: http://www.samhsa.gov (accessed April 2010).
National Institute on Drug Abuse: http://www.nida.nih.gov (accessed April 2010).
National Institute on Alcohol Abuse and Alcoholism: http://www.niaaa.nih.gov (accessed April 2010).
Chestnut Health Systems/Lighthouse Institute: http://www.chestnut.org/LI/index.html (accessed April 2010).

REVIEW QUESTIONS

1. Which of the following are *DSM-IV* substance-use disorder diagnoses?
   a. Abuse
   b. Misuse
   c. Dependence
   d. a and c
   e. All of the above

2. Regarding the assessment of substance-use behaviors in adolescents, which of the following is *not* true?
   a. The domain model allows for comprehensive assessment of adolescent functioning
   b. Screening should not take place unless a urine drug screen is positive
   c. The CRAFFT is a screening instrument for adolescents for use by primary care physicians
   d. A primary health care provider will often have to screen for depression and suicidal behavior in adolescent displaying substance use

3. Medications can be used for which of the following problems related to substance use or SUDs in adolescents?
   a. Withdrawal/detoxification
   b. Substitution therapies
   c. Coexisting psychiatric disorders
   d. All of the above

4. Which of the following is not an evidence-based practice for the treatment of SUDs in adolescents?
   a. AA/NA
   b. Motivational interviewing
   c. Cognitive–behavioral therapy
   d. Family therapy

5. Following treatment, what do adolescents generally do?
   a. Return to some substance use/abuse
   b. Show reductions in substance use and related problems over the short and long term
   c. Continue to show greater problems compared to youth in the community
   d. All of the above

Answers: 1-d, 2-b, 3-d, 4-a, 5-d

CHAPTER

7

Gail A. Bernstein, MD,
and Andrea M. Victor, PhD

Pediatric Anxiety Disorders

Introduction

Anxiety disorders is one of the most common categories of child and adolescent psycho-pathology. Although anxiety disorders are common during childhood and adolescence, many children do not gain access to services due to the difficulty in identifying internalizing symptoms. Therefore, it is critical for clinicians to develop an understanding of the presentation of anxiety disorders in children and adolescents and differentiate normal fear from anxiety disorders. Once anxiety disorders are identified, psychosocial treatments and medications have been shown to be beneficial in treating pediatric anxiety disorders.

History of Pediatric Anxiety Disorders

The primary anxiety disorders diagnosed during childhood and adolescence include separation anxiety disorder (SAD), generalized anxiety disorder (GAD), social phobia (SP), specific phobia, and panic disorder (PD). With the exception of SAD, these disorders are included in the "Anxiety Disorders" section of the *Diagnostic and Statistical Manual of Mental Disorders, Fourth Edition, Text Revision* (*DSM-IV-TR*) and are diagnosed across the lifespan. SAD is included in the "Disorders of Infancy, Childhood, and Adolescence" section of the *DSM-IV-TR* and requires that symptoms be present prior to 18 years of age.

GAD and SP are relatively new diagnoses in children and adolescents. Prior to the *DSM-IV*, GAD and SP were not diagnosed in youth. In the past, the diagnostic criteria for GAD required a minimum of 18 years of age. During that time, children with excessive anxiety were diagnosed with overanxious disorder (OAD), which was removed from the *DSM-IV* once the age requirement for GAD was discontinued. Similarly, youth who reported anxiety about or avoided engaging with unfamiliar people were typically diagnosed with avoidant disorder of childhood and adolescence. That diagnosis was removed from the *DSM-IV*, and those children are now commonly diagnosed with SP.

The essential *DSM-IV-TR* criteria of anxiety disorders included in this chapter are listed in Table 7-1. When evaluating anxiety disorders in youth, it is crucial that developmental considerations are taken into account. There are some essential differences between adult and youth criteria, which are outlined in the table.

Developmental Considerations

Anxiety is part of normal development; therefore, it is important to be cautious in distinguishing clinical anxiety from normal worry, which is estimated to occur in approximately 70% of children and adolescents. Normal fear is defined as an adaptive reaction to a real or imagined threat, whereas anxiety disorders are based on unrealistic and maladaptive reactions.

TABLE 7-1	Essential Symptoms of Anxiety Disorders and Unique Criteria for Youth	
Anxiety Disorder	**Essential Symptoms**	**Unique Youth Criteria**
Separation anxiety disorder	Developmentally inappropriate and excessive anxiety about separation from home or from attachment figures that lasts at least 4 weeks and is characterized by three or more of the following: • Excessive distress when separation occurs or is anticipated • Worry about loss or harm to an attachment figure • Worry about permanent separation from attachment figures • School refusal due to fear of separation • Fear of being alone at home and in other settings • Refusal to go to sleep alone or away from home • Nightmares about separation • Somatic complaints (e.g., headaches, stomachaches, nausea, or vomiting) when separation occurs or is anticipated	
Generalized anxiety disorder	Excessive worry in many domains that is difficult to control and occurs more days than not for at least 6 months. Worry is associated with at least three of the following symptoms: • Restlessness or feeling on edge • Fatigue • Difficulty concentrating • Irritability • Muscle tension • Sleep difficulties	Requires one associated symptom in children versus three in adults.
Social phobia	Marked and persistent fear for at least 6 months of at least one social or performance situation in which there is exposure to unfamiliar people or scrutiny by others. Primary worry is about doing something embarrassing or humiliating. Exposure to the feared situation almost always provokes anxiety. There are two types of social phobia: • Generalized: fears include most social situations • Specific: fears are about one specific social situation	Youth must have the ability to develop normal peer relationships. Must exhibit anxiety with peers, as well as adults. Children may show anxiety by crying, tantrums, freezing, or avoiding social situations. Youth are not required to recognize their fear is excessive or unreasonable.
Specific phobia	Excessive and unreasonable fear of a specific object or situation. Real or anticipated exposure to the phobic stimulus almost always provokes an anxious response.	Youth may demonstrate anxiety through crying, tantrums, freezing, or clinging.

(continued)

TABLE 7-1	Essential Symptoms of Anxiety Disorders and Unique Criteria for Youth (*continued*)	
Anxiety Disorder	**Essential Symptoms**	**Unique Youth Criteria**
	Types of phobias include: • Animals • Natural environment (e.g., storms, heights, and water) • Blood-injection-injury • Situational (e.g., airplanes, elevators, and bridges) • Other (e.g., costumed characters, choking, vomiting, and loud noises)	Youth may not recognize that the fear is excessive or unreasonable.
Panic disorder	Recurrent unexpected panic attacks that are followed for at least 1 month by one or more of the following: • Persistent fear about having another panic attack • Worry about the implications or consequences of the panic attack (e.g., losing control or going crazy) • Significant change in behavior due to the panic attacks Agoraphobia is characterized by the following: • Anxiety about being in places or situations in which escape may be difficult or humiliating (e.g., crowded place or public place) • The situations are avoided or endured with significant distress. Panic attack is characterized by a discrete period of intense fear or discomfort during which four or more of the following symptoms occur abruptly and peak within 10 minutes: • Palpitations or increased heart rate • Sweating • Shaking • Shortness of breath • Feeling of choking • Chest pain • Abdominal discomfort • Dizziness • Feelings of unreality or detachment from oneself • Fear of losing control or going crazy • Fear of dying • Numbness or tingling sensations • Chills or hot flushes	Youth may express panic attacks by crying, tantrums, freezing, or clinging.

Adapted from American Psychiatric Association. *Diagnostic and Statistical Manual of Mental Disorders, Fourth Edition, Text Revision.* Washington, DC: Author; 2000.

There is a developmental progression in common fears during childhood and adolescence. Infants and preschool-aged children typically have fears regarding concrete and specific situations, such as strangers, separation from caretakers, loud noises, and harm to self. Children more commonly endorse fears related to social, evaluative, and anticipatory experiences. With cognitive maturation, adolescents tend to demonstrate more global fears, which may include concerns about world affairs. It is necessary to understand the development of normal fears in order to assess anxiety disorders. Compared to normal fears, clinical anxiety is age and stage inappropriate, persistent, and impairing.

Epidemiology

Prevalence estimates of childhood anxiety disorders vary based on the type of epidemiologic study conducted. Higher prevalence rates result from studies with multiple assessment points, longer assessment intervals, and clinical samples. Epidemiologic studies that estimate the prevalence of any anxiety disorder during childhood show 3-month rates that range from 2% to 8% and 6-month rates that range from 5% to 18%. When estimating lifetime prevalence in retrospective studies with older adolescents and adults, the rates are even higher and range from 8% to 27%.

The prevalence rate of each anxiety disorder in youth has also been examined in epidemiologic studies. When considering nonclinical samples, there are some differences in prevalence rates and patterns of prevalence across pediatric anxiety disorders. SAD and specific phobia are more likely to be diagnosed during childhood versus adolescence. SAD has a prevalence rate of approximately 3% to 5%. Prevalence rates of specific phobia in youth range from 2% to 9%, with an average of approximately 5% across samples.

In contrast, GAD, SP, and PD are more likely to occur during adolescence compared to childhood. It is difficult to estimate the prevalence of GAD in children since it is a relatively new diagnosis in the pediatric age group. OAD, the previous diagnosis used for children with excessive worry, was estimated to occur in approximately 3% of youth. Lifetime prevalence rate of GAD in individuals who range from 15 to 54 years of age is estimated to be around 5%. SP is estimated to occur in approximately 5% of youth, with lifetime prevalence in adolescents estimated to be 16%. PD is relatively rare in youth, with a lifetime prevalence rate in adolescents estimated to be approximately 0.5%. Panic attacks seem to be significantly more common (18% prevalence rate) than a diagnosis of PD.

Etiology

There are many factors that have been identified in the etiology of childhood anxiety disorders. Etiology is often viewed within an integrated model that takes into account several factors and their relations to each other. These factors place children at a greater risk for developing an anxiety disorder, and the interplay of the factors tend to determine the presentation of the anxiety disorder.

Genetic Factors

Genetics

Genomic studies of childhood anxiety disorders have been initiated due to the belief that genetic factors impact the presentation of childhood anxiety disorders based on heritability estimates. Genetic studies provide evidence that specific genomic regions are likely related to the development of anxiety disorders; however, few studies have been completed for specific disorders, and the results are inconsistent. Linkage studies have located possible chromosomal regions, and candidate gene studies have identified possible genes associated with anxiety disorders. These studies have focused primarily on PD, SP, specific phobia, and obsessive–compulsive disorder. It is difficult to identify specific genes related to anxiety disorders due to the complexity of the disorders. It is likely that many genes play a role in the presentation of anxiety disorders.

Temperament

Behavioral inhibition, a genetically based, temperamental trait, is often associated with anxiety. It refers to the child's reaction to novel and unfamiliar stimuli. Children with behavioral inhibition have a tendency to respond to novel situations with restraint, distress, and avoidance. Studies have found that toddlers with behavioral inhibition compared to those without behavioral inhibition are more likely to develop an anxiety disorder during childhood and adolescence.

Attachment

Parent–child attachment is also related to the etiology of childhood anxiety disorders. Secure attachment with a primary caretaker may alleviate a child's risk for an anxiety disorder. Research has shown that infants with an insecure attachment, particularly an anxious-resistant attachment, are more likely to develop an anxiety disorder by 17 years of age.

Parental Impact

Parental Anxiety

Children are more at risk of developing an anxiety disorder when a parent has an anxiety disorder. Studies have shown that children of parents with an anxiety disorder are two to five times more likely to have an anxiety disorder compared to children of parents with substance abuse and children of parents without a history of an anxiety disorder and/or substance abuse.

Parenting Style

There are three aspects of parenting style associated with childhood anxiety: low acceptance, excessive control, and modeling of anxiety. These are conceptualized as moderators of childhood anxiety and not direct predictors. Acceptance is characterized by warmth and responsiveness in parent–child interactions. Parents who are low on acceptance tend to demonstrate more criticism and rejection. Control refers to the degree parents regulate their children's activities, thoughts, and feelings. When parents use excessive control, children do not learn mastery of their environment. Finally, parents who exhibit anxious behaviors (i.e., avoidance, catastrophic thinking, and poor problem solving) often impart negativity and poor coping skills to their children.

Clinical Syndromes

Separation Anxiety Disorder

Clinical Presentation

Separation anxiety from primary caregivers is a developmentally normal response in infants and young children up to 30 months of age. It typically decreases between 3 and 5 years of age as children's cognitive maturation allows them to understand that separation from a caregiver is temporary. SAD is more common in children than in adolescents and typically has an age of onset between 7 and 9 years.

The key theme of SAD is extreme anxiety and distress about separation from primary attachment figures (e.g., parents, siblings, and grandparents). Children with SAD fear that harm will come to them or their attachment figures when they are separated. Other symptoms of SAD are listed in Table 7-1. To meet *DSM-IV-TR* criteria for SAD, the symptoms must be more intense and impairing than expected for the child's developmental level, be present for a minimum of 4 weeks, and have an onset before age 18. A distinguishing feature of SAD is that the anxiety abates when the child is with his or her parent, which is not the case with GAD or SP.

Clinical Course

The course of SAD may be short lived or chronic and persistent. A study prospectively followed children in an anxiety disorders clinic for 3 to 4 years and reported that SAD had the highest remission rate (96%). Another longitudinal study was completed with 3-year-old children with clinical, subclinical, or nonclinical level of separation anxiety. The children were evaluated at baseline and 3.5 years later. At baseline, children with clinical SAD were more likely to have comorbid diagnoses, greater severity of anxiety, somatic complaints, internalizing symptoms, and parents with internalizing symptoms. Many children with SAD did not have a stable diagnosis, with their symptoms moving toward subclinical or nonclinical status at follow-up. Predictors of persistent SAD were family and parent variables (e.g., inconsistency in limit setting).

A community-based sample of 8- to 17-year-old twins with SAD was followed for 18 months. Only 20% had persistence of the SAD diagnosis at 18-month follow-up. Baseline factors predicting persistence of SAD were oppositional defiant disorder, impairing symptoms of attention-deficit hyperactivity disorder (ADHD), and maternal marital dissatisfaction. Youth with persistent SAD were significantly more likely to develop a depressive disorder at follow-up.

Participants from the Oregon Adolescent Depression Project were assessed twice as teenagers and twice as adults. Many of the teenagers with a history of SAD developed new disorders during the follow-up period. The most common outcomes for teenagers with a history of SAD were depression in 75% and PD in 25%. This study suggests a specific link between SAD in childhood and PD in adulthood; however, several other studies suggest that SAD is a risk factor for a number of different anxiety disorders in adulthood, not only PD.

Comorbidity

Common comorbid conditions include GAD, SP, specific phobia, and ADHD. Children with SAD were found to have a greater number of comorbid diagnoses compared to those with GAD or SP. However, children with SAD were least likely to have a comorbid mood disorder.

Generalized Anxiety Disorder

Clinical Presentation

GAD presents as children with multiple areas of worry. These worries are excessive, difficult to control, and impede the youth's daily functioning. The worries must have at least one associated symptom (i.e., restlessness, easily tired, difficulty concentrating, irritability, muscle tension, and/or sleep difficulties).

Since all children worry, it is critical to differentiate children with normal worry from those with GAD. Children with GAD endorse a higher number of worries and more intense worries compared to children with other anxiety disorders and healthy control children. The content of worry in children with GAD is also important to consider. Worry about health of self and of significant others has been shown to be the most predictive of a GAD diagnosis. Other common worries include school performance, appearance, and family issues (e.g., divorce and finances). The presence of associated symptoms (e.g., restlessness and difficulty concentrating) also differentiates children with GAD from other children. The number of associated symptoms seems to increase with age. Studies showed that children with GAD endorsed an average of 3.4

associated symptoms, and found that restlessness was the most common and muscle tension was the least common.

Clinical Course

GAD in youth tends to follow a chronic course with waxing and waning of symptoms and a greater degree of comorbid psychopathology compared to adult-onset GAD; therefore, early identification is beneficial. A comorbid diagnosis of depression in children with GAD usually results in a poorer prognosis, increased symptom severity, and lengthier duration of symptoms.

Since GAD and depression often co-occur and there is significant overlap in symptom constellations, there is a question as to whether these should be considered two distinct disorders. There are conflicting arguments among researchers regarding the relation between GAD and major depressive disorder (MDD). Some researchers propose that GAD is a subsyndrome to MDD because it typically occurs before the onset of MDD. This is referred to as "sequential comorbidity." In contrast, others propose that GAD and MDD typically do not occur in a predictable order. This is referred to as "cumulative comorbidity." Studies support both sequential and cumulative comorbidity. These concepts are continuing to be examined to develop a better understanding of the association between GAD and MDD.

Comorbidity

The majority of children with GAD have a comorbid diagnosis. The most common comorbid diagnosis is another anxiety disorder. Depression is also a common comorbid diagnosis in clinical samples. Only 4% of children with GAD from a nonclinical sample had a comorbid depressive disorder, whereas 66% of children with GAD from a clinical sample had a comorbid depressive disorder.

Social Phobia

Clinical Presentation

SP typically presents in children and adolescents as significant anxiety of social and/or performance situations due to fear they will act in an embarrassing manner. Common social situations that are feared by children with SP include speaking in class, talking on the phone, and interacting with peers. Feared social situations provoke an anxious response and are avoided or endured with marked distress.

There is increasing evidence that selective mutism, a consistent failure to speak in specific social situations (e.g., school and playdates), is related to SP. There is debate as to whether selective mutism should be conceptualized as a subtype of SP due to the significant overlap between the cardinal symptoms of the two disorders. Both disorders include a marked fear of social and/or performance situations, avoidance of those feared situations, and often a lack of anxiety when the child is in the home environment.

The argument to include selective mutism as a subtype of SP is based primarily on three reasons. First, children with selective mutism often endorse high rates of social anxiety, shyness, and avoidance of social situations. Second, children who are diagnosed with selective mutism commonly continue to struggle with social anxiety throughout adolescence and adulthood even after the mutism is gone. Third, children with selective mutism have relatives with high rates of anxiety disorders. Although there is evidence to support selective mutism as a subtype of SP, there is concern that there is more to the etiology of selective mutism than just social anxiety. Children with selective mutism have higher rates of language impairments and problematic interactions with peers, which are not included in the diagnostic criteria for SP.

There are some differences in presentation of SP in children and adolescents compared to adults. It is necessary to assess the youth's ability to engage in age-appropriate social relationships, which is required for a diagnosis of SP. Furthermore, the child's social anxiety must occur during interactions with peers, not only with adults. Children do not need to recognize that their social fears are unreasonable, as is required to make a diagnosis in adults.

Clinical Course

The onset of SP typically occurs during early adolescence. This is likely due to the youth's increased awareness of others' perceptions. Youth with SP report increased overall anxiety, depression, and loneliness. Children with SP also have low social acceptance and difficulty with social skills, which may be related to their avoidance of social situations. An increase in severity of SP symptoms in children seems to be related to an increase in deficits in social skills and leadership skills, attention difficulties, and learning problems based on teacher report.

The occurrence of SP during childhood or adolescence is a risk factor for the development of psychiatric disorders in adulthood, particularly GAD and depression, as well as ongoing SP. SP is a unique risk factor for the later onset of cannabis and alcohol dependence in adulthood. Due to the chronic course of SP, it is commonly associated with social, educational, and occupational impairment.

Comorbidity

Children with SP often have comorbid psychiatric disorders. In a recent study, all 45 children with SP in a nonclinical sample had at least one comorbid disorder, with 84% meeting criteria for at least one other anxiety disorder (73% had GAD, 51% had SAD, and 36% had specific phobia). There is an increase in comorbid depression and substance abuse in adolescents with SP compared to children with SP.

Specific Phobia

Clinical Presentation

Specific phobia refers to a persistent and unreasonable fear of a specific object or situation that leads to distress and/or avoidance. The fear is so intense that it causes interference in the child's daily functioning. There are five main types of specific phobias: animal, natural environment, blood-injection-injury, situational, and other. It is common for a child to have more than one type of specific phobia. A fear is typically classified as a specific phobia when it is excessive, persistent over time, and not specific to the child's age and/or developmental level.

The different types of specific phobia have slightly different clinical presentations, which should be considered during assessment and treatment. Typically, the feared stimulus of specific phobias provokes sympathetic activation (i.e., racing heart, sweating, trembling, etc.) and heightened arousal. In contrast, the blood-injection-injury phobia produces parasympathetic activation (i.e., slowing heart) and may be associated with fainting. Additionally, children with environmental and/or situational phobias are more likely to endorse anxious predictions (e.g., "I am going crazy.") and misinterpret their bodily symptoms (e.g., "I am going to die.").

Clinical Course

Many specific phobias develop during childhood and adolescence; however, the symptoms are often not assessed until adulthood. Specific phobias tend to have the lowest rate of heritability compared to other anxiety disorders and the highest environmental influences. Specific phobia tends to be a relatively stable disorder, and about 30% of children continue to have specific phobias for a duration of 2 to 5 years. Girls and younger children are more likely to endorse specific phobia symptoms compared to boys and older children.

There are several theories regarding the development of specific phobias. It is predicted that the development of a specific phobia likely stems from one of three associative pathways: direct negative experiences with the feared stimulus, observation of others' reactions to the feared stimulus, and learning negative information about the feared stimulus. A nonassociative theory speculates that the development of a specific phobia may not be due to experiences, and instead is due to a spontaneous, innate reaction to evolutionary cues. Finally, others hypothesize that some children have a genetic vulnerability that places them at risk for developing maladaptive fears. Then factors related to the environment, developmental fears, and genetic vulnerability interact to produce specific phobias. Cognitive biases maintain the specific phobia.

Comorbidity

Comorbidity rates of specific phobia seem to be markedly different based on the type of sample. Community samples show that youth with specific phobias are less likely to have comorbid disorders compared to youth with other anxiety disorders. In contrast, clinical samples show that 72% of youth with specific phobia have at least one comorbid diagnosis. Common comorbid disorders include an additional specific phobia, SAD, OAD, and ADHD.

Specific phobia is often comorbid with depression in adulthood, with the onset of specific phobia typically prior to depression. The National Comorbidity Survey data assessed this diagnostic association in individuals ranging in age from 15 to 54 years and found that individuals diagnosed with specific phobia were significantly more likely to have a comorbid lifetime diagnosis of depression compared to individuals without a diagnosis of specific phobia. Two other studies that examined this relationship in adolescents with specific phobia showed that specific phobia did not increase the risk for depression during adolescence.

Panic Disorder

Clinical Presentation

Panic attacks are defined in *DSM-IV-TR* as discrete episodes of intense fear or discomfort with at least four physiologic and cognitive symptoms that occur abruptly and peak in 10 minutes or less. If recurrent and spontaneous (i.e., uncued) panic attacks occur and are associated with persistent concern of having more panic attacks, worry about the consequences of the attacks, or behavioral changes due to attacks, the criteria for PD are met.

While PD is rare in childhood, cued panic attacks may occur in children in association with SAD, SP, or GAD. Panic attacks may be precipitated by separation from attachment figures in children with SAD and by social or performance situations in children with SP. Since panic attacks in children with SAD, SP, or GAD are usually cued, they do not support a diagnosis of PD, which requires spontaneous panic attacks.

Hayward and colleagues found that 5% of a large sample of girls (10 to 15 years) reported a history of at least one four-symptom panic attack. The frequency of panic attacks correlated positively with Tanner stage of pubertal development. As Tanner stage increased, there was a greater likelihood of having experienced panic attack(s). This finding suggests that biologic changes are associated with the onset of panic attacks.

Physiologic symptoms reported by children during panic attacks include heart racing, shortness of breath, sweating, weakness, and faintness. Symptoms that emerge in adolescents are chest pain, flushing, trembling, headache, and vertigo. Cognitive symptoms begin later than physiologic symptoms. The fear of dying is typically the first cognitive symptom reported by children and young adolescents with the fear of going crazy, derealization, and depersonalization presenting later.

Clinical Course

A community sample of 2246 high school students was followed by Wilson and Hayward prospectively over 4 years to identify vulnerabilities for differential clinical courses after initial panic attacks. Average age at onset of panic attacks was 16.8 years, and 28% described spontaneous panic attacks. Behavioral inhibition in childhood, anxiety sensitivity, negative affect, and severe uncued panic attacks were predictors of later depressive symptoms and agoraphobia. For most youth, the course of PD appears to be chronic with waxing and waning of symptom severity. Agoraphobia is one of the most impairing sequelae of PD. It does not necessarily accompany PD and may occur without PD.

Comorbidity

Common comorbid conditions include GAD (74%), agoraphobia (56%), specific phobias (56%), and depression (43%).

Assessment of Childhood Anxiety Disorders

A comprehensive assessment of the youth's psychiatric symptoms should be completed during the initial evaluation appointment. The essentials for the assessment of pediatric anxiety disorders are presented in Table 7-2. It is recommended that the evaluation include a clinical interview with the child and parents, as well as objective rating scales completed by multiple informants (e.g., child, parents, and teacher). During the clinical interview it is important to assess severity of symptoms, complete a risk assessment (i.e., suicidal ideation, self-injurious behavior, and homicidal ideation), and rule out other psychiatric and medical conditions. Medication side effects, medical conditions (e.g., hyperthyroidism, migraine, and asthma), excessive caffeine use, and drug use may emulate an anxiety disorder.

Several standardized instruments are helpful as a supplement to a comprehensive clinical interview. The Anxiety Disorders Interview Schedule (ADIS) for *DSM-IV* child version is the state-of-the-art semi-structured interview for the assessment and diagnosis of anxiety disorders and common comorbid disorders. The ADIS evaluates children's symptom severity and degree of interference in functioning, and is a helpful way to differentiate among specific anxiety disorders and comorbid diagnoses. It may be helpful to primary therapists but is too long and time consuming for a primary care office. For the latter, and to complement the ADIS in the therapist's office, objective rating scales are often helpful in further assessing children's current symptoms, including to establish symptom severity and to establish a baseline against which to assess progress in treatment. Table 7-3 provides a summary of selected instruments.

TABLE 7-2   Essentials for the Assessment of Pediatric Anxiety Disorders

- It is critical to collect information from the youth, as well as other sources (i.e., parents, other caretakers, teachers, and pediatrician).
- Assess and rule out medical causes, including hyperthyroidism, medication side effects, caffeine use, and substance abuse.
- Complete a risk assessment to assess safety of patient (e.g., suicidal thoughts and intent).
- Consider the youth's developmental level. Younger children may be better at expressing themselves through drawings and play rather than by verbal means.
- Identify the antecedents that trigger the anxiety, which may help in differential diagnosis.
- Determine the environmental (e.g., stress at home or in school) and familial (e.g., family mental health history and parental reaction to anxiety) factors that may contribute to the youth's anxiety.
- Evaluate comorbid psychiatric disorders, particularly mood and disruptive behavior disorders.
- Consider the use of a semi-structured interview and standardized rating scales to further assess symptoms.

TABLE 7-3	Rating Scales Used in the Assessment of Anxiety Disorders	
Rating Scale	**Informant(s)**	**Description**
To evaluate anxiety		
Multidimensional Anxiety Scale for Children (MASC)	Child	Four domains: physical symptoms, social anxiety, harm avoidance, and separation/panic. Respond using a Likert scale.
Screen for Child Anxiety Related Emotional Disorders (SCARED)	Child, parent	Evaluates symptoms of SAD, GAD, SP, panic disorder, and school phobia. Respond using a Likert scale.
To evaluate multiple emotional and behavioral domains		
Behavior Assessment System for Children, Second Edition (BASC-2)	Child, parent, teacher	Assessment of externalizing problems, inattention and hyperactivity, internalizing problems, school problems, adaptive skills, and personal adjustment. Respond using true/false and a Likert scale.
Child Behavior Checklist (CBCL)	Child, parent, teacher	Evaluation of externalizing and internalizing behaviors, with subscales of withdrawn, somatic complaints, anxious/depressed, social problems, thought problems, attention problems, delinquent behavior, and aggressive behavior. Respond using a Likert scale.

Treatment

Cognitive–Behavioral Therapy

Cognitive–behavioral therapy (CBT) has consistently been shown to be an effective treatment for childhood anxiety disorders. A recent review showed that CBT is probably efficacious based on the rigorous review of 32 treatment studies of pediatric anxiety disorders. CBT is effective with youth of all ages in individual, group, and school settings, with and without a parent/family component. The success of CBT is demonstrated immediately following treatment and at long-term follow-up assessments. Although treatment studies consistently show that CBT results in symptom improvement, there are still questions as to *how* CBT is effective and how it can be *more* effective.

CBT focuses on the child's behavioral avoidance and cognitive distortions related to anxious responses. Table 7-4 presents specific components that are important to the structure of CBT. CBT typically offers education to the youth and parents about anxiety, which then allows better understanding of the rationale for treatment. Psychoeducation can identify and address misconceptions children and adolescents and their parents have about the nature of anxiety, as well as help families develop a language to talk about anxiety. Prior to engaging in exposure activities, it is often important for youth to learn and practice anxiety management strategies including somatic management and cognitive modification. Somatic management teaches children and adolescents the connection between physiologic arousal and anxiety. Youth are then taught relaxation strategies to better manage their physiologic arousal and break the connection between arousal and anxiety. Cognitive modification requires children and adolescents to reflect on internal processes and identify irrational thoughts related to anxiety. Once irrational thoughts are identified, they are challenged through rational thinking and

TABLE 7-4	Primary Components of Cognitive–Behavioral Therapy for Pediatric Anxiety Disorders
Component	**Goal**
Psychoeducation	Provide information about anxiety and the treatment of anxiety.
Emotion identification	Practice identifying and differentiating emotions.
Somatic management	Address the connection between physiologic arousal and anxiety.
Cognitive modification	Identify distorted thoughts related to anxiety. Challenge these thoughts and develop alternative, more accurate thoughts.
Problem solving	Teach and practice problem-solving strategies, in which several solutions are identified, the best solution is implemented, and the outcome is evaluated.
Exposure	Gradual exposure to feared situations during which the child remains in the situation using anxiety management strategies until the anxiety diminishes.
Contingency management	Offer children rewards for successful completion of exposures to help motivate the youth's completion of the exposures.
Relapse prevention	Review anxiety management skills that were learned and practiced during therapy. Identify possible problematic situations that may occur in the future. Encourage less reliance on the therapist and caretakers and empowerment of the youth.

replaced with more adaptive and helpful thoughts. Children are encouraged to use these anxiety management strategies to successfully complete exposures.

Exposures require youth to confront an anxiety-provoking situation until their anxiety diminishes. Exposures are typically completed in a hierarchical manner, in which the child starts with less anxiety provoking situations and then gradually proceeds to more anxiety provoking situations. Children and adolescents often benefit from a contingency management system, in which they earn rewards for successful completion of exposure exercises. In order for CBT to be successful, children and their parents must practice these strategies between sessions. Relapse prevention is another important aspect of CBT, since many children will continue to experience anxiety throughout their lifespan. Manualized CBT interventions for pediatric anxiety are commercially available, such as the Coping Cat by Kendall.

Although CBT has primary components, it cannot be done using a cookbook approach. When conducting CBT, it is crucial to consider the child's developmental level, verbal skills, comorbid disorders, and parental involvement in the maintenance of the child's anxiety. CBT must be modified to successfully meet the youth's and parents' needs. Parents are often involved in the treatment; however, the degree of parent involvement depends on the child's developmental level. When treating preschool and early elementary school children, parents have a larger role in treatment. As children get older, parents typically have a smaller role in treatment. Parents benefit from psychoeducation regarding anxiety, as well as learning the anxiety management coping skills to help coach their children during the treatment period. Comorbid disorders need to be considered and prioritized in the treatment process. Nonanxiety comorbid disorders often make the treatment process more complicated.

Medication

Selective Serotonin Reuptake Inhibitors

The hallmark Child–Adolescent Anxiety Multimodal Study (CAMS) examined the effectiveness of sertraline (25 to 200 mg/day), 14 sessions of CBT, sertraline plus CBT, and pill placebo over 12 weeks in treating youth with moderate to severe GAD, SAD, and/or SP.

At posttreatment, 55% on sertraline, 60% who participated in CBT, 81% in the combination group, and 24% on placebo were rated as much or very much improved on the Clinical Global Impressions Improvement scale. Demonstrating the benefit of combination treatment is valuable because previous studies showed that monotherapy with selective serotonin reuptake inhibitors (SSRIs) or CBT is effective in only 40% to 50% of child participants. In addition, CAMS found no increased risk of suicidal or homicidal ideation in children who received sertraline compared to those who received placebo.

The clinical implication of CAMS is that anxious children who receive combination treatment have the best chance of a positive outcome. However, any of the three active treatments (SSRI, CBT, or SSRI plus CBT) can be recommended, taking into account family preference, availability of specific treatments, cost, and time constraints.

Five earlier randomized clinical trials supported the efficacy of SSRIs in treating youth with anxiety disorders. Two of these studies treated children with SAD, GAD, and SP, two included children with SP only, and one included children with GAD only. Medications included fluvoxamine, fluoxetine, paroxetine, and sertraline. There have been no head-to-head trials directly comparing different SSRIs in the treatment of children and adolescents with anxiety disorders.

Practical Considerations in Prescribing SSRIs

The selection of a specific SSRI is guided by the properties of the drug, including the side effects profile, half-life of the drug, potential drug–drug interactions, and the history of positive response to a specific SSRI in a first-degree relative. Common side effects include motor activation (i.e., hyperactivity), stomachaches, and insomnia. Motor activation is more likely to occur with initiation of the SSRI or an increase in dose in young children with a history of ADHD. This side effect can usually be managed by decreasing the dose. Other side effects may include headache, behavioral changes, sexual dysfunction, and bipolar switching. Some side effects are linked to specific SSRIs; for example, sedation is common with citalopram. Therefore, citalopram is a good choice for a child with insomnia when it is dosed at bedtime. The other SSRIs are usually given as one morning dose.

Most of the SSRIs have a short half-life, which means that withdrawal symptoms are common if they are discontinued abruptly. Due to its longer half-life compared to other SSRIs, fluoxetine is a good choice for a noncompliant teenager. If doses of fluoxetine are missed, withdrawal symptoms are unlikely. However, the longer half-life can be a disadvantage if a serious side effect occurs (e.g., bipolar switching) because it takes up to 1 month after discontinuation to clear fluoxetine and its metabolites from the body.

Potential drug–drug interactions, especially with other psychotropic medications, need to be considered in selecting a specific SSRI. For example, fluoxetine and paroxetine inhibit 2D6 cytochrome P450 enzyme pathways in the liver. This increases the levels of drugs that are metabolized at 2D6 (e.g., aripiprazole, risperidone, and tricyclic antidepressants [TCAs]).

The approach to dosing is to start low and gradually titrate up while monitoring for clinical response and side effects. In the CAMS, sertraline was administered using a fixed-flexible schedule starting with 25 mg/day and gradually increasing to a maximum of 200 mg/day by week 8. Medication was advanced if participants were evaluated as mildly ill or worse and showed minimal side effects. The mean final daily dose was 146 mg in the sertraline plus CBT group and 134 mg in the sertraline group. Serum levels of SSRIs are not routinely monitored. In patients who develop signs and symptoms of toxicity on low doses of SSRIs (possible slow metabolizers) and in those who show few or no side effects and lack of efficacy on normal or high doses (possible rapid metabolizers), consideration should be given to drawing blood for evaluation of genetically based P450 enzymatic defects in the liver that alter the metabolism of drugs.

In a review article, it is recommended that SSRIs be continued for approximately 1 year after remission of anxiety symptoms. Subsequently, during a low-stress period, the medication can be gradually tapered and discontinued. If anxiety symptoms recur during the taper-down or following discontinuation, it is suggested that the SSRI be reinitiated.

Although short-term studies show benefits of SSRIs over placebo, a substantial number of youth remain impaired after treatment. Options in these cases include a longer duration of drug treatment, higher dosage, augmentation with another drug, combination treatment (i.e., SSRI plus CBT), or changing to a different medication.

Other Medications

An alternative choice to an SSRI is venlafaxine, a serotonin-norepinephrine reuptake inhibitor (SNRI). Randomized controlled trials support the efficacy of extended-release venlafaxine in youth with GAD and SP. Venlafaxine has the potential for increase in diastolic blood pressure, pulse, and skin rashes. It requires a very gradual taper-down before discontinuation to prevent withdrawal symptoms.

TCAs have largely been replaced by the SSRIs due to TCAs having a less advantageous side effects profile, serious toxicity in overdose, and the lack of consensus regarding their efficacy for treating anxiety based on several placebo-controlled trials. TCAs are a second-line choice for treating anxiety in youth. The presence of a comorbid diagnosis, such as ADHD or enuresis, is one factor that may support the trial of a TCA. Monitoring of TCAs requires electrocardiograms due to the potential effects of TCAs on cardiac rate and rhythm, as well as blood draws to assure that a therapeutic serum level is achieved. Side effects of TCAs may include dry mouth, lightheadedness, constipation, sedation, weight gain, and urinary retention.

There are no adequately powered placebo-controlled trials of benzodiazepines that support their benefit in treating youth with anxiety disorders. Nevertheless, benzodiazepines may be used on a short-term basis (up to several weeks) in combination with an SSRI or a TCA to facilitate rapid reduction in anxiety symptoms in youth with severe anxiety disorders. Due to the possibility of dependence, benzodiazepines should be prescribed cautiously and are contraindicated in adolescents with substance abuse. Benzodiazepines can also be used in the treatment of specific phobia—situational type, such as specific phobia of flying on airplanes. In this situation, the benzodiazepine is taken 30 to 45 minutes prior to boarding the airplane.

TABLE 7-5	Psychotropic Medications in the Treatment of Pediatric Anxiety Disorders
First line: *SSRIs*—start low and go slow. Strong scientific evidence for their efficacy.	
Second line: *SNRIs*—extended-release venlafaxine has been shown to be efficacious for treating GAD and SP in youth in two studies.	
Second line: *TCAs*—require electrocardiograms and serum levels for monitoring. Consider if comorbid enuresis or ADHD is present.	
Others: *Benzodiazepines*—may be used for up to several weeks in combination with an SSRI or a TCA while waiting for the SSRI or TCA to work. Taper gradually prior to discontinuation to avoid withdrawal symptoms. *Buspirone*—does not have addictive potential. Generally well tolerated.	

SSRI: selective serotonin reuptake inhibitor; SNRI: serotonin-norepinephrine reuptake inhibitor; TCA: tricyclic antidepressant; GAD: generalized anxiety disorder; SP: social phobia; ADHD: attention-deficit hyperactivity disorder.

TABLE 7-6	Essentials in the Treatment of Pediatric Anxiety Disorders

- Complete a thorough clinical assessment prior to providing treatment.
- Consider the impact of comorbid disorders on the treatment plan. Prioritize symptoms and treatment goals.
- Provide psychoeducation about anxiety and anxiety management to child and primary caretakers.
- CBT alone, or in conjunction with medication, should be the first-line treatment.
- SSRI is the first-choice medication in the treatment of pediatric anxiety disorders.

CBT: cognitive behavioral therapy; SSRI: selective serotonin reuptake inhibitor.

Potential side effects of benzodiazepines include sedation, decreased mental acuity, and behavioral disinhibition, and if stopped abruptly, withdrawal symptoms may occur.

Buspirone is a nonbenzodiazepine anxiolytic. There are no published controlled trials in youth with anxiety disorders to support its efficacy. Unlike the benzodiazepines, buspirone does not have addictive potential. Side effects are usually mild and may include lightheadedness, nausea, and headache. This medication's onset of action is 2 to 4 weeks or longer. It is dosed two or three times per day, which may impact compliance. Table 7-5 provides a summary of the psychotropic medications commonly used. Table 7-6 provides a summary of the essential components of the psychosocial and medication treatment of pediatric anxiety disorders.

The Multimodal Treatment Study of Children with ADHD (MTA) found that approximately one third of youth diagnosed with ADHD also suffered an anxiety disorder. Many of these youth responded well to a stimulant medication. However, some anxious children are "activated" by, or their anxiety worsens on, a stimulant. For children diagnosed with both an anxiety disorder and ADHD, a stimulant may be tried alone, or an SSRI and a stimulant may be tried together, but in both cases with the caveat of "start low and go slow." Some, but not all, clinicians endorse atomoxetine as a treatment to consider for comorbid anxiety and ADHD, although controlled trials are lacking.

Conclusions

Pediatric anxiety disorders are prevalent and place youth at risk of developing social, academic, and family difficulties. Anxiety disorders are often difficult to identify in youth due to the internalizing nature of the symptoms. Therefore, it is important to conduct a multimodal assessment with multiple reporters when evaluating anxiety disorders in children and adolescents. There are several types of anxiety disorders that have unique features. Once an anxiety disorder is identified, there are effective psychosocial treatments and psychotropic medications that target anxiety symptoms. CBT, medication, and a combination of CBT and medication should be considered as treatment options for children and adolescents diagnosed with anxiety disorders.

CLINICAL VIGNETTES

VIGNETTE 1: DISTINGUISHING ANXIETY FROM ADHD

Jim is a 10-year-old boy referred by his pediatrician. He was having trouble at home and school with concentration, hyperactivity, and insomnia. His pediatrician gave him a provisional diagnosis of ADHD and initiated a trial of stimulant medication. Subsequently, Jim's parents noticed that he was more anxious. He was expressing multiple worries and seeking frequent reassurance from his mother for his worries. Jim estimated that he was spending most of his time worrying. For 6 months prior to the stimulant trial, Jim reported worries that were mildly impairing, but manageable.

Child psychiatric evaluation revealed a boy with multiple areas of worry. Jim described worrying about his schoolwork, whether the children at school liked him, his health (e.g., he was concerned about catching colds and had headaches that he believed were serious), the health of his grandfather, who was a smoker, and family issues (whether his parents had enough money to pay the bills and if his parents might get divorced). Jim stated that he could not "turn off" his worries. When Jim worried, his parents reported that he seemed restless, he jiggled his leg and squirmed in his chair, and he had difficulty concentrating. Jim said he felt tense and jittery when worrying. Bedtime was difficult because Jim could not settle down, and he reported trouble falling asleep due to his worries.

There was no history of abuse. Examination by the pediatrician was normal. Jim was on a stimulant and no other medications. He lived with his biologic parents and 13-year-old sister. Family history was positive for ADHD in father and GAD and MDD in mother. Jim's sister had a history of school refusal in first grade secondary to SAD.

Jim was diagnosed with GAD. The stimulant was discontinued. CBT alone and sertraline plus CBT were considered as treatment options. The latter option was chosen due to severity of symptoms and related impairment. Jim was started on 12.5 mg sertraline, which was increased weekly by 12.5 mg. On 37.5 mg, he developed motor activation, which was managed successfully by decreasing the dosage. Jim and his parents participated in CBT. They were initially provided psychoeducation about anxiety and the impact anxiety has on Jim's thoughts, behaviors, and feelings. Jim and his parents were then taught coping strategies (e.g., thought identification and cognitive modification) to identify his anxious thoughts, challenge those anxious thoughts, and identify more helpful, alternative thoughts. Over time, the frequency and intensity of Jim's worries decreased and he was able to fall asleep within 30 minutes. Concentration improved. Mood was less worried. With anxiety in control, the parents described Jim as a different child. He was more outgoing. He was making some new friends and was more willing to try new things. There were occasional worries, but Jim and his parents were better equipped to deal with them.

VIGNETTE 2: YOUNG TEEN WITH SOCIAL PHOBIA

Susie is a 13-year-old girl who presented for evaluation of school refusal. She was in the seventh grade and had recently started junior high school. Junior high had the added demands of changing teachers and classrooms for each subject. During the first 2 months of school, Susie missed 15 days for stomachaches and headaches. Anxiety about attending school and somatic complaints occurred in the mornings on school days. If Susie was successful in convincing her mother to let her stay home, the physical complaints disappeared. There were no somatic symptoms on weekends.

Susie had a long history of difficulties in social and performance situations. She was uncomfortable talking to new peers and speaking to adults. She became very anxious when called on in class, fearing that she would give the wrong answer and other students would laugh at her. She was often absent when scheduled to read in front of the class or give an oral report. Susie had a history of panic attacks that were precipitated by speaking in front of her classmates. The attacks were described as 5 to 10 minutes of shortness of breath, heart racing, flushing, and dizziness. Susie did not experience bullying at school.

Developmental history was remarkable for a toddler who was reticent, avoidant, and needed much reassurance in new situations. Susie was shy and had only a few friends. She did not join any clubs or participate in team sports. She took piano lessons but would not perform in the recitals due to fear of "messing up" and being embarrassed. Family history revealed a mother with SP who had selective mutism as a child.

Diagnosis of SP was made. Due to the marked degree of functional impairment, SSRI medication and weekly CBT were recommended. CBT addressed Susie's anxious beliefs about making a mistake and feeling embarrassed. Additionally, Susie completed an exposure hierarchy related to her SP to decrease her avoidance and promote her understanding that she could handle anxiety-provoking situations. The interventions were beneficial, and Susie was attending school regularly within 8 weeks. Her parents no longer allowed her to stay home for minor physical ailments. She started going to movies and basketball games with girlfriends and was preparing for a piano recital.

BIBLIOGRAPHY

Achenbach TM, Rescorla LA. *Manual for the ASEBA School-age Forms & Profiles*. Burlington, VT: University of Vermont Research Center for Children, Youth, and Families, 2000. Available at: http://www.aseba.org.

Achenbach TM, Rescorla LA. *Multicultural Supplement to the Manual for ASEBA School-Age Forms & Profiles*. Burlington, VT: University of Vermont, Research Center for Children, Youth, and Families, 2007. Available at: http://www.aseba.org.

American Academy of Child and Adolescent Psychiatry. Practice parameter for the assessment and treatment of children and adolescents with anxiety disorders. *J Am Acad Child Adolesc Psychiatry*. 2007;46:267–283.

American Psychiatric Association. *Diagnostic and Statistical Manual of Mental Disorders, Fourth Edition, Text Revision (DSM-IV-TR)*. Washington, DC: Author; 2000.

Beesdo K, Bittner A, Pine D, et al. Incidence of social anxiety disorder and the consistent risk for secondary depression in the first three decades of life. *Arch Gen Psychiatry*. 2007;64:903–912.

Bernstein GA, Bernat DH, Davis AA, et al. Symptom presentation and classroom functioning in a nonclinical sample of children with social phobia. *Depress Anxiety*. 2008;25:752–760.

Birmaher B, Khetarpal S, Brent D, et al. The Screen for Child Anxiety Related Emotional Disorders (SCARED): scale construction and psychometric characteristics. *J Am Acad Child Adolesc Psychiatry*. 1997;36:545–553.

Bittner A, Goodwin RD, Wittchen H, et al. What characteristics of primary anxiety disorders predict subsequent major depressive disorder? *J Clin Psychiatry*. 2004;65:618–626.

Bridge JA, Iyengar S, Salary CB, et al. Clinical response and risk for reported suicidal ideation and suicide attempts in pediatric antidepressant treatment: a meta-analysis of randomized controlled trials. *JAMA*. 2007;297:1683–1696.

Buckner JD, Schmidt NB, Lang AR, et al. Specificity of social anxiety disorder as a risk factor for alcohol and cannabis dependence. *J Psychiatr Res*. 2008;42:230–239.

Choy Y, Fyer AJ, Goodwin RD. Specific phobia and comorbid depression: a closer look at the National Comorbidity Survey data. *Compr Psychiatry*, 2007;48:132–136.

Ferrell CB, Beidel DC, Turner SM. Assessment and treatment of socially phobic children: a cross cultural comparison. *J Clin Child Adolesc Psychol*. 2004;33:260–268.

Foley DL, Pickles A, Maes HM, et al. Course and short-term outcomes of separation anxiety disorder in a community sample of twins. *J Am Acad Child Adolesc Psychiatry*. 2004;43:1107–1114.

Gosch EA, Flannery-Schroeder E, Mauro CF, et al. Principles of cognitive–behavioral therapy for anxiety disorders in children. *J Cogn Psychother*. 2006;20:247–262.

Hayward C, Killen JD, Hammer LD, et al. Pubertal stage and panic attack history in sixth- and seventh-grade girls. *Am J Psychiatry*. 1992;149:1239–1243.

Jensen PS, Hinshaw SP, Kraemer HC. ADHD comorbidity findings from the MTA study: comparing comorbid subgroups. *J Am Acad Child Adolesc Psychiatry*. 2001;40(2):147–158.

Kearney CA, Sims KE, Pursell CR, et al. Separation anxiety disorder in young children: a longitudinal and family analysis. *J Clin Child Adolesc Psychol*. 2003;32:593–598.

Kendall PC, Muniya C, Hudson J, et al. *The C.A.T. Project Manual for the Cognitive Behavioral Treatment of Anxious Adolescents*. Ardmore, PA: Workbook Publishing; 2002.

Last CG, Perrin S, Hersen M, et al. A prospective study of childhood anxiety disorders. *J Am Acad Child Adolesc Psychiatry*. 1996;35:1502–1510.

Layne AE, Bernat DH, Victor AM, et al. Generalized anxiety disorder in a nonclinical sample of children: symptom presentation and predictors of impairment. *J Anxiety Disord*. 2009;23:283–289.

Lewinsohn PM, Holm-Denonma JM, Small JW, et al. Separation anxiety disorder in childhood as a risk factor for future mental illness. *J Am Acad Child Adolesc Psychiatry*. 2008;47:548–555.

Lichtenstein P, Annas P. Heritability and prevalence of specific fears and phobias in childhood. *J Child Psychol Psychiatry*. 2000;41:927–937.

March JS. *Manual for the Multidimensional Anxiety Scale for Children (MASC)*. North Tonawanda, NY: Multi-Health Systems, 1997. Available at: http://www.mhs.com.

Masi G, Millepiedi S, Mucci M, et al. Generalized anxiety disorder in referred children and adolescents. *J Am Acad Child Adolesc Psychiatry.* 2004;43:752–760.

Moffitt TE, Caspi A, Harrington H, et al. Generalized anxiety disorder and depression: childhood risk factors in a birth cohort followed to age 32. *Psychol Med.* 2007;37:441–452.

Muris P, Schmidt H, Merckelbach H. The structure of specific phobia symptoms among children and adolescents. *Behav Res Ther.* 1999;37:836–868.

Ollendick TH, King NJ, Muris P. Fears and phobias in children: phenomenology, epidemiology, and aetiology. *Child Adolesc Ment Health.* 2002;7:90–106.

Pina AA, Silverman WK, Alfano CA, et al. Diagnostic efficiency of symptoms in the diagnosis of DSM-IV: generalized anxiety disorder in youth. *J Child Psychol Psychiatry.* 2002;43:959–967.

Pine DS, Cohen P, Gurley D, et al. The risk for early-adulthood anxiety and depressive disorders in adolescents with anxiety and depressive disorders. *Arch Gen Psychiatry.* 1998;55:56–64.

Reynolds CR, Kamphaus RW. *Behavior Assessment System for Children – Second Edition manual.* Circle Pines, MN: American Guidance Service Publishing, 2004.

Silverman WK, Kurtines WM, Ginsburg GS, et al. Treating anxiety disorders in children with group cognitive–behavioral therapy: a randomized clinical trial. *J Consult Clin Psychol.* 1999;67:995–1003.

Silverman WK, Pina AA, Viswesvaran C. Evidence-based psychosocial treatments for phobia and anxiety disorders in children and adolescents. *J Clin Child Adolesc Psychol.* 2008;37:105–130.

Velting ON, Setzer NJ, Albano AM. Update on and advances in assessment and cognitive–behavioral treatment of anxiety disorders in children and adolescents. *Prof Psychol Res Pr.* 2004;35:42–54.

Verduin TL, Kendall PC. Differential occurrence of comorbidity within childhood anxiety disorders. *J Clin Child Adolesc Psychol.* 2003;32:290–295.

Walkup JT, Albano AM, Piacentini J, et al. Cognitive behavioral therapy, sertraline, or a combination in childhood anxiety. *N Engl J Med.* 2008;359:2753–2766.

Weems CF, Silverman WK, La Greca AM. What do youth referred for anxiety problems worry about? Worry and its relation to anxiety and anxiety disorders in children and adolescents. *J Abnorm Child Psychol.* 2000; 28:63–72.

Wilson KA, Hayward C. A prospective evaluation of agoraphobia and depression symptoms following panic attacks in a community sample of adolescents. *J Anxiety Disord.* 2005;19:87–103.

Wood JJ, McLeod BD, Sigman M, et al. Parenting and childhood anxiety: theory, empirical findings, and future directions. *J Child Psychol Psychiatry.* 2003;44:134–151.

SUGGESTED READINGS

Practice Parameter for the Assessment and Treatment of Children and Adolescents with Anxiety Disorders.
J Am Acad Child Adolesc Psychiatry
2007;46:267–283.

Childhood Anxiety Disorders: A Guide to Research and Treatment
Authors: Deborah Beidel and Samuel Turner
Publisher: Brunner-Routledge, 2005
Hardcover 368 pages

Treating Anxious Children and Adolescents: An Evidence-Based Approach
Authors: Ronald Rapee, Ann Wignall, Jennifer Hudson, and Carolyn Schniering
Publisher: New Harbinger Publications, 2000
Hardback 195 pages

Parenting Your Anxious Child with Mindfulness and Acceptance: A Powerful New Approach to Overcoming Fear, Panic, and Worry Using Acceptance and Commitment Therapy
Author: Christopher McCurry
Publisher: New Harbinger Publications, 2009
Paperback 228 pages

What to Do When You Worry Too Much: A Kid's Guide to Overcoming Anxiety
Author: Dawn Huebner
Publisher: Magination Press, 2006
Paperback 80 pages

SUGGESTED WEBSITES

American Academy of Child and Adolescent Psychiatry: http://www.aacap.org/
United States Department of Health and Human Services, Substance Abuse and Mental Health Services Administration: http://mentalhealth.samhsa.gov (accessed April 2010).

REVIEW QUESTIONS

1. According to research, which of the following classes of psychotropic medications is the first-line treatment for pediatric anxiety disorders.
   a. SNRI
   b. Benzodiazepine
   c. SSRI
   d. Buspirone
   e. TCA

2. Which of the following anxiety disorders is characterized by a fear of doing something embarrassing or humiliating?
   a. Social phobia
   b. Generalized anxiety disorder
   c. Major depressive disorder
   d. Panic disorder
   e. Separation anxiety disorder

3. According to research, which of the following is the most effective psychosocial intervention in the treatment of pediatric anxiety disorders:
   a. Psychodynamic therapy
   b. Family systems therapy
   c. Cognitive–behavioral therapy
   d. Play therapy
   e. There is no effective psychosocial treatment

4. Generalized anxiety disorder in children and adolescents requires that they endorse at least how many associated symptoms?
   a. Two
   b. Three
   c. Zero
   d. Six
   e. One

5. Which of the following anxiety disorders is not classified as an anxiety disorder in the *DSM-IV*?
   a. Generalized anxiety disorder
   b. Social phobia
   c. Separation anxiety disorder
   d. Panic disorder
   e. Simple phobia

Answers: 1-c, 2-a, 3-c, 4-e, 5-c

CHAPTER

8

Toi Blakley Harris, MD
and John Sargent, MD

Trauma and Associated Disorders

Introduction

Millions of youth are exposed to traumatic events every year. Some are exposed to a singular event, whereas others have histories of multiple traumatic events. In Neria et al.'s 2007 systematic review of post-traumatic stress disorders (PTSDs) following disasters, they reported that greater than two thirds of the population will experience some form of traumatic event during their life span. Children and adolescents experience potentially traumatic events of varying degrees. These events may be secondary to man, nature, or medical illness. They may be intentional or unintentional, singular or repetitive. The National Child Traumatic Stress Network and others have identified traumatic stress associated with the following events: terrorism, natural disasters, refugee and war-zone trauma, medical trauma, community and school violence, domestic violence, traumatic grief, complex trauma, sexual abuse, physical abuse and neglect, and psychological maltreatment.

Since the 1980s, there has been an increased emphasis on evaluating the impact of trauma experienced during childhood and adolescence. Childhood trauma may lead to subsequent medical and psychiatric comorbidity. Examples of psychiatric comorbidity following childhood trauma include behavioral and psychological maladaptation with strongest links to anxiety and depressive disorders. Although there are a host of psychiatric conditions that may be the sequelae of childhood trauma, this chapter reviews the concepts of traumatic stress and relates them to the development of PTSD and acute stress disorder (ASD).

Background

Historically, traumatic events experienced by youth were not felt to lead to long-term adverse psychological or physical sequelae. In 1980, the term PTSD was first described by the *Diagnostic and Statistical Manual of Mental Disorders* (DSM). However, it was not until 1987 that the DSM discussed PTSD with specific reference to children victimized by trauma. Since that time, researchers have proposed additional classification systems for PTSD applicable for children, as discussed later in this chapter.

Following a traumatic event, acute and chronic physiological changes can develop. Bell has asserted that understanding these findings can assist clinicians to conceptualize how traumatic stress and PTSD can form a "biopsychosocial trap" that may result in permanent change of the neurobiological system. As a result, the literature has documented negative impacts on emotions, learning, attention, memory, and the ability to sustain life. Whether or not a child progresses to develop short- or long-term psychological ill effects after trauma is not only related to the specifics of traumatic exposure, but also to individual, family, and social–cultural or community factors.

Culture has been documented to influence the individual and collective response to trauma. Marsella and Christopher also note that culture influences the meaning of a traumatic event, subsequent symptom formation, and help-seeking behaviors. Although childhood traumatic experiences have been linked to a multitude of psychiatric disturbances and impaired legal, social, vocational, and relationship outcomes, this section will focus on ASD and PTSD.

Clinical Features and Diagnosis

Pathophysiology

Bell has reviewed the neurobiology of trauma and described the effect of trauma on multiple domains: the catecholamine system, hypothalamic–pituitary–adrenal axis (HPA), hypothalamic–pituitary–gonadal axis (HPG), and neuropsychiatric status. Increased reactivity of the sympathetic nervous system has been reported in chronically traumatized children and has manifested as physiological hyperarousal and hyperactivity. Studies have documented chronic stress alteration of the HPA system and subsequent neuroendocrine disturbances (i.e., corticosteroid and thyroid) in sexually abused girls. Additionally, research has shown the relationship between aggressive behaviors in males as the result of the HPG's response to trauma that affects cortisol, testosterone, dehydroepiandrosterone, and androstenedione. In sexually abused females, clinical observation has linked early physical maturation to a neuroendocrine response to trauma. Adult studies have examined the hippocampal volumes of adult survivors of childhood abuse with PTSD and found a smaller left hippocampal volume in comparison to matched controls. These alterations in neuroendocrine and neurocircuitry domains can manifest on physical examinations, neuroimaging, and laboratory data collection.

Clinical Evaluation

Primary care providers are frequently the first to encounter and evaluate maltreated children and adolescents. Clinical presentations following childhood traumatic experiences may vary depending upon the proximity of the event, the developmental level of the child, and cultural influences. Authors have discussed the impact of an individual's developmental level on trauma symptom formation. In 2003, Terr described four distinct features of childhood trauma: (1) "strongly visualized or otherwise repeatedly perceived memories," (2) "repetitive behaviors," (3) "trauma-specific fears," and (4) "changed attitudes about people, aspects of life, and the future." Clinically, these types of trauma patterns have different presentations.

The *Diagnostic and Statistical Manual,* 4th Edition-Text Revision (DSM-IV-TR) delineated criteria for PTSD and ASD. Following an event that included threatened serious harm or death or threat to the bodily integrity of others and or self, youth may exhibit re-experiencing, avoidance, or hyperarousal symptoms. Temporal relationships and duration and intensity of features are used to differentiate ASD from PTSD, as noted in Table 8-1.

Authors have delineated trauma types and clinical presentations based upon trauma-related factors that manifest differentially through pathophysiologic, neurocircuitry, and neuroendocrine mechanisms. Terr and the AACAP suggested that type I trauma results from a singular traumatic event and leads to the traditional DSM symptoms of PTSD (i.e., re-experiencing, avoidance, and hyperarousal). However, type II trauma or complex trauma, as described by Cook, Spinazzola, and colleagues, is due to multiple and ongoing events, and does not necessarily solely manifest as "classic" PTSD symptoms. Type II or complex trauma presents with difficulties with self-regulation in behavioral and affective domains along with physiological, cognitive/perceptual, relational, and self-attributional aberrancies. This can manifest in many variations that include mood dysregulation, aggression, dissociation, numbing, and denial. Clinical features of these forms of trauma will be highlighted later in this chapter.

TABLE 8-1   ASD and PTSD Criterion Symptoms

Symptoms	Acute Stress Disorder	Post-traumatic Stress Disorder
Re-experiencing Recurrent images, thoughts, dreams, illusions, flashback episodes, or a sense of reliving the experience; or distress on exposure to reminders of the traumatic event	One or more symptom	One or more symptom
Avoidance Avoidance of stimuli that arouse recollections of the trauma	One symptom of avoidance	Three symptoms of avoidance
Dissociative Subjective sense of numbing, detachment, or absence of emotional responsiveness; reduction in awareness of his or her surroundings, derealization, depersonalization, dissociative amnesia	Three or more symptoms	May experience dissociative flashback episodes
Hyperarousal Difficulty with sleeping, irritability, poor concentration, hypervigilance, exaggerated startle response, motor restlessness	Symptoms of anxiety or hyperarousal	Two or more symptoms
Onset of symptoms	2 days to 4 weeks	Acute if < 3 months Chronic if >3 months
Duration of symptoms	Up to 4 weeks	More than 1 month

Adapted from American Psychiatric Association. *Diagnostic and Statistical Manual of Mental Disorders, Fourth Edition (Text Revision).* Washington, DC: Author, 2000.

DSM-IV-TR utilized alternative descriptors for children while evaluating for PTSD or ASD. Children may not have the capacity to verbalize horror, fear, or helplessness and may exhibit agitated or disorganized behavior following a traumatic event. During evaluation for re-experiencing symptoms, children may display repetitive play, trauma-specific re-enactments, and have dreams without clear or recognizable content.

Although the DSM-IV-TR made reference to some differences in the clinical presentations involving young children, more scientific rigor is needed to differentiate diagnosis based upon the trauma survivor's developmental level. Lubit has noted key differences between youth and adults that make the diagnosis of PTSD problematic. Because of these challenges, children and adolescents often fail to meet full criteria for PTSD. Children's verbal abilities often render them incapable of articulating their thoughts and feelings. They may also fluctuate between numbing/withdrawal and hyperarousal symptoms.

Other authors have proposed modified criteria for PTSD that do not require the child to endorse helplessness, fear, or horror following the traumatic event and require only one symptom in the avoidance and hyperarousal categories to meet diagnostic criteria for youth. These authors have suggested these revised criteria be employed while assessing children for PTSD.

Culture influences the meaning of the traumatic event and symptom formation for the individual and the family. Researchers in the field of trauma and cross-cultural psychiatry have contributed to our understanding of this influence. Marsella and Christopher explored how cultural internal and external representations have a bearing on traumatic responses to disasters. These representations define "the way they experience the nature, meaning, and content of reality." As delineated in DSM-IV-TR, cultural variables may have a role in symptom expression and the outline for cultural formulation and culture-bound syndromes are steps to increase the clinician's understanding of the interface between culture and mental health. Within these syndromes are symptoms that overlap with criteria for many psychiatric disorders including ASD and PTSD. For example, re-experiencing symptoms such as flashbacks may be perceived as "visions." Dissociation could be seen as "spirit possession." Hyperarousal symptoms may be viewed as "ataque de nervios" depending upon an individual's cultural background and/or acculturation to western views of psychological disturbance. The interpretation of a child's response to a traumatic event determines the caregiver's response and whether subsequent assistance outside of the family system will be sought and accepted.

Epidemiology

Primary care physicians frequently encounter children and adolescents who have been traumatized. The agents of childhood and adolescent trauma may be multifactorial. These sources of trauma are due to man, nature, medical illness, or combinations. Evidence has suggested that traumatic events that were interpersonal in nature, recurrent, or those that involved a life threat carried a greater risk for psychological distress including PTSD than other sequelae of trauma.

According to the United States Department of Health and Human Services, more than 3.5 million children and adolescents received evaluations by children's protective services for suspected neglect or abuse in 2007; 794,000 of these youth were determined to have experienced maltreatment. During 2007, Child Protective Services reported the following data regarding youth maltreatment in the United States: 59% neglect, 10.8% physical abuse, 7.6% sexual abuse, 4.2% psychological maltreatment, 4.2% "other" maltreatment (abandonment, threats to the child, congenital drug addiction), <1% medical neglect, and 13.1% multiple maltreatments.

According to the literature, the population sampled and the criteria used to define a traumatic event each has bearing on the prevalence rates. There are no available data on the lifetime prevalence of ASD. Studies conducted with children exposed to traumatic injuries did not support childhood ASD as a predictor for subsequent PTSD. These studies did not demonstrate significant clinical correlations between those who met criteria for ASD at 1 month follow-up, 8–10%, and those with PTSD diagnosed between 3 and 6 month follow-up visits, 6–25%. Acute stress reactions where dissociation was not present proved to be a stronger prediction of PTSD.

A review of the PTSD prevalence literature found that 16–43% of rural youth and 39–75% of urban youth had exposure to the type of a traumatic event described as "actual or threatened death or serious injury, or a threat to the physical integrity of self or others," prior to the age of 16. Furthermore, up to 68% of youth in a primary care setting have reported being exposed to potentially traumatic events and greater than half of these youth encountered multiple such events. As a result, 25% of exposed youth met full or partial criteria for PTSD. Data also suggest that the likelihood of developing PTSD and other mental health disorders increases with each traumatic exposure.

Comorbidity and Differential Diagnosis

As discussed previously, children and adolescents exposed to traumatic events may develop a myriad of psychological sequelae and psychiatric disorders. They may present to primary care offices with high-risk behaviors such as sexual acting out, self-harming behavior, or externalizing disorders that manifest as aggression towards others. In addition to screening for ASD and PTSD, youth who are traumatized have an increased risk for frequently occurring comorbid psychiatric disorders. Therefore, it is prudent that they are screened for high-risk behaviors such as sexual acting out, self-harming behaviors, and the following diagnostic groups: (1) other anxiety disorders, (2) mood disorders (major depressive disorder, dysthymia), (3) disruptive behavior disorders (attention-deficit hyperactive disorder subtypes, oppositional defiant disorder, and conduct disorder), (4) substance-use disorders, (5) somatoform disorders, (6) eating disorders, and (7) borderline personality disorder.

Risk-Resilience Factors

As described above, all youth exposed to a traumatic event do not go on to develop adverse psychological sequelae. Collingshaw and colleagues studied resilience, defined as "positive adaptation in the face of adversity." In this study of individuals who experienced repeated sexual and or physical abuse, 44.5% were found to not develop psychiatric disorders or suicidality over a 30-year period. Similar rates of resilience were found by DuMont who identified 48% without difficulties during adolescence. Almost 33% were found to manifest resilience in adulthood despite prior trauma histories.

Protective circumstances that contribute to a child's or adolescent's resilience appear to include genetic, biological, cognitive, interpersonal, and social factors. Individual attributes that promote resiliency include intelligence, easy or positive temperament, internal locus of control, effective coping strategies, a secure attachment relationship, special talents, and spirituality. These strengths often recruit adults to be engaged with and support youth in adverse circumstances.

Sources of resilience that are external to the trauma survivor are also essential in the mitigation against adversity. Those cited included the availability of adults who provide parental warmth, affection, and acceptance. Additionally, the role of supportive networks or "villages" was also noted as an important external support to buffer against traumatic exposures and an individual's premorbid risk factors.

Researchers have also delineated risk factors that lead to maladaptation following a traumatic event and increase the likelihood that PTSD will develop. Vulnerability factors can be classified as individual, family, cultural/environmental, or trauma-related. According to studies, having these attributes places individuals at risk: a genetic predisposition for anxiety disorders, temperamental behavioral inhibition, having a prior anxiety disorder, female gender, and limited cognitive abilities. Kassam-Adams and colleagues noted that an early postinjury elevated heart rate can be seen as an early physiological marker of hyperarousal predictive of full or partial PTSD.

The data regarding the impact of family characteristics on later maladaptation to traumatic events has been mixed. The association of parental post-traumatic stress symptoms (PTSS) to child PTSS was found to occur not only in the face of parental distress. A myriad of factors were reported to be involved that included impaired modeling of adjustment to trauma that could directly alter the youth's avoidance behaviors, genetic vulnerabilities, and underlying poorly perceived parental care.

A recent review outlined evidence supporting the heritability of PTSD. Studies involving 11 twin subjects have shown three major findings that support the role of genetics in PTSD.

The first one involves the *gene–environment correlation* that points to how an individual selects his/her environment and thus potential exposure to traumatic events. Prior longitudinal studies have shown that childhood adaptation and personality characteristics (i.e., neuroticism) are predictive of future stressful life events. Twin studies also suggest that genetics could partially account for the susceptibility to develop PTSD among adults. Lastly, limited evidence from twin studies has shown "the majority of the genes that affect risk for PTSD also influence risk for other psychiatric disorders and vice versa." The disorders mentioned in this review were major depression, generalized anxiety disorder, panic disorder, alcohol, drug, and nicotine dependence.

Caregivers who are not in tune with their child's psychological distress, either due to their own personal psychological distress or due to their lack of capacity to provide emotional validation or to psychologically support their child further inhibit the trauma victim's ability to adapt.

Trauma-related factors predictive of PTSD involve the nature of the traumatic event and frequency of traumatic events. Traumatic events due to *interpersonal traumatic events* appear more likely to result in PTSD in comparison to *accidental events*. Chronicity versus a singular exposure to a traumatic event increases the likelihood that PTSD will ensue. Moreover, if an individual is closer in proximity to the traumatic event, the risk for psychological maladaptation is higher. These individual, family, and environmental factors determine whether trauma exposure will lead to maladaptation and subsequent psychological problems or post-traumatic growth.

Ko from the National Child Traumatic Stress Network discussed how some minority youth are at increased risk for PTSD due to a variety of political, social, and economic factors. Many minority immigrant youth are at increased risk for exposure to traumatic stress resulting from war-related violence experienced in their countries of origin and or as a result of traumatic events during immigration to the United States. Other ethnic minority youth have increased rates of violence in their communities and a disproportionate number of these youth are involved with gangs and/or impacted by gang-violence. Although all ethnic groups have children and adolescents who are maltreated, disproportionate amounts of African-American, Latino, Native American children have been placed in foster care following substantiated maltreatment. Increased rates of exposure to traumatic events are compounded by decreased access to early and accurate intervention. Inadequate responses to acute stress reactions can result from mental health disparities, and from decreased access to available social, mental health and health services following disasters/traumatic events. This further increases the likelihood of long-term adverse psychosocial adaptation to traumatic events.

Because traumatized youth rarely seek mental health intervention on their own and families often do not recognize the signs and symptoms associated with ASD and/or PTSD, pediatricians and other primary care providers are poised to screen for traumatic exposure within the context of their working relationship with children, adolescents, and their families. This trusted therapeutic partnership represents an extraordinary opportunity for pediatricians and primary care physicians to identify and refer youth for mental health treatment if needed.

Clinical Course

The Adverse Childhood Experiences (ACE) study documented the association between childhood adverse events and negative adult outcomes. Individuals who experience traumatic events in childhood and adolescence are at risk for medical complications, psychiatric disturbances, and impaired social functioning as they develop and in adulthood. In particular, survivors of complex trauma that occurs early in life and is multiple and or chronic and prolonged have been shown to have the maximum risk for adverse outcomes. Repeated experience of victimization may occur with chronic medical conditions, but most often occurs due to interpersonal factors through maltreatment. This results in the interference with secure attachment formation and normative neurobiological processes that allow for optimum cognitive development, for an individual to acquire the ability to modulate his/her emotions in response to stress, establish a positive self-concept, form interpersonal relationships, and then acquire the ability to effectively solve problems. As a result, complex trauma survivors are at risk to develop psychological disturbances that overlap with anxiety, mood, disruptive, cognitive, and substance misuse disorders.

Terr's review presents clinical correlates of differing types of trauma. Youth who sustain single-event traumas are more likely to develop symptoms characteristic of PTSD, remember detailed information about the trauma, and manifest "omens" and perceptual difficulties. If the trauma occurred after the age of 36 months, they are able to provide clear details of the event with occasional misperceptions and worries about future traumas. However, children and adolescents with prior histories of complex trauma manifest varied symptom patterns of denial, numbing, self-hypnosis, dissociation, and rage that may be confused with the following diagnoses: conduct disorder, attention-deficit hyperactivity disorders, depression or dissociative disorders.

Various studies show that exposure to at least one traumatic event in childhood can lead to PTSD in 14.5–25% of individuals. Others exposed to trauma may have symptoms of ASD. In this review, 88% of children admitted to hospital following motor vehicle accidents and 83% of their caregivers recorded symptoms in one or more of the four ASD domains (hyperarousal, re-experiencing, dissociation, and avoidance). Arousal was most often identified by parents, whereas children were more likely to endorse symptoms of dissociation.

In addition to short- and long-term psychological sequelae of childhood trauma, adverse medical outcomes for these youth have been described, such as high health care use, increased risk for many causes of early death in adulthood, increased rates of asthma, allergy, gastrointestinal disturbance, and headaches. Along with these medical concerns, primary care physicians are also called to treat medical conditions that are the direct result of maltreatment, accidents, disasters and or acts of terrorism. These medical disorders may require acute, brief care, or longer term management which may involve several providers within a multidisciplinary team.

Assessment

Trauma screening procedures for primary care physicians and other frontline clinicians have been recommended by several authors. Multiple informants should be interviewed to obtain the most accurate information. It is important to assess the current level of safety of the traumatized child or adolescent as well as determine the level of support available to that youth. This will greatly affect the manner and location of mental health services provided.

As the youth's clinician, there is a dual role as a mandated reporter of suspicion of child abuse or neglect. Conflicted feelings may ensue for the clinician about contacting childhood-protection agencies and legal authorities with maltreatment allegations if a long-standing relationship with the child and or family exists. However, as a mandated reporter, clinicians serve as the frontline protection for children and adolescents who may be experiencing psychological, medical, physical, and or sexual abuse and neglect. Information received during history gathering or on physical examination that points towards maltreatment must be documented and reported. Prior to reporting, it is recommended that the process be explained to the caregivers and child in a compassionate manner.

The clinician should work toward maintaining a therapeutic alliance with a patient and family subsequent to reporting. The relationship has a greater likelihood of being preserved when information is presented in a caring and informative way highlighting the legal obligation to act in the child's "best interest" and to ensure the child's safety. If the legal authorities must be contacted, this is done in conjunction with the physical and psychological trauma evaluations. Additionally, the child and family members require psychoeducation and support during and after this time of disclosure.

At times, the clinician has the suspicion or knowledge that the perpetrator of the abuse is a parent or caretaking adult. In these instances it is important for the clinician to be particularly sensitive to the child's safety. If the clinician is particularly concerned, an emergency child welfare consultation can be called and the child welfare professional can be advised of the clinician's acute concern and a determination of the child's immediate safety can be conducted. This most often will occur in the emergency room or on an inpatient ward but can also occur in the clinician's office. In these instances, the parent or caretaker can become aggressive and can be threatening. The clinician should know how to alert security or the police if he or she feels threatened. The clinician should maintain a calm and compassionate approach but also know how to maintain safety and order.

General considerations for the primary care clinician while conducting an assessment for trauma include monitoring vital signs, weight, and other physical signs associated with trauma and maltreatment including injuries and bruises. Post-trauma, youth may show elevated heart rates that have been associated with the development of PTSD. It is unclear whether this sign is a state or trait phenomenon of PTSD. Further investigation should clarify this. Children who have been maltreated may also have been neglected and may show signs of malnutrition. A history of sexual abuse warrants detailed physical examination of genitalia and laboratory examination for pregnancy and sexually transmitted diseases.

While screening youth for a history of trauma, it is important to have an open dialog privately with the child and or adolescent about his or her traumatic experiences. The practice parameter for the assessment and treatment of youth with PTSD published by the American Academy of Child and Adolescent Psychiatry notes many reasons why clinicians have not explored trauma details: avoidance of difficult topics, "fear of tainting the child's description of the trauma" for court testimony, etc. Experts have countered that it is crucial to allow the youth an opportunity to discuss trauma details. This will be beneficial therapeutically and will also assist with the diagnosis of any psychiatric disorders, such as ASD and PTSD. The clinician should never become an interrogator. That is not his or her role. The clinician should let the child know that he is being heard and that the clinician will act to ensure his or her safety. The goal of this discussion is to have enough information to file a child-protection petition and to reassure the child. This will further the relationship between the clinician and the child and help the child feel that his experience is being validated.

Developmental considerations must be applied throughout the evaluation and treatment process. Several authors and professional groups have suggested guidelines and diagnostic parameters, as described in Table 8-2.

If a youth discloses trauma exposure, several standardized measures are available to assess symptom severity during the clinic visit. These PTSD screening instruments can be sorted into two categories: semistructured interviews and self-report measures, as summarized in Table 8-3.

Prior to entering the formal mental health treatment phase, the initial stages of psychological care begin with a complete mental health evaluation of the child and his or her context. History gathering must be done in a caring and sensitive manner so as not to retraumatize the youth. Collateral reports from educators, family, and other key figures in the child's life can provide critical details that will assist in the evaluation process.

Before the child is evaluated by a mental health professional, primary care physicians can lay the foundation for a successful transition. Many families maintain stigma about mental illness and seeking care from mental health providers. The clinician can describe the youth's symptoms in terms of 'warning signs' or areas of concern (i.e., disrupted sleep, nightmares, fearfulness, avoidance of certain activities) that will educate the family about symptoms associated with maladaptive responses to traumatic experiences and emphasize the need for further evaluation and possible treatment.

TABLE 8-2	Essentials of Assessment for Trauma and Associated Symptomatology: Developmental Diagnostic Tips
Age	**Diagnostic Considerations**
0–6 years	Children less than 36 months will most probably have difficulty verbalizing information related to the trauma and/or symptoms Trauma re-enactment through play and repetitive behaviors may occur in children 12 months or older; post-traumatic play is "compulsively repetitive, represents part of the trauma, and fails to relieve anxiety" Between the ages of 3 and 4 years, children's sleep architecture permits dreaming to occur regularly. These dreams may be frightening. However, verbal abilities may also impact the recall of dreams Generalized anxiety symptoms Avoidance of scenarios with and without a specific connection to prior trauma Preoccupation with particular symbols or words with and without a specific connection to prior trauma Disordered sleep patterns Difficulties with separation from parents
6–11 years	Cohen et al. (2008) suggests asking children older than 8 years "Since the last time I saw you, has anything really scary or upsetting happened to you or your family?" If the child is younger than 8 years, it was recommended that the caregiver and the child be queried It is important to question children and adolescents separately if physical examination findings and or clinical observations warrant child maltreatment concerns School-age children may present with school and social difficulties related to motoric hyperactivity, impaired concentration, and behavioral problems (forms of avoidance, or numbing)
11 years+	Acutely, adolescents have been reported to experience invasive images, restlessness and aggression, difficulty sleeping, difficulty concentrating, loss of interest in activities, social withdrawal, and alterations in opinions and attitudes Chronically, teens may manifest aggression, mood instability, detachment, restricted affect, numbing, sadness, dissociative symptoms, and self-injury

Primary care providers who collaborate with psychiatrists, psychologists, and social workers on a regular basis can model for families the need for a multidisciplinary team in the trauma-recovery process. Establishing a systematic referral mechanism and methods of communication will ensure effective continuity of care and increase the likelihood of adherence. The partnership between primary care and mental health is essential for ongoing identification, monitoring, and treatment of traumatized youth.

A mental health referral is initiated to evaluate the psychological well-being of the traumatized child or adolescent. In addition to referrals for traumatized youth, the primary clinician may recommend a parent or caretaker be evaluated by a mental health professional. By improving the caretaker's emotional stability, the child will have more favorable long-term outcomes.

Treatment

Psychosocial Treatments

The goals of treatment are to reduce the severity of symptoms, assist the youth's return to safe development and functioning, and to prevent relapse and/or the emergence of comorbid psychiatric conditions. This will require the family, other key adult figures, and social-cultural

TABLE 8-3	Screening Instruments for Children and Adolescents with Trauma Exposure			
	Instrument	**Acronym**	**Age Range (years)**	**Administration Time (minutes)**
Semistructured interviews	Child and Adolescent Psychiatric Assessment: Life Events Section & PTSD Module	CAPA-LES	9–17	10–60
	Children's PTSD Inventory	CAPA-PTSD		
Self-report measures	Children Post-traumatic Stress	CPTSDI	7–18	5–20
	Reaction Index	CPTS-RI	8+	20–45
	Trauma Symptom Checklist for Children	TSCC	8–16	15–20
	Child PTSD Symptom Scale	CPSS	8–18	15
	Screen for Child Anxiety Related Emotional Disorders	SCARED	7–19	15–20

From Spates RC, Waller S, Samaraweera N, et al. Behavioral aspects of trauma in children and youth. *Pediatr Clin North Am.* 2003;50:901–918.

supports and networks to collaborate with treatment to promote optimum development and adaptation.

Several mental health and health entities such as the American Academy of Child and Adolescent Psychiatry, the American Psychiatric Association, the American Psychological Association, and the National Child Traumatic Stress Network, have educational tools and information available that will inform children and caregivers of the effects of trauma and the strategies to decrease potential adverse effects and foster resiliency. Basic points highlighted in these references include information about restoring sleep hygiene, consistency and predictability in the child's daily routine, exercise, care for their current caregivers, utilization of existing social, cultural, and religious supports, etc. It is advisable to have these materials available during your discussions with traumatized youth and families. Depending upon the family's religious affiliation, collaboration with members of the faith community might also lend further support in this process.

Following acute trauma associated with either man-made or non-man-made events, Sargent described the treatment process in a series of eight steps which are summarized in Table 8-4. These stages are applicable in the acute treatment of children after traumatic injury and acute abuse as well as in treatment of children with PTSD and children who have experienced repeated trauma and evidence complex traumatic stress.

TABLE 8-4	Eight Steps in Traumatic Stress Treatment

(1) Ensuring safety
(2) Ensuring availability of basic needs
(3) Building child and family knowledge about the trauma and its effects
(4) Reinforcing normative behavioral routines
(5) Identifying and supporting the child's emotional states
(6) Supporting those who support the child
(7) Building the child's trauma narrative and helping the child to share the narrative with important others
(8) Building a compassionate and healing response to the trauma (in family, community, and wider society)

From Sargent J. Eight guides to the treatment of traumatic stress in children and adolescents. *Psychiatric Times.* 2009;26:9–13.

During these eight steps of child trauma treatment, Sargent recommends that safety and basic needs are attended to at the onset of treatment. This is followed by education about the potential impact of the traumatic event and subsequent psychological and physical impairments while encouraging caregivers and families to restore daily routines to promote a sense of normalcy for the traumatized youth. Supporting the emotional states of the child and caregivers was recommended as an essential phase of treatment prior to assisting the trauma survivor with the development of a trauma narrative to integrate the adverse event(s). The final stage of Sargent's treatment model includes the mobilization of the survivor's support system, community, and larger society to promote healing.

When encountering a youth who has been victimized with multiple and chronic traumatic events, the National Child Traumatic Stress Network's Complex Trauma Workgroup has delineated six components for complex trauma intervention and treatment. The first phase of this treatment process includes two features. The first step would be to establish *safety* in the home, school, and neighborhood community. Situations that are complicated by intimate partner violence or neighborhood violence require a careful clinical approach. When intimate partner violence has occurred, the clinician can stress his or her concern about the safety and well-being of the child and offer the family information about dealing with such violence including the national domestic violence hotline phone number and support from community workers who deal regularly with domestic violence. When neighborhood violence is severe, social service support may be offered to assist the family as they consider ways to ensure safety at home. Treatment must aim to establish and maintain expectations of safety and predictability. Secondly, facilitation of the youth's capacity for *self-regulation* and management of his/her arousal and re-establishment of self-control is next. During this phase, clinicians work to assist the youth with regulation of physiology, mood, behavior, cognition, and interpersonal encounters.

As the youth's ability to recognize, modulate, and correctly verbalize thoughts and feelings improves, treatment can progress to the second phase which includes *self-reflective information processing, relational engagement, and positive affect enhancement.* Self-reflective information processing entails assisting the youth construct self-descriptions of the trauma(s) or narratives while reflecting on experiences and developing competencies in problem-solving and planning.

Relational engagement focuses on helping the youth form proper attachments to those with whom he/she currently interacts. With treatment, youth would receive specific instruction on how to improve interpersonal skills such as "assertiveness, cooperation, perspective-taking, boundaries and limit setting, reciprocity, social empathy and the capacity for physical and emotional intimacy." While relational engagement targets interpersonal interactions, *positive affect enhancement* aims to improve the youth's personal sense of self-worth and value. This is accomplished by identifying an individual's sources of strengths or resiliency, promoting achievement competence, imagination, creativity, mastering seeking, community building, and the capacity to experience pleasure.

The final phase of *traumatic experiences integration* is generally not recommended until after a substantial period of stabilization. Some trauma experts note it may be beneficial for some youth impacted by complex trauma to process their traumatic memories; however, others suggest clinicians who work with these individuals "foster integration of traumatic experiences through a focus on recognizing and coping with present triggers within a trauma framework."

Clinical evidence is limited with the treatment of ASD but has shown that psychotherapy, psychoeducation, and pharmacotherapy (if the degree of psychological distress is not relieved with nonpharmacological strategies) have been helpful. Engaging the parents and youth in the treatment process is fundamental to the success of the treatment. As discussed above, education about the impact of trauma as well as providing useful parent-management strategies can also be an important adjunct to the immediate recovery process following acute trauma.

Cohen and colleagues' review of evidence-based treatments for pediatric PTSD found: (1) child–parent psychotherapy, (2) trauma-focused cognitive behavioral therapy (TF-CBT), (3) cognitive behavioral interventions for trauma in schools (CBITS), (4) cognitive-based cognitive behavioral therapy, and (5) brief psychoanalytic psychotherapy were proven effective in at least one randomized controlled treatment trial. These therapies are summarized in Table 8-5. Primary care clinicians can make sure that the mental health professionals to whom they refer trauma victims for follow-up care know, and can utilize, one of these treatment modalities.

There are other forms of treatment for traumatized youth that either have no proven efficacy or have been found to be dangerous. Psychological debriefing immediately after a traumatic event was shown in a randomized trial to be neither harmful nor beneficial. Types of nonstructured therapy (i.e., nondirective play) have been proven to be less effective than other methods discussed previously. Restrictive holding or rebirthing treatment modalities in which the child is restricted, bound, with water or food withheld has been associated with death and is not recommended.

Psychopharmacologic Treatments

As described previously, biological alterations occur as the result of trauma. Monitoring nutrition and sleep are frequently crucial aspects of treatment of both acute and chronic traumatic stress. Pharmacotherapy to address sleep, anxiety, mood dysregulation, agitation, and comorbid psychosis is also often useful. Although traumatized youth often show other co-morbid psychiatric disturbances, this section will focus on psychopharmacological interventions utilized to treat ASD and PTSD.

The literature has limited evidence to support the use of pharmacotherapy in the pediatric population. Most of the data are derived from adult trials and case reports. Currently, the Food and Drug Administration (FDA) has not approved any medications for children or adolescents with ASD or PTSD. The following categories of medications have been utilized to treat youth with ASD and PTSD: (1) antidepressants, (2) adrenergic agents, (3) atypical antipsychotics, (4) anticonvulsants, and (5) benzodiazepines.

Antidepressants have been used widely in clinical practice to treat PTSD symptoms in children and adolescents. A randomized trial of children with severe burns proved lower rates of ASD in those who received imipramine versus chloral hydrate. Despite the proven efficacy of imipramine in this study and amitriptyline in other findings, these medications should be used with caution due to risk of cardiotoxicity. Selective serotonin reuptake inhibitors (SSRIs) are widely used in the pediatric population for the treatment of PTSD. SSRIs have been proven in adults to reduce the core symptoms of re-experiencing, avoidance/numbing, and hyperarousal. However, only paroxetine and sertraline have FDA indications for PTSD in adults. Selective serotonin–norepinephrine reuptake inhibitors (SNRIs) and SSRIs have evidence to support treatment of noncombat PTSD. The monoamine oxidase inhibitors phenelzine and brofaromine have limited evidence for efficacy in the treatment of ASD and PTSD. The FDA's black box warning on antidepressants mandates that they be prescribed only after appropriate informed consent and monitoring for suicidal behavior and ideation. Authors have summarized clinical guidelines for pharmacotherapy options utilized in childhood trauma survivors based on adult and pediatric literature, and are summarized in Table 8-6.

Thus, many classes of pharmacologic agents have been utilized for the treatment of PTSD in youth. The SSRIs can be used quite effectively by primary care physicians to treat

TABLE 8-5	Evidence-Based Psychotherapies for Childhood Trauma Survivors		
Name	**Age Group**	**Description**	**Number of Sessions**
Child–parent psychotherapy	Up to 6 years	Focus on addressing maladaptive interactions between parent–child; regulation of affect, behavior, and restoration of biological rhythms	40–50
Trauma-focused Cognitive Behavioral Therapy (TF-CBT)	3–17 years	Essential components of TF-CBT: psychoeducation, parenting skills to address the youth's symptoms, individual relaxation skills, affective modulation techniques, and cognitive coping strategies Second phase of treatment focuses on the development of a trauma narrative Child–parent sessions are held to improve communication within the relationship, to discuss the youth's trauma narrative, increase resilience, and plan for safety	
Cognitive behavioral intervention for trauma in schools (CBITS)		The cognitive-based cognitive behavioral therapy resembles TF-CBT except it does not have particular anxiety reduction strategies or a relaxation component. There is an affective modulation facet that targets "activity scheduling and reclaiming life." Detail is given to cognitive restructuring with "reliving the trauma" and to discern between harmless and harmful environmental cues Limited caregiver component; however, teachers participate	10
Brief psychoanalytic psychotherapy		The key components of this form of treatment included engagement, exploration of topics brought up by child in play, "re-working of key topics," and treatment termination. Caregivers also participate to address trauma history, safety, and behavioral concerns	30

From Cohen JA, Kelleher KJ, Mannarino AP. Identifying, treating and referring traumatized children: the role of pediatric providers. *Arch Pediatr Adolesc Med.* 2008;162:447–452.

anxiety and mood problems associated with traumatic stress in the pediatric population. Monitoring recommended by FDA guidelines can be done in collaboration with mental health providers if warranted. It is advisable that primary care physicians work closely with child and adolescent psychiatrists to manage the use of other psychopharmacologic agents. In all situations the use of psychopharmacologic treatment should be integrated with psychosocial support for the child and family and with the evidence-based psychosocial treatments discussed above.

TABLE 8-6	Clinical Guidelines for Pharmacotherapy for Childhood Trauma Survivors	
Medication Category	**Description**	**Adverse Effects**
Antidepressants	First line for noncombat PTSD, reduced core symptoms of PTSD, FDA approved for adult PTSD (paroxetine and sertraline) Venlafaxine and mirtazepine were found to be superior over placebo in trials for treatment of PTSD	Black-box warning for suicidality
Adrenergic Agents	Alpha agonists clonidine and guanfacine have both been reported as effective in open trial studies for the treatment of PTSD in pediatric populations Alpha$_1$ antagonist prazosin with preliminary findings to improve symptoms of PTSD particularly in combat-related PTSD Beta-adrenergic blocking agent propranolol has been recorded as mixed results in literature for the symptom of hyperarousal No FDA approval	Cardiac effects (i.e., hypotension, bradycardia)
Atypical Antipsychotics	Reserved for youth who are not responsive to other medications or if psychosis is present. During the acute phase of treatment, atypical antipsychotics have been beneficial when psychosis, affective dysregulation, agitation, and dissociation are present No FDA approval	Black-box warning for suicidality Prolongation of QTC interval Extrapyramidal symptoms Metabolic syndrome
Anticonvulsants	Carbamazepine (CBZ) and valproic acid (VPA) used in youth with chronic symptoms of PTSD. VPA may reduce avoidance symptoms in PTSD. CBZ has been shown to decrease re-experiencing symptoms No FDA approval	Black-box warning hepatotoxicity (VPA). Suicidality risk for all anticonvulsants Polycystic ovary syndrome (VPA), Pancreatitis (VPA), Steven–Johnson Syndrome (CBZ).
Benzodiazepines	Benzodiazepines have been used clinically to reduce anxiety and improve sleep. No efficacy with core PTSD symptoms. Not recommended as monotherapy No FDA approval	Dependence Increased PTSD symptoms after early treatment; worsening PTSD symptoms after withdrawal

Conclusions

Many children and adolescents are exposed to potentially traumatic events each year. Based upon individual, family, and trauma-related risk and protective factors, the individual may or may not progress to develop adverse psychological and or physical sequelae. In order to lessen the possibilities of negative outcomes, authors have provided clinical guidelines to be employed acutely to ensure safety, basic needs, and psychological support while conducting a thorough clinical evaluation.

Medical and mental health professionals who interface with children and families have been confronted with the challenges of providing a holding environment for traumatized youth. Throughout the evaluation process and possible treatment phase, collaboration with educators, extended family, and other areas of identified support are crucial elements in promoting resiliency in the face of adversity. Evidence-based psychotherapies and pharmacotherapy regimens according to described clinical guidelines have been utilized successfully to address negative psychological sequelae of childhood trauma. Systematic and coordinated approaches to reduce the potential for traumatic exposure, and increased access to care for populations at risk for traumatic events are warranted to globally prevent the long-term emotional and behavioral consequences of childhood trauma.

CASE VIGNETTES

VIGNETTE 1: SCHOOL-AGED GIRL WITH EXTERNALIZING SYMPTOMS FOLLOWING TYPE I TRAUMA

Khalie is an 8-year-old African American female who was evacuated from New Orleans three days after Hurricane Katrina struck her home in New Orleans. Khalie, her 5-year-old sister, her mother and maternal grandmother had temporary shelter in the Superdome while awaiting transport to public housing in Houston, Texas.

Prior to Katrina, Khalie was an eager and enthusiastic third-grade student. She had excelled academically and demonstrated leadership skills in school. Previously, Khalie did not have a history of defiance, difficulty sustaining attention in class or problems with completing her assignments. Since beginning school in Houston several months ago, her mother has received numerous phone calls from Khalie's teacher regarding her "lack of focus, poor academic performance and defiance in the classroom." In addition to her school adjustment problems, Khalie began having problems sleeping after the hurricane and now needs to sleep with her mother in order to initiate sleep onset. Her mother has sought help for Khalie through a local church community they have recently joined.

Key features: Khalie's history is characteristic of type I trauma and PTSD related to the "shock" of the natural disaster Hurricane Katrina and subsequent disruptive events. Following the hurricane, she has experienced sleep disruption, and a decline in academic performance due to inattention, irritability, and defiance. Attention-deficit hyperactivity disorder-combined type and oppositional defiant disorder were both considered in the differential diagnosis. However, the origin of these symptoms in close proximity to the traumatic event and prior history of excellent premorbid functioning at school and home pointed the diagnosis toward symptoms related to type I trauma (hyperarousal, and suspected re-experiencing symptoms). Her symptoms of post-traumatic stress have persisted for several months without formal mental health intervention. However, recently, her mother has sought assistance via her faith-based community. Many institutions of faith provide psychological support for their congregants via religious counseling and or have licensed mental health professionals co-located in their religious institutions. It is important to respect this form of counseling and for health and mental health professionals to work in collaboration with clergy to improve both continuity of care and outcomes. For additional information about the provision of mental health and faith-based collaboration in hurricane affected disaster populations that are diverse, refer to the All Healers' Mental Health Alliance.

VIGNETTE 2: AN ADOLESCENT MALE WITH MULTIPLE LIFE TRAUMAS

James is a 17-year-old Caucasian male who was hospitalized for pulmonary complications related to cystic fibrosis. Upon admission, his respiratory status was severely compromised which required intubation for a short time period. During his hospital stay, members of the primary service became concerned about his emotional state. The nurses noted James frequently stayed up all night, intermittently fluctuated between sadness and irritability, and appeared "on edge." Although he did not have a prior psychiatric history, a psychiatry consult was requested to assess for psychiatric disturbance.

During the evaluation process, James' mother confided in the team in a separate interview that their family moved six months ago due to job loss and financial instability. She reported that over the last month he had begun to associate with gang-members in their community. During the two weeks prior to admission, he began to display changes in sleep and mood. Following several days of consistent contact, James relayed to the psychiatry team that he had been initiated into a local gang for "protection." Since that time, he has witnessed and participated in numerous episodes of interpersonal violence.

Key features: James' symptoms are acute in nature and most likely the result of multiple traumatic events that have occurred in association with his medical care and through recent exposure to of community (gang and interpersonal) violence. Although his symptoms are impairing his functioning, they do not meet the criteria for ASD or PTSD. Because of the clinical impairment, he warranted psychosocial and pharmacological interventions to restore sleep, stabilize his mood, and decrease anxiety symptoms. James was at risk for comorbid anxiety disorders, mood disturbance, and substance-related disorders and required ongoing mental health follow-up. Leaders in his treatment team explored his desire to continue gang participation. Because he sought assistance from the team to terminate his relationship with the gang, the team accessed support for him via contacting law-enforcement agencies and local community groups with a long-standing history of successful gang termination. For additional information about youth gang membership refer to the National Gang Crime Research Center at www.ngcrc.com.

BIBLIOGRAPHY

American Academy of Child and Adolescent Psychiatry. Practice parameters for the assessment and treatment of children and adolescents with posttraumatic stress disorder. *J Am Acad Child Adolesc Psychiatry*. 1998;37:4S–26S.

American Psychiatric Association. *Diagnostic and Statistical Manual of Mental Disorders DSM-IV-TR Fourth Edition (Text Revision)*. Arlington, VA: American Psychiatric Publishing, Inc; 2000.

Bell C. Cultivating Resiliency in Youth [online]. Available at: http://www.giftfromwithin.org/html/cultivat.html.

Bendek DM, Zatzkick D, Ursano RJ. American Psychiatric Association Practice Guidelines: Practice Guidelines for the Treatment of Patients with Acute Stress Disorder and Posttraumatic Stress Disorder. Guideline Watch March 2009 doi 10.1176/appi.books.9780890423479.156498.

Bendek DM, Zatzkick D, Ursano RJ. Guideline Watch (March 2009) *Practice Guidelines: Practice Guidelines for the Treatment of Patients with Acute Stress Disorder and Posttraumatic Stress Disorder*. Arlington, VA: American Psychiatric Association, March 2009. Available at: http://www.psychiatryonline.com/pracGuide/loadGuidelinePdf.aspx?file=AcuteStressDisorder-PTSD_GuidelineWatch.

Bryant R, Salmon K, Sinclair E, et al. The relationship between acute stress disorder and posttraumatic stress disorder in injured children. *J Trauma Stress*. 2007;20:1075–1079.

Chavez B. A Review of Pharmacotherapy for PTSD. U.S. Pharm, 2006:31–38.

Cohen JA, Kelleher KJ, Mannarino AP. Identifying, treating and referring traumatized children: the role of pediatric providers. *Arch Pediatr Adolesc Med*. 2008;162:447–452.

Collingshaw S, Pickles A, Messer J, et al. Resilience to adult psychopathology following childhood maltreatment: evidence from a community sample. *Child Abuse Negl*. 2007;31:211–229.

Cook A, Spinazzola J, Ford J, et al. Complex trauma in children and adolescents. *Psychiatr Ann*. 2005;35:390–398.

De Bellis M, Van Dillen T. Childhood post-traumatic stress disorder: an overview. *Child Adolesc Psychiatr Clin N Am*. 2005;14:745–772.

DuMont KA, Widom CS, Czaja SJ. Predictors of resilience in abused and neglected children grown up: the role of individual and neighborhood characteristics. *Child Abuse Negl.* 2007;31:255–274.

Kassam-Adams N, Winston FK. Predicting child PTSD: the relationship between acute stress disorder and PTSD in injured children. *J Am Acad Child Adolesc Psychiatry.* 2004;43:403–411.

Kassam-Adams N, Garcia-Espana, F, Fein JA, et al. Heart rate and posttraumatic stress in injured children. *Arch Gen Psychiatry.* 2005;62(3):335–340.

Ko S. Culture and trauma briefs: promoting culturally competent trauma informed practices. In: *National Center for Child Traumatic Stress*, Vol 1, No. 1, 2005.

Koenen KC, Nugent NR, Amstadter AB. Gene-environment interaction in posttraumatic stress disorder: review, strategy and new directions for future research. *Eur Arch Psychiatry Clin Neurosci.* 2008;258:82–96.

Lubit R. Posttraumatic stress disorder in children: Overview. In: *eMedicine* http://emedicine.medscape.com/article/918844-overview, 2008.

Marsella AJ, Christopher MA. Ethnocultural considerations in disasters: an overview of research, issues, and directions. *Psychiatr Clin N Am.* 2004;27:521–539.

Neria Y, Nandi A, Galea S. Post-traumatic stress disorder following disasters: a systematic review. *Psychol Med.* 2008;38:467–480.

Pine D, Cohen, JA. Trauma in children and adolescents: risk and treatment of psychiatric sequelae. *Soc Biol Psychiatry.* 2002;51:519–531.

Sargent J. Eight guides to the treatment of traumatic stress in children and adolescents. *Psychiatric Times.* 2009;26:9–13.

Scheeringa M, Zeanah CH, Drell MJ, et al. Two approaches to diagnosing posttraumatic stress disorder in infancy and early childhood. *J Am Acad Child Adolesc Psychiatry.* 1995;34:191–200.

Scheeringa M, Zeanah CH, Myers L, et al. New findings on alternative criteria for PTSD in preschool children. *J Am Acad Child Adolesc Psychiatry.* 2003;42:561–570.

Shalev AY. Treatment failure in acute PTSD. Lessons learned about the complexity of the disorder. *Ann NY Acad Sci.* 1997;821:372–387.

Spates RC, Waller S, Samaraweera N, et al. Behavioral aspects of trauma in children and youth. *Pediatr Clin North Am.* 2003;50:901–918.

Stover CS, Berkowitz S, Marans S, Kaufman J. Posttraumatic stress disorder. In: Martin A, Volkmar FR, eds. *Lewis' Child and Adolescent Psychiatry: A Comprehensive Textbook*. Philadelphia, PA: Lippincott Williams & Wilkins; 2007:701–711.

Terr LC. Childhood traumas: an outline and overview. *Focus.* 2003;1:322–334.

Ursano RJ, Bell C, Eth S, et al. Practice guideline for the treatment of patients with acute stress disorder and posttraumatic stress disorder. *Am J Psychiatry.* 2004;161(suppl):3–31.

van der Kolk B. Developmental trauma disorder toward a rational diagnosis for children with complex trauma histories. *Psychiatr Ann.* 2005;35:401–408.

SUGGESTED READINGS

A Practical Guide to the Evaluation of Child Physical Abuse and Neglect, 2nd ed.
Angelo P. Giardino, Michelle A. Lyn, Eileen R. Giardino
Springer (Available February 2010)
Hardcover 400 pages

Collaborative Treatment of Traumatized Children and Teens: The Trauma Systems
Therapy Approach
Glenn Saxe, B. Heidi Ellis, Julie B. Kaplow
Guilford Press (2006)
Hardcover 338 pages

Effective Treatments for PTSD: Practical Guidelines from the International Society for Traumatic Stress Studies, 2nd ed.
Edna B. Foa, Terence M. Keane, Matthew J. Friedman, Judith A. Cohen
Guilford Press (2009)
Hardcover 658 pages

Trauma and Recovery
Judith Lewis Herman
Basic Books (reprint 1997)
Paperback 304 pages

Treating Trauma and Traumatic Grief in Children and Adolescents
Judith Cohen, Anthony Mannarino, Esther Deblinger
Guilford Press (June 2006)
Hardcover 256 pages

SUGGESTED WEBSITES

All Healers Mental Health Alliance (http:www.ahmha.net)
American Academy of Child and Adolescent Psychiatry (http:www.aacap.org)
American Psychiatric Association (http:www.psych.org)
American Psychological Association (http:www.apa.org)
National Child Traumatic Stress Network (http:www.nctsn.org)
National Gang Crime Research Center (http:www.ngcrc.com)

REVIEW QUESTIONS

1. Type I. traumas are consistent with the following:
   a. They are due to singular, unexpected events
   b. They are the result of chronic stressors
   c. They do not lead to characteristic PTSD symptoms
   d. All of the above
   e. None of the above

2. Which of these factors mediate the development of post-traumatic stress disorder in youth?
   a. Severity of the trauma exposure
   b. Parental trauma-related distress
   c. Temporal proximity to the traumatic event
   d. A and C are correct
   e. All of the above

3. According to the DSM IV TR, which of the following occur in children who have PTSD?
   a. Symptoms last longer than 4 weeks
   b. Repetitive play may count as a re-experiencing phenomenon seen with children
   c. Children may experience frightening dreams without dream content that might have an obvious link to the trauma
   d. A,B,C are correct
   e. None of the above

4. Children and adolescents with PTSD often have comorbid:
   a. Mental retardation
   b. Dysthymia
   c. Pervasive developmental disorder
   d. A,B,C are correct
   e. None of the above

5. In clinical practice, the following medications have been effectively utilized to reduce PTSD symptoms:
   a. Dexedrine
   b. Clonidine
   c. Daytrana
   d. A,B,C are correct
   e. None of the above

Answers: 1-a, 2-e, 3-d, 4-b, 5-b

Obsessive–Compulsive Disorder

Introduction and Background

Symptoms of obsessive–compulsive disorder (OCD) were described as far back as 1467, though in the frame of reference of that time, these symptoms were considered evidence of possession by the devil. Religious texts in the 1600s described "scrupulosity," excessive devotion, and extremes of religious doubting. Pioneers in psychiatry began studying the phenomenon as early as 1838. Sigmund Freud noted obsessions and compulsions early in his professional career, and Anna Freud proposed that ego deficits and conflicting drives led to obsessional neuroses. For many years it was thought that environmental factors, and especially family problems, played a major role in the development of OCD, leading to blaming and guilt during psychoanalytic treatment, which was the predominant treatment for many years. However, the ineffectiveness of psychoanalytic treatment for OCD has led to newer conceptualizations and treatments for this serious and tenacious disorder that frequently has its onset during childhood.

Since the 1980s there has been an explosion of research in OCD related to the discovery that the serotonin-specific reuptake inhibitors (SSRIs) can help many patients with OCD. The development of techniques like the magnetic resonance imaging (MRI) to better examine brain structure, as well as positron emission tomography (PET) and single photon emission computed tomography (SPECT) scanning to study brain metabolism and function, has played important roles as well. Studies regarding the prevalence of OCD have found that it is neither as rare as was once thought nor as prevalent as initially reported. Recent research has found evidence of genetic transmission of OCD, and possibly an infective etiology. Thus, work over the past two decades has increased the understanding and treatment of children and adolescents with OCD.

Clinical Features

Definition

In the *Diagnostic and Statistical Manual of Mental Disorders, Fourth Edition* (*DSM-IV*), OCD is defined as one of the anxiety disorders. Individuals with OCD experience certain states of mind as anxiety provoking and distressing in ways that are similar to the other anxiety disorders, but with *obsessions* and attempts to alleviate the obsessional anxiety with *compulsive behaviors*. Obsessions are defined as recurrent and persistent ideas, thoughts, impulses, or images that are experienced as intrusive and inappropriate and cause marked anxiety or distress. They are more than simply excessive worries about real-life problems as the individual recognizes that they are the product of his or her own mind, and tries to ignore or suppress them. Compulsions are defined as repetitive behaviors or mental acts that the individual feels driven to perform and are aimed at preventing distress or some dreaded event. They are not realistically connected with what they are designed to prevent or are clearly excessive. Compulsions differ from stereotypies often observed in youth with mental retardation or pervasive developmental disorders (PDDs) in that they are complex, are aimed at neutralizing an obsession, and usually serve a clear purpose unlike nonfunctional stereotypic behaviors (e.g., rocking or head-banging).

OCD requires either obsessions *or* compulsions accompanied by marked distress, consuming more than 1 hour per day, or interfering with functioning. At some point the individual recognizes that his or her symptoms are excessive or unreasonable, though *DSM-IV* notes that this criterion does not apply to children. Symptoms should not be due to a substance or a general medical condition. If another diagnosis is present, the content of the obsessions should be different from the symptoms typical of the comorbid disorder, for example, more than food and eating obsessions in an eating disorder and more than hair-pulling in trichotillomania.

OCD Symptoms

The presentation of OCD can vary widely. For those children that are secretive about their difficulties, the presenting parental concerns may be temper tantrums, decreased school performance, food restrictions, or dermatitis rather than OCD. Temper tantrums in children with OCD tend to occur when their compulsions are prevented or interrupted. Decreased school performance occurs for a variety of reasons, for example, due to redoing work until some impossible level of perfection is reached, or the child will often refuse to turn in his or her work if it is not perfect, or classes may be missed while performing bathroom rituals at school or other rituals like repeatedly going in- and outdoors or up- and downstairs even to the point of missing classes altogether. Food refusals or restrictions may be based on obsessive fears about contamination, about becoming fat, ordering rituals about food placement on the plate, or intolerance of foods touching one another. Dermatitis can result from washing compulsions. Sometimes cleaning compulsions can present as a toilet stopped up from repeated wiping after defecation, or with high-volume use of soap, water, towels, or excessive clothing changes.

Systematic studies have shown heterogeneity in the onset and course of children's illness, as well as age at onset, comorbid diagnoses, and accompanying neurologic symptoms, such as tics, or choreiform movements. The typical presentation includes obsessions *and* compulsions, often multiple; however, having *only* obsessions may be more common. This presentation can include all the symptoms of obsessions but without the compulsions, so that these children present with the internal distress and anxiety characteristics of obsessions but without the repetitive habits characteristic of compulsions. If children have insight, that is, they have an understanding that their thoughts are unusual or irrational and/or that there is something wrong with them and they can report their distress, this diagnosis is not difficult to make. However, if children lack insight, that is, they do not feel there is anything wrong with them, or perhaps feel that others are unreasonable, or they are unable to describe their inner distress, the diagnosis can be difficult. Over time, the objects and content of obsessions and compulsions may change. Most patients in one long-term study endorsed all of the common symptoms at some point during the course of their illness.

In an adolescent study, the most common categories of *obsessions* were contamination fears, fears regarding safety of themselves or loved ones, exactness or symmetry, and religious scrupulousness. Less common were concerns regarding bodily functions, lucky numbers, and sexual or aggressive preoccupations. In adults, aggressive and sexual preoccupations are more common. Obsessional slowness is a potentially disabling presentation in which a child moves dramatically slowly. Careful assessment may reveal preoccupation with multiple mental rituals that interfere with normal activities.

The most common *compulsions* in an adolescent study, in descending order of frequency, were cleaning rituals, repeating actions (doing and undoing), and checking rituals. Less common were rituals to protect themselves/others from illness or injury (e.g., avoiding "contaminated" objects), ordering maneuvers, and counting behaviors. Although some compulsions are tied to a specific worry/obsession, many consist of repeating an action until it "feels right." For example, these youth may go in and out through a door, or up- and downstairs, until they "get it right." The sense of closure or completion that the child seeks may require symmetry, such as repeating an action with both left and right hands or repeating actions an odd or even number of times. Compulsive rereading or rewriting can interfere with school performance. Mental rituals may consist of silent praying, repetition, counting, or having to think about or look at something in a particular way until it feels "right." Children with OCD are less able than adults to specify what their rituals are intended to avert, beyond a vague idea of something bad happening.

Compared to the general clinical population, children with OCD may be more selectively impaired. On the surface, they may appear to function well. School and social performance may be preserved until the symptoms become quite severe. This is partly due to awareness that their thoughts/symptoms are odd or unusual, so they can be quite embarrassed and secretive about the severity of their impairment. They often engage their families in assisting them in their rituals such as cleaning or checking for them, or "covering" for them, such as making excuses if they miss school. Some patients can accept that something is done "right" if the parent does it for them. The child may become angry with the parents for trying to seek assistance for the problems. The parents want to believe that the symptoms are "just a phase." Often by the time they come to clinical attention, the whole family revolves around the child and his or her symptoms, often not realizing how much time or money they spend supporting the child's symptoms, for example, by doing many loads of laundry, using numerous bars of soap, and paying increased water bills for a child with contamination fears. Frequently, the initial manifesting symptoms can be perceived as adaptive, such as thinking that cleanliness is good, perfect homework is a good thing, and organizing is a positive behavior. The child does not always share the disturbing thoughts with parents, so well-meaning clinicians sometimes reassure parents that all is well/"normal" without asking all the right questions. Parents often prefer to accept reassurances rather than accept that there is something wrong with their child.

Epidemiology

As with any disorder presenting in childhood, the context of what is "normal for age" must be understood. Mild or transient obsessions and compulsions are common in the general population. A survey mailed to parents of children less than 6 years old found that urges to make things "just right" and preoccupations with symmetry and rules are very common in this group. A recent study of nonclinical samples found that 60% of fourth graders reported preoccupations with guilt about lying, as well as engaging in checking behaviors, while 50% reported contamination and germ fears.

The difficulty in assessing the prevalence of OCD comes in distinguishing the *disorder* from *symptoms* that occur as common experiences and as developmental phenomena. Screening tools used in various population studies throughout the years have varying levels of sensitivity and appear to differ greatly from clinical assessment tools, making it difficult to compare prevalence rates across studies.

The first prevalence reports for childhood OCD ranged from 0.2% to 1.2%. A rigorous study of a general adolescent population in 1988 reported a weighted point prevalence of 1% with lifetime prevalence of 1.9%. Many investigators have used the term *subclinical* OCD to describe subjects reporting substantial symptoms without the severity needed to meet the full OCD criteria. Depending on the definition used, prevalence estimates of subclinical OCD in adolescence range from 4% to 19%.

Males and females appear to be equally affected though male patients may have an earlier age of onset. In a 1991 study, 35% of adult males reported that they had onset of their symptoms between the ages of 5 and 15 years, compared with 20% of females. In another study, boys were more likely to have early onset and a family member with OCD or Tourette syndrome, while girls were more likely to have adolescent onset. There do not appear to be any differences in prevalence based on race/ethnicity or geography.

Etiology and Pathogenesis

Genetic studies show evidence for a genetic component in OCD. Concordance rates are elevated in monozygotic twins compared to dizygotic ones, and higher rates for OCD are seen among first-degree relatives of clinical patients with OCD. An additional finding was that earlier age of onset was associated with greater "familiality," that is, a greater likelihood of OCD among relatives.

Elevated rates of OCD among patients with Tourette syndrome, and elevated occurrence of tics and a family history of tics among OCD patients, suggest that the two disorders may have a similar genetic origin.

A number of structural and functional neuroimaging studies have examined patients with OCD compared to never-ill controls, both adults and adolescents. While studies are not conclusive yet, several computerized tomography (CT) studies in the 1980s and structural MRI studies of the 1990s suggested abnormalities in the frontal cortex and the caudate nuclei of patients with OCD. Functional studies using PET reported increased activity in the orbital gyri and the caudate nuclei, which reversed with medication treatment. A functional MRI study in 1996 pointed to elevated activity in the frontal cortex, the caudate and lenticular nuclei, and the amygdala. Finally, functional magnetic resonance spectroscopy studies in 2000 found elevated glutamate levels in the caudate nuclei of 11 treatment-naïve pediatric subjects. After treatment with paroxetine, levels were equivalent to those in normal controls.

Pediatric autoimmune neuropsychiatric disorders associated with streptococcal infections (PANDAS) may be an important mechanism in the development of OCD in 10% to 20% of OCD patients. Typically, symptoms arise, or exacerbate, acutely after a streptococcal infection, often accompanied by the development of tics. This phenomenon may be related to obsessive–compulsive symptoms seen in Sydenham's chorea. Similar to rheumatic carditis, there is some evidence that antineuronal antibodies formed against group A beta-hemolytic streptococcal cell wall antigens cross-react with caudate neural tissue. Reviewing numerous studies that have been done in the last decade looking at PANDAS, the findings are equivocal. Therefore, it appears that treatment geared toward curbing immunologic responses, such as plasmapheresis or immunoglobulin therapy, is worth considering only for acute infection-related onset or severe exacerbation of symptoms.

Differential Diagnosis and Comorbidity

There are many disorders that either coexist with OCD or have obsessions or compulsions as part of their manifestation. Some authors argue that to organize a whole group of heterogeneous disorders and comorbid features under the term OCD based on the presence of a single symptom seems arbitrary. There is also some evidence for various "types" of OCD, such as tic related versus non–tic related.

Care must be taken not to equate *subclinical* obsessions and compulsions with OCD, especially in adolescents who may be demonstrating signs and symptoms of obsessive–compulsive personality disorder (OCPD) (Table 9-1).

Obsessive–Compulsive Personality Disorder

OCPD is, as the name suggests, a personality disorder that is coded on Axis II of the *DSM-IV* nomenclature. Because OCPD is a personality disorder, its symptoms represent a stable characteristic pattern of daily functioning, as opposed to the waxing and waning symptoms of OCD, which appear to represent an illness superimposed on an individual's personality. These

TABLE 9-1 *DSM-IV-TR* Diagnostic Criteria, Comparison of OCD with OCPD

Obsessive–Compulsive Disorder (OCD)	Obsessive–Compulsive Personality Disorder (OCPD)
Recurrent and persistent thoughts, impulses, or images that are experienced at some time during the disturbance, as intrusive and inappropriate, and that cause marked anxiety or distress	Preoccupied with details, rules, lists, order, organization, or schedules to the extent that the major point of the activity is lost
Obsessional thoughts, impulses, or images are not simply excessive worries about real-life problems	Shows perfectionism that interferes with task completion (can't complete a task because overly strict standards are not met)
Person with obsessions attempts to ignore or suppress such thoughts, impulses, or images, or to neutralize them with some other thought or action	Excessively devoted to work and productivity to the exclusion of leisure activities and friendships (not accounted for by obvious economic necessity)
Obsessional person recognizes that the obsessional thoughts, impulses, or images are a product of his or her own mind (not imposed from without as in thought insertion)	Overconscientious, scrupulous, and inflexible about matters of morality, ethics, or values (not accounted for by cultural or religious identification)
Repetitive behavior like hand washing, ordering, checking, praying, counting, repeating words silently, which the person feels driven to perform in response to obsession or according to rules that must be applied rigidly	Unable to discard worn-out or worthless objects even when they have no sentimental value
Compulsive behaviors or mental acts are aimed at preventing or reducing distress or preventing some dreaded event or situation; however, these behaviors either are not connected in a realistic way with what they are designed to neutralize or prevent or are clearly excessive	Reluctant to delegate tasks or to work with others unless they submit to exactly his or her way of doing things
At some point during the course of the disorder, the person recognizes that the symptoms are excessive or unreasonable (note this does not apply to children)	Reluctant to delegate tasks or to work with others unless they submit to exactly his or her way of doing things
Obsessions or compulsions cause marked distress, are time consuming (use at least 1 hour a day), or significantly interfere with the person's normal routine or usual social activities	Rigidity and stubbornness

two disorders do not appear to represent a simple continuum of obsessive–compulsive symptomatology, and some investigators have bemoaned the similar terminology. Patients with OCPD do not usually experience their obsessional and compulsive behaviors as egodystonic; that is, the symptoms do not provoke anxiety in them, and ordinarily the symptoms do not result in significant functional impairment, except perhaps in social or intimate relationships. OCPD does tend to exacerbate with an individual's level of stress, but persists at some level all the time. Most patients with OCD do not exhibit OCPD, but it does appear to be more common among patients with OCD and their relatives than in the general population, especially among those with hoarding symptoms. This may reflect a spectrum of conditions with vertical transmission.

Tic Disorders

At least 50% of children and adolescents with Tourette syndrome develop obsessive-compulsive symptoms or disorder by adulthood. Conversely, a personal or family history of tics is found in nearly 60% of children and adolescents seeking treatment for OCD, ranging from simple, mild, and transient tics up through Tourette syndrome. Recent studies suggest a difference in clinical presentation, neurobiology, and responsiveness to pharmacologic interventions between tic-related and non-tic-related OCD. Though there is significant overlap, these two possible subtypes appear to differ in gender ratio, age at onset, and the number and nature, but not severity, of symptoms. Some investigators have described these subtypes as early onset versus pubertal onset. Tic-related OCD appears to have earlier onset and to occur more frequently in boys than in girls, as well as a generally less satisfactory response to treatment with an SSRI. While it is clearly important to assess for tics in a patient with OCD due to a high rate of comorbidity, the importance of such assessment will likely increase even further as more is learned about potential subtypes of OCD and differential treatment protocols.

Anxiety and Mood Disorders

One third to one half of children with OCD have a current or past history of another anxiety disorder, commonly generalized anxiety disorder (GAD) or separation anxiety disorder (SAD). Children with GAD worry about many issues that are generally realistic but excessive. They do not demonstrate odd irrational thoughts, nor do they demonstrate compulsive behaviors intended to manage their intrusive irrational thoughts. GAD may coexist with OCD. Such children show baseline worry and hyperarousal in addition to their specific obsessive–compulsive symptoms. Anxiety associated with SAD is specific to separation from the attachment figure, generally the mother, and is relieved by being in that person's presence. Such youth may have major tantrums upon separation, and these tantrums may be difficult to differentiate from the tantrums associated with OCD.

Depressive disorders are also commonly comorbid with rates reported from 20% to 73%. Many depressed children demonstrate irritability as their core mood symptom, rather than a depressed mood or anhedonia. As irritability is also a common symptom of OCD, other symptoms of depression should be examined to either confirm or eliminate depressive disorders in the differential.

Pervasive Developmental Disorders

Children with PDDs, like autism or Asperger disorder, often have repetitive behaviors and routines, as well as unusual preoccupations with inanimate items such as fans, maps, or numbers, which caregivers may describe as obsessive–compulsive. Though these characteristics can cause functional impairment or be disturbing to others, the cognitive and language delays typical of these disorders make it difficult to assess whether the child finds these symptoms distressing, that is, whether they are anxiety provoking for the child. Typically, their rigid insistence on routines is part of a larger difficulty making transitions, as well as a need for sameness and structure, or more simply perseveration. While the diagnosis of OCD may not be completely applicable to these children, the obsessive–compulsive symptoms appear to share common features with uncomplicated OCD, such as high rates of OCD in first-degree relatives and potential responsiveness to SSRIs. Finally, PDD and OCD can co-occur. In this case, children must demonstrate the core PDD symptoms of deficits in interpersonal relatedness in addition to criterion symptoms of OCD.

Trichotillomania

This disorder is defined as persistent hair-pulling to the point of alopecia, and is classified in *DSM-IV* as an impulse-control disorder, not an anxiety disorder. However, many investigators now think of trichotillomania as part of an "obsessive–compulsive spectrum disorder" as it shares similarities with OCD in being a repetitive behavior associated with specific "urges" or "need" to perform the behavior. Many children and adolescents with trichotillomania do not manifest any other OCD symptoms, but the rate of OCD is elevated in this population and their first-degree relatives.

Disruptive Behavior Disorders

Most children with OCD are neat, overly compliant, or attentive to detail only within the context of their symptoms. For example, children that are perfectionistic about their schoolwork may have an extremely messy bedroom. Indeed, they may be irritable or impulsive, and as many as half of the children with OCD may meet criteria for a disruptive behavior disorder like attention-deficit hyperactivity disorder (ADHD) or oppositional defiant disorder. This particular comorbidity makes it difficult to determine the relative mix of compulsiveness versus being oppositional or inattentive in any particular behavioral incident. Previously well-behaved children may become defiant, demanding, and even assaultive in the desperate drive to perform their compulsion. On the other hand, children with oppositional tendencies frequently learn to claim their OCD as the basis for all their misbehavior.

Other Disorders

Obsessive–compulsive symptoms and disorder are common in patients with anorexia or bulimia nervosa. While obsessions related to food, exercise, or body image would be subsumed within the eating disorder diagnosis, symptoms can extend to the full range of obsessions and compulsions including symmetry, doubting, contamination, checking, counting, and ordering. In the latter case it would then be appropriate to make a separate diagnosis of OCD.

Body dysmorphic disorder is characterized by an obsessional preoccupation with an imagined or slight defect in appearance. This is frequently accompanied by obsessive grooming or mirror-checking rituals. It is not yet clear what relationship this disorder has to OCD.

Because of the bizarre nature of their behavior and their thought processes, childhood OCD can be mistaken for a psychotic disorder. If the child is unable to consider the possibility that his or her symptoms originate in the mind, that is, the child lacks insight, or if there is a dramatic deterioration in functioning, psychosis should be considered. In most cases of OCD, thinking remains reality based except for the area of obsessional concern, and the content of the "bizarre" thoughts is related to the obsessional theme and is not generalized; unless there are hallucinations, psychosis would not be an appropriate diagnosis. However, schizophrenia can also co-occur with OCD or present with OCD symptoms and should be considered in older children and adolescents with psychotic features.

In 2008, a study by Storch and colleagues found that sleep-related problems were quite common in children with OCD and correlate with OCD symptom severity. Since sleep problems may contribute to morbidity of many types, treatment of the sleep problem may be important.

As noted in Table 9-2, several medical conditions or medication side effects can induce OCD symptoms, but this would preclude the diagnosis of OCD.

There are a large number of children with poor social skills, low frustration tolerance, cognitive unevenness, and problems with mood, anxiety, and/or attention that do not fit easily into any single diagnostic category. They are often irritable, perseverative, overfocused on specific topics, unable to shift tasks easily, and insistent that things be done "just right," with intense outbursts resulting if they are denied. Authors have used various descriptors for this group of children, depending on their theoretical or professional background. More research is needed with this group of children to delineate their relationship to OCD.

TABLE 9-2	Differential Diagnosis for Obsessive–Compulsive Disorder	
Psychiatric Differential Diagnoses	**Medical/Organic Differential Diagnoses**	
Obsessive–compulsive personality disorder	Medical conditions	
Tic disorder/Tourette syndrome	Carbon monoxide poisoning	
Mood disorders (depression/bipolar)	Tumors	
Other anxiety disorders (panic disorder/phobias/PTSD)	Allergic reactions to wasp sting	
Pervasive developmental disorders	Postviral encephalitis	
Trichotillomania	Traumatic brain injury	
Disruptive behavior disorders (ADHD/ODD)	Sydenham's chorea	
Eating disorders (anorexia/bulimia)	Prader–Willi syndrome	
Body dysmorphic disorder	Medication side effects	
Psychosis/schizophrenia	Dopamine agonists (in animal studies)	
Hypochondriasis/somatoform disorder	High-dose stimulants (in children)	

Clinical Course

The onset of OCD may occur quite early; there are case reports of children as young as 5 years, and the modal age of onset in one study was 7 years, while the mean age of onset was 10.2 years. This may imply the existence of an early-onset as well as an adolescent-onset group.

Symptoms may exist an average of 5 to 8 years before patients reach clinical attention. This may be due to secretiveness, as most patients recognize their symptoms as unusual and so hide them, or lack of awareness about the disorder and treatment availability. Parental perception of the severity of the child's symptoms plays a major role when the child is brought to treatment. Often parents have spent years learning to accommodate the child's symptoms, erroneously believing that the child is just "going through a phase" or that by aiding the child in his or her compulsions they are helping relieve the child's anxiety. They will sometimes minimize the severity of the symptoms and the amount of time the family and/or child spends coping with the symptoms. If the parents have any symptoms themselves, their recognition of the abnormality of their child's symptoms will frequently be impaired. Teachers, pediatricians, and primary care physicians are frequently the people responsible for initiating an assessment.

OCD in children and adolescents appears to be a chronic condition with a waxing and waning course. In a large systematic follow-up study of pediatric OCD, 54 patients at NIMH were evaluated 2 to 7 years after treatment. At follow-up, 43% still met diagnostic criteria for OCD, with only 6% reportedly symptom free.

Early outcome studies in children and adolescents did not reveal any demographic factors promoting recovery or persistence of OCD. Patient age, sex, and socioeconomic status failed to predict response to treatment or relapse in two different studies. However, a study published in 2008 showed that children with disruptive behaviors, tics, higher levels of symptom severity, and family dysfunction did show a poorer response to treatment. Children who acknowledge the senselessness of their obsessions and are distressed by their rituals, that is, they have insight, may be more motivated to participate in treatment, though insight is not a prerequisite for treatment effectiveness. Situations complicated by disruptive behavior and/or high family dysfunction may make treatment more challenging as illustrated by one finding that high "expressed emotion" may exacerbate OCD, while a calm, supportive family may improve the outcome. Children with OCD and hoarding may have less insight and more anxiety and aggression.

Assessment

Evaluation of any child or adolescent must consist of gathering as much information as possible from as many sources as appropriate. This always includes the child and his or her primary caregiver, as well as other sources that might be able to assist in the development of a complete picture of the child and his or her difficulties. These other sources could include a teacher, a noncustodial parent, extended family members, a daycare provider, a former foster family, and previous treatment providers. A thorough assessment is the only way to distinguish normal developmental variations, subclinical symptoms, differential diagnoses, and comorbidities, as well as examine any psychological problems that might be supporting the symptoms or otherwise complicating the clinical picture. A comprehensive evaluation of the child's development, social and academic functioning, and medical and family histories is essential, including a careful assessment of current and past symptoms and any comorbid conditions. A family assessment is an important part of the evaluation, not only for the information the family can provide about the patient, but also to assess their understanding of their child, their responses to the child's behaviors, and their ability to participate in their child's treatment (potential parental psychopathology). Family history of OCD, tic disorders, or anxiety disorders should be assessed since these are often familial and can impact the child's treatment.

As previously discussed, some repetitive, perfectionistic or ritualistic behaviors are common in children at various stages of development. Thus, in an assessment, it is important not only to identify specific symptoms but also to assess their context and frequency and the severity of associated distress and dysfunction. It is also important to note the child's efforts to resist the obsessions and compulsions and his or her success in these efforts. Determining the child's ability to resist gives some idea of the child's insight and motivation for therapy.

Over time a child's OCD may manifest in many different ways, and the clinician should inquire about all the various categories of obsessions and compulsions. Some typical obsessions and compulsions are summarized in Table 9-3.

If the family presents for evaluation using the terms "obsessions" or "compulsions," it is important to ask them to describe the behavior as such terms can vary greatly from family to family. Once the potential diagnosis of OCD is suspected, instruments such as the Children's Yale–Brown Obsessive Compulsive Scale (CYBOCS) can be used to rate and record symptom severity. The CYBOCS was developed as a clinician-administered interview, and as such it can require considerable time to complete. However, some clinicians forego the formal interview format, instead using it to summarize areas to be assessed. There is also a brief self-report screening version that patients can fill out to give clinicians some guidelines for further intervention. The Children's Version of the Leyton Obsessional Inventory (CV-LOI) is also useful to assess children older than 10 years. A major advantage of the CV-LOI is that it has population norms

TABLE 9-3	Types of Obsessions and Compulsions
Types of Obsessions/Fears	**Types of Compulsions/Behavior**
Aggressive	Cleaning/washing
Contamination	Checking
Sexual	Repeating rituals
Hoarding/saving	Counting
Religious/scrupulosity	Ordering/arranging
Need for symmetry	Hoarding/collecting
Somatic	Miscellaneous
Miscellaneous	

and includes obsessive–compulsive personality traits. Based on several studies from 2006, a subscale for obsessive–compulsive symptoms can be derived from the Child Behavior Checklist (CBCL) and may serve as an effective screening tool for OCD.

Given the close association between tic disorders and OCD, specific assessment of any history of motor or vocal tics should be conducted. More complex tics, such as tapping and touching patterns, may be difficult to distinguish from compulsive behavior as both may be preceded by premonitory physical sensations, urges, and mental perceptions that persist until the action is completed. In general, if there is no history of simple tics, then complex tics can be ruled out, thereby increasing the likelihood that such behaviors represent a compulsion. When tics are present, one should inquire whether they are accompanied by specific fears or a vague discomfort that something bad might happen if the behaviors are not completed, which also would increase the likelihood that the behavior is a compulsion. Clinicians should also inquire about compulsive habits, such as nail biting, hair-pulling, or skin-picking. Generally, tics, perseverative or stereotyped behaviors, and habits are not as complex as compulsions, are not aimed at neutralizing an obsession, and are usually nonfunctional (rocking or head-banging).

There are no pathognomonic laboratory findings in OCD. Any laboratory evaluations should be based on the findings of the comprehensive evaluation. Baseline electrocardiogram (EKG), complete blood count (CBC), electrolytes, liver function tests, and renal function tests may be necessary before beginning medications. If tics, chorea, or psychotic symptoms are present, measurements of serum copper for Wilson disease should be considered. CT or MRI scanning is necessary only if focal neurologic findings are found. An electroencephalogram is indicated only if a seizure disorder is suspected.

A child with acute onset of tics and/or OCD symptoms needs careful consideration of medical illnesses during the preceding months. A throat culture and an antistreptolysin O or antistreptococcal DNAase B titer may be worth considering.

Psychological tests such as the Wechsler Intelligence Scales for Children, fourth edition (WISC-4) can help to assess concerns with intellectual function, while symptom-based rating scales and personality tests can assess the severity of associated symptoms and the child's internal stressors or defense mechanisms. Behavior rating scales such as the CBCL could be useful in screening for comorbid conditions or evaluating behavioral problems. The essential aspects of assessing a child for OCD are summarized in Table 9-4.

TABLE 9-4	Essentials of Assessment of Obsessive–Compulsive Disorder

- Since some repetitive, perfectionistic, or ritualistic behaviors are common in children at various stages of development, identify symptoms, their frequency, severity, and context within a developmental framework.
- A comprehensive evaluation should include the child's development, social and academic functioning, and medical history along with a careful assessment of current and past OC symptoms and comorbid conditions.
- Family history of OCD, tic disorders, or anxiety disorders should be assessed as these disorders are often familial, can impact the child's treatment, and may guide treatment decisions.
- As a child's OCD may manifest in many different ways, the clinician should inquire about the major categories of obsessions and compulsions.
- In order to determine severity, assess symptom context, frequency, and associated distress/dysfunction, as well as the child's efforts to resist the obsessions and compulsions and their success in these efforts.
- Instruments such as the Children's Yale–Brown Obsessive Compulsive Scale can be used to rate and record symptom severity, and can be helpful to summarize the areas to be assessed.
- Given the association between tic disorders and OCD, assessment for motor or vocal tics should be conducted.
- Any laboratory or other evaluations should be based on the findings of the clinical evaluation.
- Neuroimaging does not currently have a role in the diagnosis of OCD.

Treatment

Each child presenting with obsessive–compulsive symptoms requires an individualized, comprehensive assessment and treatment plan. The nature and severity of obsessive–compulsive symptoms, the range of comorbidities, and the functional level of each child and his or her family can vary significantly and impact treatment planning. While family psychopathology is neither necessary nor sufficient for the onset of OCD, family members affect and are affected by the disorder. Parents or siblings can become involved in the patient's rituals; they may have difficulty dealing with aggressive or sexual content of obsessions, or have differences of opinion about how to respond to the patient's symptoms. To foster compliance in treatment, both the patient and the family need to participate as much as possible in the development of the treatment plan. Family involvement can be especially important for younger patients.

Two types of treatment have been studied systematically and have shown specific efficacy for the core symptoms of OCD: cognitive-behavioral therapy (CBT) and pharmacotherapy. Although psychodynamic psychotherapy may be useful as an adjunctive treatment to teach coping skills, increase the child's sense of mastery, treat comorbid anxiety or depression, and improve peer and family relationships, it does not appear to impact the core obsessive–compulsive symptoms of OCD.

For patients with mild to moderate symptoms, CBT would ideally be the first-line treatment of choice due to potential side effects of medication. If the patient is not rapidly responsive, or if symptoms are more severe or accompanied by a significant depression, then early treatment with medication would be indicated. Some patients and their families will prefer to begin with CBT in the hopes of avoiding medication and potential side effects, while others will choose medication first, trying to avoid the time, effort, and anxiety associated with cognitive-behavioral interventions. In 2004, the Pediatric OCD Treatment Study (POTS) provided evidence that combination treatment is the most effective, with a larger magnitude of symptom improvement and lower relapse rates than when medication or CBT is used alone. This combination method allows the use of the lowest possible dose of medication over time, and may improve both short- and long-term outcome in an illness that tends to be chronic, especially for the population that requires pharmacotherapy.

Follow-up studies from POTS indicate that children with comorbid tics or disruptive behavioral problems have a poorer treatment response to medication, but not to CBT. For these children CBT alone or in combination with medications should be the primary treatment modality. The children with higher baseline symptom severity or more severe family dysfunction had poorer response rates to CBT, indicating that medications or combination therapy may be most beneficial.

Psychosocial Interventions

The use of CBT in children and adolescents with OCD has been studied systematically and has been found to be an effective treatment method, either alone or in conjunction with medication" to avoid the construction. Additionally, a 2006 study has shown preliminary support for treatment of PANDA-related OCD symptoms with CBT. Treatment generally consists of a three-stage approach, beginning with information gathering followed by therapist-assisted exposure with response prevention and homework assignments. The hallmark of CBT is "exposure with response prevention" (E/RP). This consists of real or imagined exposure to a feared object or situation without being able to perform the accompanying compulsion. The exposure portion of this treatment depends on the fact that anxiety will decrease after prolonged exposure with the feared stimulus and repeated exposure is associated with decreased anxiety across exposure trials until the child no longer fears exposure. This can be done in a gradual way, termed graded exposure, or through flooding, with the process under either patient or therapist control. In graded exposure, the therapist helps the patient make a list of his or her fears using a hierarchy from easiest to hardest to tolerate, with exposure beginning with the easiest fears. In contrast, flooding involves prolonged exposure to the most anxiety provoking stimulus on the hierarchy. While flooding may shorten the duration of the treatment, it is frequently not well tolerated by young people, and if failed may reinforce their anxiety and/or disrupt the therapeutic relationship. Children and adolescents are often more compliant with a treatment if they are given as much control as possible. For this reason, it is recommended that graded E/RP be used, with targets chosen by the patient guided by consultation with the therapist, but with the understanding that the child must make progress.

Response prevention involves blocking the performance of rituals or stopping avoidance behavior. For a child with contamination fears, this would involve refraining from washing after an exposure until his or her anxiety decreases, or not going out of the way to avoid exposure. As many exposures happen naturally during the day, response prevention can be selected independently of a scheduled exposure protocol. For instance, a child would normally encounter "unclean" situations in a school environment. Not avoiding bathrooms, or refraining from excessive washing rituals after exposure would be noncontrived, or naturalistic, response prevention.

Manuals are available to guide the clinician in implementing OCD treatment for children. However, a major limitation to this type of treatment is its relative lack of availability outside academic research centers with anxiety-disorder subspecialty clinics.

Medications

Of all childhood psychiatric disorders, OCD has the best evidence-based data supporting pharmacologic treatment and the largest number of medications approved by the Food and Drug Administration (FDA) for use in children. Even so, the best studies find approximately 42% of patients "respond" to first-time single-agent treatment with a reduction of 25% to 40% in severity of symptoms. While this represents a significant improvement in functional level and subjective distress, the majority of patients continue to experience some symptoms of OCD and more than half may not respond to the initial treatment trial. It is best to have a discussion of this issue during the initial treatment consent process so that the patient's expectations of treatment will not be unreasonable.

In order to decide whether a patient is a "responder," an adequate dose must be given for a sufficient time period. Several studies have shown that OCD response rates continue to increase for up to 12 weeks and that OCD may require higher doses of medication than would typically be used to treat depression. An adequate trial has been given when the patient receives the maximum allowable dose or the maximum dose the patient can tolerate for no less than 12 weeks. Response, or lack of response, to one medication does not predict response to another, nor do side effects with one agent predict side effects to another. Before moving on to polypharmacy, it is important to give adequate trials of at least two single medications for a sufficient period of time.

The most thoroughly studied medications in the treatment of childhood OCD are the SSRIs and the related serotonin reuptake inhibitors (SRIs). Blinded, placebo-controlled studies have been conducted with fluoxetine, fluvoxamine, sertraline, and clomipramine. The SSRIs fluvoxamine, fluoxetine, and sertraline are FDA approved for treatment of OCD in children down to the ages of 8, 7, and 6 years, respectively. Clomipramine, an SRI, has shown efficacy in the treatment of OCD in children and is FDA approved down to age 10, but due to its side-effect profile is generally considered a second-line treatment, for use primarily in patients with treatment-resistant OCD. Other SSRIs such as citalopram or escitalopram are

TABLE 9-5	Psychotropic Medications for Obsessive–Compulsive Disorder				
Medication	Dose Range	Pill Sizes Available	Cost (from www.drugstore.com)	Benefits	Common Potential Side Effects
Fluvoxamine (Luvox)	25–200 mg/day, once a day	25, 50, 100 mg tablets	$91–98 for 30 tabs, any strength	Lower sexual side effects	Nausea, lethargy, insomnia
Sertraline (Zoloft)	25–200 mg/day, once a day	25, 50, 100 mg tablets, 20 mg/ml liquid	$70–73 for 30 tabs, any strength, liquid 60 ml for $62	Fewer drug–drug interactions	Nausea, insomnia, agitation, tremor
Fluoxetine (Prozac)	10–60 mg/day, once a day	10, 20, 30, and 40 mg capsules, 20 mg/5 ml liquid, 10 and 20 mg tablets	Available in generic form, $34 for 30 tabs or caps of 10 or 20 mg, $68 for 30 caps of 40 mg, liquid 120 ml for $73	Comes in many forms, generic available	Agitation, anorexia, insomnia, dizziness, dry mouth
Clomipramine (Anafranil)	25–250 mg/day (3–5 mg/kg/day)	25, 50, 75 mg capsules	Available in generic form, $27 for 60 caps of 25 mg, $34 for 60 caps of 50 mg, $39 for 60 caps of 75 mg	May have higher antiobsessional effect size	Anticholinergic: dry mouth, constipation, urinary retention, dizziness; EKG changes, tachycardia; most toxic in overdose

in general clinical use based on extrapolating from safety and efficacy data in adult studies of OCD or in open trials with children. Escitalopram did receive FDA approval for the treatment of major depressive disorder down to age 12 but has not yet been approved for OCD. Since all of the medications show similar response rates, the choice of medication is frequently based on side-effect profile, or the patient's comorbidities, as shown in Table 9-5. For instance, an overweight and sluggish child might respond best to fluoxetine due to its potential side effects of decreased appetite and increased energy, while a teenaged boy may be more compliant with fluvoxamine due to its lower potential for sexual side effects.

Treatment-resistant patients are those that fail to respond to two adequate trials of a single medication or have only a partial response at the maximum tolerable dose of the medication. For these patients, consideration must be given to polypharmacy, as well as intense CBT. If the patient has a partial response to his or her current medication, the first choice would be to augment with the addition of a second SRI with a different mechanism of action. Small-scale studies suggest that the addition of clomipramine may be especially useful in these circumstances as it has noradrenergic qualities like the tricyclic medications, which makes clomipramine a unique agent among the SRIs, although it also increases the side-effect profile. The primary consideration in this instance must be avoiding potential drug–drug interactions, especially since increased side effects and even toxicity can result when mixing medications. For this reason, when adding a second agent it is best to start with a low dose and increase carefully. For those patients without a partial response to first-line treatment, clomipramine may be considered as a single agent.

For patients with Tourette syndrome, tics, or a family history of tics who are refractory to single-agent treatment, several studies have shown benefit from augmentation with risperidone, olanzapine, haloperidol, or pimozide. These agents may also be useful as an augmentation strategy for the treatment-resistant patient, especially those with lack of insight or any psychotic symptoms. Alpha 2a agonists, such as clonidine and guanfacine, may also be helpful for augmentation in patients with tics as they appear to have some benefit in reducing tics and can also be helpful with rage episodes. Clonazepam can be useful in the patient with high levels of comorbid anxiety or panic, but side effects of sedation and cognitive problems may complicate treatment with this agent. Some authors would argue that due to potential side effects, augmentation with CBT, or a change in CBT if previously initiated, should be tried prior to augmentation with medication in the case of treatment-refractory OCD. As practitioners trained to administer quality CBT become more available, this would certainly be desirable.

Treatment of children with comorbid OCD and ADHD can be particularly complicated due to the risk of developing tics/Tourette syndrome as a third comorbidity. Due to the high rate of comorbid tic disorders in OCD, a child with OCD should be considered at risk for the iatrogenic development of tics, especially if treated with a stimulant medication. In some children with OCD, or other anxiety disorders, stimulants can exacerbate their anxiety symptoms, especially at higher doses. This makes treating an OCD patient with ADHD somewhat more difficult. While stimulant medications are considered the first-line treatment for ADHD, if a child already has tics or if he or she has OCD and could be at risk for the development of tics, alternative medications for treating ADHD should be considered. Atomoxetine is a nonstimulant medication with an FDA indication for the treatment of ADHD that may be particularly relevant in the OCD population as there has been some evidence that it may also be beneficial for the treatment of anxiety and depression, but certainly because it is unlikely to precipitate tic disorders or exacerbate anxiety symptoms. As stimulants are the most effective treatment for ADHD, some authors argue that unless there are tics currently in evidence, or family history of tics, that stimulants are still the treatment of choice for ADHD in OCD children, and that atomoxetine should be reserved for those children that cannot tolerate stimulants. There are some children with tic disorders with severe ADHD that clearly respond better to stimulants than to the alternatives. These children can sometimes use low-dose stimulants without exacerbating their tic disorders, but careful discussion of risks versus benefits must be undertaken, and the decision be made carefully on a case-by-case basis. Bupropion (Wellbutrin) is another alternative to stimulants for treating children with comorbid ADHD and OCD. Although not as effective as stimulants, bupropion has been systematically investigated and found to be efficacious for ADHD children.

Discontinuation of medications should primarily be considered after the patient has been optimally treated and stable for 12 to 18 months. It is best accomplished in a gradual manner, both to decrease potential withdrawal side effects and to prevent severe deterioration if symptoms re-emerge with decreased doses. It would also make sense to choose a time when any symptom re-emergence would be the least disruptive, that is, during school breaks. A common strategy is to reduce the maintenance dose by 25% initially and maintain this for several weeks before making further decreases to allow for any symptom re-emergence. Sometimes there will be an initial mild increase in anxiety as a withdrawal side effect that calms down over time, depending on the elimination half-life of the particular medication and its active metabolites. Long-term medication treatment should be considered if several withdrawal trials have failed. If CBT is available, a CBT "tune-up" should be considered when decreasing medications and/or prior to reinstituting the previous dose of medications, depending on the severity of symptom re-emergence. The essentials of treating OCD are summarized in Table 9-6.

TABLE 9-6	Essentials of Treatment for Obsessive–Compulsive Disorder

- For patients with mild to moderate symptoms, CBT is the treatment of choice.
- If the patient is not responsive to CBT in a reasonable time period, or if symptoms are severe or accompanied by a major depression, treatment with an SRI/SSRI is indicated.
- A combination of both medication and CBT is more effective than either therapy alone.
- As pharmacotherapy is only 50% effective in first trials, review treatment response during the consent process so that the family's expectations will not be unreasonable.
- During the consent process, review current warnings about treating youth with SSRIs.
- An adequate medication trial consists of the highest recommended and tolerated dose of an SSRI for at least 3 months.
- Start with a low initial medication dose and increase as needed/tolerated until symptoms are significantly relieved or the patient experiences adverse effects.
- If the patient has minimal response or is intolerant to the first medication trial, switch to a different SSRI.
- If nonresponsive to a second single SSRI trial, consider a trial of clomipramine alone. If partially responsive, consider augmentation strategies based on the patient's comorbidities (clomipramine if depressed; antipsychotic if PDD, tics, or psychosis; atomoxetine or bupropion versus stimulants with ADHD).
- If the patient achieves only a partial response, consider further CBT, consultation with a child and adolescent psychiatrist, and/or referral to a specialty/research center.
- If the patient achieves adequate response and is stable for 12–18 months, consider gradual medication taper during the summertime (minimizes school disruption).

Finally, comment is warranted regarding recent concerns about the SSRIs precipitating suicidal thinking in children and adolescents. Such a reaction is a genuine concern, likely due to the "activating" effects of SSRIs. The FDA has issued a warning about the use of SSRIs at any age, and now mandates such disclosure on bottles of these medications. However, the occurrence of such SSRI-related suicidality appears low, around 3% of youth taking an SSRI, and no completed suicides have been reported. Clearly, families need to be apprised of this risk. A thoughtful informed consent must be conducted with emphasis on safety as well as the relative benefits and risks of using an SSRI for OCD. A multicenter randomized controlled trial of sertraline published in 2006 produced a positive benefit–risk ratio for child and adolescent OCD. This study produced a number needed to treat (NNT) of 2 to 10 and a number needed to harm (NNH) of 64 or greater. Currently, most child and adolescent psychiatrists continue to judiciously use the SSRIs with appropriate monitoring.

Conclusions

Though much has been learned about OCD in the past few decades and pharmacologic and psychosocial treatments have expanded, there is still much work to be done. Research with children and adolescents still lags behind the adult literature, where further research is also needed. Even with optimal current treatment, up to 40% of patients do not achieve adequate symptom control. Epidemiologic studies remind us that most persons with OCD have not sought treatment and continue to suffer in secret. While awareness regarding the benefit of CBT has increased, there are still far too a few providers trained in its administration, especially for children and adolescents. As advocates for our patients and their families, we must continue to support ongoing research and education regarding this interesting and challenging disorder.

CASE VIGNETTES

VIGNETTE 1: 11 YEAR OLD BOY WITH IRRATIONAL FEARS

BD is an 11-year-old male with an intact family. He presents to an outpatient clinic with symptoms of anxiety and school refusal. He was previously a very good student, behaviorally and academically, and a fairly compliant child in the home. Recently, his grades have decreased, he has been losing weight, and parents have been struggling to get him ready for school on time, despite getting him up earlier every morning. Teachers describe BD as being unable/unwilling to turn in his homework because it is "not good enough," and they have observed him becoming frustrated as he repeatedly completes assignments and then destroys them. BD recently became resistant to attending school due to being upset about his inability to perform. This has resulted in conflict with the parents as they attempt to get him to school. Parents describe that BD has not been eating recently because he cannot decide what to eat, and BD describes worries about eating the "right" foods. With further questioning he describes intrusive thoughts that if he eats the "wrong" things and gains weight, his increased weight could disturb the earth's orbit and destroy the laws of gravity, ending with his family/loved ones flying off into outer space. He was hesitant to describe this thought process because he realized that it "sounds crazy" but it still impedes his ability to eat and has led to his recent weight loss. This also involves the family in endless discussions, trying to persuade the patient that various foods are "safe" or that his thoughts are illogical and his fears will not happen (which he understands but is unable to believe strongly enough to overcome his fears). Parents and BD describe past distressing intrusive thoughts and compulsive habits, but they were not overly concerned about those at the time because they had not been "severe enough" to seek treatment.

Treatment options were discussed, but because of concerns with decreased nutritional status and severe disruption of school performance, medication was recommended as the first line of treatment and the patient was started on fluoxetine 10 mg each morning. He tolerated the medication without adverse effects, and clear benefit was seen after 1 to 2 weeks even at the initial dose. However, in order to get optimum symptom control, his dose was gradually increased to 40 mg each morning. With each dose there was further improvement. When he was stable on 40 mg, he experienced minimal anxiety and was able to participate in activities that he was never comfortable enough to participate in previously. BD and his parents remarked that they had not realized how restricted his activities had become until he started feeling better. Over time, BD did well and remained fairly stable though he and his parents noted that if he missed a dose or two of medication (accidentally), he would experience an increase in his anxiety symptoms. On a yearly basis, the psychiatrist would discuss with the family a trial of reducing the medication. However, due to symptom recurrence with missing a dose or two, coupled with the patient's happiness with his stability and lack of adverse side effects, they were unwilling to consider this. The option of CBT was discussed as a way to reduce the medication dose, but BD and his family were unwilling to make the time commitment due to concern that it would be disruptive to their schedules. Also, they were not particularly concerned about reducing the dose of medications as he was doing so well. It was left as an option for the future should the patient's symptoms re-emerge or his desire to reduce medication become more urgent.

VIGNETTE 2: CULTURAL DIFFERENCES COMPLICATE TREATMENT

Peter is a 14-year-old Eastern European male with a long history of severe obsessions and compulsions. His non-English-speaking parents lost custody when the local child protective services investigated allegations made by a neighbor, who thought his family was starving Peter to death. The sight of a skeletal Peter through a window horrified the neighbor. To the child protective services investigator, Peter indeed appeared to be severely emaciated and was immediately placed in a hospital for refeeding. The admitting pediatrics team discovered that Peter would not eat any meals. Peter complained germs contaminated his food. Speaking through an interpreter, his parents confirmed a history of progressive food refusal for the past several months. His parents also described his refusal to bathe, use toilet paper, and get dressed. He could stand for hours in his room without getting dressed. His religious parents thought he was being punished for his "sinful" behaviors since moving to the United States. According to his parents, he was constantly watching television shows depicting "amoral sexual activity." A psychiatric consultation was obtained and a diagnosis of OCD was made. Peter was transferred to a psychiatric residential program where he responded to treatment with an SSRI. Consent had been obtained by his local county caseworker who at the time had temporary custody. Upon discharge, however, Peter was released back to the physical custody of his parents. Several weeks later his parents called the residential program complaining that Peter had relapsed. They had stopped his medications because of their religious beliefs. He was readmitted to the residential program. During this admission he was assigned an individual therapist who received ongoing training in the use of CBT for OCD. After 3 months of treatment he was much less symptomatic. He was consistently eating, dressing, and bathing, albeit with constant coaching by staff. He was discharged to his parent's home, and again several weeks later his parents called complaining Peter had had another relapse. His parents stopped taking him to his outpatient therapist because he had improved so much. This time after a short stay in the residential program, his discharge plan included intensive outpatient treatment services that included an in-home skills trainer with an interpreter for Peter's parents. The skills trainer initially received weekly supervision from a psychiatrist in the use of exposure and response prevention. With this aftercare program, Peter has been successful in the community and has not needed a residential level of care. In contrast to the previous vignette, these parents did not want their child on medications and preferred nonmedical interventions for him. Fortunately, CBT is effective in the treatment of OCD without medication, but does need to be administered by well-trained and skilled therapists. In this case, parental education and involvement was critical in providing successful treatment.

BIBLIOGRAPHY

Cohen DJ, Leckman JF. Developmental psychopathology and neurobiology of Tourette's syndrome. *J Am Acad Child Adolesc Psychiatry*. 1994;33:2–15.

Cook EH, Wagner KD, March JS, et al. Long-term sertraline treatment of children and adolescents with obsessive-compulsive disorder. *J Am Acad Child Adolesc Psychiatry*. 2001;40:1175–1180.

DeVeaugh-Geiss J, Moroz G, Biederman J, et al. Clomipramine in child and adolescent obsessive-compulsive disorder: a multicenter trial. *J Am Acad Child Adolesc Psychiatry*. 1992;31:45–49.

Evans DW, Leckman JF, Carter A, et al. Rituals, habit, and perfectionism: the prevalence and development of compulsive-like behavior in normal young children. *Child Dev*. 1997;68:58–68.

Flament MF, Whitaker A, Rapoport JL, et al. Obsessive-compulsive disorder in adolescence: an epidemiological study. *J Am Acad Child Adolesc Psychiatry*. 1988;27:764–771.

Geller D, Biederman J, Griffin S, et al. Comorbidity of juvenile obsessive-compulsive disorder with disruptive behavior disorders: a review and report. *J Am Acad Child Adolesc Psychiatry*. 1996;35:1637–1646.

Geller DA, Doyle R, Shaw D, et al. A quick and reliable screening measure for OCD in youth: reliability and validity of the obsessive compulsive scale of the child behavior checklist. *Compr Psychiatry*. 2006;47:234–240.

Geller DA, Hoog SL, Heiligenstein JH, et al. Fluoxetine treatment for obsessive-compulsive disorder in children and adolescents: a placebo-controlled clinical trial. *J Am Acad Child Adolesc Psychiatry*. 2001;40:773–779.

Ginsberg GS, Kingery JN, Drake KL, et al. Predictors of treatment response in pediatric obsessive-compulsive disorder. *J Am Acad Child Adolesc Psychiatry*. 2008;47(8):868–878.

Grados MA, Riddle MA, Samuels JF, et al. The familial phenotype of obsessive-compulsive disorder in relation to tic disorders: the Hopkins OCD family study. *Biol Psychiatry*. 2001;50:559–565.

Leckman JF, Grice DE, Barr LC, et al. Tic-related vs non-tic related obsessive-compulsive disorder. *Anxiety*. 1995;1:208–215.

Leonard HL, Goldberger EL, Rapoport JL, et al. Childhood rituals: normal development or obsessive-compulsive symptoms? *J Am Acad Child Adolesc Psychiatry*. 1990;29:17–23.

Leonard HL, Lenane MC, Swedo SE, et al. Tics and Tourette's syndrome: a 2- to 7-year follow-up of 54 obsessive-compulsive children. *Am J Psychiatry*. 1992;149:1244–1251.

Leonard HL, Swedo SE, Lenane MC, et al. A 2- to 7-year follow-up study of 54 obsessive-compulsive children and adolescents. *Arch Gen Psychiatry*. 1993;50:429–439.

Liebowitz MR, Turner SM, Piacentini J, et al. Fluoxetine in children and adolescents with OCD: a placebo-controlled trial. *J Am Acad Child Adolesc Psychiatry*. 2002;41:1431–1438.

March JS. Cognitive-behavioral psychotherapy for children and adolescents with OCD: a review and recommendations for treatment. *J Am Acad Child Adolesc Psychiatry*. 1995;34:7–18.

March JS, Franklin ME, Leonard H, et al. Tics moderate treatment outcome with sertraline but not cognitive-behavior therapy in pediatric obsessive-compulsive disorder. *Biol Psychiatry*. 2007;61:344–347.

March JS, Leonard HL. Obsessive-compulsive disorder in children and adolescents: a review of the past 10 years. *J Am Acad Child Adolesc Psychiatry*. 1996;35:1265–1273.

Pauls DL, Alsobrook JP II, Goodman W, et al. A family study of obsessive-compulsive disorder. *Am J Psychiatry*. 1995;152:76–84.

Pediatric OCD Treatment Study (POTS) Team. Cognitive-behavior therapy, sertraline and their combination for children and adolescents with obsessive-compulsive disorder: the Pediatric OCD Treatment Study randomized controlled trial. *JAMA*. 2004;292:1969–1976.

Rasmussen S, Eisen J. The epidemiology and clinical features of obsessive-compulsive disorder. *Psychiatr Clin North Am*. 1992;15:743–758.

Riddle MA, Scahill L, King RA, et al. Obsessive-compulsive disorder in children and adolescents. *J Am Acad Child Adolesc Psychiatry*. 1990;29:766–772.

Scahill L, Riddle M, McSwiggin-Hardin M, et al. Children's Yale-Brown obsessive compulsive scale: reliability and validity. *J Am Acad Child Adolesc Psychiatry*. 1997;36:844–852.

Storch EA, Lack CW, Merlo LJ, et al. Clinical features of children and adolescents with obsessive-compulsive disorder and hoarding symptoms. *Compr Psychiatry*. 2007;48:313–318.

Storch EA, Murphy TK, Geffken GR, et al. Cognitive-behavioral therapy for PANDAS-related obsessive-compulsive disorder: findings from a preliminary waitlist controlled open trial. *J Am Acad Child Adolesc Psychiatry*. 2006;45:1171–1178.

Storch EA, Murphy TK, Lack CW, et al. Sleep-related problems in pediatric obsessive-compulsive disorder. *J Anxiety Disord*. 2008;22(5):877–885.

Swedo SE, Leonard HL, Garvey M, et al. Pediatric autoimmune neuropsychiatric disorders associated with streptococcal infections (PANDAS): clinical description of the first fifty cases. *Am J Psychiatry*. 1998;155:264–271.

Thomsen PH, Ebbesen C, Persson C. Long-term experience with citalopram in the treatment of adolescent OCD. *J Am Acad Child Adolesc Psychiatry*. 2001;40:895–902.

Towbin KE, Riddle MA. Obsessive compulsive disorder. In: Lewis M, ed. *Child and Adolescent Psychiatry: A Comprehensive Textbook*. 3rd ed. Philadelphia, PA: Lippincott Williams & Wilkins; 2002:834–847.

Zohar AH, Pauls DL, Ratzoni G, et al. Obsessive-compulsive disorder with and without tics in an epidemiological sample of adolescents. *Am J Psychiatry*. 1997;154:274–276.

SUGGESTED READINGS

OCD in Children and Adolescents: A Cognitive-Behavioral Treatment Manual
Authors: John March and Karen Mulle
Publishers: Guilford Press, 1998
(For clinicians this manual outlines this current psychotherapeutic standard of care)

Freeing Your Child from Obsessive-Compulsive Disorder: A Powerful, Practical Program for Parents of Children and Adolescents
Author: Tamar Chansky
Publisher: Three Rivers Press, 2001
(For parents this volume provides both practical understanding and advice for OCD children)

The Boy Who Couldn't Stop Washing: The Experience and Treatment of Obsessive Compulsive Disorder
Author: Judith Rapoport
Publisher: New American Library, 1997
(A *New York Times* bestseller for lay populations filled with many vignettes from the family, patient, and treating clinician points of view)

SUGGESTED WEBSITES

Anxiety Disorders Association of America: http://www.adaa.org (accessed April 2010).
Obsessive Compulsive Foundation: http://www.ocfoundation.org (accessed April 2010).
National Institutes of Mental Health: http://www.nimh.nih.gov (accessed April 2010).
Information about medications: http://www.parentsmedguide.org (accessed April 2010).

REVIEW QUESTIONS

1. Common comorbidities with OCD include:
   a. Tic disorders
   b. Mood disorders
   c. Other anxiety disorders
   d. Disruptive behaviors
   e. All of the above

2. Which of the following medications have not been approved for treatment of OCD in children?
   a. Fluoxetine (Prozac)
   b. Atomoxetine (Strattera)
   c. Sertraline (Zoloft)
   d. Clomipramine (Anafranil)

3. Principles of CBT include all of the following except:
   a. Psychodynamic psychotherapy
   b. Graded exposure or flooding
   c. Ranking anxieties according to a hierarchy from easiest to most anxiety provoking
   d. Prevention of the compulsion/ritual

4. The true statement about OCD is:
   a. The diagnosis requires that children recognize their symptoms as excessive or unreasonable.
   b. It is common for children to have OC symptoms that don't significantly interfere with functioning.
   c. Parents' concerns about their child's symptoms are accurate reflections of the child's inner world.
   d. Symptoms of OCD are usually apparent to the casual observer.

5. Which of the following obsessions are less common in adolescents than in adults?
   a. Contamination fears
   b. Sexual/aggressive preoccupations
   c. Symmetry/exactness
   d. Safety concerns

6. Common features of the family of an OCD child include all of the following except:
   a. The family often assists the child in their rituals.
   b. The family wants to believe that the child's symptoms are "just a phase."
   c. The family should not be involved in the child's treatment.
   d. The family may minimize the child's symptoms or the amount of time spent coping with them.

7. Characteristics of OC personality include all of the following except:
   a. Symptoms don't seriously impair daily functioning though they may be annoying.
   b. People with OC personality do not experience their symptoms as problematic or anxiety provoking.
   c. Symptoms are a stable chronic pattern of functioning, often experienced as rigid or demanding by others.
   d. They recognize their symptoms are excessive or unreasonable.

Answers: 1-e, 2-b, 3-a, 4-b, 5-b, 6-c, 7-b

10

Ajit N. Jetmalani, MD

Tourette Syndrome

Introduction

In 1884, the French neurologist Gilles de la Tourette described nine patients who suffered unusual repetitive motor movements and vocalizations of childhood onset, without associated cognitive impairment. Dr. Tourette's mentor, Jean-Martin Charcot, suggested the eponym "Gilles de la Tourette Syndrome" to this newly described malady. These clinicians were drawn by the profound externalizing symptoms, including profane utterances and complex motor behaviors that seemed involuntary and caused great shame. For many decades, the disorder remained unresearched, poorly understood, and relegated to curiosity and psychogenic causation. In 1968, Dr. Arthur and Dr. Elaine Shapiro reinvigorated scientific inquiry into Tourette syndrome through a series of provocative papers suggesting that it was an organic disorder. Previously, Tourette syndrome had been conceptualized as a psychodynamic disorder with unconscious processes fueling the plethora of complex behaviors and offensive verbalizations. The Shapiros, however, demonstrated the efficacy of haloperidol in ameliorating the motor symptoms of Tourette syndrome. In the ensuing years, research has led to major advances in understanding of Gilles de la Tourette syndrome as a complex neuropsychiatric illness.

This chapter reviews tic disorders with a focus on the most severe variant, Tourette syndrome. The nosology of this condition is evolving. Although the *Diagnostic and Statistical Manual,* 4th Edition (DSM-IV) uses the term *Tourette disorder (TD),* this chapter utilizes *Tourette syndrome* (TS) to avoid the abbreviation TD commonly used for tardive dyskinesia.

Clinical Features and Diagnostic Criteria

Clinical Features

The sudden repetitive muscular contractions and vocalizations cataloged by Dr. Tourette are called tics. These motoric events commonly last a second or less, and represent *voluntary* action that may be anticipated and often suppressed. Severely affected patients, however, experience barrages of motor and cognitive impulses, which overwhelm their conscious ability to suppress. Accompanying comorbid conditions, behavioral, emotional, and academic challenges may cause greater morbidity than the tic symptoms. Generally, tics are not painful and do not occur during sleep.

Over time, as noted by Leckman and colleagues, tics tend to display a rostral to caudal progression, with eye blinking as a most common beginning. At times, the anatomic origin is limited to a few muscle groups (*simple tic:* eye blinking, jaw thrusting, throat clearing), or multiple organized contractions which mimic contextual speech or movement (*complex tic:* obscene gestures such as "the finger" [copropraxia], obscene utterances [coprolalia], or repetition of others' speech and movement [echolalia, echopraxia]). The quality of obscene

TABLE 10-1	Comparison of Tic Disorders Described in *DSM-IV*	
Disorder	**Type of Tic**	**Duration of Symptoms**
Tourette syndrome	Motor *and* one or more vocal tics at some point in the illness but not necessarily concurrently	Nearly every day for more than a year with no greater than 3 months tic free
Chronic motor or vocal tic disorder	Motor *or* vocal tics	Nearly every day for more than a year with no greater than 3 months tic free
Transient tic disorder	Motor *or* vocal tics	Between 4 weeks and one year

For diagnosis, tics should cause marked distress or impairment socially, occupationally, or in other ways.
Onset is before age 18 years.
Tics should not be secondary to ingestion of drugs or medications or due to a primary medical condition.

utterances and behavior is that of a rapid usually noncontextual explosion of words or actions, not to be confused with angry or antisocial statements of a frustrated or acting out child. TS patients often experience premonitory awareness of the onset of a tic. Attempts at suppression or alteration of tics may then present as a collection of odd voluntary motions or vocalizations meant to mask the underlying episode. These behaviors may phenomenologically overlap with symptoms of obsessive–compulsive disorder (OCD) as the child repetitively takes suppressive action to relieve tic tension. This is different from the pattern noted in OCD in which the action is often accompanied by thoughts related to symmetry, counting, phobic avoidance, or ritual. For patients with tic disorders and without OCD, the behaviors are not associated with well-formed ideas; rather, there is a feeling of physical tension resulting in an ameliorative action.

Diagnostic Criteria

Multiple classifications of tic disorders are available and overlapping in detail. The DSM-IV is selected for this text. DSM-IV divides tic disorders into three categories: TD, chronic motor or vocal tic disorder, and transient tic disorder. The diagnostic criteria are quite simple considering the complexity of this condition, and are summarized in Table 10-1. For a diagnosis of TD, vocal and motor tics must be present although not necessarily at the same time, during one year of history, without a reprieve longer than three months. For the diagnosis of chronic motor or vocal tic disorder, symptoms should be present for at least one year, without a reprieve longer than three months, but without both vocal and motor subtypes. For transient tic disorder, symptoms should be present for no longer than one year. In all categories, the onset should occur before the age of 18, and the symptoms should be severe enough to intrude on functioning.

While DSM-IV criteria focus on motor findings, TS patients frequently present with additional features of OCD, and attention-deficit hyperactivity disorder (ADHD). Thus, one should consider the triad of tics, OCD, and ADHD in all patients presenting with tics. In addition, tics are present in many children with pervasive developmental disorders (PDD), particularly those with Asperger syndrome. These and other comorbid conditions are discussed throughout this chapter, and by other authors in this text.

Epidemiology

Prevalence studies of tics and tic disorders show wide-ranging results. Tics may not be associated with functional impairment, therefore, identification is highly variable and thresholds for diagnosis are inconsistent. A broad overview of epidemiologic studies by Kenn-Kim and

Freimer, revealed the following range of findings: approximately 0.1% to 1% of the population suffers from TS. The estimated prevalence of Chronic Tic Disorders is much higher ranging from 2% to 5%, and 10% to 15% of children during their school years. Boys are substantially more likely to suffer tics and TS, at 2 to 10 times the frequency of girls.

Clinical Course

Peterson and Leckman note that tics tend to occur in bouts during time increments that are clustered during a few minutes in a day, and/ or days of intensity, and/or weeks or months of waxing and waning. Because tics are suppressible to a varying degree, some children and adults will successfully "hide" their tics at school or work, and then have explosive bouts of tics at home. In addition, stress and anxiety may affect the frequency and intensity of tics. Typically, tics onset at age 5 or 6, with peak intensity at age 10 to 12, and tic reduction around the age of 15 to 17. Many patients will experience substantial or near-complete resolution of tics following adolescence.

Differential Diagnosis

Other Movement Disorders

Jankovic has reviewed other hyperkinetic movement disorders, including stereotypic behaviors, dystonias, choreiform disorders, and myoclonus which may be confused with tics.

Stereotypic behaviors: These are repetitive actions that are complex in nature and consistent over long periods. There may be a ritualistic and/or self-soothing quality to these behaviors. For example, autistic and mentally retarded patients often rock or pace for long periods of time. Rapid hand rubbing is a common finding in this population, as well, and a prominent diagnostic finding specifically in Rett syndrome. These phenomena differ from tics in their consistency and seemingly self-soothing quality.

Dystonias: These movements are often sustained contractions that are observed as abnormal postures of the head and neck (torticollis), or extremity and are frequently painful. As a rule, tics do not cause pain, unless the frequency and intensity cause repetitive strain. Sometimes, the movements are rapid and tic-like in quality. In dystonias, however, the anatomic location is often less fluid than in tic disorders.

Choreiform disorders: This collection of disorders manifests as rapid motor movements, which may begin with "piano playing" finger movements evident upon finger extension. In severe syndromes (Huntington chorea, Sydenham chorea), fulminate total body jerking may render the patient incapacitated. The early presentation is easily confused with tics, family history (Huntington chorea), streptococcal episode (Sydenham chorea), and appropriate serum and/or genetic studies assist in the differential diagnosis.

Myoclonus: This is characterized by "lightning bolt" fast muscle contractions alternating with relaxation of large muscle groups. Myoclonic movements are also common and normal during early stages of sleep.

Infectious Etiology

In 1998, Swedo and colleagues wrote about a series of patients who suffered OCD and/or tics in the context of documented infection with group A beta hemolytic streptococcus (GABHS). These researchers hypothesized GABHS induced immune-mediated injury to the basal ganglia. This was consistent with the pathophysiology of Sydenham chorea (OCD in Sydenham's patients initiated this research), and these patients were added to the "pediatric autoimmune neuropsychiatric disorders associated with streptococcal infection" (PANDAS) spectrum. Recent research, however, found that "no correlation was identified between clinical exacerbations and autoimmune markers." Their work looked at antineuronal antibodies

TABLE 10-2	Differential Diagnosis of Tics

PRIMARY

Chronic motor and vocal tics: Tourette syndrome

    Chronic motor or vocal tics

    Transient motor or vocal tics

SECONDARY

Inheritable syndromes:

    Huntington chorea

    Wilson disease

    Hallervorden–Spatz

    Tuberous sclerosis

    Neuroacanthocytosis

Infections:

    PANDAS (pediatric autoimmune neuropsychiatric disorder associated with streptococcal infection), acute viral encephalitis

    Chronic encephalitis (HIV, Creutzfeldt–Jakob disease)

Toxins:

    Medications and Drugs of Abuse (partial list): Amphetamines, methylphenidate, tricyclic antidepressants, L-DOPA, carbodopa, carbamazepine, cocaine, antipsychotic medication (withdrawal)

    Environmental: carbon monoxide, organopesticides, and volatile aromatic compounds

Others:

    Mental retardation/developmental delay

    Autism

    Head trauma

    Stroke

    Tumor

    Multiple sclerosis

and cytokines and utilized diagnostic criteria for PANDAS outlined by Swedo and others. While this controversy continues, PANDAS should be considered in the following situations: DSM-IV diagnosis of a tic disorder or OCD; prepubertal onset; episodic presentation with abrupt onset and gradual spontaneous reduction of symptoms ("saw tooth" symptom pattern); subtle neurologic findings; choreiform movements, handwriting deterioration; GABHS infection temporally during symptom exacerbation. Further considerations in the differential diagnosis of tics are summarized in Table 10-2.

Comorbid Disorders

As previously noted, children with TS have a high frequency of comorbid ADHD and/or OCD. When evaluating a child with tics, it is critical to consider the triad of tics, ADHD, and OCD, as suffering from multiple conditions substantially increases morbidity. Furthermore, ADHD and OCD may not be as apparent as tics in the office, requiring directed inquiry and data gathering. While less well researched, it is also common to see children suffering from the combination of autistic spectrum disorders and tics or TS.

Attention-Deficit Hyperactivity Disorder

Multiple studies have supported a high co-occurrence of TS and ADHD. On average, 50% of TS patients meet criteria for ADHD, and 30% to 40% of children diagnosed with ADHD have tics or TS. Children with both disorders have a much greater risk of conduct disorder, depression, and overall dysfunction, than children with TS only. Children with TS and ADHD also suffer much higher rates of cognitive disturbances and learning disabilities (LD) than children with TS alone whose rates of LD approach normal controls.

Obsessive–Compulsive Disorder

Phenomenologic, neurologic, and genetic overlap of TS and OCD has led many investigators to suggest that these two syndromes are part of the same illness. OCD is a condition in which patients describe unwanted disturbing, intrusive and often nonsensical worries, accompanied by behaviors which are meant to temporarily diminish their emotional discomfort. At times, OCD patients will describe sudden intrusive thoughts and equally sudden reactive behaviors. Patients with tics often report or are aware of cognitive or emotional elements to their movement symptoms. Some TS patients will describe "thought tics" which are different from obsessions as the thoughts are instantaneous, and may not be associated with anxiety or with a desire to carry out a behavior. Interestingly, selective serotonin reuptake inhibitors (SSRIs) effectively treat OCD, but not tics. Conversely, alpha-2a agonists treat tics but not OCD. Overall, history gathering and examination will assist in differentiating obsessions, compulsions, and tics.

Other Anxiety Disorders

Children with TS may experience substantial social stigma due to the overt symptoms of their illness. For some children, social avoidance and anxiety may lead to avoidance of public places, or public performance. Social phobia and performance anxiety are common in this population, either as primary or secondary conditions.

Autistic Spectrum Disorders

A number of authors have documented the co-occurrence of tic disorders and ASD. ASD patients have a host of movement disorders including stereotypies which are at times difficult to differentiate from tics. The clustering of ADHD, tics, OCD, and ASD suggest the variable expression of shared underlying neurodevelopmental anomalies.

Etiology and Pathogenesis

Genetics

Tourette syndrome is pervasive in family systems; the rate of TS in relatives of affected individuals is 10% to 15% and the rate of tics approximates 20%. Family studies reveal that the TS concordance rate in monozygotic (MZ) twins is greater than in dizygotic (DZ) twins reaching 70% versus 9% concordance for TS and 77% versus 23% concordance for chronic motor tics respectively. Importantly, however, the rate of concordance in DZ twins is higher than in the general population, and the severity of illness within MZ pairs is variable. Mutations involving the *SLITRK1* gene have clearly been identified in a small number of people with Tourette syndrome. This gene involves functions within the neurocircuitry attributed to TS. Recent analyses of this gene's role are complicated by various technical challenges. The definitive contribution of mutations at *SLITRK1* and other loci continue under active study. TS certainly involves an interplay of genetic and epigenetic influences leading to various phenotypic outcomes.

Environmental Factors

Severe maternal nausea, low birth weight, and forceps delivery are statistically associated nonspecific findings in patients with TS, as well as with many other neuropsychiatric conditions. Clinically, stress may herald the onset and exacerbate symptom intensity in affected patients.

Neuropathology

The neurochemical and anatomic abnormalities in tic disorders are not definitively deter-mined. Postmortem studies are rare, as this is not a fatal syndrome, and severe symptoms in many individuals dissipate early in life. Harris and Singer note that analysis of parallel disease models (Huntington, Parkinson, Sydenham chorea), lesion studies, neuroimaging studies, animal models, and limited neuropathologic and empiric findings support a primary disturbance in the corticostriatothalamocortical circuitry (CSTC) and limbic system. This "motor–limbic interface" is represented in Figure 10-1.

Cortical and subcortical structures interact normally to produce desired movement (voluntary cortical discharges), affect, and cognition. Primary neurotransmitters in the system include gamma-amino-butyric-acid (GABA), glutamate, dopamine, acetylcholine, enkephalin, substance P, and other protein messengers.

The balance of stimulation and inhibition provides smooth wanted movement. In TS, ab-normalities in the complex cycling cascade of dopaminergic neuronal functions and influences

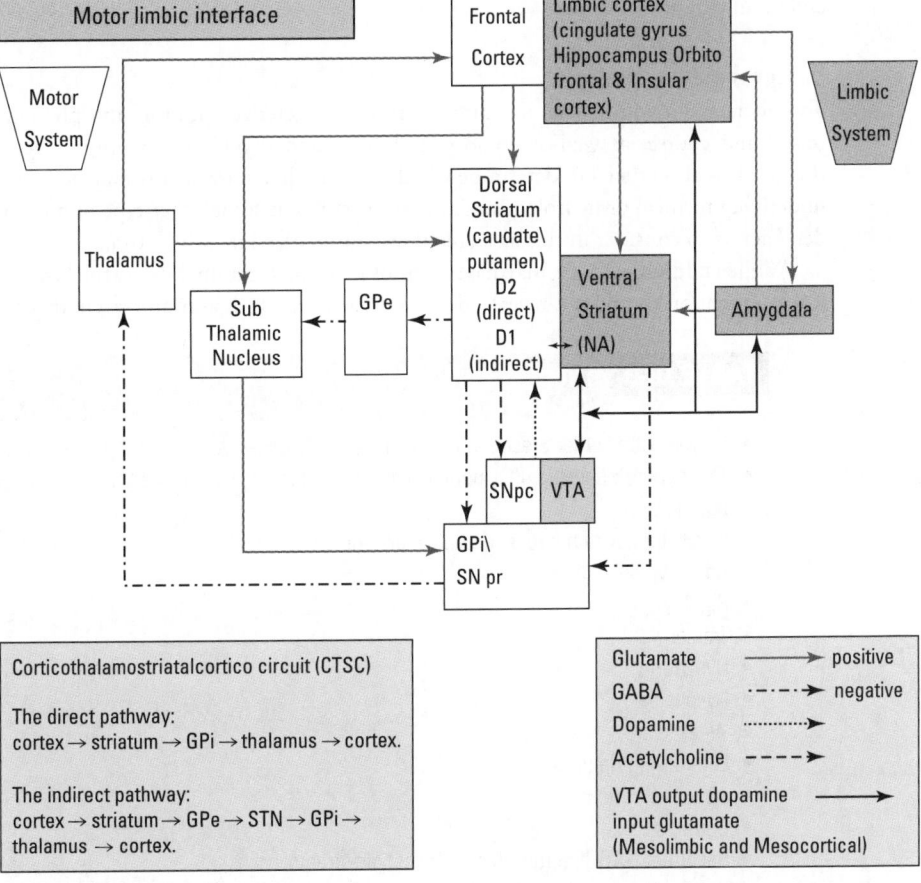

FIGURE 10-1. Schematic diagram of the motor–limbic interface. Note that these parallel systems converge in the striatum where motor and affective discharges are interactively modified. Proposed neuropathologic mod-els of Tourette syndrome (TS) suggest anomalies in the functions of cortical and subcortical structures which function normally to modulate desired movement (voluntary cortical discharges), affect, and cognition. In TD, abnormalities in the complex cycling cascade of dopaminergic neuronal functions and influences are believed to be central in causation and potential intervention. Serotonin which is not represented here, has a modula-tory role in CSTC circuits through limbic influence.

are believed to be central in causation and potential intervention. Cross activation of the limbic system may account for dysregulation of affect and control of rage in some patients, as well as the premonitory sensations and subjective experiences of tic episodes and interepisode states. Dysfunction in the striatum is also associated with the pathogenesis of OCD, ADHD, and an aspect of the neuropathology of Asperger syndrome (sensorimotor gating).

Assessment

Chief Complaint

Tics may rarely cause *pain* if the repetitive movements are unusually frequent, cause *dysfunction* due to interruption of normal activity such as reading and writing, and/or considerable social *stigma*. For many patients, attentional deficits, academic difficulties, depression, or obsessive–compulsive symptoms may accompany tic symptoms. The family member's chief concerns may be different from the child's, because the subjective experience of tics may not correlate with the observed severity. For this reason, it is important to explore the concerns of both the child and parent.

Comprehensive History

To understand a youth's tics, the clinician must characterize symptom morphology, intensity, onset, and course, as well as comorbid physical and psychiatric symptoms accompanying the tics. It is also crucial to determine whether the tic-like movements may be secondary to an underlying medical or neurological disorder or represent some other type of movement disorder. Factors to consider in this assessment are summarized in Table 10-3.

While children with TS may have signs of neuromaturational delay, the history and physical examination should not reveal a decline in functions such as motor strength, coordination,

TABLE 10-3	Factors Suggesting Other Movement Disorders

- Movement disorder presenting in mid to late adolescence
- Temporal relationship of symptom onset to head injury, illness, medication, or drug use
- Family history of neurodegenerative disorders
- Cognitive decline
- Rigidity
- Tremor
- Dysarthria
- Dysphagia
- Weakness
- Lateralizing findings
- Abnormal reflexes
- Seizures
- Recurrent GABHS (group A beta hemolytic streptococcus)
- Substantial symptoms during sleep
- Abrupt and severe onset
- Perceived as purely involuntary
- Nonsuppressible motor symptoms
- No family history of tic disorder
- Child has no premonition of tic
- Movements are painful

or sensation. The onset of primary tic disorders occurs in the context of normal continued developmental gains. When gathering history, parents and children may not have an adequate vocabulary to describe motor findings. It is helpful to ask the parent or child to demonstrate the symptom, or to bring a videotape of the movements at home. It is also difficult for a parent and child to objectively note declines in cognitive or motor functions. Questions about academic and athletic performance may reveal useful information regarding the child's overall symptom profile. Finally, handwriting is a sensitive measure of motor and cognitive decline and it is helpful to obtain samples of work completed premorbidly and currently.

Developmental History

There are no consistent specific findings expected in the early developmental history of children with tic disorders. Common early findings, particularly in children also diagnosed with ADHD, include sensory overstimulation noted in arching behaviors when held, or tactile and auditory sensitivity. There may be delays in fine and gross motor development, although *early* gross motor development is often noted in hyperkinetic children. Later, substantial academic difficulties often accompany tic and ADHD symptoms. Learning may be impaired by developmental abnormalities in reading, math, writing or language acquisition, or secondary to ADHD, OCD, or the interference of tics in the mechanics of reading and attention. Accompanying interpersonal and metacognitive deficits may be part of a broader diathesis consistent with a diagnosis of PDD.

Family History and Functioning

As noted earlier, family history is often positive for ADHD, OCD, and tics in first and second-degree relatives. Frequently, the clinician may note undiagnosed tics in a parent or sibling of the patient. It is critical to ask about other movement disorders to assist in the diagnosis.

Family structure and functioning will, of course, influence symptom tolerance, management, and treatment outcome. With chaotic or highly stressed family systems, the management of this syndrome will require collaboration with mental health providers. With a highly anxious parent, minor tics may become a major focus, as the parent overattends to symptoms. In addition, these families may transfer their anxious energy or irritation to the child who may then develop increased behavioral or emotional symptoms. The pressure to use medication, or too rapidly titrate dosing, is greater under these circumstances. Education and open, respectful discussion of these concerns may improve parental tolerance of symptoms. This in turn may help the child feel less anxious, and may improve stress and tic intensity. Conversely, further discussion may clarify that the tic disorder is more severe than the clinician realized.

Examination of the Child

A screening neurological examination should be conducted that includes assessment of coordination, motor overflow, strength, reflexes, tone, balance, and untoward motor movement. A mental status examination should focus on mood, affect, language, intelligence, cognitive processes, thought content, attention, orientation, insight, and judgment. As part of a routine general examination, special attention should be paid to skin lesions that may suggest other causes of movement disorder (neurofibromatosis, streptococcal infections/scarlatina rash, thyroid disturbances).

Tics do not warrant routine serum screening, neuroimaging, or electrical studies, unless secondary tics or differential concerns are raised by history or examination. Pharmacologic intervention will also dictate possible baseline laboratory studies. Essential aspects of evaluating the child with tics are summarized in Table 10-4.

TABLE 10-4	Assessment Essentials

- The chief complaint should be obtained from the child *and* guardian to guide a successful postevaluation discussion and treatment plan formulation.
- History gathering should include questions that differentiate tics from other movement disorders, and tics secondary to streptococcal infection.
- A directed interview will include questions intended to reveal comorbid conditions, with particular emphasis on symptoms of OCD, ADHD, and learning problems.
- The physical examination should focus on cutaneous abnormalities, infectious conditions, and the general neurologic exam.
- Neuroimaging should occur in patients with movement disorder inconsistent with tics (not necessary in tic disorders).
- Laboratory testing should occur when considering possible metabolic or infectious causes of movement disorder (not in tic disorders unless PANDAS is suspected).

OCD, obsessive–compulsive disorder; ADHD, attention-deficit hyperactivity disorder; PANDAS, pediatric autoimmune neuropsychiatric disorders associated with streptococcal infections.

Treatment

Behavioral Intervention

Many older children and adolescents with tic disorders have premonitory urges and can anticipate a tic. Over time with support, they may be able to suppress or substitute alternate actions that may be more socially acceptable than the original motor event. Cataloging and becoming aware of one's tic types and patterns may be followed by a reduction in overall tics, or the ability to suppress the tics until privacy allows expression, that is, a delay of symptoms.

Habit Reversal Training (HRT) is a specific and evidence-based behavioral technique used to reduce repetitive behavior by a cooperative and invested subject. The protocol is well described by Piacentini and Chang. There are a number of essential components:

- Tic description
- Awareness of tics through feedback, videotape, etc.
- Acknowledging tics when they happen, by documenting or labeling with a letter T verbalized after each tic
- Learning a competitive response, that is, a motor behavior that is close to the opposite of the muscle contractions, that occur in the tic, and rehearsing it with the therapist
- Learning relaxation techniques, such as breathing techniques and/or muscle relaxation techniques, to assist in carrying out a competitive response
- Applying the competitive response when the patient feels a tic coming or for 1 to 2 minutes after a tic or series of tics
- Great praise for the child when he/she follows through with the process; feedback to the child regarding observed improvements

Tics and TS, like most neuropsychiatric conditions, exacerbate with stressors such as family problems, academics, environmental events, lack of adequate sleep, excessive caffeine, etc. Stress reduction in the form of appropriate and predictable parenting, stable housing, academic support, and peer support will improve symptoms and reduce variables in management.

Pharmacological Interventions

General Comments

The medical treatment of tics should only occur in the context of significant secondary functional impairment. Mild tics may be perceived as severe and severe tics as mild by individual children and their families. It is important to try to support children and parents to tolerate mild tics due to the relative risks of medical management and the lack of curative options.

The pharmacologic treatment of chronic tic disorders is clinically challenging. Initiation of medical intervention and assessment of medication response necessitates consideration of whether any positive change in the course of tics is due to the medication or due to the naturally waxing and waning course of the tics. The decision to treat tics and comorbid conditions mandates a comprehensive discussion with the family about the natural course of tics and the risk of treating versus not treating the condition. The clinician and family must commit to a goal of gradual changes in dosing, up or down, and patience with exacerbation of tics. Rapid dose changes may cause excessive secondary side effects and receptor oversensitivity and reactivity. One may easily enter a complex cycle of clinically incomprehensible volatility in symptoms and medication management.

Successful pharmacologic reduction of tics appears to occur via the modification of the CSTC at various levels. Antipsychotics act primarily via direct blockade of dopamine receptors. Alpha-2a agonists such as guanfacine and clonidine indirectly diminish dopamine levels and stimulate cortical functions that are inhibitory. Serotonin reuptake inhibitors do not generally affect tics but modify comorbid OCD symptoms via influence on the limbic system.

Table 10-5 includes a list of agents used in the treatment of tics. Swain and colleagues utilized criteria from the International Psychopharmacology Algorithm Project (IPAP) to rank empiric support for medications as category "A," two or more placebo-controlled studies showing efficacy and safety, and "B," one such study. Medications for tics are listed in this table according to these guidelines. Pimozide (Orap) and haloperidol (Haldol) are the only FDA-approved drugs for tics in youth.

Most clinical studies of pharmacotherapy report average rates of tic reduction from 30% to 60%. It is rare to achieve greater than 50% *sustained* reduction in tics in a moderate to severely affected child. A baseline review of severity and use of tic rating scales are critical in the analysis of outcome. The Yale Global Tic Severity Scale is an effective standardized tool. It is

TABLE 10-5	Medications in the Treatment of Tourette Syndrome
Target Symptoms	**Medication**
Tics: (Swain et al. 2007) A: good evidence of efficacy B: fair evidence of efficacy	Nonantipsychotics clonidine, guanfacine (B) Antipsychotics haloperidol, pimozide, risperidone (A) fluphenazine, tiapride, ziprasidone (B)
ADHD (in recommended categorical order)	Atomoxetine, guanfacine Stimulants: Long acting Adderall XR, Concerta, Ritalin LA, Metadate CD, Focalin XR, Daytrana (patch) Stimulants: Short acting Dextroamphetamine, methylphenidate, dexmethlyphenidate Tricyclic antidepressants Imipramine, nortriptyline
OCD	SSRIs Fluoxetine, fluvoxamine, sertraline, escitalopram, citalopram TCAs Clomipramine

Note: Refer to Chapter 25 for precautions and dosage recommendations.

also reasonable to develop a personalized 1 to 10 rating of intensity, frequency, embarrassment level, functional impairment at baseline, and follow-up titration points. Careful pretreatment goal setting will provide a stronger alliance with the family and improve satisfaction with the likelihood of incomplete symptom response. The clinician is cautioned to seek the lowest effective dose when initiating psychotropic treatment of any pediatric patient. For most medications, dosage adjustment should occur at a frequency of no less than five days.

Treatment of Tics without Substantial Comorbid Condition

Clinicians and researchers have found three categories of modestly effective medications in the treatment of tic disorders: alpha-2a agonists (guanfacine, clonidine) typical neuroleptics (pimozide, haloperidol, fluphenazine), and atypical neuroleptics (risperidone, olanzapine, ziprasidone). Risk–benefit analysis may lead most physicians and patients to begin with the alpha-2a agonists. These agents act at the alpha-2a presynaptic receptor, which diminishes release of norepinephrine. This effect is central and peripheral, impacting neurologic and cardiovascular functioning. The direct effects of agonist action, that is, diminished norepinephrine release, include vasomotor relaxation, diminished anxiety, increased sedation, and smooth muscle relaxation which results in decreased salivation, and decreased bladder outlet control. The mechanism of tic reduction does not involve direct manipulation of dopamine and is not completely understood. One theory is that modulation of norepinephrine reduces the subject's response to stress, which in turn modifies the stress-based discharge of dopamine. Stimulation of the alpha-2a receptor also improves the inhibitory capacity of the frontal cortex, perhaps improving voluntary control of tics.

Clonidine is more sedating than guanfacine and is often used as a sleep agent. Some patients, however, may experience mid-phase rebound insomnia as well as nocturnal enuresis with guanfacine and clonidine. Clonidine is helpful in the reduction of aggression and hyperactivity but is neutral or negative on measures of attention. The combined use of clonidine and methylphenidate (Ritalin, Concerta, Metadate) became a concern several years ago due to case reports of sudden death in a small number of pediatric patients taking this medication combination. It was thought that the usually mild cardiovascular effects of both medications could be cardiotoxic in combination. However, this theory was never further investigated, and stimulants and alpha-2a agonists continue to be widely prescribed. A history of ventricular or trioventricular node dysfunction, known cardiac disease, or family history of sudden premature death probably warrants alternate or noncombined therapy. The American Heart Association Guidelines for pediatric stimulant prescribing are reviewed in the psychopharmacology chapter in this text, and apply whenever utilizing stimulants in the pediatric population. Guanfacine is less sedating and may be effective in the treatment of ADHD. It has a longer half-life allowing for improved compliance. The actions of these alpha-2a agonists are gradual, at times causing improvement two to three weeks after each adjustment. Because sudden withdrawal of alpha-2a agonists may cause life-threatening rebound hypertension, families who are variably compliant with care are poor candidates for these medications.

Typical neuroleptics such as pimozide (Orap), and haloperidol (Haldol) were mainstay treatments for tic disorders prior to the discovered efficacy of alpha-2a agonists. The mechanism of action, postsynaptic dopamine receptor blockade, directly addressed the presumed pathology in the basal ganglia; excessive dopaminergic activity. These agents provide the greatest tic-suppressing effect, and can be quite dramatic in their impact in the medication-naïve patient. Unfortunately, dopamine blockade may lead to receptor hypersensitivity in the basal ganglia with resulting TD and withdrawal dyskinesias. Furthermore, imbalances in the dopamine–acetylcholine pathways produce pseudoparkinsonian effects and akathisia, excessive frontal lobe inhibition causing cognitive and affective blunting. Other side effects include de novo separation anxiety, pituitary dysregulation such as gynecomastia, galactorrhea, weight gain, and cardiac conduction delays with a widened QTc. Treatment with these agents warrants pre and concurrent ECG monitoring, metabolic monitoring of glucose, triglycerides, and cholesterol, nutritional and weight counseling, and recognition of confounding disorder versus medication-related movement abnormalities. Rapid dosage adjustments increase the risk of dyskinesias, rendering the family and clinician unable to differentiate side effect from natural tic vacillations.

Many clinicians consider atypical neuroleptics such as risperidone (Risperdal), olanzapine (Zyprexa), and ziprasidone (Geodon) second-line agents after alpha-2a agonists and before "typical" neuroleptics. The relative advantage over typical neuroleptics is the reduced risk of TDs and other dopamine-receptor blockade side effects. Unfortunately, there are other substantial side effects to consider. Both olanzapine and risperidone may cause dramatic weight gain in the pediatric population. In addition and not necessarily correlated to weight gain, both of these agents may cause metabolic dyscrasias. Insulin resistance is a well-documented potential side effect of these agents. Baseline evaluation of fasting blood sugar and triglycerides is recommended. Ziprasidone is associated with QTc changes and bradycardia, especially in pediatric patients. Titration of this drug should occur slowly, with the monitoring of pulse rate and periodic EKGs. However, to date there have been no reports of cardiac fatalities or episodes of Torsade de point with the administration of ziprasidone.

Treatment of Tics with Substantial Comorbid Condition

TS patients may suffer symptoms of anxiety, depression, OCD, and ADHD. With the exception of ADHD, the pharmacologic treatment of comorbid conditions is similar to treating patients without TS. Refer to specific chapters in this text for guidance as well as dosing guidelines for the drugs discussed below.

In TS patients with co-occurring ADHD, the onset of ADHD symptoms usually precedes the onset of tics. This natural history with the initial onset of ADHD, treatment with stimulants, and then the evolution of tics leads to consideration of the impact of stimulant medication on the onset or exacerbation of tic disorders. While studies addressing this issue provide mixed data, stimulants should be considered as known to initiate or to exacerbate tics in some patients. Stimulants, therefore, should be used with caution in a patient with a family history of tics, a patient history of previous transient tic disorder, or an existing tic syndrome. Stimulant medications are the most effective drugs for ADHD, and many patients with TS have severe ADHD. When nonstimulant approaches to ADHD fail, the clinician and family must consider risk and benefit in eventually committing to stimulant use. In addition to tic exacerbation, stimulants may cause growth suppression, loss of appetite, and sleep disturbance. Stimulants are not active for 24 hours, leaving periods of inattention or hyperactivity at both ends of a day. Some investigators suggest that long-acting stimulant preparations (Concerta, Metadate CD, Adderall XR, Daytrana [patch], Focalin XR) are less neurologically noxious in the patient with tics. These preparations are, therefore, preferred if using stimulants for a patient with tics.

The norepinephrine drug atomoxetine (Strattera), is FDA-approved for children aged 6 and older, is effective in ADHD. Tic exacerbation, agitation, and suicidality are potential effects of this drug in the pediatric population. A similar but less-effective drug for ADHD, bupropion (Wellbutrin) shares the same risk profile. Both atomoxetine and bupropion are capable of causing irritability, sometimes referred to as "activation," or exacerbating bipolar disorder, but do not affect growth, appetite, or sleep, and are active for 24 hours.

Tricyclic antidepressants, now in disfavor due to case reports in the late 1980s and early 1990s of sudden death following the use of desipramine, are effective in ADHD, and are thought to rarely exacerbate tics. Cautious use of tricyclic agents (other than desipramine) may yet have a role, particularly in patients for whom all else has failed.

When to Refer to a Specialist

Uncomplicated tic disorders can be managed in the primary care office. Of course, practice patterns vary by community, training, and interest. Specialty referral is indicated in moderate to severe TS, in tic syndromes with substantial comorbid conditions or if the patient has a tic syndrome not responsive to an initial trial of an alpha-2a agonist.

Child and adolescent psychiatrists provide comprehensive evaluation and clarification of diagnostic issues, comorbid conditions, and treatment recommendations. They often provide ongoing care, including psychotherapy and medication management, or are useful for periodic consultation supporting primary care management. Referral for neurologic evaluation is recommended if the patient presents with findings suggesting a secondary movement disorder or for pharmacologic treatment of moderate to severe tics not responsive to alpha-2a agonists. Family systems in chaos will limit the already complex challenges of treating tic disorders, supporting referral for a family-therapy approach. Children with comorbid conditions may warrant individual and family approaches for effective and potentially nonmedical management of symptoms. Referral to a psychologist is recommended for cognitive and academic testing or for *cognitive behavioral therapy* (CBT) for OCD symptoms and HRT for tic suppression. Finally, occupational therapy (OT) referral may be helpful for youth with prominent handwriting deficits, sensory defensiveness, or late gross motor development. In particular, sensory motor integration therapy may provide substantial relief of irritability and inflexibility in affected children. The essentials of treatment are summarized in Table 10-6.

Conclusions

Children with tic disorders experience a primary neuropsychiatric disorder, frequently accompanied by complicating comorbidities, that presents clinical challenges requiring a combined approach of patient and family education, behavioral therapies, and medical intervention. Successful outcomes depend on attention to alliance building as well as setting realistic goals for the family and clinician. These disorders overtly bridge neurology and the behavioral sciences, undermining the artificial split of brain and mind while encouraging an integrated conceptualization and treatment approach.

TABLE 10-6 Treatment Essentials

- Inform the family and child of the waxing and waning course of tics.
- Support acceptance of tics in the family through reassurance and education.
- Treat tics with medication only if there is pain, physical dysfunction, or marked social impact.
- Set realistic targets and goals prior to beginning medical treatment.
- If medication is used, start low and go slow; consider the natural flux in tics, and medication side effects when evaluating titration outcomes (including discontinuation rebound symptoms).
- Comorbid conditions or psychological issues may cause greater dysfunction than tics, and should be weighted accordingly in the treatment plan.

CASE VIGNETTES

VIGNETTE 1: YOUNG BOY WITH TICS, ADHD, AND POSSIBLE PANDAS

Tony was a 6-year-old boy brought to his pediatrician for evaluation of a dry cough. His mother, in particular, was initially concerned and then annoyed with his repetitive coughing that seemed different from an ordinary cough ("it's as though he's forcing it to happen or something"). This had been going on for weeks at a time and then he would quiet down for a while. There did not seem to be an association with febrile illness or other symptoms of an upper respiratory infection. Tony was also very active. He had visited the pediatrician for a laceration to his occiput when he fell off a stool (no concussion observed) one month earlier. A long string of mild injuries, family exasperation, and complaints from his kindergarten led the pediatrician and family to consider medical treatment of hyperactivity, but they decided to wait until first grade. Sometimes Tony got stuck on projects and would protest at times of transition. He wore sweats at all times and was very annoyed with tags on his clothing. He flapped his arms when he was excited about something, but had no other repetitive behaviors or movements. Tony loved to tell "knock–knock" jokes and enjoyed pretending that he was a dog or a Power Ranger.

He was the product of a normal pregnancy and delivery and met developmental milestones on time or early. His past medical history included recurrent otitis media with bilateral tubes, two episodes of streptococcal pharyngitis, chronic intermittent rhinitis, and multiple injuries without loss of consciousness or concussion. He had no other history of surgery, seizure, hospitalization or ongoing medication, or exposure to heavy metals. No history of psychiatric evaluation or exposure to psychotropic medications was noted.

His family history was positive for ADHD in his father and paternal uncle, but negative for tics. His paternal grandmother was a "control freak" who did not let anyone sit on the white furniture in the living room. No psychiatric diagnoses were noted in the maternal family.

On examination, Tony was a well developed and nourished 6-year-old, who was curious about many things in the office, and had a knack for precarious acrobatics in the waiting room and the examination room. He had a difficult time leaving a toy in the waiting room. He had no overt genetic stigmata. He seemed to have normal articulation and language development and appeared to have at least a normal intelligence. He displayed a forceful dry cough of which he appeared oblivious. He also displayed frequent bilateral eye blinking in spurts. He had a normal skin examination. He denied sore throat or eye irritation. He was afebrile. Tympanic membranes were scarred but not inflamed, and his oropharynx revealed enlarged tonsils bilaterally, with clear postnasal excretions, without erythema or exudates. Lung and cardiac exam was normal, as was the remainder of his general examination. Neurologically, he showed normal strength, reflexes, and gross motor coordination. He did display substantial motor overflow and mirroring during rapid alternating hand movements. The examiner noted that the father displayed subtle sniffing and eye blinking tics.

Discussion: Tony was a hyperkinetic and impulsive little boy presenting with waxing and waning motor and vocal tics. While he was developing normally, he had tactile defensiveness and had a typical history of frequent upper respiratory illnesses, including streptococcal infection. Motor overflow and mirroring movements are normal until the age of 8 or 9 years. Tony's arm flapping with excitement appeared to be motor overflow not associated with autistic spectrum disorder, as he had the capacity for interpersonal engagement, fantasy play, joke telling, and normal language development.

The examiner should further detail the history of tic exacerbation, to rule out correlation with streptococcal infection and a diagnosis of PANDAS. In this case, careful history taking did not reveal injury, illness, or medications temporally related to the course of illness. His father's apparent tics, the family history positive for ADHD, school problems, and obsessive traits fit with probable TS. At this stage, with less than a year of symptoms, Tony's diagnosis is transient tic disorder. He also meets criteria for ADHD, predominantly hyperkinetic type.

While Tony's family is troubled by his coughing behaviors, his greatest functional difficulties are hyperkinesis, attentional deficits, and inflexibility. The family's concerns may respond to education regarding the waxing and waning nature of tics, the risk of escalation with stimulant medication and indications for treatment of tics (social and academic dysfunction) that are not met in this case. A treatment plan might include the following:

1. Education about TS if tics persist beyond a 12-month period. Possible referral to the local chapter of the *Tourette Syndrome Association* (TSA).
2. Recommend school-based evaluation and educational support, possibly with an Individual Education Plan (IEP) or a 504 plan, based on the diagnosis of tic disorder, and ADHD, and to rule out specific learning disabilities. Recommend school evaluation for OT services based on sensory defensiveness and soft neurologic signs.
3. Behavioral structure and support plan at home for ADHD symptoms, including: diminishing overstimulation; providing organized and predictable schedules, clear social rules and expectations, opportunities for "noncontingent" positive regard and engagement.
4. Pharmacologic intervention: guanfacine or clonidine that may address hyperkinesis and tics, or atomoxetine for the treatment of ADHD (as it has not been reported to exacerbate tics). The use of stimulants warrants caution, as exacerbation of tics must be weighed against the potential benefit and alternatives.

VIGNETTE 2: SCHOOL-AGED BOY WITH TRIAD OF TOURETTE SYNDROME, ADHD, AND ANXIETY

Tom is a 9-year-old brought to the child psychiatry service with a history of Tourette syndrome diagnosed by a neurologist 2 years ago. His severe tics are now under good control with haloperidol increased to 1.0 mg daily 2 months ago. Recently, he has had increasing problems with night-time fears and going to school becoming tearful and defiant. He has ongoing struggles with severe ADHD symptoms, combined type (hyperactivity, impulsivity, and inattention) and school is a real struggle. Parents are exasperated with Tom's bedtime and school struggles and the whole family is locked into heated and at times explosive battles. The school is concerned about attendance and the capacity of their small self-contained classroom to manage Tom's impulsive and disruptive behavior and is considering a day treatment program.

The child psychiatrist performs a thorough history, talks to the school, and has a play evaluation session with Tom. She is satisfied that the diagnosis is correct, that this is a competent but overwhelmed family. She does not find any other developmental or environmental issues. The school is well engaged with Tom and has a good understanding of some learning issues and basic management techniques for children with ADHD. The play session reveals that Tom is indeed hyperactive and impulsive but a sweet, well-related child with many fears of separation in his play. Based on these findings she develops the following formulation.

Tom is a child with well-established diagnosis of Tourette syndrome and a severe comorbid diagnosis of ADHD. He also has a new onset of separation anxiety. These issues are overwhelming an otherwise competent family and school and Tom is receiving increasingly negative engagement with his parents and his school. There is a risk of placement in a more restrictive educational setting if his ADHD does not come under better control. Anxiety was not a prominent feature of Tom's past history. While the struggles with ADHD in the classroom may be inducing anxiety about school, the recent increase in haloperidol is temporally related to the onset of separation anxiety and is known to induce separation anxiety.

Recommendations:

1. Following a thorough family cardiac history and assurance of normal vital signs and cardiac exam, a cross taper off haloperidol and onto guanfacine was initiated. This was expected to eliminate the issue of neuroleptic-induced separation anxiety and potentially treat tics and ADHD with one medication.

2. Trials of a low dose of long-acting stimulant (Concerta) or Strattera were recommended if guanfacine was not adequate for the control of ADHD symptoms with discussions around the potential of Tic exacerbation.

3. The family was recommended *The Explosive Child* by Ross Greene to help develop ways to de-escalate conflict at home.

BIBLIOGRAPHY

Harris K, Singer HS. Tic disorders: neural circuits, neurochemistry, and neuroimmunology. *J Child Neurol.* 2006;8:678–689.

Jankovic J. Treatment of hyperkinetic movement disorders. *Lancet Neurol.* 2009;9:844–856.

Keen-Kim D, Freimer NB. Genetics and epidemiology of Tourette syndrome. *J Child Neurol.* 2006;21(8):665–671.

Lechman JF, Bloch MH, King RA, et al. Phenomenology of tics and natural history of tic disorders. In: Walkup JT, Mink JW, Hollenbeck PJ, eds. *Advances in Neurology, Vol 99: Tourette Syndrome.* Philadelphia, PA: Lippincott Williams & Wilkins; 2006.

Leckman JF, Riddle MA, Hardin MT, et al. The Yale Global Tic Severity Scale: initial testing of a clinician-rated scale of tic severity. *J Am Acad Child Adolesc Psychiatry.* 1989;4:566–573.

Leckman JF, Zhang H, Vitate A, et al. Course of tic severity in Tourette syndrome: the first two decades. *Pediatrics.* 1998;102:14–19.

Miranda DM, Wigg K, Kabia EM, et al. Association of SLITRK1 to Gilles de la Tourette syndrome. *Am J Med Genet B Neuropsychiatr Genet.* 2009;150B(4):483–486.

Pauls, DL, et al. Genome scan for Tourette syndrome in affected-sibling-pair and multigenerational families. *The American Journal of Human Genetics.* 2007;80(2):265–272.

Peterson BS, Choi HA, Hao X, et al. Morphologic features of the amygdala and hippocampus in children and adults with Tourette syndrome. *Arch Gen Psychiatry.* 2007;11:1281–1291.

Peterson BS, Leckman JF. The temporal dynamics of tics in Gilles de la Tourette syndrome. *Biol Psychiatry.* 1998;44:1337–1348.

Piacentini J, Chang S. Habit reversal training for tic disorders in children and adolescents. *Behav Modification.* 2005;6:803–822.

Ringman JM, Jankovic J. Occurrence of tics in Asperger's syndrome and autistic disorder. *J Child Neurol.* 2000;15(6):394–400.

Shapiro AK, Shapiro E. Treatment of Gilles de la Tourette's syndrome with haloperidol. *Br J Psychiatry.* 1968;114:345–350.

Singer HS, Gause C, Morris C, et al. Serial immune markers do not correlate with clinical exacerbations in pediatric autoimmune neuropsychiatric disorders associated with streptococcal infections. *Pediatrics.* 2008;6:1198–1205.

Swain JE, Scahill L, Lombroso PJ, et al. Tourette syndrome and tic disorders: a decade of progress. *J Am Acad Child Adolesc Psychiatry.* 2007;8:947–968.

Swedo SE, Leonard HL, et al. Pediatric autoimmune neuropsychiatric disorders associated with streptococcal infections: clinical description of the first 50 cases. *Am J Psychiatry.* 1998;155:264–271.

Yoon DY; Gause CD; Leckman JF, et al. Frontal dopaminergic abnormality in Tourette syndrome: a postmortem analysis. *J Neurological Sci.* 2007;1(2):50–56.

SUGGESTED READINGS

Greene R. *The Explosive Child.* 3rd ed. New York, NY: Harpers Collins; 2005.

Walkup JT, Mink JW, Hollenbeck PJ. *Advances in Neurology, Vol 99: Tourette Syndrome.* Philadelphia, PA: Lippincott Williams & Wilkins; 2006.

SUGGESTED WEBSITE

Official website of the Tourette Syndrome Association: http://www.tsa-usa.org.

REVIEW QUESTIONS

1. Tics may be differentiated from other movement disorders as they are frequently painful.
   True/False

2. Common reasons to treat tics:
   a. Impaired ambulation
   b. Parental frustration
   c. Sleep interruption
   d. Functional impairment

3. Neuronal structures implicated in Tourette syndrome:
   a. Parietal cortex
   b. Basal ganglia and cerebellum
   c. Temporal lobe and corpus callosum
   d. Basal ganglia, frontal cortex, and limbic system

4. PANDAS patients share the following features:
   a. Rapid onset
   b. Handwriting deterioration
   c. Separation anxiety
   d. Erythema multiforme
      1. A
      2. A and D
      3. D only
      4. ABC
      5. All of the above

5. Known cardiac conduction delay would lead to preferential use of pimozide (Orap) and ziprasidone (Geodon) in a patient with tics.
   True/False

Answers: 1-False, 2-d, 3-d, 4-4, 5-False

CHAPTER 11

Elizabeth McCauley, PhD, ABPP,
Gretchen R. Gudmundsen, PhD,
Carol Rockhill, MD, PhD, MPH,
and My Banh, PhD

Child and Adolescent Depressive Disorders

Introduction

It is now recognized that depressive disorders represent a serious mental health risk for children and adolescents. Depression can present along a wide continuum stretching from brief episodes of low mood, which resolve spontaneously, to a disabling complex of symptoms that persist over time. Community-based research suggests that 20% of youth report having experienced a clinically significant depressive episode by age 18, while 65% of adolescents report experiencing transient or less severe depressive symptoms. Even subclinical levels of depressive symptomatology can, however, derail the normal developmental process, interfering with academic and social functioning and increasing risk for both substance use and suicide. Moreover, the sequelae of early-onset depression include a host of later psychosocial deficits, including poor global and adaptive functioning, academic and occupational impairment, disrupted interpersonal relationships, early childbearing, reduced life satisfaction, and substance abuse or dependence. These far-reaching consequences underscore the importance of improving our ability to identify and intervene with depressed youth.

Given the scope of the problem of depression in children and adolescents, the lack of adequate mental health resources, and the issues of stigma, clinicians in a variety of community settings including primary care offices and schools are faced with taking increasing responsibility for detection and management of these mental health problems. When symptoms of depression occur, youth and families are likely to turn first to known providers or institutions for direction and support. In many cases, primary care medical providers are contacted first as for many children and adolescents somatic complaints may be the first signs of depression and less stigma is attached to seeking medical rather than mental health care. In other cases, school-based care providers are called upon for help as declines in school performance and attendance may herald the onset of depression.

Evidence-based guidelines for the management of depression across the severity continuum within community-care settings underscore the need for varied approaches that range from "watchful waiting" in youth with mild symptoms to multimodal interventions in more severe cases. Determining how best to recognize each child's level of need remains a challenge. This chapter will summarize recent findings about depressive disorders in children and adolescents and review practical strategies that can be used to provide effective identification, assessment, and management within primary care or community-based settings.

Background

Historically, depression was considered a phenomenon that only adults experienced. Before the 1980s children were seldom given a diagnosis of depression as it was widely believed that they were not cognitively or emotionally mature enough to experience or comprehend the sense of loss or the internalization of aggression that many thought were essential elements underlying a clinically significant depressive reaction. Young people, especially preadolescent children, also tended to present with a mixture of mood-related symptoms like sadness coupled with somatic symptoms and/or noncompliance and acting out. In the late 1970s, the term "masked depression" was coined and used to describe youth whose clinical presentation included a variety of mood and behavioral disorder symptoms, but depression was thought to be a central component of the underlying problem.

During this time, efforts were being made to standardize the diagnostic process to provide a reliable method to ascertain a diagnosis across research groups and parts of the country. In this context, semi-structured diagnostic interviews were developed, which outlined strict criteria for making a diagnosis. This movement began with studies of adult psychopathology but soon trickled down to work with children and adolescents. In 1980, two landmark studies presented data indicating that using structured diagnostic interviewing and the existing adult criteria (*DSM-III*) was a valid way to diagnose depression in children. With this, masked depression fell by the wayside and a new wave of research on the development, course, and treatment of depression in children and adolescents was ushered in. This research has confirmed that children and adolescents experience a range of depressive disorders that are qualitatively similar in nature to those experienced by adults. Ironically, we have now come full circle as today we recognize that depression in young people typically presents as part of a complex constellation of emotional and behavioral problems, with anxiety and disruptive behavior disorders frequently presenting along with depressive symptoms.

Clinical Features

Depressive disorders involve individuals experiencing a change from their normal mood (euthymia) to a depressed state. These episodes may vary in number, type, and duration of depressive symptoms. Developmental level accounts for some differences in symptom presentation. Anhedonia, or the lack of enjoyment of activities, is a hallmark symptom of depression in very young children. Preadolescents are also more likely to report somatic complaints such as stomachache or headache more frequently than adolescents who report more hopelessness, fatigue, weight loss, and suicidal ideation and attempts.

The current psychiatric diagnostic manual, the *Diagnostic and Statistical Manual, Fourth Edition, Text Revision* (*DSM-IV-TR*), discusses a number of depressive diagnoses, as described in Table 11-1, that can be useful when assessing children and adolescents with major depressive disorder (MDD), dysthymic disorder (DD), depression not otherwise specified (NOS), and depression secondary to a general medical condition. Diagnostic criteria for core depressive disorders for youth parallel adult criteria, with a few exceptions. In youth MDD, irritability can be the primary emotion rather than sadness, and a child or an adolescent who experiences depressive symptoms for 1 year qualifies for a diagnosis of DD, whereas a 2-year duration of symptoms is required for adults.

Depressive disorder NOS best characterizes young people who report periods of low mood accompanied by low self-esteem or loss of interest in normally enjoyable activities, but either do not demonstrate all of the symptoms necessary to warrant a diagnosis of MDD or show a relatively recent onset of difficulties with depressed mood. In some cases their periods of low mood wax and wane. This diagnosis can be useful as a "working diagnosis" when depressive symptoms are present, but the potentially causal role of an underlying medical condition is still being evaluated.

Within the diagnosis of MDD, some young people have variant presentations. Specifically, adolescents, more frequently than adults, present with what has been termed "atypical depression." This variant of MDD is characterized by increased reactivity to rejection, lethargy, increased appetite, craving for carbohydrates, and hypersomnia. Some children and adolescents present with

TABLE 11-1	Characteristics of *DSM-IV* Depressive Disorders
Diagnosis	**Key Clinical Features**
Major depressive disorder (MDD)	• Depressed, sad, or irritable mood or anhedonia • One cardinal symptom (listed above) in concert with at least four additional symptoms • All symptoms must be present during the *same* 2-week period and must represent a change from previous functioning
Dysthymic disorder (DD)	• Depressed, sad, or irritable mood for most of the day for more days than not for 1 year (must not have gone for more than 2 months without experiencing two or more symptoms) • More protracted, less severe course than MDD (mean episode length of 33–48 months) • Heightens risk for development of MDD
Depressive disorder not otherwise specified (NOS)	• Depressed, sad, or irritable mood or anhedonia, but mood disturbance does not meet *DSM-IV* criteria for full episodes
Depression secondary to a general medical condition	• Depressed or irritable mood or anhedonia in most or all activities • Symptoms are determined to be directly related to the presence and physiologic consequences of a medical condition.

Adapted from American Psychiatric Association. *Diagnostic and Statistical Manual of Mental Disorders, Fourth Edition (Text Revision)*. Washington, DC: Author, 2000.

psychotic symptoms. In young children these tend to be brief, transient auditory hallucinations in which the child may hear a voice telling them to hurt themselves or others. Delusional thinking is more common in adolescents who may be troubled by persistent and intrusive beliefs that they are dying or controlled by some outside power. Efforts to clearly identify a group of young people with seasonal mood disorder have met with mixed results. Because the shorter, darker days of northern climates correspond with the school year, it can be difficult to disentangle the stressors related to school from the impact of reduced light exposure. Other variants in the presentation of depression may reflect ethnocultural differences; for instance, Asian American girls are more likely to describe depression as part of a relational problem (e.g., being misunderstood), having low self-esteem (e.g., "feeling insecure, useless, and insufficient"), and feeling stressed.

Many youth also present with depressive symptoms in the context of significant or chronic health conditions. When depressive symptoms appear only in the context of significant illness, a diagnosis of depression secondary to a general medical condition should be used. Many of these youths have no history of mental health concerns prior to the onset of their illness but become overwhelmed or demoralized in the face of loss of function, pain, and in some cases life-threatening circumstances. For others, significant depressive symptoms may have predated their health concerns or have been significant even when physical symptoms are in remission, suggesting the need for a diagnosis of depression independent of their medical diagnosis.

Differential Diagnoses

Given the variability in how depression can present, it is critical to consider whether there is another more central problem to address. Thus, whenever considering a depression diagnosis, the first step is to rule out the presence of an underlying medical condition (see the section "Assessment") with care to also determine whether the young person is exhibiting depressive symptoms secondary to another emotional or behavioral disorder. In addition, youth with undetected eating disorders (bulimia, early stages of anorexia nervosa) and anxiety sometimes first present with depressive symptoms.

Severity Continuum

It is also useful to categorize depressive disorders by levels of severity as this helps guide immediate treatment planning. Categorization is based on the presence or absence of the nine key symptoms (depressed mood/irritability, anhedonia, as well as difficulties with fatigue, sleep disturbance, appetite disturbance, thoughts of death or suicide, decreased concentration, self-blame/hopelessness/down on self, and psychomotor retardation/agitation) coupled with duration of symptoms and degree of impairment in psychosocial functioning. Thus, mild depression is defined as five to six or fewer symptoms of short duration with limited impairment, moderate depression as seven to eight symptoms of longer duration with moderate impairment, and severe depression as persistent presentation of most symptoms with marked impairment. If impairment is marked and suicidal ideation or psychotic symptoms are present, the depression is considered severe regardless of the number of symptoms present.

Epidemiology

Depression can vary in terms of severity, but most of the epidemiologic research has focused on clinically significant depression, or MDD with a subset of studies including youth with DD as well as those with MDD. Few epidemiologic studies have included very young children, but an epidemiologic study completed in the 1980s identified nine young children who met criteria for MDD from a community sample of 1000 preschoolers. More recently, Luby and her research team have conducted a series of studies to validate developmentally modified criteria for depression in preschool-aged children, which should lay the groundwork for further epidemiologic work with this age group.

Within the diagnostic context outlined earlier in the text, in 2002 the National Institutes of Mental Health estimated that approximately 6 million children and adolescents between the ages of 9 and 17 experience an episode of clinically significant depression over the course of their childhood and adolescent years. MDD is considered somewhat rare in children, with a 12-month prevalence of less than 3% in the sixth- to ninth-grade years. However, as reviewed by Hankin and colleagues, the rate of depressive disorders escalates over fivefold in the adolescent years reaching 17% during the 18th year of life, while 65% of adolescents report experiencing transient or less severe depressive symptoms. While rates of depression increase during this period for both boys and girls by middle to late adolescence, depressed females outnumber depressed males by a ratio of 2 to 1. A growing body of research suggests some variation in prevalence of depression across different ethnocultural groups, with Hispanic American youth demonstrating higher rates of depression and Asian American reporting lower levels of depression. Finally, between 5% and 10% of young people present with subsyndromal symptoms that do not meet criteria for MDD or dysthymia, but are associated with concerning outcomes, including considerable psychosocial impairment and increased risk for suicide and the development of more significant depression.

Risk Factors

Depression is most likely to develop when a number of risk factors converge. Inherited or biologic vulnerabilities may contribute to risk for depression. Family and twin studies suggest heritability estimates for depression of up to 50%, and descriptive research indicates that having a parent with depression is one of the strongest and most reliable risk factors for depression in children. Children may also learn depressive coping styles from observing a depressed parent and being exposed to more stressors when living with a depressed parent. Young people may also inherit temperamental qualities such as sensitivity to negative emotions, which can contribute to risk for depression.

It is widely believed that depression affects a vulnerable person (based on biologic, cognitive, or a combination of risk factors) when he or she is faced with stressful life events. For young people, major life events such as parental separation or divorce or exposure to abuse or neglect as well as peer and school pressures, loss of a friendship or romance, or a geographic move can trigger depression. Depression that first presents in childhood has been strongly associated with exposure to stressful environments. Goodyer and colleagues suggest that depressed youth may be born with dysfunctional neuroregulatory mechanisms or develop atypical responses when exposed to early stressors. In their studies, youth with hypersecretion of stress-related hormones (salivary cortisol and dehydroepiandrosterone) and recent losses were the most likely to develop a depressive disorder.

Although heritability estimates are high, researchers consistently underscore the importance of the gene–environment interaction in the development of depressive disorders. For example, there is a wealth of evidence implicating dysfunction in serotonergic signaling in depression, a process controlled in part by the serotonin transporter (SERT) gene. Initial studies suggested that the 5-HTTLPR polymorphism of SERT coupled with exposure to stress during childhood increased the risk of depression in adulthood. Although a recent meta-analysis by Risch and colleagues casts doubt on the specific role of the 5-HTTLPR polymorphism of SERT in mediating depression, the SERT gene itself remains an important candidate gene for depression.

Comorbidities

Having a "pure" form of a single psychiatric disorder is uncharacteristic of the majority of children with mental health conditions. Among depressed youth, the frequency of having a comorbid psychiatric diagnosis ranges across studies from 40% to 90%. The most common co-occurring problem is anxiety. Youth with a depressive disorder are up to eight times more likely than youth without depression to have a co-occurring anxiety problem. Longitudinal studies document that anxiety typically precedes the onset of depression and that anxious symptoms in childhood serve as an independent risk factor for depressive symptoms in adolescence. Significant separation anxiety in early childhood is commonly reported when gathering history of youth with comorbid depression and anxiety. Generalized anxiety disorder symptoms are most typical, as panic disorder is less common in both children and adolescents than in adults. Posttraumatic stress disorder can be associated with both generalized anxiety and depressive symptoms. Anxiety symptoms typically persist even after the depressive symptoms become apparent. In addition, McCauley and colleagues have found that depressive and anxiety disorders are more common in young people with chronic illness and add to symptom burden and functional impairment.

Depression also frequently co-occurs with externalizing behavioral problems. Clinically depressed youth are 5.5 times more likely to have attention-deficit hyperactivity disorder (ADHD) and 6.6 times more likely than youth without depression to meet the criteria for conduct disorder (CD) or oppositional defiant disorder (ODD). Externalizing behavior problems tend to be present before depressive symptoms are apparent, and persist even while depressive symptoms wax and wane. A "dual failure" model has been proposed to explain the co-occurrence of depressive and conduct problems. This model posits that the repeated academic and social failures experienced by youth with ADHD and conduct problems (ODD and CD) lead to moodiness and poor emotional control, thereby increasing vulnerability to depression.

Comorbidity with substance use or abuse is also common as youth move into adolescence. In one study, Rohde and colleagues reported a depression prevalence of 47.9% among high school students with alcohol abuse or dependence compared to about 20% in abstainers, experimenters, or social drinkers. A negative affect pathway in which youth turn to alcohol or other drugs to alleviate psychological distress has been proposed, but efforts to test this model have resulted in inconsistent findings. Depression typically precedes adolescent substance use and abuse, but substance use also exacerbates depression.

Clinical Course

Depressive episodes in children and adolescents can persist for a significant period of time with mean length of episode across samples ranging from 9 to 17 months. The persistence of depression over this kind of time period can clearly alter the developmental process. Depression is associated with a high recurrence rate, with between 40% and 69% of adolescents experiencing a relapse within 2 to 5 years.

Differential outcomes have been associated with age of onset. Depression that first presents during childhood appears to increase the risk for a number of behavioral problems later in life including both conduct- and mood-related difficulties. In contrast, depression that first presents in adolescence has been more strongly associated with a family history of depression and follows a course similar to that observed in adults, with increased risk for recurrence of depressive disorders over time.

Developmental Considerations

Recent research led by Joan Luby has documented that even preschool-aged children experience depression. In infants and toddlers, depression is most frequently associated with deprivation and can take the form of failure to thrive. In preschoolers, anhedonia or loss of interest in activities has been identified as a "highly specific symptom of depression" based on parental interviews, observations of play, and alterations in stress cortisol reactivity. While large-scale studies of the prevalence of depressive disorders are not available for very young children, they appear to be rare. As noted earlier in the text, the prevalence of depression remains fairly low in childhood but increases markedly as youth move through adolescence.

Neurologic development, physical growth, and sexual maturation are factors thought to contribute to the increased risk for depression observed during adolescence. Changes in emotions and behavior (changes in sleep, increases in moodiness, emotional intensity, romantic interests, and risk taking) are observed at the time of pubertal development. Sexual maturation and the intensification of emotions occur while the adolescent's nervous system is also undergoing a number of structural changes (completion of brain cell genesis, nerve myelination, and dendrite pruning in the frontal cortex) that lay the foundation for more sophisticated cognitive skills. These cognitive skills (inhibitory control, problem solving, and long-term planning), however, only become operational as the adolescent matures and gains experience. Because there is typically a developmental lag between the onset of the emotional and behavioral activation of early puberty and the mastery of cognitive and emotional coping skills, problems with affect regulation intensify during the early adolescent period. For example, because they have not mastered the cognitive and coping skills needed to handle strong emotions, adolescents are prone to biased interpretations of experiences, self-criticality, and low inhibitory control. They also use coping mechanisms that are emotion focused, such as talking about problems with friends or wishful thinking, strategies that often do not result in problem solving and can exacerbate risk for depression or prolong an existing depression.

Assessment

Screening and Symptom Assessment

The US/Canadian and British guidelines for management of depression in young people stress the importance of early identification of at-risk youth with subsequent monitoring for the development of a depressive disorder. As part of every contact, including well-child or problem-focused medical visits, the guidelines recommend that patients and parents complete a brief screening tool that covers symptoms of depression including thoughts of self-harm and suicide, to allow the care provider to carry out a rapid check for depression and to track changes in symptom presentation over time. Screening tools flag youth in need of more follow-up

TABLE 11-2 Screening and Interview Measures		
Measure	Informants	Number of Items
Depression measures		
Moods and Feelings Questionnaire (MFQ; Angold and Costello 1987)	Youth (age 8–18) and parent version	32 items (complete form); 13 items (short form)
Patient Health Questionnaire (PHQ-9; Kroenke, Spitzer, and Williams, 2001)	Adolescents	9 items
Childhood Depression Inventory (CDI; Kovacs, 1992)	Youth (age 7–17)	27 items
Reynolds Child Depression Scale (RCDS; Reynolds, 1989)/Reynolds Adolescent Depression Scale (RADS; Reynolds, 1987)	Youth–Child (8–12)/ Adolescent (13–18)	30 items
Beck Depression Inventory (BDI; Beck and Steer, 1993)	Adolescents	21 items
Broadband measures		
Achenbach System of Empirically Based Assessment (Achenbach and Rescorla, 2001): Youth Self-Report (YSR); Child Behavior Checklist (CBCL)	Youth (age 11–18) and parent (regarding youth age 5–18)	118 items
Semi-structured interview guidelines		
HEADDSSS psychosocial interview for adolescents (Goldenring and Cohen, 1988; Goldenring and Rosen, 2004)	Adolescents	Domains: home, education/ employment, activities, diet, drugs, sexuality, suicidality/depression, safety

while also communicating to the young person that concerns about mood and feelings are legitimate topics for discussion. There are a number of patient/parent self-report scales and clinician's interviews that can be incorporated readily into routine practice (Table 11-2).

As outlined in Table 11-3, a brief psychosocial assessment should be built into each medical clinic or community-care visit, via the inclusion of brief but routine questions that ask about home, school, and social functioning.

As with a screening questionnaire, asking key questions about social and emotional adjustment communicates to the child or adolescent that these are legitimate topics to bring up and opens the door for further discussion if/when concerns arise. Inclusion of the parents' perspective in evaluating depressive symptoms is essential for young children and useful at all ages. Assessment of adolescents, however, requires a private interview with the adolescent to discuss issues such as substance abuse and sexual activity and to assess risk for self-harm and suicidal ideation that may be difficult for the teen to reveal in front of their parents. A review of confidentiality and its limits should lead off this interview process. When assessing for self-harm risk, it is essential to ask specifically about thoughts of suicide and engagement in risky or self-harming behaviors. If the youth indicates that he or she has been thinking about suicide, determining whether he or she has a specific plan or access to means (e.g., are there guns in the home) is essential. Inclusion of a safety plan that covers who the youth can turn to for support, ways to manage stressors (e.g., listen to music and take a run), and identification of something the youth has to live for is an effective way to draw this evaluation, no matter how brief to a close. Assessment of co-occurring problems is also essential to assure a clear understanding of

TABLE 11-3	Essentials of Assessment for Child and Adolescent Depression

- Physical examination, review of systems, and laboratory testing are included to rule out possible medical etiologies including neurologic, systemic, and substance-induced disorders. Common medical conditions that produce symptoms similar to depression include anemia or disorders related to thyroid and hormone functioning.
- A structured or semi-structured clinical interview involving both the youth and at least one parent facilitates proper diagnosis and case conceptualization, including making appropriate differential diagnoses, such as bipolar disorder, and identifying comorbid disorders, such as an anxiety disorder.
- Ideally, the assessment should include time with the youth and parent together, as well as time with just the youth and just the parent(s) to ensure all parties have had sufficient opportunity to speak candidly about their concerns. With the youth alone, it is important to assess suicidality, substance use, sexual behavior, and other high-risk behavior.
- Gather information about the child's previous course of the depression, including duration, prior episodes, and age of onset.
- Assess key symptoms, including suicidal ideation, psychotic symptoms, and manic behaviors.
- Collect history of the youth's development, general medical history, family history of psychopathology, and overall functioning across school, home, and social domains.
- Assess significant stressors and traumas, including both episodic and ongoing stress.
- Evaluate the youth's and family's history of previous treatment, including psychosocial and pharmacologic intervention.

the issues the young person is coping with and identifying what kind of interventions may be needed. Some of the self-report/parent report scales described in Table 11-2 are a good way to track a wide range of problem areas as well as the brief review of current status vis-à-vis substance use and trouble at home, at school, or in the community.

Medical Assessment

Screening positive for depressive symptoms can result from numerous causes, including medical conditions. Thus, it is important to include a medical screen when assessing depressive symptoms, given the overlap of depression with medical problems and medication side effects. Weller and colleagues provide a comprehensive overview of medical concerns that might contribute to a presentation of depression. In particular, evaluation for substance abuse and consideration of urine toxicology are important roles for the medical provider. If a child or an adolescent is using substances, he or she should be counseled about mood-altering effects of the substance used. For example, chronic alcohol use and binge drinking both are associated with increased risk for depression as well as causing or worsening sleep disturbance; marijuana can cause amotivational syndrome; repeated cocaine or amphetamine use depletes serotonin, and postcocaine intoxication dysphoria greatly increases the risk for suicide; inhalants cause central nervous system damage that may result in reduced school performance and secondary depression (see Chapter 6 for more detail).

In addition, it is essential to review the child's medication list for agents known to have a potential for depressive or psychotic symptoms as side effects (e.g., corticosteroids, benzodiazepines, isotretinoin [Accutane], interferon therapy, barbiturates, antihypertensive agents, and some chemotherapy medications). Providers should also consider whether an infectious illness such as pneumonia, subacute bacterial endocarditis, or infectious mononucleosis could be causing malaise and masquerading as depression. For patients with prominent fatigue, at a minimum a complete blood count (CBC) should be completed, and other studies such as testing for human immunodeficiency virus (HIV) or mononucleosis should be considered.

Rare infectious risks such as encephalitis and syphilis are part of the infectious differential diagnosis.

Endocrine problems can cause depressive symptoms, and the most common offender is hypothyroidism. Testing of thyroid function at baseline is recommended, even though it is "low-yield," to avoid misdiagnosing depression while not recognizing a treatable medical illness. Pituitary, adrenal, and parathyroid diseases are much less common but should be considered if symptoms such as weakness are prominent, since fatigue but not weakness is typical of depression. Electrolyte abnormalities, anemia, autoimmune disorder, cancer, Wilson disease, and porphyria also cause prominent weakness, and testing for those disorders should be done if the history or symptoms are suggestive of these disorders. Many neurologic illnesses include a potential for overlapping symptoms with depression, including traumatic brain injury, epilepsy, and multiple sclerosis. Finally, selected vitamin deficiencies, such as vitamin D deficiency, have shown an association with depressive symptoms.

Overall, regardless of the setting of care, ongoing screening for depression in children and adolescents allows for early identification and initiation of efforts to prevent escalation of symptoms. In all situations, accurate assessment is critical to the development of an optimal treatment.

Treatment

Education about depression and careful monitoring of symptom severity are recommended as the initial steps of intervention for all cases (Table 11-4).

TABLE 11-4 Treatment Essentials for Child and Adolescent Depression

- Treatment planning should be guided by the severity of disorder, comorbid psychiatric and medical conditions, and the motivation of the youth and family.
- Early intervention is important in order to limit the duration of a depressive episode and to potentially curtail recurrence of symptoms given its significant impact on youth academic, social, and familial functioning.
- Mild to moderate depression is often well treated with an evidence-based psychosocial intervention, including either cognitive–behavioral therapy or interpersonal therapy.
- Psychotherapy is an important part of treatment with youth who have severe psychosocial stressors, poor medication compliance or refusal to take medications, suicidality or poor or limited response to pharmacotherapy alone.
- For moderate to severe depression, combined treatment involving both psychosocial and pharmacotherapeutic intervention is recommended.
- Pharmacotherapy is an important treatment choice when there is a positive family history of a mood disorder; a family history for a good response to antidepressant medications; the presence of neurovegetative signs and symptoms; severe, chronic, or recurrent depression; a poor or limited response to psychotherapy alone; or limited resources.
- SSRIs are typically the first line of pharmacotherapy given the low side effect profile. Fluoxetine (Prozac) and ecitalopram (Lexapro) are the only FDA-approved SSRIs for use with children and adolescents, although all SSRIs have the potential to be helpful.
- If SSRIs are ineffective, the next line of treatment is buproprion (Wellbutrin) or mirtazapine (Remeron).
- Providers should continually monitor the status and/or emergence of suicidality, and manic and psychotic symptoms.
- Ongoing collaboration with the school should focus on education about depression, development of an appropriate Individualized Education Plan, and assistance with behavioral management planning.

Mild depression may allow a "watchful waiting" approach as the first step as long as the youth's level of stress is assessed and support is provided via regular follow-up appointments to monitor progress. With mild depression or with families not yet ready to seek active treatment, education can focus on the importance of general health and self-care, including information about how to regulate sleep and eating patterns, encouraging increased physical activity, and engaging the youth and/or family in tracking a particular symptom or area such as sleep with a timeframe set for them to report back about what they have noticed. Primary medical care providers may need to introduce the possibility of depression to youth and parents who are seeking relief from what they see as a physical concern. This is best done by reviewing depression as one of a number of conditions that needs to be considered and evaluated further, particularly if families are focused on a medical explanation.

Beginning with a trial of psychotherapy is reasonable for children and adolescents who meet criteria for MDD or DD, but whose symptoms are mild to moderate and functional impairment is not severe and who do not have suicidal ideation or psychosis. This recommendation is based on two sets of findings. First, as reported by Rohde and his team, there is a relatively high response rate to therapy without medication in treatment of mild depression in children and adolescents. Second, since children and adolescents have a high rate of placebo response (30–60%) during antidepressant medication trials, it is difficult to evaluate whether improvement in symptoms is due to placebo response, medication effect, or concurrent therapy effects. In children or adolescents with mild depression who start with therapy, a re-evaluation should take place in 4 to 6 weeks, and if symptoms have not improved, initiation of medication intervention can be reconsidered.

For cases of moderate to severe depression, it is important for the youth and family to be connected with a mental health professional as both psychotherapy and pharmacotherapy may be indicated. In many cases, transitioning families to more formal mental health care can be challenging. Ethnic minority youth and families may be particularly reluctant to seek formal mental health services. African American and Mexican American youth, for instance, are more receptive to community-based programs such as those offered within their church or family support than formal mental health care. Asian American youth do not want to burden their parents and worry about the sense of shame associated with talking about feelings of depression. To smooth the referral process, it is helpful to focus on the functional impairment associated with depression rather than the particular depressive symptoms. Getting support to solve problems about school attendance or performance or to keep up with an activity may help facilitate the development of common goals for parents and youth in seeking help.

An informed referral also includes being mindful to educate patients and families about what further assessment is indicated and what intervention strategies are evidence based. While a specific treatment plan can be determined only once a clear case conceptualization is in hand, it is important to direct families to providers who have expertise in treating depressed youth and who are skilled in using evidence-based approaches (see later in the text for summary of evidence-based interventions for depression in young people). If a youth or family member is reluctant to seek care from a mental health specialist, providers may need to use follow-up appointments to assess ongoing function while setting up guidelines and goals so that it is clear when a transfer of care is warranted, for example, "if you are still feeling so down, when we meet again, let's talk again about how to get you more help." Many adolescents like to assert some independence in dealing with their depression, so providing self-help resources such as books or Internet-based resources (see the "Suggested Readings" and "Suggested Websites" sections) or connecting them with leadership and empowerment programs offered through the community agencies may be effective first steps in linking youth to services. Finally, failure to sufficiently integrate and address comorbid symptoms and diagnoses can interfere with treatment engagement. Treatment referral and planning should address the symptoms that most concern the child and family. Providing education that emotional and behavioral problems, even those as different as depressive and conduct problems, commonly coexist in young people is critical.

It is important for the community-based care provider to continue to play a central role in the child's care, working collaboratively with the mental health care provider. This may involve prescribing and following an antidepressant medication or working with school personnel to institute practical interventions such as development of a 504 Plan or an Individualized Education Plan, to establish accommodations to support the young person and keep them engaged in school and social activities.

Psychosocial Intervention

Of the small number of well-controlled studies of psychosocial treatments with depressed adolescents that have been conducted, cognitive–behavioral therapy (CBT) and interpersonal therapy (IPT) have been most widely investigated and demonstrate the strongest evidence base as therapeutic approaches to treating youth with depression. Both approaches were originally developed for depressed adults and were developmentally adapted for use in youth. Additionally, both approaches are typically delivered to the child or adolescent alone and focus on teaching individual skills for managing depressive symptoms. However, as with any therapy with youth, parents and family members are involved to varying degrees. In addition to individual CBT and IPT, other treatment modalities have demonstrated promise, including group and family therapy. Luby is currently testing a widely used parent-training approach adapted to address mood disorders in children as young as 3. In this approach, the parent–child interaction therapy–emotion development, the parent or caregiver is "coached" in how to intervene with the child to teach effective emotion regulation skills and to foster their ability to enjoy activities and experiences.

The core premise of CBT is that the way individuals perceive or think about situations and the way they respond, influence how they feel. For instance, when a youth is called on in class and feels unsure of how to respond, he or she may think automatically, "I'm always wrong," tell the teacher he or she does not know the answer, and feel embarrassed and like a "loser." CBT targets maladaptive thoughts and actions in order to improve and reduce symptoms of depression. It uses a variety of techniques with the goal of teaching youth how to use these skills to change their thoughts and behaviors and improve their mood when depressed, as well as preventing or curtailing future episodes of depression. The CBT therapist takes a collaborative role with the young person and applies CBT techniques by asking youth to keep track of their mood, schedule and engage in pleasant events, and make efforts to notice and change the negative thoughts that can be automatic responses to stressful or ambiguous situations. The CBT therapist also tries to help the young person identify and then gradually change the underlying core beliefs that lead to negative cognitions (e.g., I'm stupid and will never learn) to more positive and realistic ideas (e.g., These questions are difficult, but if I pay attention I'll be able to figure out the answer).

CBT was used in the most comprehensive multisite, randomized clinical trial (RCT) of adolescent depression completed to date, the treatment of adolescents with depression study (TADS), and was found to be an important part of a comprehensive treatment plan for adolescent depression with particular value with regard to its offering greater protection against suicidality as compared to pharmacotherapy. Clarke and colleagues have also demonstrated efficacy using a group CBT approach with adolescents. Additionally, CBT approaches have been used successfully with children as young as 11 and have demonstrated efficacy in the treatment of anxiety problems as well, making it a good approach for this population.

Mufson and colleagues have led efforts to modify individual IPT to treat adolescent depression. IPT focuses on addressing the adolescent's interpersonal interactions and how they affect his or her depressive symptoms, with the primary treatment goals being to decrease depressive symptoms and improve relationships and social interactions. Most work has involved adolescents, but there are current efforts under way to extend IPT with younger ages. IPT utilizes a variety of techniques, including communication analysis, role-plays, and the use of relationship. For example, if a depressed teen reports a pattern of giving others the silent treatment, an IPT therapist might conduct a communication analysis in order to identify how this pattern of behavior is related to depressed mood. In a therapy session, the therapist and teen would recreate a recent interaction in which the teen stopped speaking to someone, essentially doing a functional analysis to track and understand the impact of the teen's silent treatment on the other person and the feelings conveyed and generated by the exchange. This is typically diagrammed visually and may involve role-plays to allow the teen and therapist to get a thorough understanding of the sequence of communication. This information guides the therapist and teen with regard to what communication skills to practice in order to improve the teen's relationships and, in turn, improve depressed mood. Many of these techniques are similar to those used in other approaches; however, in IPT, the guiding principle relates to how relationships and interpersonal functioning influence mood and what social and relational changes can be made to improve mood.

Finally, both CBT and IPT group-based prevention programs have demonstrated notable success in reducing the rate of depression in youth. The most successful preventive interventions targeted participants who were at heightened risk for developing depression (e.g., reporting some depressive symptoms or living with a depressed parent), included more females and/or older adolescents, were of short duration, included at-home therapeutic tasks, and were delivered by professional clinicians.

Medication Intervention

Medication treatment has an important role in the treatment of adolescent depression. Offering medication treatment, in combination with CBT or IPT, is recommended for children and adolescents with moderate to severe major depression or dysthymia. Practice parameters for the assessment and treatment of depression have been published by Birmaher and colleagues and serve as a detailed guide to care. Studies that have evaluated the use of medication alone in comparison with medication plus therapy show that the cost–benefit analysis for treatment of children with medication only is less favorable. In addition, a consensus conference of experts in child and adolescent mood disorders was convened to synthesize research and clinical evidence to develop algorithms for the treatment of MDD in children and adolescents, resulting in the Texas Children's Medication Algorithm.

A combination of CBT or IPT and a selective serotonin reuptake inhibitor (SSRI), with specific preference to fluoxetine or ecitalopram, the two agents currently approved by the Federal Drug Administration (FDA), is the treatment of choice for moderate to severe depression. This recommendation is largely based on the strongly favorable results of the TADS study. The TADS study compared treatment with CBT alone, fluoxetine alone, the combination of fluoxetine and CBT, and placebo. An initial positive response rate (within 12 weeks) of 71.0% for a combination of CBT and fluoxetine (doses between 10 and 40 mg) and 60.6% for fluoxetine alone was found. Those on fluoxetine alone and 80% of those on combination therapy obtained a positive response by the 36th week of the study, and among positive responders in the first 12 weeks, 88.4% of those on the combination of CBT and fluoxetine and 82.5% on fluoxetine alone sustained their positive response through the 36th week of treatment. Although RCTs have shown positive results for other SSRIs, other agents have had less consistent positive results. All of the SSRIs have the potential to be helpful, as suggested by a large meta-analysis that included studies of fluoxetine (Prozac), citalopram (Celexa), sertraline (Zoloft), ecitalopram (Lexapro), and paroxetine (Paxil) conducted by Usala and colleagues. These analyses showed an overall positive effect of the medications and also that each trial showed some benefit of medications versus placebo. In children or adolescents whose major depression or dysthymia is comorbid with social phobia, separation anxiety disorder, or generalized anxiety disorder, a recent highly positive RCT showing effectiveness for sertraline (Zoloft), may move that agent to first choice. The other SSRIs with positive RCTs may be initiated first in cases where the child or adolescent has a family history of good response to a specific agent or a problematic response to fluoxetine, or may be initiated as a subsequent trial in the case of a negative fluoxetine or ecitalopram trial. Concerns about prominent withdrawal symptoms with paroxetine have limited its use in children and adolescents. Tricyclic antidepressants are generally not recommended due to a lack of evidence of effectiveness in children and adolescents and their potential for fatal overdose. However, the consensus algorithm that was developed for the treatment of MDD in children and adolescents, which was published by Hughes et al. in 1999 and updated in 2007, recommends that after two trials of SSRIs, two options are considered depending on the child's or adolescent's response to the SSRI trials. If partial response has been achieved, augmentation with lithium or buspirone is recommended. If no response has been achieved, consideration of an alternate class of medications such as buproprion, mirtazapine, nefazadone, a tricyclic antidepressant, or venlafaxine was recommended. More recently, cautions about the use of venlafaxine have emerged as discussed later in the text. If the major depression includes psychotic features, the treatment is the same except that the addition of antipsychotic medication should be considered, the role of possible substance abuse evaluated, and the increased risk of the eventual development of bipolar disorder noted.

Prior to initiating a trial of an SSRI or other antidepressant agent, it is important to discuss potential side effects, including common SSRI side effects of nausea, headache, restlessness, insomnia or hypersomnia, and sexual dysfunction. These side effects tend to be mild and to diminish in the first two weeks of treatment. However, in a small minority of patients, these side effects can be intolerable and can result in discontinuation of the medication. In addition, in children "behavioral activation" with increased energy, impulsivity, agitation and/or giddiness can occur in 3% to 8% of youth. Although medication-induced behavioral activation is distinct from bipolar disorder, it is thought to be a risk factor for the future development of bipolar disorder. Some studies have reported that children and adolescents experience shorter half-lives of antidepressant medications, so providers should be alert to withdrawal symptoms, and can consider twice-per-day dosing if needed. More rare potential side effects include serotonin syndrome, increased predisposition to bleeding, and increased suicidality. Serotonin syndrome is a rare, medically urgent event, more likely to occur in overdose than in therapeutic dose ranges, and includes tachycardia, hyperreflexia, and sweating. Patients should be sure to inform other medical providers regarding their use of an SSRI, and consider perioperative discontinuation due to the potential for increased bleeding. The potential for the development or worsening of suicidal thoughts and behaviors in depressed children and adolescents treated with medication versus without medication (i.e., with therapy alone or placebo) has been supported by a meta-analysis of all available RCTs conducted by Hammad and colleagues. The conclusions of the TADS analysis of data over 36 weeks is that "clinically significant suicidal ideation persists in a minority of patients and is significantly more common in patients treated with fluoxetine alone than with combination therapy or CBT," but they close by saying, "After taking benefit and risk into account, we conclude that the combination of fluoxetine and CBT appears superior to either monotherapy as a long-term treatment strategy for MDD in adolescents." However, patients and families need to be alerted to the possible risk of increased thoughts of suicide with a clear plan of who to call if increases in suicidality present.

Regardless of agent, re-evaluation for reduction of depressive symptoms and for side effects should be done frequently, with consideration of dosage increase at 4-week intervals. Given that adolescent compliance with medication regimens tends to be poor, it is important to include medication compliance as a goal of therapy and to discuss issues that make it difficult to remember to take medication or problematic side effects that may interfere with motivation. In addition, it can be helpful to emphasize the potential for improvement in specific symptoms identified by the adolescent as bothersome (e.g., difficulty falling to sleep) and to partner with them to track change in these symptoms. Ongoing care should include tracking of response to treatment and side effects from medications. Medication prescribers should wait a minimum of 4 weeks on a particular dose of medication, but then should move to a higher dose if no improvement is noted. According to the American Academy of Child and Adolescent Psychiatry Practice Parameter for depression developed by Birmaher and colleagues, once remission of symptoms has been achieved, continued medication treatment is recommended for 6 months to 1 year after symptoms resolve.

If no improvement is achieved after a trial at the highest recommended dose of medication, cross-tapering to a different medication in the same class is recommended. Other antidepressant agents such as buproprion (Wellbutrin) or mirtazapine (Remeron) should be considered only in treatment-resistant patients, those who cannot tolerate SSRIs, or for whom sufficient concern about the development of bipolar disorder results in reluctance to engage in a trial of an SSRI, but these agents lack effective RCT data in children and adolescents and have additional side effects. Venlafaxine (Effexor) is not recommended because it has been found to have a much higher relative risk of suicidal thoughts and behavior in children and adolescents than the SSRIs and also can cause increased blood pressure and tachycardia. Paxil is not recommended due to inconsistency between studies on the effectiveness of this medication and the potential for significant withdrawal effects in children and adolescents. For children or adolescents who have a suboptimal response to several trials of SSRIs along with CBT or IPT, alternative agents can be considered, although at that point a psychiatrist should take over prescribing, given the lack of evidence base. Psychiatrists may augment the SSRI with a different antidepressive agent or an agent from another class of medications such as atypical antipsychotic agents. Youth with a strong family history of bipolar disorder, psychotic depression, behavioral activation in response to a trial of an SSRI, or prominent mood lability have increased risk of the development of bipolar disorder. For children and adolescents who meet criteria for major depression, but have these risk factors, initiation of a mood stabilizer may be indicated. For further discussion, please refer to the chapter 12 which covers the evaluation and treatment of bipolar disorder.

There has been limited research of nontraditional intervention for youth depression. A recent review demonstrated limited support for St John's Wort, vitamin C, omega-3 fatty acids, and exercise. Vitamin D supplementation has recently been suggested for those who are deficient. Further research assessing the efficacy of these alternative treatments is needed prior to their recommended use. Bright light therapy was demonstrated to be effective for adolescents with seasonal symptoms of depression, but does not have an FDA indication for use. Consideration of electroconvulsive therapy (ECT) has had positive open-label trials, but no RCTs have been done with children or adolescents. ECT is recommended only in cases of severe depression after a lack of response to two trials of medication or when the severity of symptoms prohibits waiting for a response to medication. Transcranial magnetic stimulation (TMS) has been approved by the FDA for treatment of adults with major depression who have failed two medication trials, but no studies have yet been published on its use in children or adolescents.

Conclusions

The assessment of depression can be difficult, given that presentation can vary depending on the youth's development, unique environmental circumstances, and overall physical health. Furthermore, an underlying medical condition must be ruled out when depressive symptoms such as fatigue, trouble sleeping, or somatic complaints are central. Depression can also co-occur with other behavioral disorders that also require treatment. Once the diagnosis has been made, guidelines for treatment of depressive disorders in youth have been clearly articulated, but challenges remain in engaging families and youth in treatment and finding mental health providers training in optimal evidence-based approaches. Finding a qualified therapist and on-going monitoring for and management of suicidal ideation as well as medication compliance present the primary potential difficulties in case management. However, early detection and active intervention are effective in resolving depressive symptoms and fostering healthy growth and development.

CASE VIGNETTES

VIGNETTE 1: JOY, A PREADOLESCENT GIRL WITH AN "ANXIOUS PREDISPOSITION"

Joy is a 10-year-old girl who has been followed by her primary care physician (PCP) since infancy. In preschool she had severe separation anxiety disorder, and she still has had some observable anxiety and shyness during her well-child visits. She presents at her PCP's office for an office visit because of a recent increase in complaints about stomachaches and some requests to stay home from school because she feels like she might throw up. During the examination, her mother reports that in addition to the stomach pain, Joy has recently begun to have some academic difficulties and to talk about herself "as stupid." In talking with Joy, the PCP learns that although she has one or two close friends, she often doesn't feel like doing things with them like she did before, and when she does play with them, she reports it isn't much fun. She also comments that her weight has increased and that she now feels like she is "fat" and "ugly." She reports feeling sad some of the time, not always, but it is harder for her to pay attention in school because the teacher is "so boring," and she also gets distracted by worries about how she will ever finish all her homework.

Because of her long-standing history of anxiety and shyness and the fact that she is moving toward puberty, Joy's PCP thinks that she would benefit from a course of CBT. While he recognizes that her depression is mild now, he worries that it will intensify as she moves through puberty and hopes that she could learn some skills now that would ease her transition into adolescence. To introduce the idea, Joy's PCP first educates Joy and her mother about depression in children. He points out that many children who tend to be anxious or "worriers" can begin to feel overwhelmed as school and peer pressures increase. This in turn can trigger feelings of depression or sadness, or that things are not fun anymore. While we all get depressed or sad from time to time, like when we don't do as well on a school test as we had hoped, it is important to learn some ways to change our moods, so that feeling depressed does not get in the way of having fun and feeling good about ourselves. In this context he recommends that Joy and her mother make an appointment to see a local therapist who will teach Joy some "skills" so that she can quickly feel better when she gets down and also teach mother some ways to support Joy in this. Joy participates in a 12-session course of CBT that focuses on helping her understand what triggers her feelings of depression and anxiety and what activities help to improve her mood, including spending time with friends even though at first she might be reluctant. She also learned how her way of thinking about something can affect her mood and developed her own list of "positive phrases" to use when she would begin to feel down or stupid. Joy's mother also learned ways to support Joy by validating her feelings but then encouraging her to keep trying to stay active with friends and positive activities. With these skills on board, the stomachaches disappeared and Joy began to regain her confidence at school. Her PCP plans to keep a watchful eye on her as she transitions to middle school in case some depressive symptoms reappear.

VIGNETTE 2: JOHN, AN ADOLESCENT MALE WITH DEPRESSION AND CO-OCCURRING CONDUCT PROBLEMS

John, 17-year-old, comes in to his PCP's after his teacher reports to his mother that he has been writing "morbid stories about death and suicide." His mother describes much "bad" behavior, including smoking, drinking, and hanging out with "a bad crowd." She is overwhelmed as a single parent with three children and complains that her oldest son hardly ever helps her and gets angry if she asks for help. Alone, he admits that he is depressed and irritable, and has suicidal ideation, poor appetite, disrupted sleep, and decreased interests. He also reports feeling bad about "stressing my mom out" and acknowledges that he should do more to help her out at home but just feels overwhelmed by school and home responsibilities. He feels that he has "wasted too much time" in high school and is now worried about having the grades needed to get into any college. He reports that his new crowd "keeps my mind off of my problems." Family history is positive for depression in multiple family members.

John is reluctant to consider therapy because he does not want anyone "in my business" but wants something to help him sleep. The PCP talks about her concerns about John's risk for self-harm particularly in the context of all the stress he is trying to cope with and his use of alcohol to "chill out." She conducts a further assessment of his suicidality during which he reports no past attempts and describes the morbid stories as one way to get "out" his anger and frustration. He is willing to work out a safety plan with the PCP and mother. The PCP agrees to talk with him further about medications but only if he is willing to meet with the county's mental health treatment team and give her permission to work together with the therapist to make sure he is keeping himself safe. They also talk about the need to monitor his alcohol use as that might be exacerbating his feelings of depression and could interfere with the efficacy of any medication they might try. The PCP's office calls to set up a next-day appointment and completes a safety plan with John and his mother that identifies triggers for his depression and irritability, things he can do to distract himself when feeling upset or unsafe, things mother can do to support him, and finally a list of adults, in addition to mother, that he can call when he needs help or feels in crisis.

Over the next year, John worked with a mental health therapist for about 6 months with regular visits initially and then some "booster" sessions on a monthly basis. His difficulties with sleep persisted, and he agreed to quit drinking in order to at least see if medications would be useful. A trial of fluoxetine (Prozac) was initiated and gradually titrated to a therapeutic dose. After about 3 months of treatment, his sleep patterns had normalized and his irritability was lessened. He still had occasional thoughts about death but no ongoing suicidal ideation. He was more able to engage in school and social activities but still preferred his "wild" friends although now he was willing to respect mother's requests regarding curfews and was working on cutting back his smoking to "get my mom off my back."

VIGNETTE 3: NHI, DEPRESSION IN THE CONTEXT OF CULTURE

Nhi, a 15-year-old Vietnamese American female who had immigrated to the United States with her family at age 13, was called in to meet with her school counselor because of concerns about numerous absences and a few instances of Nhi nodding off during class. As Nhi became comfortable and realized that she was not in trouble, she disclosed that since moving to the United States, she had taken on numerous responsibilities, including caring for her three younger siblings after school while both of her parents were at work, as well as serving as an interpreter for a variety of family errands and appointments. Nhi expressed both guilt and frustration about these tasks, indicating that they got in the way of her participating in after-school academic and extracurricular opportunities, in addition to causing her to miss school when her parents needed help with translation. Nhi reported having frequent conflict with her parents regarding the added demands that they placed on her, as well as conflict with her older brother, who was not expected to aid in these family tasks. She also described feeling socially isolated due in large part to not having the time or the means to do activities with her peers due to her parents' work schedule and limited finances, as well as a lack of transportation. She noted, though, that recently she has no longer felt like engaging with friends and has even turned down opportunities she would typically enjoy. Nhi described having difficulty with concentration over the last few weeks, having headaches nearly every day, in addition to frequent difficulty with falling asleep and fatigue, often related to worrying about the family's financial situation when she went to bed. Throughout the conversation, Nhi was quite apologetic and unsure whether she should be sharing this information. She noted that she had been afraid to share her troubles with her parents because she did not want to burden them further with her problems, particularly in light of the sacrifices they had made for Nhi and her siblings.

Following their open-ended discussion, the counselor asked Nhi to complete an SMFQ, which indicated a mildly elevated SMFQ score. The school counselor gave Nhi feedback about her possibly having a depressive disorder and offered to speak to Nhi's parents in order to educate them about depression, as well as how to access appropriate services. Nhi thanked the counselor for her concern, but she adamantly refused both options. She was adamant that speaking with her parents would make things even worse as her parents did not believe in depression and felt that Nhi should be working harder rather than getting help.

Based on Nhi's presentation of mild depression, with the absence of any significant safety concerns, the counselor opted to take a "watchful waiting" approach. She deferred to Nhi's request to keep their conversation private and asked Nhi to maintain close communication if she started to feel worse. She also asked Nhi to return to her office for check-ins every other week and collaborated with Nhi to generate and implement goals that would improve her mood and comfortably allow for gradual change within the bounds of her family and culture. With Nhi's permission, the school counselor discussed her concerns about a possible depressive disorder with Nhi's PCP, and they agreed to continue to monitor her symptoms and communicate regularly about her well-being and treatment plan. This partnership allowed both the counselor and the PCP to appropriately account for cultural considerations and to creatively engage Nhi. They worked together to identify after-school resources for Nhi's siblings, as well as how to present these options to Nhi's parents, which then allowed Nhi to join the school choir and to participate in math tutoring. Over time, Nhi's symptoms began to abate and her functioning began to improve at school, at home, and with peers.

BIBLIOGRAPHY

Achenbach TM, Rescorla LA. *Manual for ASEBA School-Age Forms & Profiles*. Burlington, VT: University of Vermont, Research Center for Children, Youth, & Families; 2001.

American Psychiatric Association. *The Diagnostic and Statistical Manual of Mental Disorders. Third Edition*. Washington, DC: American Psychiatric Association; 1977.

American Psychiatric Association. *The Diagnostic and Statistical Manual of Mental Disorders. Fourth Edition*. Washington, DC: *Text Revision*. American Psychiatric Association; 2000.

Angold A, Costello E. *The Moods and Feelings Questionnaire*. Duke University Developmental Program, unpublished document; 1987.

Beck AT, Steer RA. *Manual for the Beck Depression Inventory*. San Antonio, TX: The Psychological Corporation; 1993.

Birmaher B, Brent D, Bernet W, et al. Practice parameter for the assessment and treatment of children and adolescents with depressive disorders. *J Am Acad Child Adolesc Psychiatry*. 2007;46(11):1503–1526.

Birmaher B, Williamson DE, Dahl RE, et al. Clinical presentation and course of depression in youth: does onset in childhood differ from onset in adolescence? *J Am Acad Child Adolesc Psychiatry*. 2004;43(1):63–70.

Caspi A, Sugden K, Moffitt TE, et al. Influence of life stress on depression: moderation by a polymorphism in the 5-HTT gene. *Science*. 2003;301:386–389.

Cheung AH, Zuckerbrot RA, Jensen PS, et al. Guidelines for adolescent depression in primary care (GLAD-PC): II. Treatment and ongoing management. *Pediatrics*. 2007;120(5):e1313–e1326.

Clarke GN, Hawkins W, Murphy M, et al. Targeted prevention of unipolar depressive disorder in an at-risk sample of high school adolescents: a randomized trial of group cognitive intervention. *J Am Acad Child Adolesc Psychiatry*. 1995;34:312–321.

Compas BE, Connor-Smith JK, Saltzman H, et al. Coping with stress during childhood and adolescence: problems, progress, and potential in theory and research. *Psychol Bull*. 2001;27:87–127.

Fergusson DM, Woodward LJ. Mental health, educational, and social role outcomes of adolescents with depression. *Arch Gen Psychiatry*. 2002;59(3):225–231.

Garber J, Clarke GN, Weersing VR, et al. Prevention of depression in at-risk adolescents: a randomized controlled trial. *JAMA*. 2009;301:2215–2224.

Ghaziuddin N, Kutcher SP, Knapp P, et al. Practice parameter for use of electroconvulsive therapy with adolescents. *J Am Acad Child Adolesc Psychiatry*. 2004;43:1521–1539.

Giedd JN. Structural magnetic resonance imaging of the adolescent brain. *Ann NY Acad Sci*. 2004;1021:77–85.

Glied S, Pine DS. Consequences and correlates of adolescent depression. *Arch Pediatr Adolesc Med*. 2002;156:1009–1014.

Goldenring JM, Cohen E. Getting into adolescent heads. *Contemp Pediatrics*. 1988;5:75.

Goldenring JM, Rosen D. Getting into adolescent heads: an essential update. *Contemp Pediatrics*. 2004;21:64–90.

Goodyer IM, Herbert J, Tamplin A, et al. Recent life events, cortisol, dehydroepiandrosterone and the onset of major depression in high-risk adolescents. *Br J Psychiatry*. 2000;177:499–504.

Grant KE, Compas BE, Thurm AE, et al. Stressors and child and adolescent psychopathology: measurement issues and prospective effects. *J Clin Child Adolesc Psychol*. 2004;33:412–425.

Hammad TA, Laughren T, Racoosin J. Suicidality in pediatric patients treated with antidepressant drugs. *Arch Gen Psychiatry*. 2006;63(3):332–339.

Hankin BL, Abramson LY, Moffitt TE, et al. Development of depression from preadolescence to young adulthood: emerging gender differences in a 10-year longitudinal study. *J Abnorm Psychol*. 1998;107:128–140.

Hughes CW, Emslie GJ, Crimson ML, et al. The Texas children's medication algorithm project: report of the Texas consensus conference panel on medication treatment of childhood depressive disorder. *J Am Acad Child Adolesc Psychiatry*. 1999;38:1442–1454.

Hughes CW, Emslie GJ, Crimson ML, et al. Texas Children's Medication Algorithm Project: update from Texas conference panel on medication treatment of childhood major depressive disorder. *J Am Acad Child Adolesc Psychiatry*. 2007;46:667–686.

Jorm AF, Allen NB, O'Donnell CP, et al. Effectiveness of complementary and self-help treatments for depression in children and adolescents. *Med J Aust*. 2006;185:368–372.

Keenan K, Feng X, Hipwell A, et al. Depression begets depression: comparing the predictive utility of depression and anxiety symptoms to later depression. *J Child Psychol Psychiatry*. 2009;50(9):1167–1175.

Kovacs M. *Children's Depression Inventory Manual*. North Tonawanda, NY: Multi-Health Systems, Inc; 1992.

Kroenke K, Spitzer RL, Williams JB. The PHQ-9: validity of a brief depression severity measure. *J Gen Intern Med*. 2001;16(9):606–613.

Lewinsohn PM, Clarke GN, Seeley JR, et al. Major depression in community adolescents: age at onset, episode duration, and time to recurrence. *J Am Acad Child Adolesc Psychiatry*. 1994;33:809–818.

Lewinsohn PM, Hops H, Roberts RE, et al. Adolescent psychopathology: prevalence and incidence of depression and other DSM-III-R disorders in high school students. *J Abnorm Psychol*. 1993;102:133–144.

Lewinsohn PM, Rohde P, Seeley JR, et al. Psychosocial functioning of young adults who have experienced and recovered from major depressive disorder during adolescence. *J Abnorm Psychol*. 2003;112:353–363.

Luby JL. Early childhood depression. *Am J Psychiatry*. 2009;166:974–979.

Luby JL, Belden AC, Pautsch J, et al. The clinical significance of preschool depression: impairment in functioning and clinical markers of the disorder. *J Affect Disord*. 2009;112(1–3):111–119.

March JS, Silva S, Petrycki S, et al. The treatment for adolescents with depression study (TADS): long-term effectiveness and safety outcomes. *Arch Gen Psychiatry*. 2007;64(10):1132–1143.

McCauley E, Katon W, Russo J, et al. Impact of anxiety and depression on functional impairment in adolescents with asthma. *Gen Hosp Psychiatry*. 2007;29(3):214–222.

Mufson L, Dorta KP, Moreau D, et al. *Interpersonal Psychotherapy for Depressed Adolescents*. New York: Guilford Press; 2004.

National Institute for Clinical Excellence (NICE). Depression in children and young people: identification and management in primary, community and secondary care. Available at: http://www.nice.org.uk/CG28. Accessed January 20, 2010.

National Institutes of Mental Health. *Breaking Ground, Breaking Through: The Strategic Plan for Mood Disorders.* Bethesda, MD: National Institute of Mental Health; 2002.

Reynolds WM. *Reynolds Adolescent Depression Scale: Professional Manual.* Odessa, FL: Psychological Assessment Resources, Inc.; 1987.

Reynolds WM. *Reynolds Child Depression Scale*: Odessa, FL: Psychological Assessment Resources, Inc.; 1989

Risch N, Herrell R, Lehner T, et al. Interaction between the serotonin transporter gene (5-HTTLPR), stressful life events, and risk of depression: a meta-analysis. *JAMA.* 2009;301(23):2462–2471.

Rohde P, Lewinsohn PM, Seeley JR. Psychiatric comorbidity with problematic alcohol use in high school students. *J Am Acad Child Adolesc Psychiatry.* 1996;35(1):101–109.

Rohde P, Silva SG, Tonev ST, et al. Achievement and maintenance of sustained response during the treatment for adolescents with depression study continuation and maintenance therapy. *Arch Gen Psychiatry.* 2008;65(4):447–455.

Steinberg L, Dahl R, Keating D, et al. The study of developmental psychopathology in adolescence: integrating affective neuroscience with the study of context. In: Cicchetti D, ed. *Handbook of Developmental Psychopathology.* New York: Wiley; 2006.

Stice E, Shaw H, Bohon C, et al. A meta-analytic review of depression prevention programs for children and adolescents: factors that predict magnitude of intervention effects. *J Consult Clin Psychol.* 2009;7:486–503.

The Pediatric OCD Treatment Study (POTS) Team. Cognitive–behavior therapy, sertraline, and their combination for children and adolescents with obsessive–compulsive disorder: the Pediatric OCD Treatment Study (POTS) randomized controlled trial. *JAMA.* 2004;292(16):1969–1976.

Tremblay J. Metabolism: clinical and experimental. *Metabolism.* 2005;54(5):10–15.

Usala T, Clavenna A, Zuddas A, et al. Randomised controlled trials of selective serotonin reuptake inhibitors in treating depression in children and adolescents: a systematic review and meta-analysis. *Eur Neuropsychopharmacol.* 2008;18(1):62–73.

Weisz JR, McCarty CA, Valeri SM. Effects of psychotherapy for depression in children and adolescents: a meta-analysis. *Psychol Bull.* 2006;132(1):132–149.

Weller EB, Weller RA, Rowan AB, et al. Depressive disorders in children and adolescents. In: Lewis M, ed. *Child and Adolescent Psychiatry: A Comprehensive Textbook.* Philadelphia: Lippincott Williams & Wilkins; 2002.

Young JF, Mufson L, Davies M. Efficacy of interpersonal psychotherapy-adolescent skills training: an indicated preventive intervention for depression. *J Child Psychol Psychiatry.* 2006;47:1254–1262.

SUGGESTED READINGS (FOR PATIENTS, FAMILIES, AND TEACHERS)

I Had a Black Dog, by Matthew Johnstone, Pan Macmillan, Australia, 2005.

This is a short book that describes depression, and what helps, in cartoon format. It is an excellent introduction to depression for patients and families and should appeal to wide range of people.

Journeys with the Black Dog, Edited by T Wigney, K Eyers, and G Parker, Allen and Unwin, Australia, 2007.

This book contains first-hand accounts from people who have suffered from depression.

SUGGESTED WEBSITES

Websites that provide information on depression specifically for young people

    http://www.kidshealth.org/

    http://www.thelowdown.co.nz/

    http://www.ybblue.com.au/

    http://www.sortoutstress.co.uk/

    http://moodgym.anu.edu.au/

Websites that provide more general information on depression

    www.blackdoginstitute.org.au

    http://bluepages.anu.edu.au/home/

    http://www.bluesnews.info/

    http://www.library.nhs.uk/mentalHealth/

    http://www.helpguide.org/mental/depression_teen.htm

    http://www.nasponline.org/publications/cq/cq354suicide.aspx

RESOURCES FOR PROFESSIONALS

Evidence-based Treatment for Children and Adolescents: http://sccap.tamu.edu/EST/

Society of Clinical Child and Adolescent Psychology: http://www.clinicalchildpsychology.org

GLAD-PC Toolkit: http://www.thereachinstitute.org/files/documents/GLAD-PCToolkit.pdf.

REVIEW QUESTIONS

1. What is the difference in diagnostic criteria between major depressive disorder and dysthymia?
   a. The number of symptoms required for diagnosis differs, with dysthymia requiring more symptoms.
   b. The number of symptoms required for diagnosis differs, with major depressive disorder requiring more symptoms.
   c. The amount of time that symptoms are required to be present differs between the disorders.
   d. Dysthymia does not require that the child has depressed or irritable mood.

2. When screening for depression in children and adolescents, what laboratory testing should be considered?
   a. A complete blood count can help rule out anemia.
   b. A chemistry panel can evaluate for electrolyte disturbances.
   c. Thyroid studies can rule out hypothyroid disease.
   d. Brain imaging can rule out epilepsy or traumatic brain injury.

3. The prevalence of depressive symptoms in epidemiologic studies is
   a. 30% in preadolescence
   b. 15–20% during the 18th year of life
   c. Less than 3% in the 6th to 9th grade years
   d. Larger in adolescence than in preadolescence

4. Recommended therapy for depression in children and adolescents includes all of the following except
   a. Psychoeducation about depression for the child or adolescent and family members
   b. Supportive therapy focused on understanding and supporting the child's perspective
   c. Interpersonal therapy (IPT)
   d. Cognitive–behavioral therapy (CBT) for depression

5. Medications approved by the Federal Drug Administration for treatment of depression in children and adolescents include
   a. Paroxetine (Paxil)
   b. Citalopram (Celexa)
   c. Ecitalopram (Lexapro)
   d. Fluoxetine (Prozac)

6. What is the recommended length of a trial of a dose of antidepressant medication?
   a. Two weeks
   b. Four weeks
   c. Six weeks
   d. Eight weeks

Answers: 1-b,c, 2-a,b,c, 3-b,c,d, 4-b, 5-c,d, 6-d

CHAPTER 12

Gretchen R. Gudmundsen, Ph.D.,
Stefanie A. Hlastala, Ph.D., Kathleen
Myers, M.D., M.P.H., M.S., FAACAP

Early-Onset Bipolar Disorder

Introduction

Early onset of bipolar disorder (BD), particularly during prepuberty, is one of the most controversial issues in child and adolescent psychiatry. The past decade has seen investigation into the definition of the disorder, developmentally appropriate expression of manic symptoms, comorbidities that mask mania, neuroimaging, and pharmacological treatment. Much has been learned, but much remains to be understood. This chapter will help primary clinicians to develop an index of suspicion regarding BD when youth present with mood instability and to know when to refer for further evaluation.

Background

Research in the 1980s on the early onset and longitudinal course of major depressive disorder (MDD) revealed that over 5 years 20% to 40% of these youth "switched" from MDD to BD, a rate three to five times higher than that for adult-onset MDD. Then, work in the 1990s suggested that a subset of children diagnosed with severe attention-deficit hyperactivity disorder (ADHD) suffered from BD. These studies paved the way for the investigation of mood instability in youth as many youth with severe irritability and behavioral outbursts were diagnosed with mixed episodes of BD. In an attempt to bring order to the controversy, investigators have proposed two subtypes of early-onset BD: "a narrow phenotype" and a "broad phenotype." These definitions appear to be gaining acceptance despite the absence of any research demonstrating their validity. The premature reification of these hypothesized "phenotypes" has further complicated scientific and clinical work as their implications for diagnosis, treatment, and prognosis of early-onset BD are unclear. Clinicians continue to face major challenges in diagnosing and treating youth with possible BD.

Clinical Features

The *Diagnostic and Statistical Manual*, Fourth Edition (DSM-IV), documents two major categories of mood disorders: Depressive Disorders and Bipolar Disorders. The pathognomonic feature distinguishing Bipolar Disorders from Depressive Disorders is the experience of mania or hypomania, as shown in Table 12-1.

In depressive disorders, individuals experience a change from normal mood (euthymia) to depression, while in BD moods alternate between two poles, depression and mania, in addition to euthymia. These episodes may vary in the severity and duration and be separated by months, weeks, days, or hours, in part defining the two major subtypes of BD recognized by DSM-IV and described in Table 12-2.

As noted in Table 12-2, *Bipolar-I Disorder* (BD-I) requires the occurrence of at least one manic or mixed episode with marked impairment of *at least 1 week* or requiring hospitalization.

TABLE 12-1	Characteristics of DSM-IV Manic and Hypomanic Episodes		
Type of Episode	**Duration**	**Salient/Diagnostic Symptoms**	**Differentiating Features**
Manic episode	At least 1 week, or any length if hospitalized	A *distinct period* of abnormally and persistently elevated, expansive, or irritable mood, that includes three or more of following (four if mood is mostly irritable) • increased self-esteem or grandiosity • decreased *need* for sleep • more talkative or pressure to keep talking • flight of ideas or racing thoughts • distractibility • increased goal-directed activity or psychomotor agitation • involvement in pleasurable activities with increased potential for harm.	Sufficiently severe to cause *marked* impairment in social or occupational function, or to necessitate hospitalization • May have psychosis • Should have at least one cardinal symptom of elation, euphoria, or grandiosity • In children, there are fewer distinct episodes, more rapid cycling, and/or a more chronic course
Hypomanic episode	At least 4 days	A distinct period of elevated, expansive, or irritable mood along with three of the diagnostic symptoms described above for a manic episode (four symptoms if mood is mostly irritable)	• Change in functioning, is less severe than in mania • Shorter duration than mania • No psychosis • Often perceived to be a personality style, not an illness
Mixed episode	Nearly every day for at least 1 week May occur for mania or hypomania	Criteria are met for both a Manic Episode and a Major Depressive Episode, but duration of each is very short or episodes are concurrent. Term sometimes used interchangeably with "ultradian rapid cycling"	• Sufficiently severe to cause impairment in social or occupational function, or to require hospitalization • May have psychosis • Can be difficult to distinguish from other conditions with severe irritability or other forms of affective dysregulation

The presence of psychotic symptoms mandates a diagnosis of BD-I. *Bipolar-II Disorder* (BD-II) differs from BD-I in that the manic symptoms are of shorter duration and are less severe and, thus, termed hypomanic. Hypomania may not cause marked impairment, although it is sufficiently severe to constitute a departure from normal, or to be noted by others, and often involves later regrettable behaviors.

When criteria for a manic, or hypomanic, episode and a depressive episode occur concurrently for at least 1 week, the mood episode is termed a *mixed episode*. This is generally difficult

TABLE 12-2	Characteristics of DSM-IV Bipolar Disorders	
Diagnosis	**Time Course and Relationship to Depressive and Manic Episodes**	**Differentiating Features**
Bipolar I disorder (BD-I)	• At least one Manic Episode or Mixed Episode. • May or may not have had prior Major Depressive Episode	• Thought to be the most severe form of the illness due to extremes of the mania • Cycling less evident in youth as depressive episodes may be less well developed, or short • Cycling may not be evident as children may sustain chronic manic states • The mania may be "masked" by comorbid ADHD and other disruptive behaviors • Must document the pathognomonic features of BD, such as grandiosity and hypersexuality, to distinguish from ADHD and ODD
Bipolar II disorder (BD-II)	• At least one Major Depressive Episode, and at least one Hypomanic Episode • May have multiple recurrent Major Depressive Episode with only intermittently superimposed Hypomanic Episodes • No Manic Episodes • No psychosis	• Hypomania not as severe as mania • Major Depressive Episodes as severe as in BD-I and can be more difficult to treat, increasing overall severity • May be more susceptible to antidepressant-induced "switching" • Differentiation from Personality Disorders with affective dysregulation may be difficult, for example, Borderline, Narcissistic, Histrionic
Cyclothymic disorder	• Numerous cycles of lower grade depression and hypomania • Symptoms ongoing for at least one year in children • During symptomatic period, no remission of hypomania or depression for more than 2 months at a time • No Major Depressive Episode or Mixed Episode occurs during the first year of the disturbance	• May exist as a distinct disorder, or may be prodromal to later BD-I or BD-II; or may exist intermorbidly between cycles of Major Depressive Episode and Manic Episode • May be perceived more as a personality style • Diagnosis not often used in children or adults
Bipolar disorder, NOS	• Diagnosis for individuals who have manic-like and depressive symptoms that do not meet criteria for BD-I or BD-II • Criteria for change in functioning not indicated • Variable time course • Heterogeneous samples in studies	• Examples include: recurrent Hypomanic Episodes without apparent interepisode depressive symptoms • Diagnosis has been applied to children with severe affective instability of uncertain relationship to BD-I and BD-II • Most controversial of early-onset BD diagnoses; caution in using this diagnosis

Adapted from American Psychiatric Association. *Diagnostic and Statistical Manual of Mental Disorders, Fourth Edition.* Washington, DC: Author; 2000.

to identify in children due to the co-occurrence of elation, irritability, and depression as the youth quickly cycles between moods. Additionally, if an individual experiences more than four episodes of depression or mania/hypomania in a year, a *rapid cycling* specifier is used.

Cyclothymia refers to a mood state in which individuals experience numerous periods of hypomanic and depressive symptoms that do not meet criteria for either a full manic or depressive episode, but do cause distress. For youth, these symptoms must occur over a period of at least 1 year without any symptom-free intervals lasting longer than 2 months. Individuals with BD may return to a baseline of cyclothymia much as individuals with MDD may return to a baseline of dysthymia.

Bipolar Disorder, Not Otherwise Specified (BD, NOS) allows the diagnosis of BD for individuals with more heterogeneity in presentation. For example, some youth may not meet DSM-IV criteria for BD-I or BD-II because of severity or duration criteria; but they may experience impairment due to mood instability. Unfortunately, this heterogeneity introduces laxity into the construct of BD resulting in overdiagnosis. Birmaher has proposed guidelines for standardizing the diagnosis of BD, NOS in youth, which has helped in distinguishing BD-I or BD-II from youth with disruptive disorders.

Developmental Considerations

Recent work has focused on reconciling divergent conceptualizations of how the DSM-IV criteria for BD, particularly mania, apply to youth. As noted, this controversy has led to two conceptualizations of how DSM-IV criteria apply to early-onset BD: a "narrow phenotype" and a "broad phenotype" or "severe mood dysregulation (SMD)." Liebenluft and colleagues have coined the term "narrow phenotype" to describe youth who demonstrate classic DSM-IV criteria for mania, or hypomania, that is, unmodified adult criteria. Geller and colleagues emphasize that core manic symptoms must be present to diagnose BD in children but that children express these symptoms within their developmental capabilities. They have generated examples of child-equivalent classic manic symptoms. For example, adults might run up their credit cards, become sexually promiscuous, or take on multiple new businesses. Equivalent childhood behaviors might include trying to use parents' credit card, stealing money to give away, expressing inappropriate sexual interest, speaking in an unusually loud and rapid manner, or engaging peers in grandiose activities. These manic symptoms usually occur as part of mixed episodes and must be teased out from their associated disruptive behaviors. Geller's interpretation of the proposed "narrow phenotype," then, emphasized unmodified adult criteria but with developmentally appropriate expression.

Liebenluft and colleagues have used the term "broad phenotype" to define youth with SMD evidenced by extreme irritability, anger, aggression, and explosive rages without obvious euphoria or other core manic symptoms. It is difficult to discern cycling in these youth's mood episodes and frustration seems to provoke dysregulation.

The proposal for these subtypes arises at least in part due to the "mix and match" approach of the DSM-IV nomenclature. This allows the "A criteria" to be met with a predominantly irritable, rather than a euphoric, mood. Then, the requisite four of seven "B criteria items" can be met by symptoms that overlap considerably with ADHD and do not convey the pathognomonic elation traditionally associated with BD. Thus, many investigators and clinicians contend that the "broad phenotype" represents disorders other than BD, such as severe disruptive and/or anxiety disorders. Perhaps, the greatest advantage in identifying such "phenotypes" is teasing out the "narrow phenotype" with traditional manic symptoms for future research and clinical work.

This issue may be at least partially resolved with the next revision of the DSM nomenclature, or DSM-V. Currently, there is a proposal to add a new diagnosis, "temper dysregulation disorder with dysphoria (TDD)." This disorder recognizes many of the features of SMD proposed by Liebenluft, but also recalls concepts proposed 20 to 30 years ago by Akiskal. In brief, the disorder is characterized by severe recurrent temper outbursts in response to common stressors, which are grossly out of proportion and are not appropriate to the child's developmental status. These episodes may be manifested verbally and/or behaviorally, such as in the form of verbal rages or physical aggression. They should occur at least three times per week. Mood between temper outbursts is persistently negative (irritable, angry, and/or sad). Onset must be before 10 years of age. The proposed criteria further require that in the past year there has never been a distinct period lasting more than one day during which abnormally elevated or expansive mood was present most of the day, and the abnormally elevated or expansive mood was accompanied by the onset, or worsening, of three of the adjunctive criterion symptoms, that is, grandiosity or inflated self-esteem, decreased need for sleep, pressured speech, flight of ideas, distractibility, increase in goal-directed activity, or excessive involvement in activities with a high potential for painful consequences. A draft proposal of the DSM-V was released for review and comment in 2010. It will be interesting to see how these proposed criteria are critiqued.

Epidemiology

BD-I affects approximately 1% of adults, ranging from 0.8% to 1.6% in different studies. The overall prevalence is higher if BD-II is included as it affects at least another 1% of the population. Rates in childhood have not been established and rates during adolescence have been estimated from relatively small community surveys and retrospective report. Retrospective data indicate that 40% to 60% of bipolar adults report their symptoms to have begun prior to age 19. The few available community studies have found a point prevalence of 0.6% for mania among 14 to 16 years old and a lifetime prevalence of 1% for hypomania in high school students. Interestingly, community studies of "subthreshold BD" in high school students found that 5 years later they had not converted to BD-I, questioning the stability of such diagnoses in early life.

Rates of BD in children can only be estimated. Retrospective adult studies have noted that onset before age 10 is rare (0.3% to 0.5%). Birmaher notes that the prevalence of MDD ranges from 0.4% to 2.5% in children and 0.4% to 8.3% in adolescents and that 20% to 40% will "switch" to BD within 5 years of the initial depressive episode.

Gender differences are also not well established, although prepubertal boys are diagnosed 3.85 times more often than girls. This sex pattern is typical of other early-onset psychiatric disorders. Sex rates are equal during later adolescence, similar to adult BD.

Risk Factors

Heritability
Family studies of adult twins, adoptees, and family aggregation support a genetic contribution to BD with a polygenic transmission. No specific pattern of inheritance and no gene have yet been identified. Studies of early-onset BD are consistent with adult studies indicating an increased loading for all mood disorders in family members, some specificity for increased loading of BD, and family loading that is higher for childhood-onset than for adolescent-onset BD. Earlier onset of BD in adults may further increase the risk of early-onset BD in offspring, as well as push forward the age of onset.

Neurobiology
There is no clear etiology proposed for BD. Current understanding of other psychiatric illnesses does not lend much insight into conceptualizing any neurobiological process that can account for such extreme mood swings. Many untested hypotheses exist focusing on

dysregulation of sodium ion channels, second messenger systems, excitation and inhibition of gamma-aminobutyric acid (GABA), as well as genetically regulated growth factors and neuronal plasticity.

Regarding mood disorders in general, there is evidence supporting a role of both the *long (l)* and *short (s) alleles* of the serotonin transporter gene. Preliminary findings indicate that the *s allele* may increase risk for progression toward BD in offspring of parents with BD. The *s allele* has been identified as a risk factor for suicidal behavior, which is also common in BD, and for pharmacologically induced mania. The *l allele* has been associated with prophylactic response to lithium. Additionally, preliminary analyses of adult linkage samples suggest that early-onset BD is associated with the BDNF gene, the GAD1 gene, and the dopamine transporter gene.

Imaging Studies

The role of the central nervous system (CNS) in early-onset BD has focused on both structure and functioning. Structurally, magnetic resonance imaging (MRI) scans have shown abnormalities in both cortical and subcortical regions, particularly pathways associated with emotion regulation, such as decreased volumes of the frontal lobe, amygdala, hippocampus, anterior cingulated gyrus, and the dorsolateral prefrontal cortex. One study of at-risk offsprings with subsyndromal symptoms of BD also showed decreased amygdala volume. Increased ventricular size has also been described. A functional MRI study has shown perturbations in the prefrontal-limbic system associated with misinterpretation of stimuli. Such findings suggest a neural basis for the erratic behaviors demonstrated by youth with BD. However, most of these studies have not been replicated; and, not all studies examining the same sections of the brain have found the same abnormalities. The most consistent finding has been decreased amydgala volume.

Environmental Factors

Stress and the Home Environment

While environmental factors do not cause BD, they may potentiate a genetic vulnerability. Indeed, behavioral genetic research suggests that genetically vulnerable individuals are also at greatest environmental risk. Hlastala has shown that either acute (e.g., death of a loved one) or chronic (e.g., chaotic family) stressors may worsen the course of illness in adults with BD. For example, adult patients who live with families characterized by high levels of "expressed emotion" marked by intrusiveness, hostility, and overinvolvement experience higher rates of relapse and hospitalization than patients in families with lower "expressed emotion." Recently, Kim and colleagues demonstrated similar associations between stress and changes in mood symptoms among adolescents with BD. With preadolescents, Geller has described "low maternal warmth," a parental behavioral component of expressed emotion, for youth with BD who spend more weeks ill, have higher rates of relapse, and relapse sooner. Thus, the home environment appears to affect the course of illness, providing a focus for intervention.

Circadian Rhythm Instability

In their classic textbook on manic depressive illness, Goodwin and Jamison articulated an "instability model" of the pathophysiology of BD. In this model, they postulate that circadian instability is "the fundamental dysfunction in manic depressive illness." Wehr and colleagues have also hypothesized that sleep deprivation/disruption might act as the "final common pathway" to mania, noting that episodes of mania are often preceded by life events interfering with the ability to sleep (e.g., transmeridian flights, childbirth). Malkoff-Schwartz and colleagues conducted studies demonstrating that life events involving social-rhythm disruption (events that influence sleep or wake times, patterns of social stimulation or daily routines) are strongly associated with the onset of manic episodes and more modestly associated with the onset of depressive episodes in adults with BD. Based on this line of research most psychosocial treatments for BD include some emphasis on increasing routine and attempts to minimize sleep disruption. In particular, Interpersonal and Social Rhythm Therapy (IPSRT), a psychosocial treatment that specifically targets the regularity of a bipolar patients' sleep and social routines has been proven effective in preventing recurrence of episodes of mania and depression. Furthermore, that protective effect of this treatment was directly related to the extent to which patients increased the regularity of their social rhythms.

Comorbidities

The differential diagnosis of BD in youth cannot be discussed separately from comorbidity. BD involves impaired affective regulation with deficits in processing and organizing, as well as severe emotional outbursts. Not only must BD be teased out from other causes of dysregulation, but some of these disorders may be comorbid with BD.

Mood Disorders Due to a General Medical Condition can be confused with BD especially if they involve the CNS, such as a traumatic brain injury or seizures, or systemic illness such as lupus, hyperthyroidism, or paraneoplastic syndrome. Less well recognized is that many medications may induce a manic episode, such as isoniazid, steroids, sympathomimetics, and antidepressants, as well as illicit substances such as cocaine. Careful medical examination and laboratory screening are indicated when BD is in the differential diagnosis. After medical etiologies have been ruled out, other psychiatric disorders must be considered.

Disruptive Behavior Disorders (DBD) comprise the diagnostic category most commonly needing to be differentiated from BD, as well as the most common comorbidity; and ADHD is the single most relevant of these disorders. Most prepubertal children who meet criteria for prepubertal BD also meet criteria for ADHD, while the converse is not true. Age of onset may help to discriminate between these two disorders with ADHD evident before age 7 and BD usually beginning after age 9. However, many children have prodromal symptoms early in life and age of onset is not easily determined. ADHD and BD symptoms have considerable overlap including increased motor activity, impulsivity, irritability, dysphoria, loquaciousness, poor attention, easy distractibility, and sleep disturbances. However, bipolar youth should demonstrate additional core manic symptoms that cannot be attributed to ADHD, and these symptoms should occur episodically, rather than showing a pervasive pattern as occurs with core ADHD symptoms. Youth with mania will often have middle-of-night awakening that is unusual in ADHD. If ADHD is present, symptoms should be evident after mood stabilization.

Youth with conduct disorders (CD) may have underlying BD that fuels their disruptive behaviors. These youth's conduct problems cause so much chaos that the underlying mania is not evident. In such cases, the CD should resolve with mood stabilization. It is possible to have CD independent of BD in which case the CD symptoms should persist after mood stabilization.

Youth with oppositional defiant disorder (ODD) often respond to frustration with tantrums. The occurrence of ODD with alcohol-related neurodevelopmental disorders or pervasive developmental disorder (PDD) may, in particular, confer difficulty in dealing with interpersonal demands, frustration, and other social situations that require flexibility and compromise. These youth can respond with serious and prolonged outbursts or "rages" or SMD that can be mistaken for BD.

Anxiety Disorders are common comorbidities with all mood disorders at any age, and a common differential diagnosis for BD in youth due to the severe affective dysregulation that can occur. Youth with post-traumatic stress disorder (PTSD) may dysregulate upon re-exposure to traumatizing stimuli and may report psychotic like symptoms. The history of trauma and symptom activation with re-exposure helps to tease out the diagnosis. During panic attacks, youth experience surges of anxiety and cognitive distress (decreased concentration, feelings of losing control) and irritability that lead to tantrums. The differential from mania is based on the physiologic arousal during panic and the quick escalation and defervescence of a panic attack. However, this may be more difficult to ascertain in rapid cycling BD. Separation anxiety disorder (SAD) is one of the most common misdiagnoses due to the sudden unprovoked irritability. Also, these youth often have depressive symptoms and sleep disturbances that suggest cycling. The appropriate diagnosis becomes evident when the dysregulation is linked to separation or anticipated separation. Also, the sleep disturbance in SAD usually occurs at the beginning of sleep due to worry, whereas mania is also associated with middle of the night awakening and decreased need for sleep.

Substance-use Disorders are important differential diagnoses as drugs like cocaine and stimulants have "activating" effects and can precipitate mania. The "highs" and "crashes" of amphetamines can mimic the cycling of BD and hallucinogens can mimic a manic psychosis. In these cases, the differential must be delayed until the youth has been detoxified. A time line can determine whether the bipolar symptoms started after the use of substances in which case the diagnosis would be a substance-induced mood disorder, bipolar type; or whether the bipolar symptoms started first and the youth "self-medicated" to treat mood symptoms.

Schizophrenia and Other Psychotic Disorders must be differentiated from a manic psychosis. Manic youth are more likely to experience grandiose or mood congruent delusions and do not exhibit the "negative symptoms" of schizophrenia. Of course, such symptoms must be distinguished from depressive cycles of BD. Schizophrenic youth often show prodromal schizoid traits, while bipolar youth seek others, although unsuccessfully, due to their behavioral difficulties.

Borderline Personality Disorder (BPD) has many features of BD including affective instability, poor impulse control, and interpersonal deficits, and also follows a chronic course. However, youth with BPD are more likely to have been maltreated, self-mutilate, and show a pattern of unstable relationships and disturbed self-image. This differential underscores the importance of a longitudinal perspective.

Clinical Course

BD is considered to be a chronic illness; however, outcomes are variable, with episode recovery rates ranging from 70% to 100% and relapse rates ranging from 35% to 80%. This variability is due in part to the heterogeneity in diagnosis, as well as the samples studied. Geller and colleagues have followed 89 youth aged 6 to 16 years with BD-I for 8 years into young adulthood. They found a mean length of initial episodes of 55 weeks, 88% recovery rate, but a 73% relapse rate. Subjects had a mean of two episodes of mania or mixed episodes during follow-up, but they also had very long episodes and spent many weeks ill. Recent data from the multisite "Course and Outcome of Bipolar Illness in Youth" (COBY) study of 263 youth, 7 to 18 years old, with BD-I, BD-II, or BD, NOS demonstrated similar results, with 82% of youth recovered from their index episode, but 64% had at least one recurrence. During the 2.5-year follow-up, 25% of youth with an initial diagnosis of BD-II converted to BD-I and 38% with an initial diagnosis of BD, NOS converted to BD-I or BD-II. Conversion rates in adults are lower and suggest that the diagnoses of BD-II and BP, NOS are less stable in youth. Overall, early-onset BD appears to portend a poor course, including frequent switches of polarity, mixed episodes, psychosis, comorbidity, suicide risk, and seriously impaired global functioning.

When depression is the initial presentation of BD, the "switch" into mania is obvious due to the rapid resolution of the depression and the emergence of core manic symptoms. However, if irritability is the primary presenting symptom, adults may think that the youth is just getting more moody or aggressive as part of the depression, or due to comorbid ADHD. The eventual emergence of elation, grandiosity, racing thoughts, pressured speech, and the lack of need for sleep clarifies the diagnosis. However, if the development of mania is gradual or a mixed episode comprises the first presentation, the clinical picture can be murky.

Assessment

The essentials of assessment for BD in youth are summarized in Table 12-3.

History Gathering

The American Academy of Child and Adolescent Psychiatry notes that the aims of the clinical interview are to obtain a detailed history of symptom onset, duration, and intensity; develop a time line of symptoms; perform a developmentally appropriate mental-status examination; and review the child's functioning across settings. A time line of mood symptoms using holidays and important events as anchors to assess the chronology of symptoms can help to delineate a pattern of some cyclicity. It is important to cue the family and child regarding periods of increased goal-directed activity, irritability, amount or rate of speech, excessive involvement in pleasurable activities, delusions or hallucinations, and decreased need for sleep. In addition, major changes in function, such as worsening performance at school or social isolation may elucidate mood changes. It is also important to interview the child alone about possible abuse or substance use. A complicating factor in teasing out cyclicity is that the winters are often more difficult for individuals with mood disorders but they also occur in the mid school year which is a difficult time for many youth and may suggest cycling during the winter time.

A developmental history includes a chronological picture of the child's growth and development, including early temperament that may be prodromal to BD, the need for sleep and disrupted sleep (especially waking in the middle of the night), stressors that exacerbate temperamental features, and emotional milestones that vary by childhood disorder. Assessing peer relationships and academic performance helps to determine the degree of impairment. The parents' view of the family dynamics provides context that may relate to comorbidity or the differential diagnosis, and sets the tone for interventions. Of course, a family history of mood disorders increases the suspicion of BD in the youth.

TABLE 12-3	Essentials of Assessment for Early-Onset Bipolar Disorder

- Physical examination, review of systems, and laboratory testing are included to rule out suspected medical etiologies including neurological, systemic, and substance-induced disorders.
- The clinical interview of the youth is the cornerstone of assessment for BD. Although many young patients lack insight regarding their manic symptoms, they can often describe their internal states.
- A longitudinal perspective with a time line of symptom evolution is needed to demonstrate cyclicity and understand the youth's illness.
- The child or adolescent interview should include open-ended questions and discussion of unrelated topics in order to assess thought processes.
- Always inquire about psychotic symptoms.
- Always inquire about suicidality which is a risk during both depressed and manic stages due to impaired judgment.
- For older children and adolescents part of the interview should occur without parental presence in order to assess risk-taking behavior, such as substance abuse, sexuality, and legal transgressions.
- Family members' behavioral observations provide corollary information regarding the patient's range of difficulties and comorbidity.
- School performance and interpersonal relationships should be assessed to determine the youth's functional impairment and educational needs.

Mental-Status Examination

The mental-status examination of a bipolar child in a depressed state is consistent with that of unipolar depression as described in the depression chapter of this text, although there may be more psychotic symptoms. The child in a manic state will show motor function that is hyperactive and, unlike most youth with ADHD, may describe a subjective need to move. Speech will show an increased production, rate and volume, possibly tangentiality. The youth will be difficult to redirect and will often be self-aggrandizing. Usually, the child will seem truly unable to control himself. Inappropriate sexual themes may arise, although this may not come up in the interview. The child may also display poor impulse control and can be threatening or assaultive when crossed. Insight and judgment are impaired, the degree of which will help to determine disposition, that is, the need for hospitalization.

Evaluation of the youth's mood should include observation, the parent's report, and the youth's own description. Affect is elated although this may not be initially evident, especially if the child is also irritable. The elation may be evident as the youth discusses topics that should not evince elation. Manic youth may talk about violating societal rules, knowing more than relevant adults, and describe grandiose, unrealistic plans. In the setting of a clinical interview, excessive joking, especially the use of puns can be an indicator of manic symptoms. It should be noted that euphoria and grandiosity are distinctly different from children's fantasy or tendency to become overstimulated, and from adolescents' feelings of invincibility. In a mixed state, the child may also be very irritable, contrary, bossy, demanding, confrontational, and may have a major tantrum without age-appropriate concern for what others think. However, the child may have to be "provoked" during the interview to demonstrate this mood lability. If asked, this child may endorse sadness along with all of the irritability and anger. These youth may also endorse odd perceptual alterations, if asked.

Psychotic symptoms may not be spontaneously endorsed. Parents are often unaware of these symptoms, making it important to query the youth about hallucinations and any other odd ideation. Grandiosity in delusions can be evident at all ages, although it may be more apparent for adolescents for whom fantasy is no longer age appropriate. With children, delusional thinking is less common, but when present may be grandiose with great plans or feats. Less frequently, delusions may be bizarre. Any psychotic symptoms in the presence of manic symptoms should alert the clinician to closely monitor the emergence of BD, and the risk of harm due to impaired judgment. Indeed, suicide risk must be ascertained, no matter how young the child, as bipolar youth are at risk for suicidality whether in the depressed or manic phase of illness. Youth with BD, psychosis, and suicidal behavior should be assessed for the need for hospitalization.

Screening Tools

Given the difficulty of BD diagnosis, several tools may assist in assessing the symptom severity and help to determine when a referral to a specialist is warranted. Such tools may also be used as a guide for interviewing a youth or parent regarding BD. Once a diagnosis has been made, these scales can also help to track the presence and severity of symptoms. The General Behavioral Inventory (GBI), a widely used adult self-report screening measure for mood disorders, has been modified to be administered to parents of youth aged 5 to 17 years. The Parent General Behavior Inventory (P-GBI) is designed to screen clinically referred youth for BD. The P-GBI contains 76 items that contain two mood-related subscales: one for depression and one for hypomania/biphasic. The original GBI can be used as a self-report by adolescents. The P-GBI has demonstrated good psychometric properties including good sensitivity in detecting cases of BD, as well as distinguishing between BD and ADHD. Another scale is the Young Mania Rating Scale (Y-MRS) that documents the presence and severity of manic symptomatology. The Y-MRS was developed as a brief clinician-administered scale for adults on an inpatient unit and integrates data from various sources. Gracious and colleagues have modified this scale into a parent-report version (YMRS-P). The YMRS-P has only 11 items and preliminary evidence of adequate psychometric properties. The Child Mania Rating Scale–Parent (CMRS-P) was developed specifically for parent-report of children's mood symptoms. Its psychometric data are strong and it demonstrates good clinical utility with regard to differentiating pediatric mania from ADHD. The original measure had 21 items; however, the new 10-item version shows comparable functioning.

Medical Work-Up

The first consideration is to rule out medical causes for the youth's presentation. If the patient is taking medications that may precipitate mania, they should be stopped and the youth observed for a period of time to see if symptoms resolve. A urine toxicology screen will detect amphetamines, cocaine, and phencyclidine; however, inhalants and methylenedioxymethamphetamine (ecstasy) are not tested in urine toxicology screens. A noncontrast head CT (computerized tomography), or an MRI, should be obtained for atypical cases or if there is suspicion of other etiologies. There is no role for routine scanning. If temporal lobe and partial complex seizures are suspected, for example, due to visual perceptual distortions, an electroencephalogram (EEG) should be considered a complete blood count, electrolytes, thyroid studies, liver function tests, BUN, and creatinine are part of a standard work-up for any first-episode mood disorder and to establish a baseline for monitoring. Due to the potential for hyperphagia and weight gain, most clinicians now obtain baseline glucose, hemoglobin A1c, triglycerides, and cholesterol. Further testing is individualized to the clinical findings.

Treatment

The treatment of BD requires multimodal management that extrapolates from research on adults with BD complemented by studies or case series with youth when available. Optimal treatment involves pharmacological containment of symptoms and structured psychosocial interventions to help the young person to cope with his/her illness and maximize the quality of life.

Pharmacotherapy

Pharmacotherapy remains the cornerstone of treatment for BD at any age. Early-onset BD appears to respond to pharmacotherapy more slowly and/or less adequately than does BD that onsets in adulthood. Youth who cycle between mood states will usually require medication, often more than one medication, and even polypharmacy, to reduce morbidity and prevent mortality. Furthermore, because BDs are highly impairing, life threatening, and tend to be recurrent and/or chronic, prophylaxis is generally indicated. Current guidelines are based on adult guidelines complemented by juvenile studies when available. The essentials of pharmacotherapy are summarized in Table 12-4; specific medications for BD are presented in Table 12-5.

Treatment of the Manic or Hypomanic Phase of Illness

The Child Psychiatric Workgroup on Bipolar Disorder for the American Academy of Child and Adolescent Psychiatry has developed the Practice Parameter for the Assessment and Treatment of Children and Adolescents with BD. The guidelines note that medication choice depends upon any evidence-base, subtype of BD (BD-I, BD-II, psychosis, mixed episode, rapid cycling), phase of illness (manic/hypomanic or depressed), the patient's personal history, and family history. As for adults, mood stabilizers are the primary treatment for both acute stabilization and for maintenance of euthymia. However, only 40% to 60% of youth have an adequate response to a single mood stabilizer that leads to a change in medication or augmentation with a second agent, either another mood stabilizer or a second-generation antipsychotic

TABLE 12-4	Treatment Essentials for Early-Onset Bipolar Disorder

- Mood stabilizers are the cornerstone for treatment of BD.
- Among the mood stabilizers, lithium and divalproex sodium are the first-line treatment for episodes of euphoric mania. Divalproex may be more effective for mixed or rapid cycling episodes, but caution in using with females of child-bearing age.
- Lamictal is gaining acceptance, especially for depressed phases of illness. Slow titration may limit its use as a sole agent for acute mania.
- Adjunctive antipsychotic medication can be used during acute mania to rapidly stabilize the youth, assure safety, and provide sleep. Chronic use may be needed.
- If using antipsychotic medications, establish baseline and then monitor for "metabolic syndrome" due to hyperphagia and weight gain. Establish dietary plan and exercise regimen at the start of pharmacotherapy.
- Antidepressants should be avoided; but if the youth becomes depressed and is not responsive to other pharmacotherapy, cautious use may be necessary. Carefully monitor for manic "switch".
- Consider psychotherapy for mild-to-moderate depressive symptoms as an alternative to antidepressant medication.
- Stimulants may be used to treat comorbid ADHD once the patient has been stabilized on a mood stabilizer. However, they may destabilize the patient.
- Adjunctive psychosocial treatments (e.g., psychoeducation, family therapy, individual therapy) are always indicated in the treatment of early-onset BD. At a minimum, treatment should include psychoeducation about BD, its risks, treatment, prognosis, and complications associated with medication noncompliance.
- Constant vigilance about suicide potential during any phase of BD is indicated.
- Ongoing collaboration with the school should focus on education about BD, development of an appropriate Individualized Education Plan, and assistance with behavioral management planning.

(SGA). Polypharmacy is common, and may even comprise best practice. Relapse rates are high in early-onset BD even when youth consistently comply with taking a mood stabilizer.

Lithium is approved by the Food and Drug Administration (FDA) for acute treatment of mania and for maintenance therapy in individuals over 12 years old. In a systematic study over the first month of treatment, less than 75% of youth will respond with at least partial improvement and only 26% to 46% achieve remission. A longer period may be needed to observe improvements in youth. In open trials, lithium has been effective in 63% to 81% of youth in the absence of ADHD but 57% with comorbid ADHD. Divalproex, or valproate, is a first-line agent approved by the FDA as a mood stabilizer in adults and considered equivalent to lithium in the treatment of euphoric mania, but superior if the patient experiences rapid cycling or a mixed state. Work with youth also suggests such efficacy. Adding lithium to divalproex has not shown improved response, but adding an SGA, specifically quetiapine, has. Carbamazepine is included in the recommendations by The Child Psychiatric Workgroup due to its efficacy with adults. Oxcarbazepine is widely used with youth, but a recent multicenter study found no benefit over placebo and there are limited studies with adults.

Treatment guidelines developed by the AACAP Workgroup also support a role for the SGAs as first-line agents. Open label trials and case series with several SGAs, including olanzapine, risperidone, quetiapine, ziprasidone, and aripirprazole, support their use either alone or in combination with a mood stabilizer. Improvements have ranged from 50% to 67% when used alone to 82% when used in combination with a mood stabilizer. Their rapid onset of action in controlling mania and psychosis improves safety, relieves youth's distress, and allows quicker integration back into school and activities.

The guidelines of the AACAP Practice Parameter for the treatment of the manic phase are consistent with the algorithm for adult BD-I published by the Texas Medication Algorithm

TABLE 12-5   Mood-Stabilizing Medications for Bipolar Disorder

	Putative Mechanism of Action	Average Daily Dosing	Serum Levels	Side Effects	Monitoring
Primary Mood Stabilizers					
Lithium Carbonate (150, 300, 600 mg capsule; 300 mg tablet) Lithobid-SR (300 mg tablet) Eskalith-CR (450 mg tablet)	Proposed action at various signal transduction sites beyond neurotransmitter receptors by inhibiting second messengers such as phosphatidyl inositol, and/or by modulating G proteins, and/or by interaction at sites within downstream signal transduction cascades, for example, inhibition of glycogen synthetase kinase 3. Also, thought to affect regulation of gene expression for growth factors and neuronal plasticity	***Children:*** 15–60 mg/kg/day in divided doses ***Adolescents:*** 600–1800 mg/day in three to four divided doses for immediate release or two doses for sustained release Usually start 150–300 mg b.i.d. and titrate over 2–4 weeks to serum levels between 0.6 and 1.5 mEq/L (generally upper limit is 1.2 mEq/L, but higher levels may be used as tolerated)	***Acute mania:*** 0.8–1.5 mEq/L ***Maintenance:*** 0.5–1 mEq/L Caffeine decreases lithium level; nonsteroidal anti-inflammatories increase level	***Black box warning:*** Lithium toxicity with neurological sequelae; narrow therapeutic window. ***Serious reactions:*** seizures, syncope, decreased cognitive ability, dysrhythmias, hypothyroidism, diabetes insipidus, weight gain; possible teratogenicity potential neurotoxicity with SSRIs and carbamazepine ***Common side effects:*** acne, GI intolerance, thirst, polydipsia, polyuria, tremor, fatigue, sedation	***Baseline:*** Electrolytes, TSH, renal panel, urinalysis, EKG, glucose, weight, triglycerides, cholesterol ***Follow-up:*** Lithium levels on alternate weeks until stable then every 3–6 months or if symptom breakthrough Electrolytes, TSH, renal panel, urinalysis, EKG at 1,3 and then every 6–12 months If major weight gain, also follow triglycerides, cholesterol, glucose, Hgb 1Ac, insulin levels

TABLE 12-5   Mood-Stabilizing Medications for Bipolar Disorder *(continued)*

	Putative Mechanism of Action	Average Daily Dosing	Serum Levels	Side Effects	Monitoring
Anticonvulsant Mood Stabilizers					
Sodium divalproex; valproate; valproic acid (Depakote, Depakene)	Anticonvulsant mood stabilizers, including divalproex/valproate, are hypothesized to inhibit voltage-sensitive sodium channels, VSSC (and possibly potassium and calcium channels), to enhance inhibitory neurotransmission and reduce excitatory neurotransmission of gamma amino butyric acid (GABA) Divalproex/Valproate may also regulate downstream signal transduction cascades, such as inhibiting GSK3 or activating signals that promote neuroprotection and plasticity	***Children:*** 30–60 mg/kg/day in 2–3 divided doses ***Adolescents:*** 750–2000 mg/day in 2–3 divided doses Usually start with 125–250 mg b.i.d. and titrate over 2–4 weeks to serum level of 50–100 µg/mL	***Serum level:*** 50–125 µg/mL, but typically 75–100 µg/mL Phenytoin and carbamazepine increase clearance and decrease serum levels of valproate Lamotrigine decreases valproate level approximately 25%	***Black box warning:*** *hepatoxicity:* particularly in toddlers and with multiple anticonvulsants *teratogenicity:* neural tube defects; protect females with folic acid *pancreatitis:* acutely or after years of use ***Serious reactions:*** suicidality, agranulocytosis, neutropenia, thrombocytopenia, hepatotoxicity, hyperammonemic encephalopathy, polycystic ovary syndrome, alopecia, decreased cognitive ability; salicylates may cause toxicity ***Common side effects:*** Hyperphagia, sedation, nausea, weight gain, tremor, GI upset	***Baseline:*** CBC, liver function tests (LFTs) ***Follow-up:*** Valproate serum level at 2 weeks, 1 month, 3 months, then every 6–12 months or with symptom breakthrough CBC and LFTs at 2 weeks, 1 month, 3 months, and every 6 months thereafter If major weight gain, also follow triglycerides, cholesterol, glucose, Hgb 1Ac, insulin levels If serious abdominal pain with other GI symptoms, check amylase and LFTs

Medication	Mechanism of action	Dosing	Serum level	Warnings/reactions	Monitoring
Carbamazepine (Tegretol, Carbatrol)	Carbamazepine is hypothesized to inhibit voltage-sensitive sodium channels (VSSC) perhaps at a site within the channel itself, the alpha subunit of VSSC. This proposed mechanism on the alpha subunit of the VSSC is different from the actions of valproate at this site. May also act at other ion channels, for example, potassium and calcium channels. Such interference with voltage-sensitive channels may enhance the inhibitory actions of GABA	**Children:** 10–20 mg/kg/day in 3–4 divided doses **Adolescents:** 400–800 mg/day in 2–3 divided doses	**Serum level:** 8–12 µg/mL Lamotrigine increases serum level of carbamazepine	**Black box warning:** None **Serious reactions:** Suicidality, agranulocytosis, hepatotoxicity, decreased cognitive ability, impaired coordination, slurred speech, ataxia, Stevens–Johnson Syndrome **Common side effects:** Dizziness, headache, rash, drowsiness, sedation, nausea, vomiting	**Baseline:** CBC, LFTs **Follow-up:** Serum carbamazepine level, CBC, LFTs at 2 weeks, 1 month, 3 months and then every 6–12 months
Oxycarbazepine (Trileptal) 150 mg, 300 mg, and 600 mg tablets 300 mg/5 mL suspension	Same as carbamazepine in binding to the VSSC alpha subunit	**Children and adolescents:** 8–10 mg/kg/day in 2–3 divided doses Usually initiate at 150–300 mg b.i.d. and titrate over 2–4 weeks to 1200–1800 mg/day	Serum level not generally monitored	**Black box warning:** None **Serious reactions:** Same as carbamazepine, but with less risk of neutropenia; fewer CYP 450 3A4 interactions, making it more tolerable and easier to dose; increased risk of hyponatremia **Common side effects:** Same as carbamazepine	**Baseline:** No specific recommendations as monotherapy, but consider: electrolytes, CBC, LFTs especially if used with other medications **Follow-up:** No specific recommendations, but consider electrolytes, CBC, LFTs, and serum level if no benefits, especially if used with other medications

(continued)

	Putative Mechanism of Action	Average Daily Dosing	Serum Levels	Side Effects	Monitoring
Anticonvulsant Mood Stabilizers					
Lamotrigine (Lamictal) 25 mg, 100 mg, 150 mg, 200 mg tablets Chewable tablets: 2 mg, 5 mg, 25 mg	Some similarities to carbamazepine in binding to the open channel conformation of the VSSCs, but perhaps less potently as not as effective for manic phase May act to reduce the release of the excitatory neurotransmitter glutamate which may relate to its effects in bipolar depression, unlike other anticonvulsant mood stabilizers	***Children and Adolescents:*** 12.5 mg daily for weeks 1 and 2 25 mg daily for weeks 3 and 4 50 mg daily for week 5 100 mg daily for week 6 Target dose: 100 mg to 200 mg daily, although in practice higher doses commonly used depending on response	Serum level not generally monitored as not helpful in dose adjustment for psychiatric disorders Serum level increased/doubled by valproate, so decrease lamotrigine doses by 50% Serum level decreased by carbamazepine, so increase lamotrigine doses, perhaps up to 50% Phenobarbital and primidone lower the level of lamotrigine by about 40% Estrogen-containing birth-control pills lower lamotrigine levels by up to 40%	***Black box warning:*** Stevens–Johnson Syndrome and Toxic Epidermal Necrolysis ***Serious Reactions:*** Suicidal thoughts and behaviors; agitation, decreased cognitive ability; potential teratogenicity ***Common side effects:*** rash, insomnia; headache, dizziness, diplopia, sedation, insomnia, GI intolerance, irritability	***Baseline:*** No specific recommendations as monotherapy, but consider: electrolytes, CBC, LFTs especially if used with other medications, especially valproate ***Follow-up:*** No specific recommendations, but consider electrolytes, CBC, LFTs, and serum level if no benefits, especially if used with other medications
Antipsychotics/Neuroleptics					
First-generation antipsychotics (FGAs) (all)	Hypothesized action in psychosis is blockade of the dopamine-2 (DA-2) receptors in mesolimbic tracts No clearly proposed action for mania motor side effects due to DA-2 blockade in the mesocortical and nigrostriatal pathways		Not relevant to clinical action	NMS; blockade of muscarinic cholinergic receptors; blockade of histamine receptors; akathisia, extrapyramidal effects (EPS), dystonia, tardive dyskinesia, increased appetite, constipation; emotional blunting, cognitive blunting	No serum monitoring; BP/orthostasis, QTc interval, weight, CBC, glucose, HgbA1c, LFTs, cholesterol, triglycerides, motor functioning (SAS and AIMS)

Drug	Dosing	Proposed mechanism of action	Clinical relevance	Side effects	Monitoring / comments
Haloperidol	**Children:** 0.01–0.15 mg/kg/day in 2–3 divided doses **Adolescents:** 0.25–10 mg qd				Potent with low occurrence of anticholinergic effects but increased occurrence of EPS
Molindone	**Children and adolescents:** 5–15 mg t.i.d. to q.i.d.				Possibly less weight gain than for other FGAs and SGAs
Second-generation antipsychotics (SGAs) (all)		Hypothesized action in psychosis is via serotonin 2A-DA-2 antagonism. No clearly proposed action for mania. Suggested role for the 5HT2A antagonist properties of the SGAs in reducing glutamate hyperactivity from overly active pyramidal neurons, thus reducing symptoms of both mania and depression depending on the circuit involved. Serotonin variably inhibits DA-2 transmission in selected DA pathways, with effects on the nigrostriatal and mesocortical pathways	Not relevant to clinical action	Lower likelihood of motor side effects but still capable of producing akathisia, extrapyramidal effects, dystonia, tardive dyskinesia; increased appetite, constipation	No serum monitoring; BP/orthostasis, QTc interval, weight, CBC, glucose, HgbA1c, LFTs, cholesterol, triglycerides, motor functioning (SAS and AIMS)
Risperidone	0.25–6.0 mg/day qd or in divided doses			Increased prolactin, orthostasis, QTc interval	
Olanzapine	5–20 mg qd or in divided doses			Anticholinergic effects, orthostasis	
Quetiapine	25–600 mg qd or divided doses			QTc interval, orthostasis	
Ziprasidone	20–80 mg b.i.d.			QTc interval	
Aripiprazole	5–20 mg qd			QTc interval	

TS, thyroid stimulating hormone; EKG, electrocardiogram; SSRI, selective serotonin reuptake inhibitor; GI, gastrointestinal; BP, blood pressure; CBC, complete blood count; HgbA1c, hemoglobin A1c; LFTs, liver function tests; NMS, neuroleptic malignant syndrome; SAS, Simpson-Angus Side Effects Scale; AIMS, Abnormal Involuntary Movements Scale

TABLE 12-6	Treatment of Manic/Hypomanic/Mixed Stage of BD

Stage 1A Monotherapy:
For patients presenting with euphoric mania or hypomania:
lithium, VPA, SGAs (ARP, QTP, RISP, ZIP)
For patients presenting with mixed or dysphoric hypomania or mania:
VPA, SGAs (ARP, RISP, ZIP)

Stage 1B: Monotherapy (euphoric or mixed mania or hypomania)
OLZ *or* CBZ

Stage 2: Two-drug combination therapy
lithium, VPA, SGA
choose two of these options, but not two SGAs, not ARP, not CLOZ

Stage 3: Two-drug combination with a larger set of choices
lithium VPA,, SGA, CBZ, OXC, FGA
choose two of these options, but not two SGAs, not CLOZ

Stage 4: Option of electroconvulsive treatment, clozapine, or three-drugs
ECT *or*
add clozapine *or*
Lithium + (VPA *or* CBZ *or* OXC) + SGA

ARP, aripiprazole; CBZ, carbamazepine; CLOZ, clozapine; ECT, electroconvulsive therapy; FGA, first-generation antipsychotic; OLZ, olanzapine; OXC, oxcarbazepine; RISP, risperidone; SGA, second-generation antipsychotic or atypical antipsychotic; QTP, quetiapine; VPA, valproate; ZIP, ziprsidone.

Project (TMAP). Interestingly, the TMAP group does not offer an algorithm for BD-II given the lack of sufficient evidence-based data on its treatment. In the TMAP algorithm for mania/hypomania/mixed episode, all patients are treated with an antimanic agent. If symptom improvement is inadequate or intolerable side effects occur, they then progress to another agent. In the case of partial response with good tolerance or response with residual symptoms, the recommendation is to add a medication (i.e., combination therapy) versus switching agents. If the patient is intolerant of the first agent, the recommendation is to try an alternative antimanic agent. When changing medications, the recommendation is to cross taper from one to the other medication, with eventual discontinuation of the ineffective agent. This algorithm considers the SGAs to be antimanic agents. The recently revised TMAP algorithm is presented in Table 12-6.

Olanzapine is not a first-line choice despite its FDA approval for the treatment of mania. Lamotrigine's requirement for slow titration makes it an unrealistic choice for acute stabilization. Some experts suggest stabilizing with an SGA and then slowly adding lamotrigine for ongoing maintenance treatment. The use of lamotrigine with another anticonvulsant mood stabilizer, such as carbamazepine or valproate, will necessitate dosage adjustments (see Table 12-5). Note that gabapentin and topiramate are not included here as they have been discredited as mood stabilizers in adult studies.

Algorithms represent expert opinion about "best practices" and are not mandates. Thus, the TMAP allows for clinical judgment regarding deviation from the algorithm to address an individual patient's treatment history, family history, or other specific needs.

The Depressive Phase of Illness

The AACAP workgroup declined to develop an algorithm for the treatment of the depressed phase of illness as there was insufficient evidence to support any algorithm. The traditional advice is that antidepressants should be avoided or used cautiously in BD due to the risks of

TABLE 12-7	Treatment of the Depressed Phase of BD

Stage 1: Address current mood stabilizer status
For patients currently taking lithium or another antimanic drug, or patient on no antimanic drug but with recent severe and/or recurrent mania
   Start/continue antimanic drug + LTG
For patients on no antimanic drug and without history of severe and/or recent mania
   LTG

Stage 2: QTP monotherapy
OFC combination treatment

Stage 3: Two drug combination
Lithium, LTG, QTP, OFC
Choose any two

Stage 4: {(lithium, LTG, QTP, OFC, VPA, or CBZ) + (SSRI, BUP, or VEN)}
or ECT

Stage 5: MOAIs, TCAs, other SGAs not already included, OXC, other combinations of drugs at earlier stages, inositol, stimulants, thyroid

SGA, second-generation antipsychotics; BUP, bupropion; CBZ, carbamazepine; ECT, electroconvulsive therapy; LTG, lamotrigine; MAOI, monoamine oxidase inhibitor; OFC, olanzapine/fluoxetine combination; OXC, oxcarbazepine; QTP, quetiapine; SSRI, selective serotonin reuptake inhibitors (citalopram, escitalopram, fluoxetine, paroxetine, sertraline, fluvoxamine); VEN, venlafaxine; VPA, valproate.

accelerating mood cycling and worsening the long-term course of illness, particularly for patients with rapid cycling or mixed states. However, a recent study in the *New England Journal of Medicine* found that an antidepressant combined with a mood stabilizer did not result in any destabilization, although it also did not offer any increased antidepressant effects over a mood stabilizer with placebo. The TMAP algorithm (Table 12-7) prioritizes medications that are least likely to destabilize mood. Lamotrigine has great appeal in that it does not carry such risks. Clinical lore suggests that bupropion may be less likely to destabilize moods than other antidepressants; however, the TMAP algorithm does not prioritize bupropion, perhaps due to its lack of an evidence base. The TMAP does recommend that all patients with BD in a depressed phase have mood-stabilizer treatment optimized before initiation of any antidepressant treatments.

Finally, seriously depressed youth without a prior manic/hypomanic episode but with a family history of BD should also be considered for the above algorithm, or otherwise protected against mood destabilization. If the depressive symptoms are mild to moderate, observation in psychotherapy for a while can be helpful in deciding whether a medication trial is indicated.

Treating Residual Comorbid Symptoms

Residual impairing ADHD symptoms often persist after the mood stabilization. With mood stabilizers and/or SGAs at therapeutic levels, the stimulants are putatively less likely to precipitate a manic "switch" and may improve cognitive functioning and academic performance. The pros and cons must be carefully discussed with the family prior to implementing such a course. Anxiety disorders may also persist after mood stabilization. SSRIs comprise the usual pharmacologic treatment and the same caveats apply in using them to treat anxiety as to treat the depression. An alternative may be gabapentin or pregabalin as open trials with adults suggest safety and effectiveness in treating anxiety. Psychotherapy is the preferred intervention for mild-to-moderate anxiety.

Psychosocial Interventions

According to the Practice Parameters of the American Academy of Child and Adolescent Psychiatry, a combination of pharmacology and psychosocial therapy is "almost always indicated" for early-onset BD. Recently, several adjunctive psychotherapies for BD in adults have been adapted for youth with BD, including *Family Focused Treatment* by Miklowitz and colleagues, *Interpersonal and Social Rhythm Therapy* by Hlastala and Frank, and *Cognitive Behavioral Therapy* by Feeny and colleagues. These therapies have been shown to improve the psychosocial factors implicated in the onset and maintenance of BD, speed recovery, delay relapse, and decreased symptoms between episodes in adults with BD. Other psychotherapies have also shown promise, including *Multifamily Psychoeducational Psychotherapy* by Fristad and colleagues, *Dialectical Behavior Therapy (DBT)* by Goldstein and colleagues, and *Child and Family Focused Cognitive Behavior Therapy* by Pavuluri and colleagues.

General psychosocial interventions that are indicated for early-onset BD include: psychoeducation, mood monitoring, social-skills training, strategies aimed at increasing lifestyle regularity and decreasing activities/situations that are overstimulating to the child. Parent training in behavioral interventions for dealing with problematic behaviors may also be helpful. The therapist plays an important role in helping to resolve factors in the family that might exacerbate the youth's course, such as high expressed emotion and other negativity. The therapist is also often an important liaison with school personnel, and may assist in the development of an Individualized Education Plan or other school accommodations.

As in adult treatment, psychosocial interventions should always include a strong and consistent focus on medication adherence. Strober and colleagues found that 35% of bipolar adolescents were nonadherent with their lithium regimen over 18 months. The relapse rate of youth who were nonadherent (92.3%) was nearly three times that of adolescents who continued to take their lithium (37.5%). These researchers also stated that levels of "ambient stress and interpersonal discord" were increased in the families of nonadherent patients. Therefore, psychosocial interventions that focus specifically on medication adherence, interpersonal functioning, and family stress could potentially improve the long-term outcome in bipolar youth.

Other Considerations

BD is a chronic, possibly lifetime, life-threatening illness with high rates of relapse. Subsequent as well as prior episodes may not stabilize, especially as youth enter their maximum age of risk. Thus, after the youth achieves some stability, and especially during puberty, further education becomes important. Typical topics include: the length of treatment, possible intermittent increases in medication, career goals, and family planning. Girls will need to consider their reproductive health. Valproate has been associated with polycystic ovary syndrome. Pregnancy may cause their illness to exacerbate. Pharmacotherapy during pregnancy carries risks for the fetus as valproate has been associated with neural tube defects and lithium with cardiac anomalies. The SSRIs have some risks of minor abnormalities. The SGAs may be the most benign approach during pregnancy if pharmacotherapy is required. Also, BD confers increased risk of a postpartum event that can endanger the mother and baby. Initially, these discussions might be most appropriate to have with the parents, but as girls mature, they must have the knowledge to manage their reproductive health.

Conclusions

A decade of research has established that BD can onset in children and adolescents, but there continues to be a controversy regarding how the DSM-IV criteria are expressed during development, and particularly the proposed "phenotypes." Such uncertainty must be resolved in order for studies into etiology, treatment, and prognosis to progress. In particular, it is important to determine whether the entities defined as early-onset BD are continuous with the adult disorder. Meanwhile, youth currently diagnosed with BD suffer difficulties across most domains of life and require multidisciplinary and multimodal interventions. As BD is considered a neurobiological disorder, most intervention research has focused on pharmacological treatments, but there are clearly environmental factors that contribute to the onset, perpetuation, and morbidity of this highly prevalent, and life threatening, disorder. Until there is a better understanding of early-onset BD, its underlying pathophysiology, and treatment options, clinicians and families need to collaborate to minimize secondary morbidity and optimize the lives of these young people and their families.

CASE VIGNETTES

VIGNETTE 1: MARIA, ADOLESCENT WITH BD

Maria is a 15-year-old girl who was brought in to her physician's office by her parents because of a drastic change in her behavior. She had begun to act strangely just prior to their return from their summer vacation in Spain, several time zones away from their home. During examination, Maria was agitated and pacing, yelling at her parents, "I can do whatever I want!" Her parents reported that Maria had slept only 2 to 3 hours per night for several days and not at all last night. She read the bible all night, blessed everyone in the home to "get the demons out" and described ideas that were incongruent with her family's beliefs. As the parents described their concerns, Maria made jokes.

Her mother reported that Maria had struggled with depression since the age 10, after her best friend moved away. For a year, she was bored, irritable, and hypersomnic, often missing school because she refused to get out of bed. She was tearful and wished she would not wake up in the morning. Mother wondered whether she had BD like mother's brother, and brought her to her doctor and a therapist; but they thought that Maria was being "difficult." Her therapist noted that Maria was a "lateral thinker" as she had many ideas and could go from topic to topic in conversation—"a verbally precocious girl." After 4 months of therapy, her mood, school refusal, and energy improved. At age 13, mood cycling developed. Maria struggled with depression through the winter, but then seemed "too happy" in the summer during which she slept only 4 hours/night, especially last summer after a vacation in Mexico. She was giddy as she discussed attending Harvard and becoming the ambassador to Mexico, an unlikely occurrence given her poor grades.

Given the severity of Maria's manic and psychotic symptoms, her history of recurrent depressions and hypomanias, and a family history of BD, she was diagnosed with BD-I and hospitalized. Maria's symptoms came under control with lithium carbonate and quetiapine that also regulated her sleep. Upon discharge 2 weeks later, Maria was better but still struggling with the cycling of her mood.

Maria began treatment with a psychologist who treated her with IPSRT, an evidence-based adjunctive psychotherapy for BD. They met weekly for 5 months and focused on three areas: (1) psychoeducation about BD, (2) learning skills to ameliorate the interpersonal problems associated with her illness, and (3) increasing routine and structure with an emphasis on her sleep. Maria struggled with the acceptance of her illness and the weight gain due to her medication. But, with therapy she learned to cope with an illness that severely affected her mood and behavior and to better communicate with her psychiatrist regarding adherence to her medication regimen. She established a regular schedule of rest and activity and avoided events that might disrupt her sleep. With pharmacotherapy and "booster" sessions of IPSRT, Maria avoided severe manic or depressive relapse, and managed intermittent moderate periods of depression with IPSRT. She graduated from high school and started community college.

VIGNETTE 2: SAMUEL, CHILD WITH MIXED EPISODES OF BD

Sam is a 10-year-old boy who was diagnosed at 4 years of age with ADHD and ODD. The parents worked with a therapist to develop behavioral programs to little avail. He became increasingly aggressive. At 7 years of age, his tantrums with frustration turned to threats to his peers and teacher. The school tested him for an individual education plan that documented an IQ of 132. They placed him in a self-contained classroom. He was prescribed stimulant medication that helped him to stay on task, but he required doses every 2 to 3 hours to moderate his impulsivity. At 8 years of age, he would stand up on the desk and yell commands to others. One day he hit his teacher, and another day attacked his mother. When frustrated with chores one day, he unintentionally choked his cat to death, plunging him into depression. Later, he talked of having "a good brain and a bad brain" and that "my brain makes me do bad things." Yet, Sam always seemed remorseful for his "bad" behaviors. Sam started to have middle-of-the-night awakening up to 3 hours, sometimes all night. Then, he was suspended from school for sexually harassing a girl.

At age 11, Sam became suicidal. In an interview, he noted that when angry he was also very sad. He endorsed "someone telling me to do things I know I should not do." He described that when he got angry, "I want to make someone else feel what I feel, to hurt someone, to kill someone, to throw the flames off me and onto them." He was placed on an antidepressant. A week later, he felt great remorse for threatening his mother and shot himself in the stomach with his father's gun. He was admitted to the hospital, stabilized, and transferred to a psychiatric unit.

His psychiatrist developed a time line of symptom evolution since age 3. Sam's impulsivity and anger seemed episodic, often in response to not getting his way, but often without provocation. These episodes were followed by brief periods of remorse during which he would sit in a dark room and think about dying. Sam revealed that he had been having hallucinations for as long as he could remember but that they now were threatening. His parents revealed periods when Sam talked incessantly and hectically planned reasonable activities. The staff described him as "narcissistic". Due to the mix of elevated, depressed, and irritable mood, hallucinations, and cyclicity to his increased speech and activities, Sam was diagnosed with BD-I.

Sam's medications were stopped. Risperidone was started to help him sleep and contain his hallucinations and aggression while sodium divalproex was titrated up to therapeutic levels. Over a month, he was sufficiently stable to return to outpatient care. Academic work was reintroduced, and more normative experiences at home and in the community were instituted. His parents were offered Family Focused Therapy to work on the conflicts regarding Sam's management at home and school. They refused, thinking that the medications had sufficiently treated their son.

Over the next year, Sam gained 40 pounds, his breasts were tender, his cholesterol, triglycerides, and prolactin were elevated. He could not tolerate decreases of his medication. Sam started to "cheek" his medication. After he attacked his father, he was rehospitalized. Risperidone was changed to aripiprazole with a reduced dosage, and lithium was added to aripiprazole and divalproex. This time, he and his family committed to participate in family therapy. They also agreed to a family diet and exercise program. Three months later, an amphetamine was added to help with persistent deficits in concentration. Now at 13 years of age, Sam continues to struggle with intermittent mood instability, but he has sufficiently improved and has transitioned into a regular classroom, is getting good grades, lost 10 pounds, and went to summer camp.

BIBLIOGRAPHY

Akiskal H, Downs J, Jordan P, et al.. Affective disorders in the referred children and younger siblings of manic-depressives: mode of onset and prospective course. *Arch Gen Psychiatry*. 1985;42:996–1003.

American Academy of Child and Adolescent Psychiatry. Practice parameter for the assessment and treatment of children and adolescents with bipolar disorder. *J Am Acad Child Adolesc Psychiatry*. 2007;46(1):107–125.

American Psychiatric Association. *Diagnostic and Statistical Manual of Mental Disorders*. Fourth Edition. Washington, DC: American Psychiatric Association, 1994.

Alloy LB, Abramson LY, Urosevic S, et al.. The psychosocial context of bipolar disorder: environmental, cognitive, and developmental risk factors. *Clin Psychol Rev*. 2005;25:1043–1075.

Althoff RR, Faraone SV, Rettew DC, et al.. Family, twin, adoption, and molecular genetic studies of juvenile bipolardisorder. *Bipolar Disord*. 2005;7:598–609.

American Academy of Child and Adolescent Psychiatry. Practice parameters for the assessment and treatment of children and adolescents with bipolar disorder. *J Am Acad Child Adolesc Psychiatry*. 2007;46:107–125.

Birmaher B, Axelson D, Goldstein B, et al. Four-year longitudinal course of children and adolescents with bipolar spectrum disorders: The Course and Outcome of Bipolar Youth (COBY) study. *Am J Psychiatry*. 2009;166:795–804.

Birmaher B, Axelson D, Strober M, et al. Clinical course of children and adolescents with bipolar spectrum disorders. *Arch Gen Psychiatry*. 2006;63:175–183.

Blumberg HP, Fredericks C, Wang F, et al. Preliminary evidence for persistent abnormalities in amygdala volumes in adolescents and young adults with bipolar disorder. *Bipolar Disord*. 2005;7:570–576.

Chang K, Karchemskiy A, Barnea-Goraly N, Garrett A, Simeonova DI, Reiss A. Reduced amygdalar gray matter volume in familial pediatric bipolar disorder. *J Am Acad Child Adolesc Psychiatry*. 2005;44:565–573.

Consoli A, Deniau E, Huynh C, et al.. Treatment in child and adolescent bipolar disorders. *Eur Child Adolesc Psychiatry*. 2007;16:187–198.

Danielson CK, Youngstrom EA, Findling RL, et al.. Discriminative validity of the General Behavior Inventory using youth report. *J Abnorm Child Psychol* 2003;31:29–39.

DelBello MP, Hanseman D, Adler CM, et al.. Twelve-month outcome of adolescents with bipolar disorder following first hospitalization for a manic or mixed episode. *Am J Psychiatry*. 2007;164:582–590.

DelBello MP, Schwiers ML, Rosenberg HL, et al.. A double-blind, randomized, placebo-controlled study of quetiapine as adjunctive treatment for adolescent mania. *J Am Acad Child Adolesc Psychiatry*. 2002;41:1216–1223.

DelBello MP, Simmerman ME, Mills NP, Getz GE et al. Magnetic resonance imaging analysis of amygdala and other subcortical brain regions in adolescents with bipolar disorder. *Bipolar Disord*. 2003;6:43–52.

Feeny NC, Danielson CK, Schwartz L, et al. Cognitive Behavioral Therapy for bipolar disorder in adolescents: a pilot study. *Bipolar Disord*. 2006;8:508–515.

Findling RL, McNamara NK, Youngstrom EA, et al. Double-blind 18 month trial of lithium versus divalproex maintenance treatment in pediatric bipolar disorder. *J Am Acad Child Adolesc Psychiatry*. 2005;44(5): 409–417.

Frazier JA, Ahn MS, DeJong S, et al. Magnetic resonance imaging studies in early-onset bipolar disorder: a critical review. *Harv Rev Psychiatry*. 2005;13(Suppl):125–140.

Fristad MA, Verducci JS, Walters K, et al.. Impact of multifamily psychoeducational psychotherapy in treating children aged 8 to 12 years with mood disorders. *Arch Gen Psychiatry*. 2009; 66:1013–1020.

Geller B, Cooper TB, Sun K. Double-blind, placebo-controlled study of lithium for adolescent bipolar disorders with secondary substance dependency. *J Am Acad Child Adolesc Psychiatry*. 1998;37:171–178.

Geller B, Tillman R, Bolhofner K, Zimerman B. Child bipolar I disorder: prospective continuity with adult bipolar I disorder, characteristics of second and third episodes, predictors of 8-year outcome. *Arch Gen Psychiatry*. 2008;65:1125–1133.

Goldstein TR, Axelson DA, Birmaher B, et al.. Dialectical behavior therapy for adolescents with bipolar disorder: a 1-year open trial. *J Am Acad Child Adolesc Psychiatry*. 2007;46:820–830.

Goodwin FK, Jamison KR. *Manic-Depressive Illness Bipolar Disorders and Recurrent Depression*. New York: Oxford University Press; 2007.

Gracious BL, Youngstrom EA, Findling RL, et al. . Discriminative validity of a parent version of the Young Mania Rating Scale. *J Am Acad Child Adolesc Psychiatry*. 2002;41:1350–1359.

Hlastala SA. Stress, social rhythms, and behavioral activation: psychosocial factors and the bipolar illness course. *Curr Psychiatry Rep*. 2003;5:477–483.

Hlastala SA, Frank E. Adapting Interpersonal and Social Rhythm Therapy to the developmental needs of adolescents with bipolar disorder. *Dev Psychopathol*. 2006;18:1267–1288.

Kim EY, Miklowitz DJ, Biuckians A, et al.. Life stress and the course of early-onset bipolar disorder. *J Affect Disord*. 2007;99:37–44.

Kafantaris V, Coletti DJ, Dicker R, et al. Lithium treatment of acute mania in adolescents: a placebo-controlled discontinuation study. Lithium treatment of acute mania in adolescents: a placebo-controlled discontinuation study. *J Am Acad Child Adolesc Psychiatry*. 2004;43:984–993.

Kowatch RA, Fristad M, Birmaher B, et al.. Child Psychiatric Workgroup on Bipolar Disorder. Treatment guidelines for children and adolescents with bipolar disorder. *J Am Acad Child Adolesc Psychiatry*. 2005;44:213–235.

Leibenluft E, Charney DS, Towbin KE, et al. Defining clinical phenotypes of juvenile mania. *Am J Psychiatry*. 2003;160:430–437.

Lewinsohn PM, Klein D, Seeley JR. Bipolar disorders in a community sample of older adolescents: prevalence, phenomenology, comorbidity, and course. *J Am Acad Child Adolesc Psychiatry*. 1995;34:454–463.

Malkoff-Schwartz S, Frank E, Anderson BP, et al. Social rhythm disruption and stressful life events in the onset of bipolar and unipolar episodes. *Psychol Med*. 2000;30:1005–1016.

Merikangas KR, Akiskal HS, Angst J, et al. Lifetime and 12-month prevalence of bipolar spectrum disorder in the National Comorbidity Survey replication. *Arch Gen Psychiatry*. 2007;64:543–552.

Miklowitz DJ, Axelson DA, Birmaher B, et al. Family-focused treatment for adolescents with bipolar disorder: results of a 2-year randomized trial. *Arch Gen Psychiatry* 2008;65:1053–1061.

Pavuluri MN, Graczyk PA, Henry DB, et al. Child and family-focused cognitive behavioral therapy for pediatric bipolar disorder: development and preliminary results. *J Am Acad Child Adolesc Psychiatry*. 2004;43: 528–537.

Pavuluri MN, Henry DB, Carbray JA, Sampson G, Naylor MW, Janicak PG. Open-label prospective trial of risperidone in combination with lithium or divalproex sodium in pediatric mania. *J Affect Disord*. 2004;82:103–111.

Pavuluri MN, Henry DB, Devineni B, Carbray JA, Birmaher B. Child mania rating scale: development, reliability, and validity. *J Am Acad Child Adolesc Psychiatry*. 2006;45:550–560.

Pavuluri MN, Henry DB, Moss M, Mohammed T, Carbray JA, Sweeney JA. Effectiveness of lamotrigine in maintaining symptom control in pediatric bipolar disorder. *J Child Adolesc Psychopharmacol*. 2009;19:75–82.

Perlis RH, Miyahara S, Marangell LB, et al. STEP-BD Investigators. Long-term implications of early onset in bipolar disorder: data from the first 1000 participants in the Systematic Treatment Enhancement Program for Bipolar Disorder (STEP-BD). *Biol Psychiatry*. 2004;55:875–881.

Rich BA, Vinton DT, Roberson-Nay R, et al. Limbic hyperactivation during processing of neutral facial expressions in children with bipolar disorder. *Proc Natl Acad Sci USA*. 2006;103:8900–8905.

Sachs GS, Nierenberg AA, Calabrese JR, et al., Effectiveness of adjunctive antidepressant treatment for bipolar depression. *N Engl J Med*. 2007;356:1711–1722.

Scheffer RE, Kowatch RA, Carmody T, et al. Randomized, placebo-controlled trial of mixed amphetamine salts for symptoms of comorbid ADHD in pediatric bipolar disorder after mood stabilization with divalproex sodium. *Am J Psychiatry*. 2005;162:58–64.

Stahl SM. *Stahl's Essential Psychopharmacology: Neuroscientific Basis and PracticalApplications*. Third Edition. New York: Cambridge University Press; 2008.

Strober M, Schmidt-Lackner S, Freeman R, Bower S et al. Recovery and relapse in adolescents with bipolar affective illness: a five-year naturalistic, prospective follow-up. *J Am Acad Child Adolesc Psychiatry*. 1995;34:724–731.

Taylor E. Managing bipolar disorders in children and adolescents. *Nat Rev Neurol*. 2009; 10:1038/nrneurol. 2009.117.

Tillman R, Geller B. Definitions of rapid, ultrarapid, and ultradian cycling and of episode duration in pediatric and adult bipolar disorders: a proposal to distinguish episodes from cycles. *J Child Adolesc Psychopharmacol*. 2003;13:267–271.

Tohen M, Baker RW, Altshuler LL, et al. Olanzapine versus divalproex in the treatment of acute mania. *Am J Psychiatry*. 2002;159:1011–1017.

Tohen M, Kryzhanovskaya L, Carlson G, et al. Olanzapine versus placebo in the treatment of adolescents with bipolar mania. *Am J Psychiatry*. 2007;164:1547–1556.

Wagner KD, Kowatch RA, Emslie GJ, et al. A double-blind, randomized, placebo-controlled trial of oxcarbazepine in the treatment of bipolar disorder in children and adolescents. *Am J Psychiatry*. 2006;163(7):1179–1186.

Wehr T A, Sack DA, Rosenthal NE. Sleep reduction as a final common pathway in the genesis of mania. *Am J Psychiatry*. 1987;144:201–204.

Young RC, Biggs JT, Ziegler VE, Meyer DA. A rating scale for mania: reliability, validity, and sensitivity. *Br J Psychiatry* 1978;133:429–435.

Youngstrom EA, Findling RL, Danielson CK, et al.. Discriminative validity of parent report of hypomanic and depressive symptoms on the General Behavior Inventory. *Psychol Assess.* 2001;13:267–276.

SUGGESTED READING (FOR PATIENTS, FAMILIES, AND TEACHERS)

Jamison, KR (1995), *An Unquiet Mind: A Memoir of Moods and Madness.* New York: AA Knopf. *(An excellent, best selling autobiography of a leading investigator of Bipolar Disorder chronicling her own struggle with this disorder)*

Miklowitz DJ, George EL (2008), *The Bipolar Teen: What You Can Do to Help Your Child and Your Family.* New York: Guilford Press. *(For families living with a teen with Bipolar Disorder. The author is an investigator of family processes contributing to mental illness)*

Greenberg, R (2007), Bipolar Kids: Helping Your Child Find Calm in the Mood Storm. Cambridge, MA: DeCapo Press. *(Written by a child psychiatrist with extensive clinical experience helping youth with BD).*

SUGGESTED WEBSITES

Additionally, patients and families can benefit from information and connection with support groups some of which can be found on the following websites:

National Alliance for the Mentally Ill: www.nami.org

The Depression and Bipolar Support Alliance: www.dbsalliance.org

The Child and Adolescent Bipolar Foundation: www.bpkids.org

REVIEW QUESTIONS

1. For BD-I, the first line of treatment for children and adolescents is:
   a. Carbamazepine
   b. Fluoxetine
   c. Lamotrigine
   d. Lithium

2. Adjunctive psychosocial interventions such as *Cognitive Behavioral Therapy, Family Focused Treatment,* and *Interpersonal and Social Rhythm Therapy* are indicated and recommended for youth with:
   a. BD-I
   b. BD-II
   c. Cyclothymia
   d. All of the above

3. Compared to adults with BD, youth with BD:
   a. Are less likely to switch diagnostic categories over time
   b. More frequently demonstrate mixed episodes
   c. Are less likely to evidence psychotic symptoms
   d. Are more likely to demonstrate elation and euphoria with mania rather than irritability

4. The primary difference between hypomania and mania is:
   a. Age of onset
   b. Duration and severity of symptom presentation
   c. Presence of comorbid diagnosis(es)
   d. Type of symptoms

5. The bipolar spectrum disorder that is most similar to unipolar depression is:
   a. BD-I
   b. BD-II
   c. BD, NOS
   d. Cyclothymia

6. Treatment with an antidepressant during a depressive episode of early-onset BD:
    a. Should always start with a low dose SSRI
    b. Has no clear evidence base
    c. Should always start with bupropion
    d. Is safe if there are no manic symptoms evident

7. Identification of the proposed "narrow phenotype" and "broad phenotype":
    a. Has no validity
    b. Helps to guide overall treatment decisions
    c. Has recently been shown to be reliable across multiple studies
    d. Helps to choose between a mood stabilizer and an SGA

8. The mechanism for the therapeutic efficacy of mood stabilizers in BD is:
    a. Dependent on other medications being taken
    b. Hypothesized to involve the reuptake and decreased degradation of serotonin
    c. The same as their anticonvulsant effects
    d. Hypothesized to involve second messenger systems and stabilization of voltage-sensitive ion channel

9. For mild-to-moderate depression during early-onset BD, the best approach is:
    a. Involvement in a cognitive-behavioral psychotherapy
    b. Rapid titration of lamotrigine
    c. Involvement in a dynamic psychotherapy
    d. Change of current SGA to another SGA

10. The family environment and life stressors:
    a. May cause BD
    b. Have no role in the treatment of BD
    c. May exacerbate the course and severity of illness
    d. Have not yet been studied as a focus for intervention for BD

Answers: 1-d, 2-d, 3-b, 4-b, 5-b, 6-b, 7-a, 8-d, 9-a, 10-c

Eating Disorders

Introduction

Anorexia nervosa and bulimia nervosa are two of the most challenging disorders afflicting children and adolescents, with the potential for serious impact on both physical and psychological development. Anorexia nervosa has been documented by historians for many centuries. For example, "Holy Anorexia" was used to describe the severe fasting and self-initiated purging among those aspiring for sainthood during the medieval period. In modern medical history, there is a debate regarding first descriptions of currently defined anorexia nervosa. Bulimia nervosa has been described for an even longer time than severe restricting behaviors. The ancient Egyptians purged for "health" reasons. Binge eating and purging by the Roman upper class is well documented, most notably by Emperors Claudius and Vitellius. In modern times, Gerald Russell, a British psychiatrist, first described bulimia nervosa as a distinct syndrome in 1979. Current understanding hypothesizes that broad cultural forces and social stressors meld with individual biomedical and psychological factors to put an increasing number of young women and men at risk of developing eating disorders.

Clinical Features

Signs and Symptoms

Core features that define anorexia nervosa and bulimia nervosa as defined in the American Psychiatric Association's (1994) *Diagnostic and Statistical Manual of Mental Disorders, Fourth Edition* are summarized in Table 13-1.

For anorexia nervosa, the first core feature and hallmark of the disorder is significant weight loss or failing to gain weight commensurate with height. The second core feature is an intense fear of gaining weight or becoming fat. Individuals with anorexia struggle with the idea of eating and think that anything but the most stringent control of their food intake will result in undue weight gain. The primary distortion is these youths' perceptions of themselves as overweight despite their emaciated state. Even those youth who achieve remission often continue to perceive themselves as overweight. The third core feature is amenorrhea, defined as three consecutive missed menstrual cycles, in postmenarchal women. Obviously, this last feature does not apply to premenarchal girls or to boys. Though not part of the DSM-IV criteria, rigid thinking, perfectionism, and preference for predictability are common in youth with anorexia.

Individuals with anorexia nervosa can be further classified as those who are primarily restricting, meaning that they achieve their weight loss by limiting caloric intake, and those who both restrict and engage in binge eating and/or purging. The binging and purging subtype of anorexia nervosa is distinct from the binge eating and purging of bulimia nervosa in that restricting, weight loss, and low weight are the presenting concerns. Adolescent females remain the predominant population with anorexia nervosa but males and younger children are becoming more commonly affected.

TABLE 13-1   Comparing DSM-IV-TR Diagnostic Criteria for Anorexia Nervosa and Bulimia

Anorexia Nervosa	Bulimia Nervosa
A. Refusal to maintain body weight at or above a minimally normal weight for age and height (e.g., weight loss leading to body weight less than 85% of ideal body weight or failure to make expected weight gain during period of growth, leading to less than 85% of ideal body weight)	A. Recurrent episodes of binge eating. An episode of binge eating is characterized by both of the following: (1) eating, in a discrete period of time (e.g., within any 2-hour period), an amount of food that is definitely larger than most people would eat during a similar period of time and under similar circumstances, (2) a sense of lack of control over eating during the episode (e.g., a feeling that one cannot stop eating or control what or how much one is eating)
B. Intense fear of gaining weight or becoming fat, even though underweight	B. Recurrent, inappropriate compensatory behavior in order to prevent weight gain, such as self-induced vomiting; misuse of laxatives, diuretics, enemas, or other medications; fasting; or excessive exercise
C. Disturbance in the way in which one's body weight or shape is experienced, undue influence of body weight or shape on self-evaluation, or denial of the seriousness of the current low body weight	C. The binge eating and inappropriate compensatory behaviors both occur, on average, at least twice a week for 3 months
D. In postmenarchal females, amenorrhea, that is, the absence of at least three consecutive menstrual cycles	D. Self-evaluation is unduly influenced by body shape and weight
E. Restricting type: during the current episode of anorexia nervosa, the person has *not* regularly engaged in binge-eating or purging behavior (i.e., self-induced vomiting or the misuse of laxatives, diuretics, or enemas) Binge-eating/purging type: during the current episode of anorexia nervosa, the person has regularly engaged in binge-eating or purging behavior (i.e., self-induced vomiting or the misuse of laxatives, diuretics, or enemas)	E. The disturbance does not occur exclusively during episodes of anorexia nervosa. Specify type: Purging type: during the current episode of bulimia nervosa, the person has regularly engaged in self-induced vomiting or the misuse of laxatives, diuretics, or enemas Nonpurging type: during the current episode of bulimia nervosa, the person has used other inappropriate compensatory behaviors, such as fasting or excessive exercise, but has not regularly engaged in self-induced vomiting or the misuse of laxatives, diuretics, or enemas

Adapted from American Psychiatric Association. *Diagnostic and Statistical Manual of Mental Disorders, Fourth Edition (Text Revision)*. Washington, DC: Author; 2000.

The chief differentiating factor between bulimia nervosa and anorexia nervosa is the absence of severe weight loss, that is, those with bulimia are above 85% of their ideal weight and often slightly overweight. It is estimated that approximately 50% of those with anorexia become bulimic. The diagnostic criteria for bulimia nervosa focus primarily on two components: binge eating and an inappropriate compensatory action to prevent weight gain. Binge eating is defined as eating substantially more than a regular person would eat in a 2-hour period on at least two occasions per week for 3 months. The binges may consist of any food, but tend to be of high-sugar and high-carbohydrate content, for example, cake and ice cream. These episodes of binge eating are typically associated with a sense of loss of control and often occur following an unpleasant experience involving an injury to self-esteem. The individual usually feels ashamed during a binging episode and immediately afterwards. Engagement in some other activity to "undo" the binge is common, such as self-induced vomiting and less commonly misuse of laxatives, enemas, or diuretics. For individuals with the nonpurging subtype, compensatory behaviors may include excessive exercising, subsequent fasting or restricting, the misuse of appetite suppressants or thyroid hormone to speed metabolism or, in diabetics, deliberately missing insulin doses in order to avoid weight gain.

While bulimia is predominantly found in young women, it has a higher prevalence in males than anorexia nervosa. This is thought to be attributed to male competitive sports that require specific body measures or weigh-ins (e.g., wrestling). Individuals with bulimia may have poor dentition or halitosis from repeated self-induced emesis. They may also be engaged in other pathologic behaviors that will become apparent on examination or during interview, such as substance abuse which may be identified only on urine toxicology, or self-mutilation which may be evident as scarring on the arms, abdomen, hips, or thighs (more common in women but increasingly common in males). Individuals with either bulimia or anorexia tend to avoid eating with others, preferring privacy and often provide numerous reasons for not eating with others.

Eating disorders not otherwise specified (ED NOS) comprise the largest category for eating disorders as they include all subthreshold presentations of anorexia nervosa and bulimia nervosa.

Diagnostic and Developmental Issues

It is interesting to note that anorexia nervosa, binge/purge subtype, and bulimia nervosa are separated solely by the fact that the adolescent with anorexia is underweight. Indeed, with the trend toward rethinking of psychiatric disorders on a continuum, it is likely that these nosologic categories will undergo further adjustment for the DSM-V, scheduled for publication in 2010.

The challenge of accurate evaluation and diagnosis of anorexia nervosa is compounded in younger patients by several factors. A young patient may be gaining weight, however, not at a rate appropriate to height. Anorexia nervosa in prepubertal children is further complicated by the fact that prepubertal youth have less body fat, are more prone to volume depletion, are more likely to fluid restrict, and are more difficult to engage in the interview, and in later treatment, because of their cognitive limitations. Younger girls may not have started their menses or established a routine pattern of menses. Therefore, the third diagnostic criteria of missing three menstrual periods may not always apply. Younger patients and males may also not have the same level of body distortion or intense fear of becoming fat. Thus, a developmental framework is needed when diagnosing and treating younger or male youth.

Epidemiology

Eating disorders are among the most serious psychiatric disorders in terms of morbidity and mortality. Over a 30-year period, approximately 15% to 20% of individuals with anorexia nervosa will die from the disorder. The prevalence of eating disorders has been increasing since the 1950s. These disorders typically begin in adolescence, with onset by age 20 in over 85% of patients. Among females, the lifetime prevalence of anorexia nervosa is approximately 0.5% to 1.0% and the lifetime prevalence of bulimia nervosa is approximately 2%. When anorexia nervosa occurs in younger children, it may be part of more severe psychopathology. Individuals who are afflicted at a young age, however, tend to have a better prognosis in terms of remission of the disorder. Bulimia nervosa has a slightly older profile, affecting 1% to 3% of girls during adolescence and up to 4% in young adulthood. Both anorexia nervosa and bulimia nervosa are eight to ten times more prevalent in females than in males depending on age and type of eating disorder. There is also a strong cultural component. Both disorders are more common in Western postindustrialized nations including the United States. Caucasians are more often affected than African Americans or Hispanic Americans, although the latter two groups show higher rates for obesity and binge eating. Immigrants to Western countries tend to be afflicted at a rate similar to their new society.

Differential Diagnosis and Comorbid Conditions

Ruling out medical illness is important to the diagnostic process, as anorexia and weight loss can be a presenting symptom of many medical illnesses, including: neoplasms and the associated paraneoplastic syndrome, acquired immunodeficiency syndrome (AIDS) and other infectious diseases, vascular disease (e.g., the superior mesenteric artery syndrome), metabolic abnormalities, and endocrine disease.

Other psychiatric disorders should also be evaluated both as etiologies for weight loss and as relevant comorbidities. The loss of appetite or weight occurs in major depressive disorder (MDD). The depressed individual without an eating disorder, however, will not want to lose weight and will often complain of the loss of appetite. The weight loss, therefore, should abate with successful treatment of the MDD. Treatment of MDD comorbid with anorexia nervosa may make the patient more amenable to treatment; up to 60% of those with anorexia can present with premorbid or comorbid MDD.

Changes and idiosyncrasies in eating behavior can occur in schizophrenia, however, these individuals rarely have the distorted body image demonstrated in anorexia nervosa. Obsessive compulsive disorder (OCD), body dysmorphic disorder, and social phobia share features with anorexia nervosa regarding repetitive behaviors, need for perfection, or social avoidance, but they do not usually involve weight loss. Anxiety disorders are also highly co-morbid, particularly OCD which may occur in 30% of those with anorexia. A diagnosis of OCD should be made only if the compulsive behaviors extend beyond those related to food and eating.

In adults, both anorexia nervosa and bulimia nervosa show an association with personality disorders. Features of avoidant personality disorder are especially common in individuals with anorexia while features of borderline personality disorder including impulsivity and substance-use disorders are more common in individuals with bulimia and those with the subtype of binging and purging in anorexia.

Etiology and Pathogenesis

There is no known etiology for either anorexia nervosa or bulimia nervosa. A combination of biologic, psychological, environmental, and social factors have been implicated in their patho-genesis. Once a pattern of disordered eating begins, multidetermined factors maintain and promote the dysregulated eating patterns.

While no candidate gene has been identified for either disorder, data from family and twin studies suggest heritable factors. Anorexia nervosa has a concordance rate of nearly 70% for identical twins and 20% for nonidentical twins. Bulimia nervosa also shows a higher concor-dance in monozygotic twins than dizygotic twins. First-degree relatives of those with anorexia are more likely to develop anorexia. There is also an increased prevalence of mood disorders among the first-degree relatives, particularly among the binge-purging type. Bulimia shares this same heritability profile, but has the additional vulnerability of higher rates of substance-use disorders and substance-dependence disorders in first-degree relatives. Males in particular are at higher risk if there is genetic loading in first-degree relatives.

While heritable factors are important, psychological and sociocultural factors are also important to understand in the development of eating disorders. A diathesis-stress model is helpful in understanding the interplay between genetic predisposition and vulnerability to psycho-socio-cultural influences and stressors. The large national and cultural differences in these disorders support an important role of societal preferences. Specifically, it has been hypothesized that the high rates of eating disorders in young women and men pursuing professional acting, modeling, and dancing careers and those youth who emulate media stars is secondary to the emphasis on an excessively lean appearance as a standard of attractiveness. Similarly, in athletic activities requiring a low weight, such as gymnastics and wrestling, there is also an increased occurrence of abnormal eating behaviors. Weight loss or decreased appetite as a result of illness or self-directed dieting are common gateways into eating disorders. Initial results may lead to weight loss which is almost uniformly seen and commented on positively by others lending itself to a boost in self-esteem and excessive attention to appearance. This then can lead to further restricting, exercising, bingeing, and eventually semistarvation. Because semistarvation itself can lead to many of the same cognitions and behaviors common in individuals with anorexia, it is not unusual for semistarvation to take on a life of its own that then evolves into a more classic eating disorder. Semistarvation can also mimic many of the symptoms associated with depression and anxiety or can lower the individual's resilience to warding off normal occurrences or reactions of depression or anxiety resulting in an escalation of these normal occurrences for frequency and intensity. Additionally while there is no uniform personality type for the development of an eating disorder, it is not uncommon for those with anorexia to be attractive, intelligent, possessing a preference for predictability, tendencies toward perfectionism, acutely sensitive to others, and often described as caregivers.

Clinical Course

Anorexia Nervosa

The vast majority of new cases of anorexia nervosa typically onset in mid-to-late adolescence (age 14 to 18 years) to early adulthood (approximately 25 years old) with later onset being rarer thereafter but still occurring. Its onset is often associated with a stressful life event (e.g., significant illness, school or work transitions, change in peer group, change in family configuration, trauma) or an individual's high dissatisfaction with his/her body as compared to social standards of the "perfect body." The course and outcome of anorexia nervosa can be highly variable. Some individuals recover fully after a single episode, some exhibit a fluctuating pattern of weight gain followed by relapse with eventual recovery, and others experience a chronically deteriorating course over many years. Particularly within the first 5 years of onset, up to 50% of individuals with the restricting type of anorexia nervosa develop binge eating, indicating a change to the binge eating/purging subtype. A sustained shift in clinical presentation to weight gain plus binge eating and purging may eventually warrant a change in diagnosis to bulimia nervosa. Of the remainder who do not show such a shift in presentation, many have a chronic course with high likelihood of depression and anxiety. Mortality is relatively high compared to other psychiatric disorders with estimate that approximately 6% of those with anorexia die a premature death from complications of malnutrition, bradycardia, and electrolyte abnormalities, and another 5% or higher die from suicide.

Bulimia Nervosa

Bulimia nervosa usually onsets in late adolescence. The first binge-eating episode is often preceded by dieting to address poor body image and as an attempt to lose weight. Dieting creates excessive hunger and cravings which then lead to the binge resulting in guilt or feelings of failure.

This in turn fuels further poor body image and low self-esteem which lead to purging or other compensatory behaviors to "undo" the binge and restore a sense of relief and control. This cycle repeats itself over and over again, often becoming a habitual way of living. Typically, the course is chronic, although there may be interspersed periods of remission. As the individual passes from early into middle adulthood, symptoms tend to decrease. Periods of remission longer than 1 year are associated with better long-term outcome. Mortality is rare and is usually related to underlying pathology that was exacerbated by the rigors of frequent purging.

Assessment

The essentials of assessment for eating disorders are summarized in Table 13-2. The diagnosis of anorexia nervosa and bulimia nervosa is based on the history, physical examination, psychiatric interview, and mental-status examination. Standardized assessment instruments are also helpful adjuncts to the evaluation.

Medical

The physical examination provides the first clues regarding the patient's compromised health. A flow chart should be started to determine the youth's actual growth history compared to the current and expected height and weight for age. Measures taken for the physical exam should include height, weight, orthostatic blood pressure, and heart rate and body temperature to assess for concerns of low body mass index (BMI), cardiac functioning, and hypothermia. Laboratory assessment includes: blood urea, potassium, sodium, chloride, bicarbonate, calcium, magnesium, phosphate, creatinine, full blood picture, erythrocyte sedimentation rate, electrocardiogram, urinalysis, urine pregnancy test, and dual-energy x-radiograph absorptiometry (DEXA) scan of

---

TABLE 13-2   Essentials of Assessment of Eating Disorders

- Data gathering from multiple sources as youth with eating disorders often minimize his/her symptoms and parents may not appreciate their child's pathologic eating patterns
- A medical examination to rule out medical illnesses and provide a baseline to assess progress
- Characteristic findings to look for during physical examination include:
  — Anorexia nervosa: cachexia, dry skin, lanugo, bradycardia, and hypotension
  — Bulimia nervosa: calluses on the backs of hands, decreased gag reflex, chipped teeth (moth eaten in appearance), and hypertrophy of the parotids
- A psychiatric examination to:
  — rule out comorbid disorders underlying or comorbid with the eating disorders, for example, depression, substance abuse, anxiety, and personality disturbances.
  — assess individual characteristics associated with eating disorders, such as altered body image, perfectionism, onset of puberty, sexual orientation, or gender identity
- Rating scales may screen for an eating disorder and establish severity:
  — Self-report scales:
    – Eating Attitudes Test-26
    – Eating Disorder Examination Questionnaire
    – Clinical Impairment Assessment Scale
    – Eating Disorder Inventory 3
  — Clinician interview: SCOFF
- Assess family characteristics associated with eating disorders, such as emphasis on external attractiveness and/or excellence in academics or athletics; parents' eating and/or exercising patterns; families' management of conflict and/or negative affect

the spine or hip. Bone density is often lost in the malnourished state and restoration of weight and normalized eating can help to address the loss.

History and Physical Examination

Anorexia Nervosa

Because of the special circumstances presented when assessing youth for eating disorders (e.g., their tendency to under-report their eating-disordered behaviors and symptoms, over-report their intake, and/or deny any concerns), parents can be a particularly valuable resource. Questions to ask parents include: What concerns do you have about your child's eating, weight, growth? How much do you actually see your son/daughter eat? Is he/she on a particularly restrictive diet (e.g., vegan, vegetarian, low-fat, no "junk" food) and willing to find nutritious and diverse options within these parameters? Does s/he appear to spend long times in the bathroom immediately after meals (purging)? Do food items (e.g., tubs of ice cream) disappear without explanation (binge eating)? Does your child exercise an inordinate amount on a very regular basis? Does s/he make excessive remarks about his/her body weight and shape or ask for frequent assurance regarding body weight and shape or appearance. Affirmative answers to any of these questions should guide further clinical exploration.

The medical management of the adolescent with an eating disorder requires knowledge of the physical presentations and quick attention to the medical complications that may occur. Significant weight loss by unhealthy methods establishes the first criteria for anorexia nervosa. This information is needed to make decisions about medical and nutritional management. Physical complaints and findings on examination are consistent with those of acute malnutrition. While the vast majority of these individuals will likely appear cachectic, there is a subset of teens with anorexia who, despite significant weight loss from unhealthy anorexic practices, present within the average weight range due to being previously obese. Thus, for the assessment of anorexia, what is most important is the amount and rapidity of the weight loss and methods used to achieve weight loss and not sole reliance on a cachectic appearance. Adolescents engaging in anorexic behaviors may complain of decreased cold tolerance, dysregulation in sleep/wake cycle, low energy, weakness, feeling of fullness after minimal intake, bloating, constipation, primary or secondary amenorrhea, delayed puberty, and acrocyanosis. There may be hypotension, chest pain, and/or bradycardia with associated vertigo and syncope. In terms of dermatologic findings, individuals with anorexia nervosa often exhibit hair loss, dry skin, sometimes with lanugo (fine hair) on their arms, thighs, face, or trunks and rarely a yellowing of the skin associated with hypercarotenemia. Head and neck examination may exhibit hypertrophy of the parotid glands and erosion of the dental enamel in those inducing emesis. A comprehensive evaluation of anorexia nervosa includes the consideration of medical conditions that may cause weight loss. These may include metabolic, infectious, neoplastic, and endocrine illnesses. Physiologic monitoring includes a complete blood count (CBC), electrolytes, glucose, liver function tests, and thyroid function tests. While anorexia nervosa is typically accompanied by a normal laboratory profile, some findings may be abnormal due to malnutrition (e.g., nutritional anemia) and dehydration. Typical abnormalities are included in Table 13-3.

Electrocardiographic (EKG) studies usually show sinus bradycardia and, arrhythmias are rarely observed which can be particularly malignant in the presence of hypo or hyperkalemia and this is a primary reason why medical hospitalization occurs. These laboratory values generally remain normal until the late stages of illness. Therefore, these values should not independently influence decisions about the intensity of treatment.

Finally, bone loss is common due to starvation, placing anorectic youth at risk for osteoporosis. This risk persists even after normal weight has been restored. Nonconventional approaches to increase bone density include, oral contraceptives and dihydroepiandrosterone (DHEA).

TABLE 13-3	Common Laboratory Findings in Anorexia Nervosa
Hematologic studies	Anemia Leukopenia
Blood chemistries	Hypercarotenemia Hypoproteinemia Hypercholesterolemia Low blood glucose
Endocrine studies	Decreased estrogens Decreased testosterone (in males) Immature LH pattern Decreased T3 Increased corticoids Increased growth hormone
Urinalysis	Increased or decreased osmolality, protinuria, ketoacidosis
Cardiac findings	QTC Prolongation Orthostasis in resting to standing heart rate and/or blood pressure Bradycardia Tachycardia
Electrolytes	Abnormalities in potassium, magnesium, carbon dioxide, sodium, phosphorus
DEXA scan radiology	Osteopenia or osteoporosis

DEXA, Dual-energy x-ray absorptiometry.

Both remain poorly researched and may mask the body's own ability to resume menses which is an important marker for assessing recovery and promoting bone density without the use of outside agents.

Bulimia Nervosa

Bulimia nervosa is more easily hidden on initial examination. However, the damaging effects of repeated vomiting and laxative abuse can be highly injurious and affect multiple systems. Repeated emesis may cause alkalotic conditions with low potassium and high bicarbonate levels while laxative abuse may cause acidotic conditions with high potassium and low bicarbonate. Amylase levels are occasionally high, almost always due to increased salivary, rather than pancreatic, amylase. Frequent purging can also cause hypokalemia, hyponatremia, and hypochloremia.

The physical examination of individuals with bulimia may also reveal markedly eroded tooth enamel that can predispose to frequent chipping and caries. There is often swelling of the parotid glands. Other signs of self-induced vomiting include calluses on the back of the hand, mouth sores, heartburn, chest pain, muscle cramps, weakness, bloody diarrhea (in laxative abusers), bleeding or easy bruising, irregular periods or amenorrhea. More rare but serious complications include cardiac and skeletal myopathy in patients who abuse ipecac to induce emesis, esophageal tears due to repeated vomiting, and rectal prolapse due to abuse of laxatives.

Medical Consideration for Hospitalization

The American Academy of Child and Adolescent Psychiatry recommends medical hospitalization for the following indications (see Table 13-4): weight less than 75% of ideal body weight or extreme weight loss over a short time, hypoglycemic syncope, hypothermia, severe electrolyte

TABLE 13-4	Considerations for Hospitalization

- Sinus bradycardia, rate less than 45 beats per minute
- Other arrhythmia, including prolonged corrected QT interval
- Hypothermia (temperature <97.5°F)
- Orthostatic hypotension by pulse or by blood pressure
- Precipitous weight loss in a short time period
- Severe electrolyte imbalances (potassium <3.0, phosphorus <2.0, carbon dioxide >38)
- Unable to eat or drink, acute food refusal
- Intractable vomiting
- Marked depression, with suicidal ideation and intent
- Failure to progress in outpatient treatment with continued low weight, increased medical risk, or severe bingeing and purging behaviors

imbalances, cardiac arrhythmias, severe volume depletion, marked depression with suicidal ideation or attempt, and/or failure to progress in outpatient treatment with continued low weight and medical risk.

Mental-Status Examination

During an interview, these youth may or may not have an open discussion of body image and eating habits. The openness by which individuals with eating disorders actively disclose or conceal their symptoms is often reflective of whether they are ready to receive help and engage in recovery treatment or are forced to seek treatment by a parent or court. Frequently, they feel their appearance is inadequate and they hide their body by wearing layers of over-sized clothes or conversely, they take great pride in their thinness by wearing body revealing or body hugging clothing to flaunt their skeletal figure. It also happens that they have become so accustomed and habituated to their emaciated body that they have lost all objectivity as to how they feel or how others perceive them, that is, they are alexithymic. Standard mental-status observations of the youth include appearance, relatedness, orientation, coherence, activity level, speech and thought patterns, cognitive ability, mood and affect, suicidality, and signs of psychosis and self-harm or high-risk behaviors. It is important to note that many individuals with eating disorders will endorse thoughts directly related to their eating disorder that may suggest delusional thinking related to body perception or food "safeness"; paranoia in their high distrust of parents or professionals wanting to make them "fat" or others looking at them and judging their appearance; or auditory hallucinations in which they hear a voice berating them, directing their activities around eating, restricting, exercising, or discounting the recommendations of care providers. These seeming psychotic or delusional reports must be taken as part of the eating disorder and not assumed to be a psychotic process. Only if the delusions, paranoia, and auditory hallucinations extend beyond eating-disordered and body image concerns should serious consideration be given to a separate diagnosis of a psychosis.

Assessment Instruments

Assessing eating disorders is complicated by the heterogeneity of the presentation. Several questionnaires and assessment tools may aid in diagnosis and establishing a baseline for monitoring. The most facile is the SCOFF (a mnemonic for Sick, Control, One, Fat, Food), a group of basic screening questions that can be asked during a clinical interview.

The SCOFF consists of five general questions:

- Do you make yourself *Sick* because you feel uncomfortably full?
- Do you worry that you have lost *Control* over what you eat?
- Have you lost more than *One* stone (14 lbs) in a 3-month period?
- Do you believe yourself *Fat* when others say you are thin?
- Would you say that *Food* dominates your life?

An affirmative response to *any* of these questions should raise concern about an eating disorder and lead to an in-depth evaluation.

Specific structured interviews, such as the Eating Disorder Examination are available but are of limited clinical utility with youth. Self-report questionnaires include the Eating Disorder Inventory (EDI) which has normative data for youth as young as 14 years, and the Eating Attitude Test (EAT) which has a version applicable to school-aged children. These screening questionnaires provide normative data for adolescents and adults by which to measure the irregularities in clinical populations. An eating-disorder diagnostic interview should cover the major facets of anorexia, bulimia, eating rituals and beliefs, body image distortion, readiness for change, and medical symptoms to create a comprehensive profile of the illness.

Treatment

The treatment of eating disorders usually occurs in an outpatient setting, though medically comprised patients will periodically need hospitalization. Treatment plans can include a combination of medical, nutrition, and psychosocial and pharmacologic interventions to a greater or lesser degree depending on the presentation and severity of the eating disorder, the psychotherapeutic intervention utilized, the expertise available in the community, and the availability of caregivers to engage in the recovery process. Documenting and tracking weight, BMI, body mass composition (muscle mass and fat mass), return of menses, and vital signs are used to guide both medical and psychiatric interventions, and track treatment progress from a medical perspective.

Because food is the best medicine and stabilization of nutritional status and eating patterns is critical for recovery from an eating disorder, whether in an inpatient or outpatient setting, dietary correction should be done carefully so as not to introduce "refeeding syndrome" or establish new unhealthy eating rituals. Refeeding syndrome refers to a drop in phosphate levels that occurs during increased oral intake following a period of starvation. The precipitously decreased phosphate depletes intracellular adenosine triphosphate (ATP), with resulting delirium and cardiovascular collapse. Phosphate levels should be closely monitored in the first 2 to 3 weeks of weight gain. For severely depleted youth, a typical hospital-based refeeding plan usually starts at 800 to 1000 kcal/day if intake has been extremely low, or at the starting point of current intake with an increase of 100 to 200 kcal/day or every other day, as tolerated, in order to reach a level of metabolically calculated intake for food and fluids which promotes steady weight gain and medical stability. All efforts should be made to avoid nasogastric feeds and liquid supplements, and promote active eating of real food with normal diversity of fats, proteins, and carbohydrates. The essentials of treatment for psychosocial interventions are summarized in Table 13-5.

Psychosocial Interventions

Because of the complexity of anorexia nervosa and its co-occurrence with other psychiatric conditions, it is unclear whether multiple aspects of the illness must be addressed simultaneously, or in sequence, or whether by addressing the malnourished state all presenting problems will resolve. A primary example is the extent to which youth with eating disorders need to be medically stable and cognitively intact before psychotherapy interventions can be utilized or

TABLE 13-5	Treatment Essentials for Eating Disorders

- Therapists should advise their patients to be medically supervised by a physician with expertise in treating patients with eating disorders
- Nutrition should be applied at a judicious pace so as to avoid "refeeding syndrome"
- Implement clear recovery goals and steps toward specific behavior changes
- Psychoeducation for the youth and parents to promote understanding regarding the medical, nutritional, and psychosocial aspects of the eating disorder and the recovery process
- Psychotherapy to focus on:
  — Family-based therapy for anorexia nervosa and bulimia nervosa
  — Narrative therapy that conceptualizes the eating disorder as separate from the individual and provides alternate internal "dialogues" to challenge the "voice" of the eating disorder
  — Interpersonal therapy that promotes realistic interpersonal relationships to replace the youth's relationship with the eating disorder
  — Cognitive behavioral therapy for eating disorders for older adolescents to establish new measures of success for self-esteem, challenges maladaptive beliefs regarding body image, and promotes affective awareness and tolerance of negative affect
  — Cultivating parents as healthy role models regarding eating, exercise, stress management, and communication skills
  — Developing a balanced lifestyle of work/school, recreation, social relationships, and community involvement
- Treat comorbid psychiatric disorders (e.g., depression, anxiety, self-harming behaviors)
- Medications have a limited role and should be reserved for:
  — Severe anxiety in the face of eating and weight gain
  — Premorbid or persistent comorbid psychiatric conditions, for example, depression
  — Fluoxetine for reducing bulimic symptoms.
  — Fluoxetine for maintaining weight gain after refeeding goals have been achieved.
  — Antipsychotic medications for refractory body image distortions that impede treatment
- Hospitalization for severe and life-threatening medical complications

whether the primary intervention is refeeding that is charged to caregivers (parents or professionals). Therapists often employ an eclectic approach to treatment and work closely with medical and nutrition providers. Treatment provision may be influenced by the apparent suitability of the individual taking into account his/her age, understanding, intellectual ability, availability, and appropriateness for caregiver involvement, and the appropriateness of language-based or more abstract therapies. Psychosocial interventions rely on multiple factors, including: psychological awareness of underlying concerns, empathy with the patient's struggle, respect for the patient and family, consistent adherence to safety and treatment goals to move patients toward healthy eating, realistic body image, and improved coping strategies to address stressors associated with developmental expectations for maturation, personal growth, and independence.

With the exception of family-based interventions, there is little research to support the efficacy of the more commonly used treatment approaches described below for anorexia nervosa in adolescents. Despite the lack of a well-informed research literature, these interventions are reported by both clinicians and clients to be useful and are summarized here.

Psychoeducation

Psychoeducation is based on the assumption that eating-disordered adolescents possess misconceptions about the factors that lead to and maintain the illness. The goal is to reduce the resistance to treatment by increasing the adolescent's awareness of the scientific evidence regarding factors that perpetuate eating disorders and to secure the engagement and partnership of the teen for changing his/her behaviors. Psychoeducation is a preliminary step for enhancing the understanding of eating disorders and is considered an integral component of cognitive behavioral therapy (CBT). Information is offered on the multiple causes of eating disorders, cultural influences, physiology of body weight, effects of starvation, the importance of restoring normal eating patterns, the ill effects of vomiting, laxatives, and other weight-controlling substances or practices, medical and physical complications, determining a healthy body weight and muscle to fat body composition, and relapse prevention. Parents can also benefit from psychoeducation about eating disorders and can use this information to be more accepting, patient, and understanding of their child and facilitate their child's recovery.

Family-Based Intervention

Considerable work has been carried out on family-based intervention for the treatment of adolescent anorexia nervosa. Families with an adolescent with anorexia nervosa traditionally have been viewed to have a high level of closeness that typically involves the youth and a parent, usually the mother, hidden but ongoing conflict between the parents, and a lack of expressed warmth and emotion in the families. As new research emerges, for example, regarding the genetics of eating disorders (particularly anorexia nervosa), these formulations must be understood within the context of the teen's genetic vulnerability. New family-based interventions do not look for family pathology, but instead focus on family strengths to promote their teen's recovery. This new perspective on family strengths has produced a specific intervention approach that includes a clear role for parents with directive elements and avoidance of blaming the parents for creating eating disorders in their children. Empirical research is emerging to support this approach. Specifically, family interventions that focus on the parents' guiding their adolescent to eat more have been associated with more rapid improvement than individual psychological treatments or no intervention. Most youth (70%) made good progress as defined by achieving healthy weight by the end of treatment over 12 to 15 months. Improvement in some studies occurred not only in weight but also eating attitudes and mood, in the absence of specific therapies targeting these areas. There is improvement in family relationships involving both the parents and the youth, and the relationship between the parents during the course of therapy. Families with high conflict show better results when parents and youth are separated for the family therapy. Treatment manuals for family-based therapy to address anorexia and bulimia are now available. Additional research is ongoing with multifamily interventions.

Meal-Support Therapy (MST)

MST is well suited to a family-based therapy approach as it provides families with a framework by which to structure meals, set expectations for meal completion, and provide support and assurance to their teen during meal times. MST can be defined as a combination of social modeling, psychoeducation, and cognitive behavioral techniques that are aimed at stabilizing and normalizing eating behaviors in individuals with eating disorders. Additionally, MST is a present-oriented intervention to be used "in the moment" with adolescents struggling to eat during a meal. Key therapeutic elements for MST are the supervision, emotional support, reassurance, distraction, education, and anxiety reduction offered in order to help the teen complete each meal or snack. The rationale of MST is to provide this structure and encouragement through modeling, CBT techniques, and family therapy approaches to stabilize and normalize eating behaviors in order to facilitate further treatment and recovery. Parents are provided a number of key instructions that emphasize the importance of their own emotional regulation, helpful engagement with their teen, and being appropriate role models for eating.

Skills-Based Interventions

Cognitive behavioral Therapy, Narrative Therapy, Interpersonal Psychotherapy, and Dialectical Behavior Therapy were all developed to address psychiatric symptoms or behavioral concerns other than eating disorders. However, each is used in the treatment of eating disorders as they all allow for a generalization of their core techniques to address the anxiety associated with body distortion, weight restoration, and normalizing eating patterns. The commonality among these approaches is that they all encourage an objectification of the eating disorder which allows for a separation of the person with the disorder and associated fears and anxiety. By objectifying the eating disorder, the individual can then create multiple internal contrary dialogue retorts to the often incessant critical "voice" of the eating disorder, understand triggers which ignite fear and anxiety leading to eating-disordered behaviors, build a repertoire of coping strategies to manage the anxiety, and present contrary evidence to the "false promises" which often drive the destructive eating patterns and associated eating-disordered behaviors. They also encourage improved interpersonal relationships and renewed sense of self not defined by the eating disorder. These skill-based interventions are paired with ongoing psychoeducation.

The challenge of using these skill-based interventions with clients with anorexia nervosa is that they often lack motivation for weight gain and this must be addressed first in the initial phase of treatment in order to cultivate and sustain motivation for change. In cases where there is a lack of motivation, the use of motivational interviewing can be very helpful to move the youth from stages of precontemplation or contemplation or preparation to action and maintenance of recovery behaviors. Clients with bulimia nervosa do not necessarily require weight gain as a sign of successful outcome, but rather, ending the binge/purge behaviors and engagement in skills-based interventions may be easier for them. CBT for Eating Disorders (CBT-ED), an adaptation of CBT techniques for behaviors and cognitions specific to eating disorders, has shown good outcomes for adults across all eating-disorder diagnoses (transdiagnostic). Studies are now underway to assess the efficacy of CBT-ED in older adolescents.

Body Image Therapy

Body image distortion and overemphasis of self-worth being dependent on body image are hallmark diagnostic criteria of eating disorders. Adaptation of body image therapy is a systematic approach to transforming the teen's relationship with his/her body from a self-defeating struggle to an experience of self-acceptance and enjoyment. Body image therapy is best utilized as an adjunct intervention to treatments that directly address the primary symptoms of the eating disorder.

Exercise and Physical Activity

Exercise and physical activity can be helpful to ease the anxiety associated with increased intake and weight regain, restore bone density, improve mood, and restore a healthy perspective on the role of exercise and physical activity in one's general well-being. However, exercise is often overused by individuals with anorexia to reduce their weight or sabotage weight gain or by those with bulimia to compensate for binges. Studies are equivocal as to whether exercise can benefit the recovery from anorexia nervosa though there is growing evidence that introducing light exercise even at the early stages of recovery may be beneficial if monitored and done correctly. Until further evidence is available, it is suggested that only moderate levels of exercise should be part of the treatment plan as weight is clearly improved by starting slowly and closely monitoring for any regression in medical stability or excessive use.

Nutrition Counseling

The goal of nutrition counseling is to provide individualized assessment and treatment regarding the physiologic aspects of an eating disorder. These aspects include: metabolic needs, energy needs for growth and development, activity needs, food and nutrition needs, effects of semistarvation, body composition, and body image. The nutritionist facilitates the teen's understanding of what he/she needs from a physiologic standpoint and how to apply this knowledge to his/her own body. The goal is to normalize the teen's food intake so as to achieve normal hunger and satiety signals to fuel him/herself adequately in order to support health and achieve life goals. Nutritional counseling is not a primary treatment, but rather an important component for a comprehensive treatment plan. As a counterpoint, there are evidence-based treatments for eating disorders (e.g., the Maudsley Family-Based Treatment or Fairburns' CBT-ED) that do not include nutritional counseling as a component to the recovery process. They rely instead on the parents' or their child's inherent knowledge of what the teen needs to eat in order to gain weight and, therefore, focus on fear reduction and rehabituation of eating.

Psychopharmacologic Management

There is no clear role for pharmacotherapy in the treatment of children and adolescents with eating disorders. Some gains have been made in the treatment of adults with bulimia nervosa and binge-eating disorder, but their relevance to youth remains unclear. Yet, for anorexia nervosa at any age, no medication has been shown to restore weight or reduce body image distortions during the acute phase of illness and there is only equivocal evidence that the selective serotonin reuptake inhibitors (SSRIs) help to prevent relapse after remission of anorexia nervosa. Many classes of medications have been tried in open trials and a few randomized studies, but results have been disappointing. Thus, it is not possible to recommend a medication trial for core anorectic symptoms.

The reasons for the lack of effectiveness likely relate to the starvation state itself. Neuroimaging and cognitive studies demonstrate alterations in central nervous system functioning, putatively due to the lack of nutrients needed to synthesize neurotransmitters required for medication response and to promote synaptogenesis. Adolescence is an important phase of synaptogenesis and pruning which are thought to affect the integration of emotion and cognition. It has been hypothesized that the limbic system is especially vulnerable to the negative effects of malnutrition at this time. Other explanations may relate to the need for dual-medication therapy to affect multiple receptor systems, similar to the treatment of bipolar disorder.

Despite the lack of efficacy, youth who do not respond to psychological and behavioral interventions to regulate their oral intake often receive a medication trial. The American Psychiatric Association has developed guidelines for care, including medication trials.

When instituting a medication trial, it is important to identify whether the treatment targets are the core deficits in eating disorders or associated symptoms, such as depression and anxiety. If the target is core symptoms, weight gain and stabilization may be the goal, but a medication trial should not be deemed a failure without considering other symptoms, such as greater flexibility in food choices or decreased negative cognitions regarding body image, as these changes may precede regulation of oral intake. If associated symptoms of depression and anxiety are the target, then a time line should establish their onset in relation to the eating disorder. Symptoms that emerge as a direct result of the eating-disordered behaviors often respond to weight gain. But, if these symptoms do not abate with improved health, or if they developed premorbidly, then a medication trial is reasonable.

The most commonly prescribed medications are the SSRI antidepressants which target both core symptoms of rigid thinking and perfectionism and associated depression and anxiety. In particular, fluoxetine appears effective in the treatment of adolescents with major depression and/or anxiety disorders, although benefits with children have not been substantiated and there are no controlled trials for either of these disorders comorbid with anorexia nervosa. Also, in open trials of the SSRI citalopram, the condition of some patients with anorexia nervosa deteriorated. For adult patients with bulimia nervosa, substantial evidence exists for the benefit of SSRIs in decreasing binge eating and purging activity. Youth appear to tolerate robust doses, up to 60 mg/day. Other antidepressants have been even less well investigated. There is one specific caveat. Bupropion must not be used with individuals suffering eating disorders due to the increased risk of seizure.

Some investigators report that in the presence of very high levels of anxiety, particularly at mealtimes, medications may be used to reduce anxiety. Benzodiazepines have shown uneven success and there are no data on the use of buspirone, the non-benzodiazepine anxiolytic. As many youth with bulimia nervosa have comorbid substance-abuse problems, benzodiazepines should be approached cautiously. If a benzodiazepine is used, the long-acting agent clonazepam is most often chosen to avoid the peaks and valleys in anxiety control which can lead to increasing ad lib doses.

Atypical antipsychotics may have a role in treating children and adolescents with anorexia nervosa. Multiple single case studies and a few controlled trials of olanzapine have shown clinical improvement in alleviating body image distortions, reducing rigid and obsessive thinking about food and eating, and increasing the rate of weight gain. This rationale is similar to the use of antipsychotics in cases of mood disorders or posttraumatic stress disorder that are accompanied by disturbances in thinking and do not respond to usual treatments. The sedating properties of many neuroleptics also improve the insomnia that often accompanies the starvation of anorexia nervosa. Because patients with anorexia are vulnerable to hypotension, caution is warranted with the use of antipsychotics, particularly quetiapine.

Another rationale sometimes offered for the use of neuroleptics is their propensity for hyperphagia and weight gain. Youth knowing this side effect may resist taking these medications. However, patients with anorexia nervosa do not consistently experience these effects for unclear reasons. Therefore, in discussing the benefits and side effects of the neuroleptics, the main focus should be on their role in reducing the anxiety in eating and tolerating weight gain, in allaying the thought disturbances regarding food and body image, as well as restoring sleep. Such discussions can nicely be integrated in Narrative Therapy or in CBT as these medications can be conceptualized as agents against the intruding disease. There is currently no role for these neuroleptics in the treatment of bulimia nervosa.

In summary, the role for medication in the treatment of eating disorders in youth is limited and discouraging, particularly for anorexia nervosa. SSRIs may be helpful in treating bulimia nervosa and for treating anxiety and depression comorbid with an eating disorder. Atypical antipsychotics may help with the core cognitive symptoms that interfere with eating and may improve weight gain. Physicians participating in the treatment of youth with eating disorders should approach medication trials cautiously due to the risks of side effects in these medically compromised patients. But, they should not deny a medication trial to youth who cannot achieve self-efficacy in establishing appropriate eating habits.

Levels of Care

As in many other areas of medicine and psychiatry, the role of hospitalization in the treatment of eating disorders is limited, particularly for bulimia nervosa. Youth with bulimia are hospitalized only for severe electrolyte imbalance such as life-threatening hypokalemia or volume depletion. By contrast, adolescents with anorexia may be so medically and psychiatrically compromised that mortality from starvation, electrolyte imbalance, bradycardia, or suicide is a much higher risk thus warranting a more intensive treatment setting. When the youth with an eating disorder is hospitalized, inpatient treatment requires a multimodal team approach. The team usually includes an adolescent medicine provider, psychiatrist, therapist, nutritionist, and nursing staff all specifically trained to treat eating disorders. Inpatient treatment should include a comprehensive psychiatric and medical evaluation with appropriate laboratory monitoring. Severe cases of anorexia nervosa may require rapid refeeding or use of nasogastric feeding methods until more normalized oral intake can be re-established. Patients who have been discharged from the hospital medically stabilized but still at a low weight tend to have a poor prognosis, as they are less psychologically amenable to outpatient psychosocial interventions and tend to lose weight rapidly necessitating rehospitalization.

One option that can be particularly useful for patients with anorexia with a history of repeated acute hospitalizations is a "partial hospitalization program (PHP)." These programs allow patients to receive hospital-based treatment during the day and then return home in the evenings. Attendance is individualized from 4 to 7 days per week. PHP is often undertaken as an intermediate step between inpatient and outpatient care. PHP may be used to prevent acute hospitalizations or as a step-down for patients from inpatient to outpatient treatment. Similar to inpatient programs, most PHPs provide multimodal treatments including: individual, family, and group therapy, usually with a behavioral or cognitive behavioral orientation. Medical care, medication management, and nutritional counseling are also included. Patients are typically ready for discharge to outpatient care when they are within 5% of their target weight, are medically stable, able to tolerate eating at the intake level prescribed with a diversity in the foods they eat, and a significant decrease in ritualized eating and purging behaviors.

Long-term residential programs continue to be a popular treatment option for the intervention for eating disorders. However, these programs traditionally have lengths of stay of several months, and, in some cases, over a year. Reintegration into the family and peer group can be more challenging due to the long separation and only periodic contact with family and friends. Because of their high cost and lack of long-term evidence-based outcome to support their effectiveness, these programs are reserved for most of the treatment-resistant cases. They are often not comprehensively covered by commercial insurance.

Conclusions

Eating disorders in children and adolescents are severe, life-threatening illnesses with major medical and psychiatric morbidity and one of the highest rates of mortality among psychiatric disorders. While eating disorders traditionally have been conceptualized as a chronic medical-psychiatric disorder, new evidence-based treatment approaches specific to eating disorders are bringing an optimism for full recovery if diagnosed and treated early after onset. Treatment often requires a team of providers experienced in treating eating disorders and who are committed to the coordination of care among themselves and with the family. Family-based treatment appear to be the most effective approach for youth with anorexia nervosa. There is no established role for medication in the treatment of core anorexic symptoms. In contrast, there is an evolving evidence base supporting the use of family-based therapy, skills-based interventions, other psychosocial interventions and psychotropic medications in the treatment of bulimia nervosa. Psychiatric medications may be helpful in treating comorbid psychiatric problems in both anorexia and bulimia. Clearly, much more research is needed to develop effective treatments for youth suffering with an eating disorder. Professionals trained in the treatment of eating disorders remain a limited resource, therefore, in the absence of a widespread clear evidence base to guide treatment, interventions should follow community standards of care that emphasize multimodal and interdisciplinary treatment approaches to refeeding to restore and maintain optimal health status, and to address underlying factors that may have contributed to the onset of the eating disorder.

Acknowledgment

The assistance of Kathleen Myers MD, MPH in preparation of the medication section of this chapter is greatly appreciated.

CASE VIGNETTES

VIGNETTE 1: YOUNG TEEN WITH ANOREXIA NERVOSA AND OBSESSIVE COMPULSIVE DISORDER

Jane is a 13-year-old girl in the eighth grade of a suburban middle school. She has always excelled academically, is involved in ballet, and is a talented musician. While she appears attractive to her peers, she has always disparaged her appearance while striving to be more perfect in her many activities. During the course of a viral illness she lost 8 pounds. Her friends commented about how good she looked and she perceived more attention from boys. She began to cut back on her food intake, initially insisting on a strict vegetarian diet and then on a vegan diet. Mealtime became a time of anxiety for her and she avoided eating in public. Over the next 4 months she lost an additional 15 pounds and stopped menstruating. Some friends asked if she was anorectic, but she usually humorously replied, "I wish." Secretly, though, she sometimes felt as though the other students in the cafeteria were watching her eat. At those times she could almost hear them thinking "Jane is such a pig." Her parents repeatedly confronted her about her weight loss, but she could not quite believe their concern. She trusted their sincerity but also believed that she would be better off losing further weight and that she would "balloon up" if she ate the regular family diet. She was referred by her family practitioner to a child and adolescent therapist. Family-based therapy was initiated focusing on the parents assuming the responsibility for providing, structuring, supervising all meals and snacks to initiate and promote refeeding and provide support and reassurance to their daughter during this refeeding and weight-regain phase of treatment. As Jane's eating, weight, and medical status improved and normalized, she was gradually given back age-appropriate independence with her eating. Treatment then shifted to examining any difficulty the parents may be having in allowing Jane's individuation, Jane's frenetic attempts to excel and to please her parents, and the family's reaction to negative emotions. In family sessions, Jane revealed that she had occasionally purged. Given Jane's persistent and significant distorted perceptions of her body and anxiety with eating despite parents support, a low dose of risperidone to aid her eating patterns, body distortions, and insomnia was initiated. Jane experienced a decrease in eating-disordered symptoms. As her eating and weight normalized, symptoms of obsessive-compulsive disorder became increasingly more evident. Prozac was added to her medication regimen. Jane became increasingly more comfortable with her appearance, felt less guilty and self-conscious about her food intake, and was able to tolerate the return of her menses.

VIGNETTE 2: HIGH SCHOOL STUDENT WITH BULIMIA NERVOSA AND SELF-MUTILATION

Vicki is a 17-year-old high school junior. She comes from an upper middle class family and is a good student and successful in both athletics (gymnastics) and academics, with aspirations to attend an Ivy-league college. Last year, she lost her spot in the gymnastics lineup. Her coach told her that her technique needed improvement and that she "may want to trim down a little." She began a crash low-calorie diet. She soon regained her spot in the lineup, but her weight continued to drop from the initial of 120 pounds, to 108 pounds. Her parents became concerned and discussed the matter with Vicki at length, but she denied any problem. She began to eat more at meals, but also started to sneak boxes of cookies into her room and gorge them in one sitting at night. She felt anxious and disgusted after these episodes and began to induce emesis.

Over the next few months she binged and purged 6 to 8 times per day. She withdrew from her friends and became depressed. She was finding school increasingly unpleasant and felt bored much of the time. Her relationship with her boyfriend deteriorated and he broke up with her. In a fit of anger she cut her upper arm several times. During a visit to her primary care physician, the light scars on her arm, calluses on the back of her hand, enlarged parotid glands, halitosis, and precipitous weight loss aroused her physician's suspicions. He asked about her mood. She reluctantly admitted to being depressed and that she hated her body. After consultation with a child and adolescent psychiatrist, Victoria was prescribed fluoxetine. She also began psychotherapy and adopted some behavioral techniques to help her curb her binge eating, purging, and self-mutilation. Later, she developed techniques to tolerate the discomfort of eating and to reduce the anxiety leading to binging. She developed a therapeutic alliance with her therapist and was eventually able to explore her feelings of emptiness, alienation, and need for others' approval. Her parents engaged in family therapy to examine the role that parental conflict and eating styles played in Victoria's difficulties. After 12 months of treatment, Victoria's depression abated as her eating became increasingly normalized and her weight restored. She still binges on occasion, feels guilty afterwards, but does not purge or self harm. She remains in psychotherapy, but now is focusing on individuation as she prepares to transition to college.

BIBLIOGRAPHY

American Psychiatric Association. Treatment of patients with eating disorders, third edition. *Am J Psychiatry.* 2006;163(suppl):4–54.

American Psychiatric Association. *Diagnostic and Statistical Manual of Mental Disorders.* 4th ed. Text Revision. Washington: American Psychiatric Association; 2000.

Bacaltchuk J, Hay P. Antidepressants versus placebo for people with bulimia nervosa. *Cochrane Database Systematic Review*, CD003391. Oxford: Update Software Ltd; 2003.

Barbarich NC, Kaye WH, Jimerson D. Neurotransmitter and imaging studies in anorexia nervosa: new targets for treatment. *Curr Drug Targets CNS Neurol Disord.* 2003;2:61–72.

Bellodi L, Cavallini MC, Bertelli S, et al. Morbidity risk of obsessive-compulsive spectrum disorders in first-degree relatives of patients with eating disorders. *Am J Psychiatry.* 2001;158:563–569.

Boachie A, Goldfield GS, Spettigue W. Olanzapine use as an adjunctive treatment for hospitalized children with anorexia nervosa: case reports. *Int J Eat Disord.* 2003;33:98–103.

Brumberg JJ. *Fasting Girls: The History of Anorexia Nervosa.* New York, NY: Vintage Books, a division of Random House; 1988.

Bulik CM. Eating disorders in adolescents and young adults. *Eat Disord Child Adolesc Psychiatr Clin N Am.* 2002;11:201–218.

Connan F, Murphy F, Connor SE, et al. Hippocampal volume and cognitive function in anorexia nervosa. *Psychiatry Res.* 2006;146:117–125.

Crow SJ, Mitchell JE, Roerig JD, et al. What potential role is there for medication treatment in anorexia nervosa? *Int J Eating Disord.* 2009;42:1–8.

Dennis K, Le Grange D, Bremer J. Olanzapine use in adolescent anorexia nervosa. *Eat Weight Disord.* 2006;11:e53–e56.

Fairburn CG, Cooper Z, Shafran R. Cognitive behaviour therapy for eating disorders: a "transdiagnostic" theory and treatment. *Behav Res Ther.* 2003;41:509–528.

Fairburn CG. *Cognitive Behavior Therapy and Eating Disorders.* New York: Guilford Press; 2008.

Frank GK, Bailer UF, Henry S, et al. Neuroimaging studies in eating disorders. *CNS Spectrums.* 2004;9:539–548.

Godart NT, Flamant MF, Lecrubier Y, et al. Anxiety disorders in anorexia nervosa and bulimia nervosa: co-morbidity and chronology of appearance. *Eur Psychiatry.* 2000;15:38–45.

Golden NH, Katzman DK, Kreipe RE, et al. Eating disorders in adolescents: position paper of the Society for Adolescent Medicine. *J Adolesc Health.* 2003;33(6):496–503.

Gowers S, Bryant-Waugh R. Management of child and adolescent eating disorders: the current evidence base and future directions. *J Child Psychol Psychiatry.* 2004;45:63–83.

Hall D, Leichner P, Calderon R, et al. *Meal Support Manual: Introduction for Parents, Friends & Caregivers.* Vancouver, BC, Canada: British Columbia Children's Hospital; 2004.

Halmi KA. Anorexia nervosa and bulimia nervosa. In: Lewis M, ed. *Child and Adolescent Psychiatry, A Comprehensive Textbook*. 3rd ed. Philadelphia, PA: Lippincott, Williams and Wilkins; 2002:692–699.

Herpertz-Dahlman B. Eating disorders and obesity. *Child Adolesc Psychiatr Clin N Am*. 2009;18(1):31–48.

Hodes M, Calderon R, Breuner C, et al. Treatment of eating disorders in children and adolescents. In: Tyrer P, Silk K, eds. *Cambridge Textbook of Effective Treatments in Psychiatry*. New York: Cambridge University Press; 2008:841–854.

Kafantaris V, Leigh E, Berest A, et al. Pilot Study of Olanzapine in the Treatment of Anorexia Nervosa. American Academy of Child and Adolescent Psychiatry 54th Annual Meeting Poster Presentation, 26 October 2007, Boston, MA.

Keys A, Brozek J, Henschel A, et al. *The Biology of Human Starvation*. 2 vols. Minneapolis, MN: University of Minnesota Press; 1950.

Kotler LA, Devlin MJ, Davies M, et al. An open trial of fluoxetine for adolescents with bulimia nervosa. *Child Adolesc Psychopharmacol*. 2003;13:329–335.

Lock J, Le Grange D, Agras WS, et al. *Treatment Manual for Anorexia Nervosa. A Family Based Approach*. New York: Guilford; 2001.

Maisel R, Epston D, Borden, A. *Biting the Hand That Starves You: Inspiring Resistance to Anorexia/Bulimia*. New York: Norton Press; 2004.

McGivern RF, Andersen J, Byrd D, et al. Cognitive efficiency on a match to sample task decreases at the onset of puberty in children. *Brain Cogn*. 2002;50:73–89.

Mitchell JE, de Zwaan M, Roerig JL. Drug therapy for eating disorders. *Curr Drug Targets CNS Neurol Disord*. 2003;2(1):17–29.

Mondraty N, Birmingham CL, Touyz S, et al. Randomized controlled trial of olanzapine in the treatment of cognitions in anorexia nervosa. *Australas Psychiatry*. 2005;13:72–75.

Olfson M, Shaffer D, Marcus S, et al. Relationship between antidepressant medication treatment and suicide in adolescents. *Arch Gen Psychiatry*. 2003;60:978–982.

Reinblatt SP, Redgrave GW, Guarda AS. Medication management of pediatric eating disorders. *Int Rev Psychiatry*. 2008;20(2):183–188.

Robb AS, Dadson MJ. Eating disorders in males. *Child Adolesc Psychiatr Clin N Am*. 2002;11(2): 399–418.

Rosenblum J, Forman S. Management of anorexia nervosa with exercise and selective serotonergic reuptake inhibitors. *Curr Opin Pediatr*. 2003;15:346–347.

Shapiro JR, Berkman ND, Brownley KA, et al. Bulimia nervosa treatment: a systematic review of randomized controlled trials. *Int J Eat Disord*. 2007;40(4):321–336.

Walsh BT, Kaplan AS, Attia E, et al. Fluoxetine after weight restoration in anorexia nervosa: a randomized controlled trial. *J Am Med Assoc* 2006;295:2605–2612.

SUGGESTED READING

Fasting Girls: The History of Anorexia Nervosa
Author: Joan Brumberg
Publisher: Vintage, 2000
(For both clinicians and interested families, a fascinating historical look at anorexia nervosa)

Off the CUFF: A Parent Skills Book for the Management of Disordered Eating,
Author: Nancy Zucker, PhD
Publisher: Duke University, 2006
(For both clinicians and families, a useful guide for parents to develop and model appropriate emotional regulation and problem-solving skills to promote recovery in their child)

Help Your Teenager Beat an Eating Disorder
Authors: James Lock and Daniel Le Grange
Publisher: Guilford Press, 2005
(For families looking for information on eating disorders and guidance in treatment)

Treatment manual for anorexia nervosa: A Family-Based Approach
Authors: James Lock, Daniel Le Grange, Stewart Agras, Christopher Dare
Publisher: Guilford Press A Division of Guilford Publications, Inc., 2001
(For clinicians who want specifics about the implementation of family-based treatment for anorexia nervosa)

Eating Disorders, Child and Adolescent Psychiatric Clinics of North America, Volume 11, 2
Guest Editor: Adelaide S. Robb, MD
Publisher: W. B. Saunders Company, 2002

(Provides a collection of articles covering a vast range of topics related to eating disorders across childhood and adolescents)

Eating Disorders and Obesity, Child and Adolescent Psychiatric Clinics of North America, Volume 18, 1
Guest Editors: Beate Herpertz-Dahlmann, MD, Johannes Hebebrand, MD
Publisher: Elsevier Saunders
(Provides summaries of latest finding on diagnosis, treatment, genetics, and neurobiologic, and neuroimaging of eating disorders and obesity)

Life Without Ed: How one woman declared independence from her eating disorder and you can too
Author: Jenni Schaefer with Thom Rutledge
Publisher: McGraw Hill, 2004
(Offers common scenarios and tips for maintaining recovery behaviors)

Cognitive Behavior Therapy and Eating Disorders
Author: Christopher Fairburn
Publisher: Guilford Press, 2008
(A manual for clinicians to treat adults and adolescents 19 and older with eating disorders across the transdiagnostic spectrum)

Overcoming Binge Eating
Author: Christopher Fairburn
Publisher: Guilford Press, 1995
(A manual for clinicians and older adolescents and adults seeking to address binge eating)

SUGGESTED WEBSITES

Academy for Eating Disorders: www.aedweb.org
National Eating Disorders Association: www.nationaleatingdisorders.org
Something Fishy: www.something-fishy.org
National Association of Anorexia Nervosa and Associated Disorders: www.anad.org/

REVIEW QUESTIONS

1. Use of medications with adolescents with eating disorders is best targeted to address:
   a. Anorexia nervosa
   b. Bulimia nervosa
   c. Comorbid psychiatric concerns (e.g., depression, anxiety)
   d. All of the above

2. Why is a diagnostic continuum approach to understanding eating disorders useful?
   a. The vast majority of eating disorders do not meet the threshold for a classification of bulimia nervosa or anorexia nervosa, yet are serious and need to be treated
   b. The crossover from anorexia to bulimia can be as high as 50%
   c. A distinguishing factor that separates anorexia binge/purge subtype from bulimia is the person's weight
   d. All of the above

3. Family-based therapy is considered a "well-established" primary treatment for which of the following psychiatric disorder:
   a. Attention deficit hyperactivity disorder (ADHD)
   b. Anorexia nervosa
   c. Bipolar disorder
   d. Bulimia nervosa
   e. Early-onset schizophrenia

4. Sequelae of semistarvation can present as:
   a. Symptoms of depression
   b. Increased anxiety
   c. Seemingly delusional or psychotic thinking
   d. All of the above

5. The best medication for the treatment of anorexia is:
   a. An SSRI
   b. An atypical antipsychotic
   c. A short-acting benzodiazepine
   d. A combination of psychiatric medications
   e. Food

Answers: 1-c, 2-d, 3-b, 4-d, 5-e

Elimination Disorders: Enuresis and Encopresis

Introduction

Enuresis and encopresis are disorders commonly seen in primary care as well as child psychiatry settings. These disorders can be challenging to identify and treat and also place a great deal of stress on the family and child. For most children, the sequence by which the overall bowel and bladder control is obtained is very similar. Children first obtain bowel control during sleep, which is followed by bladder and bowel control during wakefulness and concludes with bladder control during sleep. When children have difficulties in any of these areas, a careful assessment is imperative to identify possible urologic, gastrointestinal, endocrinologic, developmental, psychosocial, or sleep-related etiologies for a delay or regression in this sequence. Treatment may include supportive approaches, behavioral programs, and/or pharmacotherapy. Special attention should also be given to the psychosocial consequences the symptoms have for the family and individual patient.

Historical Background

Enuresis

The symptom of bed-wetting and its treatment have existed for centuries. According to a review by Glicklich in 1951, multiple punitive treatments for enuresis have historically been tried, including electric shocks to the genitalia, penile ligation, and cautery of sacral nerves. The option of utilizing pharmacotherapy became possible after the efficacy of imipramine for the treatment of enuresis was first described in 1960. Since then, the understanding of the pathophysiology behind the symptom of enuresis and its treatment approaches has progressed substantially and appropriate diagnostic and treatment algorithms can be derived from the current knowledge.

Encopresis

Although fewer historical data are available with regard to encopresis, at least one study by Freud and Burlingham described high frequencies of children who had problems with soiling and wetting after being separated from their parents during World War II, postulating a high likelihood of psychological components to the symptom.

Clinical Features

Enuresis

When evaluating enuresis, it is important to first understand the sequential steps by which urinary and bowel continence are attained. Urinary continence involves three steps including enlarging bladder capacity, obtaining voluntary control of the sphincter muscles, and gaining voluntary control of the micturition reflex. The sensation of bladder fullness typically does not develop until the second year of life, while the ability to control sphincter muscles typically occurs by age 3.

The fourth edition of the *Diagnostic and Statistical Manual of Mental Disorders* (*DSM-IV*) defines enuresis as involuntary or intentional voiding of urine into bed or clothes at least twice per week for three consecutive months, in a child who is at least 5 years old (or equivalent developmental level). If it has been occurring for a shorter amount of time or less frequently, the child can still meet the criteria for the diagnosis if the symptoms cause significant distress or impairment in social, academic, or other areas of functioning. According to the *DSM-IV*, the symptom cannot be substance induced (e.g., a diuretic) or due to a general medical condition (e.g., diabetes, spina bifida, or seizure disorder).

Three types of enuresis exist. Nocturnal enuresis is voiding during sleep, diurnal enuresis is voiding during waking hours, and nocturnal and diurnal is a combination of the two. A further distinction is made between children who have never been consistently dry (primary enuresis) and children who have had the return of wetting after at least 6 months of dryness (secondary enuresis).

Encopresis

Acquiring fecal continence requires each child to undergo a six-step sequence, including sensing rectal fullness; constricting the external anal sphincter, puborectalis, and internal anal sphincter; having rectal contraction waves; contracting the diaphragm and abdominal muscles; increasing intra-abdominal pressure; and relaxing the sphincters. Most children are capable of acquiring fecal continence by 18 to 24 months of age.

With regard to encopresis, the *DSM-IV* definition includes the passage of feces into inappropriate places, such as in clothing or on the floor, involuntarily or intentionally. This has to occur at least once per month for 3 months in a child whose mental and chronologic age is at least 4 years. This cannot be due to the effects of a substance (i.e., laxative) or a general medical condition (except constipation). Similar to enuresis, if there has been a period of fecal continence preceding the incontinence, it is termed secondary encopresis, while primary encopresis is designated in children who have never achieved fecal continence.

Two subtypes of encopresis are recognized. The first is encopresis with constipation and overflow incontinence, commonly known as retentive encopresis. The other is encopresis without constipation and overflow incontinence, which is commonly referred to as nonretentive encopresis. Nonretentive encopresis may present in at least three different ways. One is in children with severe behavior problems who defecate deliberately in inappropriate places, even though they exhibit no problems with retention or constipation. Another is in children with an insensitivity to rectal fullness who pass feces involuntarily. And the last is a group of children who pass feces (frequently liquid) when anxious, fearful, or laughing.

Epidemiology and Clinical Course

Enuresis

The prevalence of enuresis varies for different age groups. This may, in part, be due to the spontaneous remission of enuresis in 14% to 16% of children, every year after the age of 5. Children younger than the age of 5 have a higher annual spontaneous remission rate of 30%. Spee van der Wekk and colleagues similarly found decreasing prevalence rates for nocturnal enuresis with age: 12% to 25% in 4-year-olds, 7% to 10% in 8-year-olds, and 2% to 3% in 12-year-olds. Prevalence rates of 1% to 3% have been found in the teenage years. Enuresis will also occur in greater frequency in children undergoing psychosocial stress, as shown in the 1989 Isle of Wight study by Rutter. These findings indicate that secondary enuresis is most likely to initiate in children between the ages of 5 and 7. Lastly, boys are more likely to develop secondary enuresis than girls.

Encopresis

An early study by Bellman found a prevalence rate for encopresis of 1.5% in children between 7 and 8 years of age, with a male-to-female ratio of around 3:1. The 1981 Isle of Wight study found that boys between the ages of 10 and 12 had a 1.3% prevalence rate of encopresis, while girls had a 0.3% rate. The study also noted a significant relationship between enuresis and encopresis.

A more recent study by Foreman and Thambirajah found that children with primary encopresis were more likely to have developmental delays and associated enuresis, while children with secondary encopresis were more likely to have psychosocial stressors and conduct disorder behaviors. In fact, a minority of children who have been raised in neglectful or abusive homes can exhibit severe behavioral disturbances, which include deliberately defecating in inappropriate places. When encopresis occurs under stress in normal children, however, it typically remits when the stressor is removed. Most cases of encopresis will resolve by adolescence; however, a small minority of patients may continue to have difficulties through adulthood.

Etiology and Pathogenesis

There is a large array of risk factors associated with the development of enuresis and encopresis. The major factors are summarized in Tables 14-1 and 14-2, respectively.

Enuresis

Biologic Factors

A relationship between bladder infections and enuresis has been long established and was further confirmed by Hansson in 1992. However, urinary tract obstruction is highly debated in the literature as a cause, warranting caution before recommending unnecessary surgery, especially considering that urethral dilatation and/or bladder neck repair do not appear to be effective treatments for enuresis. Circadian rhythmicity and its role in the ability for children to concentrate their urine has also been implicated. A substance called plasma arginine vasopressin (AVP) has been found to be decreased in children with enuresis and may be able to explain the ability for desmopressin (DDAVP) to help resolve enuresis. Certain medications

TABLE 14-1 Risk Factors for Enuresis	
Genetic	**Psychosocial**
Chromosomal linkage	Sexual molestation
Autosomal dominant subtype	Neglect
Family history	Poor toilet training
Sleep patterns	Emotional and/or behavioral difficulties
Difficult to arouse	**Biologic**
Narcolepsy	Bladder infections
Sleep apnea	Decreased arginine vasopressin
Developmental delay	Medications
Language	
Speech	
Motor skills	
Social development	

TABLE 14-2	Risk Factors for Encopresis
Physiologic	**Developmental**
Failure of external sphincter to relax in conjunction with rectal contraction waves	Lower intellectual abilities
	Psychosocial
Weak internal sphincter	Neglectful or abusive environments
Abdominal straining	Enuresis
Anterior location of the anus	Oppositional defiant disorder
Anal fissure	Tantrums
Anal stenosis	School refusal
Anal atresia	Fire setting
Hormonal	Parents who punish children for failing in potty training
Earlier peak and sustained elevation of postprandial pancreatic polypeptide	Parents who coerce the child to use the toilet
Lower motilin response	Parents with depression or other psychiatric disorders

are also known to cause secondary enuresis and include lithium, valproic acid, clozapine, and theophylline.

Developmental Delay

Developmental delay has been found to occur twice as often in children with enuresis as in those without enuresis in an early study by Essen and Peckham. Enuresis correlates with multiple maturational delays in the areas of language, speech, motor skills, and social development. Furthermore, delayed maturation of central nervous system functioning has been considered as a possible contributing factor after a study by Mimouni and colleagues in 1985 showed that children with enuresis lagged behind control children in bone age and height. Delayed maturation likely also contributes to the manifestation of enuresis in conjunction with behavioral disturbances. The association of enuresis with behavioral disturbance is higher in secondary enuresis and enuresis that persists into adolescence. Lastly, among adolescents, late sexual maturation has been associated with enuresis.

Psychosocial Factors

The rate of psychiatric disorders is higher in children with enuresis compared to children without enuresis; however, most children with enuresis do not show symptoms of emotional or behavioral difficulties. A recent prospective study by Zink and colleagues in 2008 found that children with voiding postponement had the highest rates of psychiatric comorbidity, while children with monosymptomatic nocturnal enuresis had the lowest rates of psychiatric comorbidity. Psychiatric disorders can occur coincidentally with enuresis or even as a result of enuresis. It is important to remember that for a small subgroup of children, however, enuresis does have a psychological etiology, which is most frequently associated with secondary enuresis that develops after a stressor. Secondary enuresis has also been reported after sexual molestation. When psychological factors are related to primary enuresis, it is typically when there has been considerable disorganization or neglect within the family so that appropriate efforts at toilet training were not made.

Genetics

Genetics plays a large role in the transmission of primary enuresis across generations. The chromosomes that have been identified include 13q, 12q, 8, and 22. In families of enuretic children, one third of fathers and one fifth of mothers were themselves enuretic as children.

A penetrance above 90% has been found in some families with an autosomal dominant mode of transmission.

Sleep Patterns

Although a sleep disorder cannot be identified as a major etiologic factor in enuresis, sleep states have long been studied in terms of their relationship to enuretic episodes. Roberts found that these episodes occur in each sleep stage, in proportion to the amount of time spent in that stage. Children with primary enuresis also appear to be more difficult to arouse during sleep compared to control subjects. Enuresis has also been reported in association with specific sleep disorders, including narcolepsy and sleep apnea syndrome. However, no specific sleep state or disorder has been found to be causal in enuresis.

Encopresis

Biologic Factors

Physiologic factors must be considered in children with encopresis. Abnormal anorectal dynamics can contribute to problems with encopresis. These include a failure of the external sphincter to relax in conjunction with rectal contraction waves, a weak internal sphincter, or abdominal straining. Anatomic causes include anterior location of the anus, anal fissure, anal stenosis, and/or anal atresia. Furthermore, a correlation has been found between children who were constipated in the first year of life and the development of subsequent encopresis. On the other hand, encopresis also arises after a bout with diarrhea or acute constipation. Constipation can cause painful defecation and can lead to anal fissures, both of which can cause children to withhold to prevent further pain, leading to chronic constipation.

Hormonal influences have also been postulated in the etiology of encopresis. Stern and colleagues speculated that postprandial levels of pancreatic polypeptide peaked earlier and remained higher, while the motilin response was lower in children with encopresis. However, the authors could not conclude whether these findings were the result or the cause of chronic constipation.

Developmental Delay

Developmental delay associated with encopresis has been shown specifically in patients with lower intellectual abilities. Fragile X syndrome and other forms of mental retardation, cerebral palsy, and hypotonia can increase the risk of fecal incontinence.

Psychosocial Factors

Parental attitudes toward toilet training play a key role in the development of fecal continence. Parents must be attuned to their child's signals and be able to remain calm when introducing their child to the toilet. They need to be encouraging and give praise when children are able to defecate in the toilet. Conversely, parents should avoid punishing children when they fail and not try to coerce children to use the toilet. Parents who are experiencing depression or other psychiatric disorders may not be fully emotionally available to assist in this process. Toilet training for fecal continence also involves a great deal of learning on the children's part. They must learn when and where it is appropriate to defecate, how to sense rectal fullness, and the process of withholding until the appropriate place to defecate is found. They also must learn to get into the right posture, relax their sphincters, and increase intra-abdominal pressure.

Children who have been sexually abused may present with fecal incontinence. Signs and symptoms that may accompany this can include sexual acting out or other regressive behaviors. Additional psychiatric disorders and/or symptoms that have been associated with encopresis include enuresis, oppositional defiant disorder, tantrums, school refusal, and fire setting. However, the degree of association between these symptoms has not yet been established, and therefore, it is undetermined whether psychological problems are causal, associated, or secondary to encopresis.

Differential Diagnosis and Comorbidity

A thorough evaluation is warranted to rule out a medical or psychological problem contributing to the symptom of enuresis and/or encopresis. Neurologic, anatomic, and endocrinologic causes should be explored.

Enuresis

Neurogenic causes of enuresis include abnormal innervation of the bladder or external sphincter, myelomeningocele, spinal cord injury, epilepsy, and spina bifida. Children with anatomic causes typically have primary enuresis and will have abnormalities such as obstruction of the bladder outlet or an ectopic ureter with insertion distal to the bladder neck. Lastly, endocrinologic disorders that can cause enuresis include diabetes mellitus and diabetes insipidus.

Encopresis

Anatomic anal causes of encopresis include anal stenosis or atresia, fissures, trauma, postsurgical repair, and anterior displacement of the anus. Smooth muscle disease and endocrine disorders (hypothyroidism, renal acidosis, lead intoxication, diabetes insipidus, and hypercalcemia) must also be ruled out as a cause for constipation. Neurogenic diseases such as spinal cord disorders, Hirschsprung disease, cerebral palsy, hypotonia, and neuronal intestinal dysplasia also can result in constipation. This wide array of medical conditions is summarized in Table 14-3. Certain medications, noted in Table 14-4, can also produce constipation. Furthermore, clinicians should rule out mental retardation, learning problems, disruptive behavior disorders, or anxiety disorders. It should be noted that some children who are impulsive or hyperactive will have encopretic episodes because they do not attend to the signs of rectal fullness until too late.

TABLE 14-3	Differential Diagnosis for Encopresis	
Anal causes	**Neurogenic causes**
Anal stenosis or atresia	Spinal cord disorders
Fissures	Hirschsprung disease
Trauma	Cerebral palsy
Postsurgical repair	Hypotonia
Anterior displacement of the anus	Neuronal intestinal dysplasia
Smooth muscle disease	**Medications**
Endocrine disorders	**Developmental delay**
Hypothyroidism	Mental retardation
Renal acidosis	Learning problems
Lead intoxication	**Psychiatric disorders**
Diabetes insipidus	Disruptive behavior disorders
Hypercalcemia	Anxiety disorders
	Impulsive disorders
	Hyperactive disorders

TABLE 14-4	Medications Associated with Encopresis	
Methylphenidate • Phenytoin • Imipramine • Phenothiazines	• Iron-containing preparations • Aluminum-containing antacids • Codeine	

Assessment

The History

The essentials of assessment of enuresis and encopresis are summarized in Table 14-5. The history should focus on every aspect of symptom expression by talking with the patient and parents individually. For both disorders, the clinician should inquire about any family or personal stressors, especially the history of any type of abuse. Specifically, clinicians should focus on the association between the onset of symptoms with regard to toilet training, any separation, or relationships the child may find emotionally stressful. It is also very important to inquire about the emotional consequences of the symptom on the patient and family and also the motivation in resolving the symptom in both parties. Associated urinary or bowel symptoms should be ascertained in addition to a detailed developmental history. Lastly, any previous interventions (i.e., therapy, medications, and/or behavioral modifications) the family and child have utilized and their efficacy or reasons for failure are important in guiding treatment planning.

Enuresis

When taking a history specific to enuresis, a review of the genitourinary and neurologic systems must be done to rule out these biologic causes of enuresis. In terms of the symptom itself, the frequency, time of day, duration, possible environmental influences, onset, and any other associated symptoms such as dribbling, dysuria, and urgency should be obtained. It can be very helpful to document a 2-week baseline record of the enuretic episodes to help measure current severity and the success of any future intervention. A family history of enuresis is important to obtain as well as the list of medications the child is taking. The sleeping conditions within the home should be assessed as well as any symptoms of sleep apnea (snoring, night waking, or upper airway obstruction). A specific etiology will be identified in only approximately one third of children with enuresis; however, the assessment will still help guide treatment approaches in those children for whom a specific cause cannot be found.

Encopresis

One of the deciding factors for how to approach the treatment of encopresis will be whether or not the child has constipation. Children with constipation will often have incontinence during sleep, while children without constipation will often have episodes during the day. Nonetheless, the interval, amount, volume, size, and consistency of bowel movements reported comprise an especially important part of the history. The type and amount of food (especially fluid and fiber) the children eat as well as any changes in their diet are important as well.

Physical Examination

Enuresis

The practice parameter for children with enuresis developed by Frtiz and colleagues for the American Academy of Child and Adolescent Psychiatry states that a thorough physical examination is necessary and should focus on ruling out any anatomic or neurologic cause of the symptoms.

TABLE 14-5	Essentials of Assessment for Enuresis and Encopresis
Enuresis	**Encopresis**
Urinary symptoms • Frequency • Time of day • Onset • Course • Environmental influences • Associated symptoms	Fecal symptoms • Stool size • Consistency • Interval • Symptom duration • Type and amount of food the child eats • Changes in diet • Urinary symptoms
Review of systems • Genitourinary • Neurologic • Sleep apnea	Review of systems • Genitourinary • Neurologic
Developmental history	Developmental history
Sleeping conditions	Family or personal stressors
Abuse history	Emotional consequences of the symptom
Family history	Family history
Previous treatment	Previous treatment
Current medications	Current medications

Physical examination
• HEENT
  • Patency of nares
  • Enlarged adenoids
  • Enlarged tonsils
• Abdominal examination
  • Bladder distension
  • Fecal impaction
• Genitourinary
  • Abnormal meatus
  • Epispadias
  • Phimosis
• Back
  • Sacral dimple
  • Spinal cord anomaly
  • Verterbral anomaly
• Neurologic
  • Spinal cord injury
	Physical examination
	• Abdominal examination
	  • Distention
	  • Suprapubic mass
	• Rectal examination
	  • Sacral dimple
	  • Position of the anus
	  • Anal fissures
	  • Anal wink
	  • Sphincter tone
	  • Rectal vault size
	  • Presence or absence of stool in the rectum
	  • Pelvic mass
	• Dsymorphic features
	• Stigmata of hypothyroidism
	• Stigmata of spinal disease
	• Complete neurologic examination

Laboratory data • Urinalysis • Urine culture	Laboratory data • Serum calcium • Thyroid hormone studies Imaging • Abdominal x-ray Psychological testing

Encopresis

A complete neurologic examination is important when evaluating encopresis, in order to rule out spinal cord abnormalities or other neurologic disorders in which constipation can occur. When evaluating encopresis, abdominal distention and/or a suprapubic mass should be ruled out. The rectal examination should be completed and note made of any sacral dimple, the position of the anus, anal fissures, anal wink, sphincter tone, rectal vault size, presence or absence of stool in the rectum, and/or any pelvic mass. A positive rectal examination will provide evidence of fecal retention, but a negative examination does not rule it out. Physicians should further look for dysmorphic features and any manifestation of hypothyroidism or spinal disease.

Laboratory Studies

Enuresis

Urinalysis as well as culture should be performed to rule out a urinary tract infection, a cause of enuresis that is easily treated. More invasive or painful studies (renal ultrasound, voiding cystourethrogram, intravenous pyelogram, or cystoscopic evaluation) should be performed with caution. However, children with daytime wetting, continuous wetting, recurrent urinary tract infections, significant findings on physical examination, positive results from the urinalysis or culture, and/or obvious disturbances of voiding are more likely to have urinary tract abnormalities and may suggest the need for more extensive and invasive evaluation.

Encopresis

Minimal laboratory data are typically required in children with fecal incontinence. Other causes may need to be ruled out with serum calcium, thyroid hormone levels, and even urinalysis and culture if the child has enuresis. The plain abdominal roentgenogram can be helpful, when the rectal examination is negative, to reveal fecal retention. When children who are constipated have been unresponsive to treatment, anorectal manometry may be helpful. Once obvious physiologic causes have been ruled out, however, the cause is more than likely psychogenic.

Psychological Testing

Psychological evaluation and testing can be important in providing a detailed picture of the child. However, psychological testing may be reserved for those cases in which no clear physiologic or psychological cause has been determined.

Treatment

Enuresis

Multiple approaches to the treatment for enuresis have been described over the past four decades, and are summarized in Table 14-6. Treatment is based on the concerns of the child and family, their collective and individual motivation, and intelligence, if no specific cause is found for which specific treatment is indicated. Not all children with enuresis need treatment, given its high rate of spontaneous resolution.

Common Sense

These approaches have not been proven interventions but have developed over time and are generally agreed upon by practitioners as noninvasive approaches to treating enuresis. Education is a powerful tool by which parents should learn how common enuresis is, the high spontaneous cure rate, and the fact the children do not do this on purpose. Children should be encouraged to keep a chart where they can document the days and/or nights when they

TABLE 14-6 Essentials in the Treatment for Enuresis

Treatment Type	Specific Treatment	Method	Mechanism of Action	Number Needed to Treat (NNT)*	Controlled Trials
Common sense	Education	Educate parents/child on prevalence, spontaneous cure rate, and unintentional aspect	Increased knowledge	Unknown	None
	Decreased fluid intake	Limit fluid/caffeine intake before bedtime	Decreased fluid to urinate	Unknown	None
	Nighttime voiding	Awaken child during the night to void	Prevents symptom from occurring	Unknown	None
Behavioral	Bell and pad	Circuit completes upon wetting, sounding alarm	Conditions child to awaken earlier in urination sequence	2	Yes
	Alarm	Set alarm for time child is most likely to urinate	Conditions child to awaken earlier in urination sequence	Unknown	Yes
	Reward contingency	Provide reward for certain number of dry nights or days	Increases likelihood of dryness as children motivated for reward	Unknown	None
	Dry chart	Children document number of dry nights/days	Increases child's awareness of success or difficulties	Unknown	None
Medications	Imipramine	1.0–2.5 mg/kg/single dose at bedtime	Unknown	6	Yes
	Desmopressin	0.2–0.6 mg at bedtime	Synthetic analogue of ADH vasopressin	7	Yes
Psychotherapy	Individual (any type)	Target behavioral or psychological component to enuresis	Increases coping skills, awareness, and motivation	Unknown	None

*NNT=14 consecutive dry nights.

are dry. They can also help by changing the bed linens or putting their clothes in the washer when they have an accident. Both of these interventions serve to raise the children's consciousness of the problem. To help decrease the volume of urine at bedtime in nocturnal enuresis, parents should be encouraged to reduce fluid intake before bedtime, especially caffeinated beverages. To attempt to prevent the symptom, the child should be awakened during the night to void. For diurnal enuresis, regularly scheduled time on the toilet to urinate should be implemented. The interval between voiding episodes can be gradually increased as the enuresis resolves.

Behavioral Methods

Behavioral methods should be considered prior to initiating pharmacotherapy, given their limited invasiveness and successful outcomes. In a meta-analysis by Houts and colleagues, conditioning methods were shown to have an initial success rate of 66%, with more than 50% of subjects showing long-term success. These methods must be taught to parents with confidence, be familiar to the person delivering them, and be explained with thoroughness. Close follow-up (i.e., monthly), family support, and the reliability of the adults to monitor the situation are all imperative for this type of treatment to provide good outcomes.

The enuresis alarm, commonly known as the bell and pad method, has been in existence for many years and is now designed as a portable transistorized alarm. When a child urinates, the moisture completes a circuit between two electrodes, setting off an alarm. Initially, the parents may need to help awaken the child to finish voiding in the toilet. The child, however, is eventually conditioned to awaken earlier and earlier in the enuretic episode until the sensation of bladder fullness awakens the child before wetting occurs. After the children have had 3 to 4 weeks of consecutive dry nights, success can be further attained utilizing intermittent reinforcement, by wearing the belt every other day before stopping use.

A similar method entails the use of an alarm clock, set at a time when the bladder is expected to be reaching maximal capacity. El-Anany and colleagues reported a success rate of 77% for this approach with a 6-month relapse rate of around 25%.

Reward contingencies can be especially motivating and satisfying for children. Utilizing a sticker chart for every dry night or day can encourage motivation, progress, and hope. Obtaining a reward such as a game played with parents, a special meal, or special outing can be exciting after a specific number of dry nights or days is achieved.

Pharmacologic Methods

Tricyclic antidepressants and desmopressin are the two medication classes shown to be effective in the treatment of nocturnal enuresis. Desmopressin, also known as DDAVP (desamine-D-arginine vasopressin), is a synthetic analogue of the antidiuretic hormone vasopressin and is available as a tablet or nasal spray. However, the nasal spray has a blackbox warning from the Food and Drug Administration. Its use is no longer recommended due to the increased risk of hyponatremic seizures. Hyponatremia is a serious side effect that must be discussed with the patient and family, even when utilizing the tablet form. In children with an illness that might affect hydration status or drug absorption, serum electrolyte levels should be monitored. Other rare side effects include headache, abdominal discomfort, nausea, and nasal congestion.

Historically, success rates for DDAVP have ranged from 10% to 65%, but relapse rates can be as high as 80%. Furthermore, in 2002 Glazener and Evans performed a systematic review of 47 randomized trials including 3448 children and concluded that desmopressin is effective in the treatment of enuresis. The starting dose for the tablet is 0.2 mg at bedtime, and this can be increased up to 0.6 mg, with a duration of action of 10 to 12 hours. No guidelines exist as to how long to continue treatment with DDAVP once a patient responds, but 3 to 6 months appears reasonable. However, Glazener and Evans found that treatment effects were rarely sustained after treatment with desmopressin and that the efficacy of desmopressin compared to tricyclic antidepressants was very similar. By contrast, a 2009 study by Marschall-Kehrel and Harms showed that a gradual decrease in dose frequency was effective in improving outcomes with the treatment of DDAVP. The outcomes in their study were, in fact, superior to alarm treatment, with a 72% response rate and 82% of those children having less than two wet nights per month at 1-month follow-up. A combination of DDAVP with the bell and pad method may provide even more successful results.

The mechanism of action of tricyclic antidepressants (e.g., imipramine, amitriptyline, and desipramine) in the treatment of enuresis is not known. The tricyclic antidepressant most commonly studied and used for enuresis is imipramine. Reduction in rapid eye movement sleep as well as the anticholinergic effects has been implicated, but has not been shown to explain its effects. Nonetheless, imipramine is effective 40% to 60% of the time, but the relapse rate can be as high as 75%. The usual dose range is 1.0 to 2.5 mg/kg/single dose at bedtime, with a maximum dose of 50 mg in children 6 to 12 years of age and 75 mg in children ages 12 and older. If effective, the treatment should be continued for 4 to 6 months. Unexpected death due to cardiac arrhythmia has been reported, so a baseline electrocardiogram with periodic monitoring is recommended. Assessment of serum levels of imipramine and its metabolite is indicated only when no effect is seen despite dosing at 2.5 mg/kg/day.

Multiple varied medications such as indomethacin, tolterodine, hyoscyamine, and oxybutynin have been tried in the treatment of nocturnal enuresis, without benefit. Interestingly, carbamazepine has shown efficacy in one randomized, double-blind, controlled trial. By contrast, anticholinergic medications may be useful in diurnal enuresis when children have daytime urgency. If these medications are used, close follow-up is recommended to monitor for the development of constipation and increased residual volume after voiding, since these adverse effects may actually worsen enuresis, according to enuresis management guidelines published in 2009 by Robson.

Psychotherapy

Psychotherapy is typically used only when secondary enuresis has occurred and a specific psychological issue is associated with the onset of the symptom. Children who may benefit from psychotherapy would include those who have had a situational reaction with prolonged regressive behaviors, a posttraumatic stress response, a separation–individuation conflict in which bed-wetting is the focus, or an impulse control disorder. Psychotherapy may also be useful for managing the behavioral disorders that accompany enuresis, but will have little effect on primary enuresis itself. Lastly, psychotherapy may help to address the low self-esteem seen as a result of primary enuresis.

Encopresis

The treatment of encopresis should include educational, physiologic, psychological, and behavioral approaches, as summarized in Table 14-7. An early study found a success rate of 78% when all of these approaches are used together. The use of laxatives in conjunction with behavior modification appears superior to behavior modification alone. Other practitioners have found complementary and alternative medicine approaches to be essential in an integrative treatment plan for patients who have had more chronic courses of the illness.

Education

Both the parent and the child should be educated about normal bowel function and the important nuances of toilet training as well as the steps children need to take to become continent. Parents should be made aware of the lengthy process it sometimes takes to resolve encopresis. Cox and colleagues describe a specific toilet-sitting routine that may be useful to utilize with parents and children.

TABLE 14-7	Essentials in the Treatment of Encopresis

Education
- Normal bowel function
- Toilet training
- Extended time for treatment

Behavioral
- Daily timed intervals on the toilet
- Rewards for successful voiding

Physiologic
- Bowel catharsis
- Daily laxative

Psychological
- Diffuse psychological tension
- Treat specific psychiatric disorder contributing to encopresis

Psychological

Clinicians will likely need to help diffuse the psychological tension within the family surrounding the encopresis. Furthermore, children may require psychotherapy to address associated disorders including disruptive behavior disorders, anxiety, and impulse control problems. If sexual abuse has occurred, a therapist or program specially trained to treat children who have encountered abuse should be utilized.

Pharmacologic

If evidence of constipation is confirmed, the child should undergo an initial bowel catharsis (utilizing a hypertonic phosphate enema or mineral oil) followed by daily doses of laxatives or mineral oil. The key to successful treatment is providing an adequate dose for an adequate period of time to achieve smaller, softer stools. Multiple laxatives are available for use and include malt soup extract, corn syrup, milk of magnesia, mineral oil, lactulose, and senna syrup. Laxative use should be continued for 3 to 6 months, and then tapered slowly until the child can maintain a daily bowel movement without pain or stool withholding.

Increasing fluid intake and dietary residue are two ways to change a child's diet to help resolve the symptoms, but are usually effective only in constipation of a short duration. Once stool withholding and retention have occurred, dietary changes are unlikely to be effective. In either case, parents should be encouraged to provide their children a well-balanced diet, which should be maintained even after encopresis has resolved. Imipramine has been used to treat encopresis, but no controlled studies are available.

Behavioral

The behavioral component to treating encopresis consists of daily timed intervals on the toilet, where the child receives a reward when successful voiding occurs. Initially, rewards should be given simply for sitting on the toilet for a designated amount of time. Loening-Baucke recommends children not be initiated on a behavioral regimen until 1 month after laxative treatment is begun so that regular bowel patterns are closer to being restored. Lastly, a 2008 study by Montgomery and Navarro indicates that stool pattern diaries may be used to track progress and help the child to see his or her improvements.

Complementary and Alternative Medicine

In 2007, Culbert and Banez suggested that children with multiple factors contributing to their symptoms of constipation and encopresis may benefit from an integrative approach, utilizing conventional methods along with alternative medicine treatments. Controlled studies have evaluated the effectiveness of biofeedback in addition to conventional treatments, with mixed results. Other strategies such as teaching children relaxation and stress management techniques and hypnosis have not been studied but seem to be logical approaches to reducing overall anxiety and stress. Some herbal medicines have reported benefits in the treatment of constipation, but none of these has been systematically studied in the treatment of constipation in children. Similarly, probiotics has been postulated to improve constipation in children, but the limited studies in this area have also shown mixed results. Other strategies that have had minimal results in reducing constipation include massage and chiropractic and osteopathic manipulation. Lastly, acupuncture has been shown to improve constipation. While there are limited data on the use of complementary and alternative medicine techniques for encopresis, these modalities may be used prior to attempting more invasive treatments. It is important to monitor children while using these techniques for any untoward adverse effects, given the limited data on their use with children.

Conclusions

Enuresis and encopresis are common psychiatric disorders that often present in the primary care setting. They can cause a great deal of stress for families and are often difficult for clinicians to treat, given the frequency of multifactorial etiologies. A thorough evaluation examining multiple possible etiologies is therefore important to assist in developing a comprehensive treatment plan. Education for the parents and children plays a substantial role in treating either enuresis or encopresis, and families often need significant support and encouragement. Multiple treatment strategies exist and should be tailored to each specific patient, frequently combining approaches for maximal treatment outcomes. Successful treatment can provide families, children, and clinicians with a sense of pride and accomplishment and may improve other aspects of the child's and family's life that had contributed to these disorders.

CASE VIGNETTES

VIGNETTE 1: 5 YEAR OLD GIRL WITH NOCTURNAL AND DIURNAL ENURESIS

Sally is a 5-year-old female who presents to clinic with secondary nocturnal and diurnal enuresis. She had been potty-trained at the age of 3, but when her parents' rights were terminated 6 months ago, and she began living with a maternal aunt, she began having daytime and nighttime enuresis. Her aunt brought her to the pediatrician to be evaluated. A thorough history provided information on Sally having urinary accidents in her seat at school, and while standing on the playground and in the corner. She was also having nighttime incontinence approximately four times per week. Physical examination and urinalysis were within normal limits. The pediatrician instituted a reward system for both daytime and nighttime dryness where Sally and her aunt would place stickers on a calendar for every night and day she remained dry. She also discussed commonsense techniques, such as limiting fluid intake near bedtime, awaking her in the night to void, and providing role play for the times when Sally needed to use the restroom at school but was unsure how to ask. Sally responded with excitement to the reward system and soon began asking the teacher in school when she had to use the restroom, and would even remind her aunt at what time she should stop taking fluids at night. She achieved total dryness within 2 months of initiating the behavioral treatment. Individual psychotherapy was recommended to continue to help address other regressive behaviors that had occurred with the transition and also to cope with the separation from her parents.

VIGNETTE 2: 8 YEAR OLD BOY WITH SECONDARY ENCOPRESIS

An 8-year-old boy was admitted to the inpatient psychiatric unit for suicidal ideations. He had expressed wishing he would die because he was embarrassed he was still wearing a diaper and children at school called him names because of this. His mother was a nurse aid at a local nursing home and had simply been dressing him in a diaper for the past year, after he began soiling his underwear. The family was becoming concerned, though, because children at school were making fun of him and he seemed to be getting more and more depressed. This patient had achieved bowel continence by the age of 4, but had had a difficult bout of constipation at about age 8 for unexplained reasons. He had been experiencing constipation for 1 year, but his biggest problem was overflow incontinence, which caused him to have to wear a diaper. The family had not tried any specific techniques to address the issue. A thorough physical examination was performed, which showed abdominal distension and fecal impaction on rectal examination. All appropriate laboratory data were performed to rule out any endocrinologic disease that could be contributing to his symptoms. An abdominal x-ray showed significant fecal retention. A bowel catharsis was performed on the inpatient unit. He was discharged after 4 days when he was expressing hope that his condition could improve and he felt he had the tools to resolve the constipation. The boy was instructed to take milk of magnesia daily until he was having regular, soft bowel movements every day. His diet was reviewed and exercise was encouraged. He and his mother were educated about the extensive time it can take for this condition to resolve. They were also instructed to have him sit on the toilet for 10 minutes every 3 hours. He was to be rewarded with playing a board game with his mother for every successful void in the toilet. Gradually, he began to have more regular bowel movements and his daily laxative was discontinued after 5 months of use. The interval at which he sat on the toilet was reduced to twice per day for 10 minutes, continuing to receive a reward for a successful void. He no longer had to wear the diaper and had much better control over his bowel functioning.

BIBLIOGRAPHY

Al-Waili NS. Carbamazepine to treat primary nocturnal enuresis: double blind study. *Eur J Med Res.* 2000;5(1):40–44.

American Psychiatric Association. *Diagnostic and Statistical Manual of Mental Disorders. Fourth Edition, Text Revision* (DSM-IV-TR). Washington, DC: American Psychiatric Association; 2000.

Bellman M. Studies on encopresis. *Acta Paediatr Scand Suppl.* 1966;170:59–70.

Broide E, Pintov S, Portnoy S, et al. Effectiveness of acupuncture for treatment of childhood constipation. *Dig Dis Sci.* 2001;46(6):1270–1275.

Cox D, Sutphen J, Borowitz S, Kovatchev, Ling W. Contribution of behavior therapy and biofeedback to laxative therapy in the treatment of pediatric encopresis. *Ann Behav Med.* 1998;20(2):70–76.

Culbert TP, Banez GA. Integrative approaches to childhood constipation and encopresis. *Pediatr Clin North Am.* 2007;54:927–947.

El-Anany FG, Maghraby HA, Shaker SE, et al. Primary nocturnal enuresis: a new approach to conditioning treatment. *Urology.* 1999;53:405–408.

Essen J, Peckham C. Nocturnal enuresis in childhood. *Dev Med Child Neurol.* 1976;18:577–589.

Feehan M, McGee R, Stanton W, et al. A 6 year follow up of childhood enuresis: prevalence in adolescence and consequences for mental health. *J Pediatr Health Care.* 1990;26:75–79.

Foreman DM, Thambirajah MS. Conduct disorder, enuresis and specific developmental delays in two types of encopresis: a case study of 63 boys. *Eur Child Adolesc Psychiatry.* 1996;5:33–37.

Forsythe WI, Redmond A. Enuresis and spontaneous cure rate. Study of 1129 enuretics. *Arch Dis Child.* 1974;249:259.

Freud A, Burlingham DT. *War and Children*. New York: Medical War Books; 1943.

Fritz G, Rockney R, Bernet W, et al. Practice parameter for the assessment and treatment of children and adolescents with enuresis. *J Am Acad Child Adolesc Psychiatry*. 2004;43(12):1540–1550.

Glazener CM, Evans JH. Desmopressin for nocturnal enuresis in children. *Cochrane Database Syst Rev*. 2002;3:CD002112.

Glicklich LB. An historical account of enuresis. *Pediatrics*. 1951;8:859.

Hansson S. Urinary incontinence in children and associated problems. *Scand J Urol Nephrol*. 1992;141:47–55.

Houts AC, Berman JS, Abramson H. Effectiveness of psychological and pharmacological treatments for nocturnal enuresis. *J Consult Clin Psychol*. 1994;62:737–745.

Jenkins PH, Lambert MJ, Nielson SL, et al. Nocturnal task responsiveness of primary nocturnal enuretic boys: a behavioral approach to enuresis. *Child Health Care*. 1996;5:143–156.

Kuhn BR, Marcus BA, Pitner SL. Treatment guidelines for primary nonretentive encopresis and stool toileting refusal. *Am Fam Physician*. 1999;59(8):2171–2178.

Levine MD, Bakow H. Children with encopresis: a study of treatment outcome. *Pediatrics*. 1976;58:845–852.

Loening-Baucke V. Management of chronic constipation in infants and toddlers. *Am Fam Physician*. 1994;49(2):397–406.

Marschall-Kehrel D, Harms TW. Structured desmopressin withdrawal improves response and treatment outcome for monosymptomatic enuretic children. *J Urol*. 2009;182:2022–2027.

Mimouni M, Shuper A, Mimouni F, et al. Retarded skeletal maturation in children with primary enuresis. *Eur J Pediatr*. 1985;144:234–235.

Montgomer DF, Navarro F. Management of constipation and encopresis in children. *J Pediatr Health Care*. 2008;22:199–204.

Nolan T, Coffey C, Debelle G, et al. Randomized trial of laxatives in treatment of childhood encopresis. *Lancet*. 1991;31:523–527.

Robert M, Averous M, Besset A, et al. Sleep polygraphic studies using cystomanometry in twenty patients with enuresis. *Eur Urol*. 1993;24:97–102.

Robson WLM. Evaluation and management of enuresis. *New Engl J Med*. 2009;360:1429–1436.

Rutter M. Isle of Wight revisited: twenty-five years of child psychiatric epidemiology. *J Am Acad Child Adolesc Psychiatry*. 1989;28:633–653.

Rutter M, Tizard J, Whitmore K. *Education, Health and Behavior*. London: Longmans; 1970.

Spee van der Wekk J, Hirasing RA, Meulmeester JF, et al. Childhood nocturnal enuresis in the Netherlands. *Urology*. 1998;51:1022–1026.

Stern HP, Stroh SE, Fiedorek SC, et al. Increased plasma levels of pancreatic polypeptide and decreased plasma levels of motilin in encopretic children. *Pediatrics*. 1995;96:111–117.

Thompson S, Rey JM. Functional enuresis: is desmopressin the answer? *J Am Acad Child Adolesc Psychiatry*. 1995;34:266–271.

US Food and Drug Administration. *MedWatch Safety Alerts for Human Medical Products*; 2007. Available at: www.fda.gov/Safety/MedWatch/SafetyInformation/SafetyAlertsforHumanMedicalProducts/ucm152113.htm. Accessed December 18, 2009.

Zink S, Freitag CM, von Gontard A. Behavioral comorbidity differs in subtypes of enuresis and urinary incontinence. *J Urol*. 2008;179:295.

SUGGESTED READINGS

Fritz G, Rockney R. American Academy of Child and Adolescent Psychiatry. Practice parameter for the assessment and treatment of children and adolescents with enuresis. *J Am Acad Child Adolesc Psychiatry*. 2004;43(12):1540–1550.

Robson WLM. Evaluation and management of enuresis. *N Engl J Med*. 2009;360(14):1429–1436.

Montgomery DF, Navarro F. Management of constipation and encopresis in children. *J Pediatr Health Care*. 2008;22:199–204.

Kuhn BR, Marcus BA, Pitner SL. Treatment guidelines for primary nonretentive encopresis and stool toileting refusal. *Am Fam Physician*. 1999;59(8):2171–2178.

Wolraich M, Tippins S. *Guide to Toilet Training*. American Academy of Pediatrics. Bantam Doubleday Dell Publishing Group Inc.; 2003.

Bennett HJ. *Waking Up Dry: A Guide to Help Children Overcome Bedwetting*. American Academy of Pediatrics; 2005.

SUGGESTED WEBSITES

Brochures from the American Academy of Pediatrics
www.aap.org (*Bedwetting and Toilet Training*)
International Children's Continence Society
www.i-c-c-s.org

University of Virginia Research Study on an Internet Enuresis Treatment Program
www.healthsystem.virginia.edu/bmc/ucp2_interest/index.htm
International Children's Continence Society
www.i-c-c-s.org
American Academy of Child and Adolescent Psychiatry Facts for Families on Bedwetting
www.aacap.org/cs/root/facts_for_families/bedwetting
American Academy of Child and Adolescent Psychiatry Facts for Families on Encopresis
www.aacap.org/cs/root/facts_for_families/problems_with_soiling_and_bowel_control
American Academy of Pediatrics Parenting Corner: Encopresis
www.aap.org/publiced/BK5_Soiling.htm

REVIEW QUESTIONS

1. Which of the following is characteristic of encopresis?
   a. Involuntary or intentional passage of feces into inappropriate places
   b. Encopretic episode at least once per month for 3 months
   c. The child is at least 4 years old
   d. All of the above

2. Which of the following has been found to be the most effective in both acute stabilization of enuresis and in long-term resolution?
   a. Desmopressin
   b. Tricyclic antidepressants
   c. Bell and pad method
   d. Limiting fluid intake before bedtime

3. Which of the following is not correct regarding enuresis?
   a. The child is at least 4 years old.
   b. Enuretic episode at least twice per week for 3 consecutive months or clinically significant distress or social/academic impairment
   c. Secondary enuresis is more common in boys
   d. None of the above

4. Which of the following should be the first approach when treating enuresis or encopresis?
   a. Pharmacotherapy
   b. Individual psychotherapy
   c. Education
   d. Punishment

5. Which of the following is true in the treatment of encopresis?
   a. Treatment is short term, typically only 2–4 weeks.
   b. Enemas should be used daily throughout the treatment.
   c. Stool softeners, laxatives, and increased dietary fiber are utilized to prevent reaccumulation of stool.
   d. The child requires no behavioral treatment in conjunction with pharmacologic approaches.

Answers: 1-d, 2-c, 3-a, 4-c, 5-c

CHAPTER

15

Stefanie A. Hlastala, PhD,
Ian Kodish, MD, and Jon M.
McClellan, MD

Early-Onset Schizophrenia and Related Psychotic Disorders

Introduction

Early-onset schizophrenia (EOS; onset prior to age 18 years) is a serious, often debilitating disorder characterized by deficits in affect, cognition, and the ability to relate socially with others. EOS is often associated with significant morbidity, chronicity, and psychosocial impairment. Although schizophrenia and other severe psychotic disorders are rarely found in children, the profoundly negative effects of these illnesses and the necessity for intensive intervention require that clinicians who work with juveniles be familiar with their phenomenology, course of illness, assessment, and treatment. This chapter will review current research findings on the etiology, illness course, diagnostic considerations, and treatment of schizophrenia and related psychotic disorders in children and adolescents.

Background

Until relatively recently, physicians were reluctant to diagnose schizophrenia and other psychotic disorders in children and adolescents. Indeed, the existence of an early onset form of schizophrenia has been debated since Kraepelin's 1919 groundbreaking descriptive work on psychotic disorders. Although Kraepelin's early descriptions of childhood-onset schizophrenia (COS) were similar to the adult form of the disorder, other descriptive psychopathologists lumped early-onset psychosis into a broader range of childhood syndromes that were defined by developmental deficits in language, social relations, perception, and movement. Psychotic speech and thought were believed to be important components of early-onset psychosis, but hallucinations and delusions were not required for a diagnosis. As a result, childhood psychoses often included a broader rubric of neurodevelopmental disorders, including autism.

It wasn't until the 1970s that EOS was demonstrated to be distinct from other developmental disorders found in children such as autism and pervasive developmental disorders (PDD). In 1980, the American Psychiatric Association revised the criteria in the *DSM-III (Diagnostic and Statistical Manual of Mental Disorders, Third Edition)* so that EOS was diagnosed using the same criteria as those used for adult-onset schizophrenia. This practice has been maintained in subsequent DSM iterations, and is widely accepted as valid. Since a large portion of past research used the term COS overinclusively to describe a broader range of severely disturbed children, older studies of EOS need to be interpreted with caution.

Clinical Features

Although EOS is a syndrome consisting of a group of varied symptoms including social withdrawal, self-care deficiencies, and bizarre behaviors, hallucinations and delusions are the characteristic symptoms of schizophrenia. Schizophrenia is usually categorized as having two broad sets of clusters, positive and negative. Positive symptoms are those that are traditionally considered to be the disorder's hallmark—florid hallucinations, delusions, and thought disorder. Negative symptoms include flat affect, anergia, and paucity of speech and thought. A third cluster, including disorganized speech, bizarre behavior, and poor attention, has been more recently discussed in the literature. A recent study of youth with early-onset psychotic disorders (including schizophrenia and bipolar disorder) found four symptom domains—positive symptoms, negative symptoms, behavioral problems, and dysphoria. Only negative symptoms were specifically associated with a diagnosis of schizophrenia. In descriptive studies, hallucinations, thought disorder, and flattened affect have been consistently found in EOS, whereas systematic delusions and catatonic symptoms are less frequent. Children with EOS exhibit low rates of incoherence and poverty of speech. When assessing a child's thinking, it is important to distinguish between psychotic thought processes and developmental delays or language disorders.

DSM-IV Criteria

According to the *DSM-IV-TR*, at least two of the following are needed for a diagnosis of schizophrenia, each present for a significant period of time during a 1-month period: (1) delusions, (2) hallucinations, (3) disorganized speech, (4) grossly disorganized or catatonic behavior, and/or (5) negative symptoms, that is, affective flattening, alogia, or avolition. Only one of the following symptoms is needed for the diagnosis of schizophrenia: the delusions are bizarre, hallucinations consist of a voice keeping a running commentary on the child's behavior or thoughts, or two or more voices are conversing with each other. For a significant amount of time since the onset of the disorder, one or more areas of social functioning, such as school functioning, interpersonal relationships, and/or self-care, are noticeably below the pre-onset level or the expected level of age-appropriate social and academic achievement. The disturbance must persist for at least 6 months including at least 1 month of active psychotic symptoms. If the duration criterion of 6 months is not met, a diagnosis of schizophreniform disorder is made.

Several different subtypes of schizophrenia are described in the *DSM-IV-TR* including paranoid, disorganized, catatonic, undifferentiated, and residual. Studies on schizophrenic children and adolescents report that the paranoid and undifferentiated subtypes are the most commonly found.

Epidemiology

Because EOS is relatively uncommon, few studies have examined incidence rates in the population. Available evidence suggests that the prevalence of schizophrenia in children is significantly lower than in adults, which is estimated to be approximately 1%. The onset rate rises dramatically during the age range of 15 to 30 years. Although the timing of disorder suggests a relationship with pubertal status, puberty has not been specifically associated with this trajectory.

In children less than 15 years of age, the prevalence rate has been estimated at 14 per 100,000. COS (very early onset—prior to age 13) is extremely rare with a prevalence of approximately 1.6 per 100,000. A Danish research study reported that only 1% of hospitalized schizophrenic youth were younger than 13 years of age and only 9% were younger than 15 years of age. COS occurs predominantly in males with ratios of approximately 2:1, but this ratio becomes closer to 1:1 as age increases. The youngest age of onset reported in the research literature is 3 years, although any case below age 8 years needs to be carefully scrutinized.

Etiology and Pathogenesis

EOS is a heterogeneous disorder with multiple potential causes. A neurodevelopmental model suggests that environmental and genetic risk factors interact to disrupt key neurobiologic pathways, ultimately resulting in the disorder.

Genetic Factors

Schizophrenia has a strong genetic component. The lifetime risk of developing the illness is 5 to 20 times higher in first-degree relatives of affected probands compared to the general population. The rate of concordance among monozygotic twins is approximately 40% to 60%, whereas the rate of concordance in dizygotic twins and other siblings is 5% to 15%. EOS may have a greater genetic risk than adult-onset schizophrenia.

However, specific genes definitely linked with schizophrenia remain elusive. Until recently, most schizophrenia genetic research was based on the common-disease common-variant model, which hypothesizes that the illness is the sum result of different susceptibility genes, with each genetic risk variant contributing only a small degree of risk. This model suggests that the combination of common risk variants and exposures to environmental risk factors ultimately leads to the illness.

Large international collaborative efforts have identified numerous candidate genomic regions and candidate genes. Some candidate genes reported in the adult literature have associated with EOS, including dysbindin, neuregulin, DAOA/G30, GAD1, and Prodh2/DGCR6. Recent genome-wide association studies implicated different variants in the major histocompatibility region. However, the search for common risk alleles in schizophrenia has been challenged by variable results, lack of replication, small diminishing effect sizes, and lack of definitive biologic significance for any given candidate mutation.

In contrast, several studies recently demonstrated that rare deletions and duplications are enriched in individuals with schizophrenia. Many rare copy number errors associated with the illness either appear to be de novo or arose in recent generations. Most of these mutations were detected at different genetic loci, and many were unique to one individual or family. However, structural mutations at genomic "hotspots," that is, 1q21, 15q13, and 22q11, may be responsible for 0.5% to 1.0% of cases.

Interestingly, many of the same genes or genomic loci that are disrupted by structural mutations in individuals with schizophrenia are also implicated for other neuropsychiatric disorders, such as autism and mental retardation. The same mutation may present variably with different neurologic or psychiatric phenotypes, or no phenotype at all. There are likely a variety of interactive factors that influence how a mutation is expressed, including the dose and timing of the impact on gene functioning as it related to neurodevelopment, gene-by-gene interactions, epigenetic regulation (e.g., imprinting), and environmental exposures.

Collectively, this emerging research suggests that rare large-effect alleles play an important role in schizophrenia and that the illness is characterized by marked genetic heterogeneity. Since the majority of human genes are expressed in the brain, there are a vast number of potential genetic mechanisms by which neurodevelopment may be disrupted, any one of which may result in a neuropsychiatric or developmental disorder. It is possible that a substantial portion of patients with schizophrenia have a different genetic cause. If so, this has enormous implications for biologic and treatment research.

Environmental Exposures

A number of different environmental factors have been variably associated with the development of schizophrenia, include in utero exposure to maternal famine, paternal age, prenatal infections, obstetric complications, marijuana use, and migrant status. Each of these factors may mediate disease risk via a number of different complex mechanisms, including direct neurologic damage, gene–environment interactions, epigenetic effects, and/or de novo mutations.

Neurodevelopmental Factors

Early neurodevelopmental problems, such as obstetric complications, minor physical irregularities, and disruption of fetal neural development during the second trimester, have been associated with the eventual development of schizophrenia. Children who later develop schizophrenia display a variety of subtle behavioral abnormalities that often remain undetected until the full onset of the disorder such as delayed motor milestones, speech problems, lower educational test scores, and/or poor social adjustment. These developmental delays have been hypothesized to represent the early neuropathologic manifestations of schizophrenia.

Neurobiologic Findings

Neuroimaging studies of adults with schizophrenia reveal significant changes in multiple brain areas. The most consistent findings are enlarged lateral ventricles and reductions in volumes of the hippocampus, cingulate and prefrontal cortex, and thalamus. These data suggest that patients exhibit abnormalities in the developmental tuning of integrative brain networks, which likely contribute to clinical and symptomatic impairments. Furthermore, studies of first-episode and medication-naïve patients suggest that anatomic changes emerge early in the course of illness, and can affect the developmental trajectory of extensive synaptic refinements occurring in adolescence and continuing into adulthood.

Studies of EOS reveal brain abnormalities similar to those reported in adult cohorts, including problems with smooth pursuit eye movements, autonomic responsivity, and regional volumetric brain changes. Rapoport and colleagues at the National Institute of Mental Health (NIMH), in a unique cohort of youth with COS, found reductions in total cerebral volume and the midsagittal thalamic areas compared to age-matched normal controls. While normal brain development proceeds by early synapse overproduction and subsequent pruning to result in programmed contraction of brain regions through late childhood and adolescence, prospective scans in EOS revealed that patients had more rapid reductions of gray matter. Furthermore, this heightened atrophy proceeded in a parietal-to-frontal pattern, consistent with greater vulnerability in highly integrative prefrontal regions that serve executive functions thought to be compromised in schizophrenia. Longitudinal data suggest that the differential atrophy may plateau in early adulthood as the volumetric reductions decelerate.

While other studies of EOS reveal variable findings in terms of regional deficits and the rate of progression, the data generally support the notion of neurobiologic continuity between EOS and adult-onset schizophrenia. An earlier age of onset may interact with normal neurodevelopmental processes, resulting in greater severity of atrophic changes early in the course of illness. Further study is needed to elaborate on regional differences in rates of developmental sculpting, the effects of genetic and etiologic heterogeneity, the relevance of neuroanatomic changes to clinical symptoms and illness course, and the implications for treatment to restore functional brain networks.

Psychological Factors

Psychological and social factors by themselves have not been found to cause schizophrenia. However, such factors potentially interact with biologic risk factors to influence the timing of onset, the course, and the severity of the illness. Chronic interpersonal stress within the family (i.e., expressed emotion) has been found to influence the onset and exacerbation of acute psychotic episodes, as well as relapse and hospitalization rates.

Clinical Course

Although often characterized as a chronic condition, schizophrenia is a phasic illness, with the course and duration of the phases varying dependent on the illness and treatment response. The phases include (1) prodrome, (2) acute, (3) recuperative/recovery, and (4) residual. The prodromal phase involves general deterioration in functioning before the onset of psychotic symptoms in the active phase. Social withdrawal, idiosyncratic or bizarre preoccupations, unusual behaviors, academic decline, deteriorating self-care, increasing anxiety, depression, somatic complaints, and/or changes in appetite and sleep are common disturbances that occur during the prodromal phase. Children in the prodromal phase of illness may also exhibit increased behavioral problems, including aggression, deceitfulness, and/or substance abuse. Such symptoms may represent a significant change from baseline functioning or a worsening of premorbid personality characteristics, which may make it difficult to identify the onset of the disorder in some children. Prodromes can vary from an acute change (days to weeks) to a more insidious, chronic impairment. Children tend to have more insidious onsets, whereas both acute (less than 1 year) and insidious onsets have been noted in adolescents.

The acute phase is marked by a predominance of positive psychotic symptoms (i.e., hallucinations, delusions, and disorganized thinking and behavior) that often shift to negative symptoms (i.e., affective flattening, avolition, and paucity of thought or speech) over time. This phase usually lasts between 1 and 6 months; however, it may last longer if the child does not respond adequately to treatment. As the acute psychosis remits, there is often a recuperative/recovery phase lasting several months where the patient continues to experience a significant degree of impairment. This is most often due to negative symptoms (flat affect, anergia, or social withdrawal), although it is common for some positive symptoms to persist. In addition, some patients will develop a postpsychotic depression characterized by dysphoria and flat affect.

The residual phase is characterized by the overall improvement of active psychotic symptoms. Generally, there is some persistence of negative symptoms, including social isolation, poverty of speech, odd beliefs/perceptions, and/or anergia. Individuals may continue to display peculiar behavior (e.g., poor hygiene and blunted or inappropriate affect) and disordered thinking (tangentiality and circumferentiality). The residual phase may last for several months or more. Some patients exhibit significant symptoms that do not respond to adequate pharmacologic and psychosocial treatment. These chronically ill patients exhibit the most severe impairment over time and require the most comprehensive treatment resources (e.g., medications combined with individual, family, and school interventions).

Differential Diagnosis and Common Comorbid Diagnoses

Several other psychiatric disorders manifest themselves with the expression of symptoms that either overlap or are easily mistaken for the primary symptoms of schizophrenia. These disorders are summarized in Table 15-1. If the symptoms of schizophrenia have not persisted for a 6-month

TABLE 15-1 Differential Diagnosis for Schizophrenia	
Psychiatric	**Medical**
• Psychotic disorder due to a general medical condition	• Substance intoxication
	• Delirium
• Bipolar disorder	• Brain tumor
• Major depressive episode with psychotic features	• Head injury
	• Seizure disorder
• Schizoaffective disorder	• Meningitis
• Psychotic disorder NOS	**Psychosocial**
• Delusional disorder	• Abuse
• Posttraumatic stress disorder	• Traumatic stress
• Obsessive–compulsive disorder	• Chaotic family environment
• Pervasive developmental disorder	
• Conduct disorder	
• Evolving borderline personality disorder	

period, a diagnosis of schizophreniform disorder should be made. In juveniles, this often ultimately develops into schizophrenia. Schizoaffective disorder and mood disorders with psychotic features need to be ruled out when diagnosing a child or an adolescent presenting with psychotic symptoms. This is especially important for adolescents with bipolar disorder, because manic episodes during adolescence often include psychotic symptoms during the acute phase of illness. In fact, research suggests that early-onset bipolar disorder is associated with higher rates of psychosis than bipolar disorder of adult onset. As a result, bipolar youths are often misdiagnosed as schizophrenic when seen during an acute manic or mixed episode.

Psychotic symptoms during the acute phase of illness in EOS and early-onset bipolar disorder have considerable overlap. However, bipolar youths tend to have more mood congruent delusions and a lower percentage of hallucinations, loosening of associations, and negative symptoms than schizophrenic children. In addition to differences during the acute phase of illness, a thorough understanding of the child's symptomatic and psychosocial history will aid in the differential diagnosis of schizophrenia and bipolar disorder. Youths with schizophrenia tend to have higher rates of premorbid social withdrawal and global impairments than bipolar youths. Further, psychotic symptoms must present only during active periods of depression or mania for a diagnosis of bipolar disorder. During euthymic periods, the bipolar patient will not experience psychotic symptoms.

Schizoaffective disorder and major depression with psychotic features may be the most difficult disorders to distinguish from schizophrenia. Negative symptoms of EOS are sometimes mistaken for depression, especially since dysphoria is commonly experienced as a part of the illness. Although an accurate picture of the temporal overlap between mood episodes and psychotic symptoms can be extremely difficult to obtain, this retrospective understanding is necessary to distinguish EOS from other psychotic disorders. For a diagnosis of depression with psychotic features, psychosis will be present only in the context of a severe major depressive episode. For a diagnosis of schizoaffective disorder, positive and negative psychotic symptoms must occur in the absence of significant mood episodes. The diagnosis of schizoaffective disorder appears to be somewhat unreliable in community settings. This is due in part to the tendency to use this diagnosis when mood and psychotic episodes co-occur (which may represent a primary mood disorder) or when an individual with schizophrenia has mood symptoms (i.e., dysphoria and grandiosity) without meeting the prerequisite mood episode criteria. Moreover, it is not uncommon in clinical settings that youth with emotional and behavioral dysregulation problems, often with traumatic histories, report psychotic-like symptoms and are diagnosed with schizoaffective disorder even though they may not actually have true psychosis.

Youths with traumatic histories, including physical, sexual, and/or emotional abuse, may report symptoms suggestive of auditory or visual hallucinations and/or paranoid delusions. However, these symptoms are generally either brief or atypical in nature, and the child does not demonstrate the other hallmark symptoms of schizophrenia. Further, some children with abuse histories may report psychotic symptoms in the context of reinforcement that occurs in a chaotic environment. Therefore, potential environmental reinforcers of psychotic behaviors should be assessed. For example, a child who reports hearing voices telling her to kill herself only when her parents are arguing (which, as a result, stops the parents from arguing because they are concerned with her behavior) is unlikely to have a primary psychotic condition such as EOS. Conversely, children with schizophrenia also may have suffered abuse; therefore, the mere presence of a trauma history does not rule out a primary psychotic illness.

Some psychoses are caused by substance intoxication or delirium. Patients with substance-induced psychosis generally present with an acute onset of psychotic symptoms that are temporally related to the intake of the drug. Psychostimulants can produce paranoid delusions and disorientation, whereas hallucinogens may produce vivid hallucinations and delusions.

Substance intoxication and/or withdrawal can also induce delirium, which is associated with fluctuating mental status, varied levels of consciousness, and altered short-term memory. Therefore, it is important to identify if the psychosis is attributable to delirium or substances, because psychoses of these etiologies often have a different clinical course from psychosis due to EOS. Some youth may present with a psychotic illness in the context of substance/alcohol abuse, leading to an uncertain diagnosis. Because substance-induced psychosis generally clears within hours to days, psychotic symptoms that persist after a significant period of detoxification indicate the possibility of an underlying primary psychotic illness that may have been precipitated or exacerbated by substance abuse.

There are other psychotic disorders that are generally rare in juveniles and have not been studied. Delusional disorder presents with nonbizarre delusions (e.g., isolated paranoid belief) without the other accompanying symptoms of schizophrenia. Brief psychotic disorder consists of schizophrenic symptoms lasting less than 1 month in duration. Such presentations warrant careful evaluation, including the possibility of an acute response to stress, intoxication, or misreporting (or misinterpretation) of psychotic symptoms. Brief psychotic episodes may also be harbingers of developing schizophrenia or a psychotic mood disorder.

Developmental disorders, especially PDD, may overlap in symptomatology with EOS. Behavioral oddities, restricted interests, and significant interpersonal deficits are often present in both EOS and PDD. However, frank psychosis is evidence of a primary psychotic condition, regardless of developmental disabilities or autistic-spectrum disorders.

A significant number of patients with transient psychotic symptoms who fail to meet full criteria for any of the primary psychotic disorders discussed earlier in the text are often given a diagnosis of psychotic disorder not otherwise specified (PDNOS). PDNOS children have been found to exhibit significant overall impairment and similar risk factor profiles and neurobiologic abnormalities as EOS children. Follow-up studies ranging from 2 to 17 years indicate that many PDNOS patients continue to have hallucinations or delusions over the long term, are chronically impaired, require residential placement, or have significant work and social difficulties as adults. Only a very small percentage of these children received a follow-up diagnosis of schizophrenia. Half of the patients in a 2001 study by Nicolson and colleagues received a later diagnosis of a psychotic mood disorder (e.g., schizoaffective disorder, bipolar disorder, and major depressive disorder with psychotic features). It is questionable whether some of the individuals actually have true psychosis, and likely include the group with subjects that at outcome have personality disorders and/or posttraumatic phenomena.

Developmental Considerations

Because it can be difficult to distinguish true psychotic symptoms in young children, clinicians should be very careful when making a diagnosis in these patients. Overactive imaginations, developmental delays, language problems, posttraumatic phenomena, and/or misperceptions of the questions being asked all may lead to misinterpretations of psychotic symptoms in youth. Furthermore, very young children's inability to apply logical reasoning to their perceptions can make it difficult to identify delusions in children younger than 5 years old.

In school-age children with psychosis, the delusional content often revolves around ideas of reference, somatic preoccupations, or delusions of persecution. Compared to delusions in psychotic adults, those in school-age children are less likely to be richly detailed or elaborate and are often nonsystematized. In fact, more elaborate descriptions of suspected psychotic phenomena should raise questions as to the validity of the report.

Most children that report psychotic symptoms do not actually have a psychotic disorder. Youth with conduct and other nonpsychotic emotional disorders may report psychotic-like symptoms, and are at risk of being misdiagnosed. In these cases the psychotic symptom reports are often atypical in nature in the following manner: (1) the reports are inconsistent, and there is no other documented evidence of a psychotic process (e.g., thought disorder and bizarre disorganized behavior); (2) the qualitative nature of the reports were not typical of psychotic symptoms, for example, greatly detailed descriptions or reports more suggestive of fantasy or imagination; and/or (3) the reported symptoms occurred only at specific times, for example, hearing voices only after an aggressive outburst. Atypical psychotic symptoms may represent a number of phenomena, including posttraumatic stress disorder (PTSD), factitious or conversion disorders, or developmental delays that interfere with the accurate reporting of internal experiences, difficulty distinguishing fantasy from reality, and/or misunderstanding the questions being asked by the clinician. Children with a history of abuse, especially those with PTSD, often report higher rates of psychotic-like symptoms than do control children. In these children, atypical psychotic symptoms may actually represent dissociative phenomena or anxiety symptoms, including intrusive thoughts/worries, derealization, and/or depersonalization. In general, it is reasonable to assume that an older adolescent presenting with psychotic symptoms is more likely to have a primary psychotic illness than a young child, although the validity of the reports in either age group needs to be carefully assessed.

Another complicating factor is the presence of developmental delays. Ten to twenty of children with EOS have IQs in the borderline–to–mentally retarded range. Because many research studies have excluded patients with mental retardation, rates may actually be higher in clinical populations. Although youth with schizophrenia are at risk for cognitive deficits, the presence of developmental delays also creates diagnostic difficulties. In these cases, reported psychotic symptoms may simply represent misunderstanding of the concepts and/or misinterpreted normal sensory phenomena.

Assessment

A complete history and physical examination, as well as psychiatric evaluation, are necessary to provide an accurate assessment of psychosis in children and adolescents. These components are summarized in Table 15-2. A careful and systematic assessment of the child's current and previous psychiatric symptoms, psychosocial functioning, and family psychiatric history is a vital source of information when making a diagnosis. Whenever possible, the history should be gathered from all available sources, including the child, his or her parents, other caregivers, teachers, treatment providers, and community support persons (e.g., case workers, probation officers, and peers). When interviewing the child and his or her parents, the psychiatric history

TABLE 15-2	The Essential Evaluation for Early-Onset Schizophrenia (EOS)

- A systematic psychiatric history focusing on a longitudinal understanding of the patient's current and past symptomatology, and any changes.
- A thorough psychosocial history including current and past academic and interpersonal functioning and current and past abuse.
- Multiple historical informants (e.g., child, parents, teachers, and past providers) to gather aforementioned history.
- A physical examination to rule out organic causes of psychotic symptoms.
- There are no specific laboratory tests or neuroimaging procedures that are yet clinically diagnostic of EOS. These tests are used to rule out other disorders, such as organic psychoses.
- There are no rating scales or psychological tests that have been established to diagnose schizophrenia.
- Baseline and follow-up rating scales that assess positive and negative symptoms and psychosocial functioning are helpful in monitoring the effectiveness of treatment.

should focus on the presenting symptomatology, the longitudinal timeline of symptom development, and associated features and/or confounding factors (e.g., mood disorders, developmental problems, and substance abuse). Because of the many phases of psychotic disorders, it is important to obtain a longitudinal understanding of the child's illness. Certain core aspects of psychotic disorders may be missed if the clinician conducts only a cross-sectional checklist of symptoms.

Questions such as "Do you hear voices, whispers or other noises that other people cannot hear?," "Do you see things other children don't see?," "Does your mind ever play tricks on you?," and "Do you ever feel that you have special abilities or powers?" can be used as preliminary probes assessing for hallucinations and/or delusions. The child's behavior, speech, and affect should also be observed closely. An actively psychotic child will have symptoms in multiple domains, including disorganized thinking, flattened or inappropriate affect, strange behavior, and significantly impaired functioning along with their reports of hallucinations and/or delusions.

A physical examination is necessary to rule out any medical causes of psychotic symptoms. Drug or alcohol intoxication, delirium, central nervous system lesions, tumors, infections, metabolic disorders, and seizure disorders are potential organic conditions that can cause psychosis. Neuroimaging, electroencephalographs, and laboratory tests are not required to diagnose primary psychotic conditions. However, such tests are often indicated based on information obtained from the history and physical examination to rule out other organic illnesses and/or to serve as a baseline for medication therapy monitoring.

An assessment of current and past psychosocial functioning is also important given the role of family support and stressors in modulating the course of illness and treatment response. Because cognitive deficits may influence the presentation and/or interpretation of psychotic symptoms, an intellectual assessment may be helpful when there is evidence of developmental delays. However, neuropsychological testing is not indicated as a method for differentiating schizophrenia from other psychiatric disorders.

Treatment

Pharmacotherapy

The short-term efficacy of antipsychotic agents for the treatment of schizophrenia in adults is well established. These medications help reduce psychotic symptoms in the acute setting, significantly reduce relapse, and can improve functioning in multiple domains. Atypical antipsychotic medications (e.g., olanzapine, risperidone, quetiapine, ziprasidone, and aripiprazole) are often considered the drugs of first choice. However, recent large comparative trials in both adults and youth have not demonstrated the superiority of the second generation from traditional neuroleptics with regard to efficacy or tolerance.

Antipsychotic agents are recommended as first-line treatment for schizophrenia spectrum disorders in children and adolescents. The only atypical antipsychotic agents currently approved by the Food and Drug Administration (FDA) for the acute treatment of EOS in children 13 and older are aripiprazole and risperidone. The FDA Psychopharmacologic Drugs Advisory Committee voted in June 2009 to approve quetiapine and olanzapine for schizophrenia in adolescents. Industry-sponsored randomized controlled trials support the efficacy of these agents for symptoms of EOS.

Older controlled studies found that loxapine and haloperidol were helpful for EOS. However, youth may also be particularly sensitive to extrapyramidal side effects. A comparative trial found that olanzapine treatment was maintained significantly longer than haloperidol or risperidone treatment in youth with broadly defined psychotic disorders. However, the proportion of responders at 8 weeks did not differ between medication groups, and side effects were common. Another open-label study of youth with various psychotic illnesses found no difference in efficacy between olanzapine, risperidone, and quetiapine.

A naturalistic follow-up study of youth with first-onset psychosis revealed treatment providers most frequently used risperidone, quetiapine, and olanzapine and that these agents did not differ in measures of symptoms reduction. Olanzapine showed the greatest weight gain, while risperidone was associated with more neurologic side effects.

A publically funded multisite randomized double-blind trial, the Treatment of Early Onset Schizophrenia and Schizoaffective Disorder (TEOSS), compared olanzapine, risperidone, and molindone. No differences were found in the response or magnitude of symptom reduction across treatment arms. Importantly, only 34% to 50% of youth responded to 8 weeks of acute treatment. Olanzapine showed the greatest weight gain, while molindone was associated with more self-reports of akathisia. Youth on molindone received prophylactic benztropine therapy, which may have mitigated differences in extrapyramidal symptom ratings. These results mirror those of large adult comparative trials and raise similar questions as to whether atypical antipsychotics truly exhibit greater efficacy compared to first-generation agents such as molindone or perphenazine.

Clozapine has been shown to be effective in the treatment of positive and negative symptoms of COS, including evidence of greater response in treatment-resistant youth, as compared to haloperidol. However, clozapine has serious potential side effects including neutropenia and seizures, which limits its use to a second-line agent for treatment refractory cases.

Thus, at this time, the EOS treatment literature supports that antipsychotic medications are superior to placebo for the short-term reduction in psychotic symptoms. Comparative trials do not support the superiority of atypical agents over traditional neuroleptics, with the exception of clozapine. The potential for side effects, and the lack of maintained long-term effectiveness, remain significant clinical challenges. There are no systematic trials that have examined combined therapies or multiple medication strategies.

Despite these limitations, antipsychotic medications remain the primary treatment of EOS, given the lack of other treatment alternatives and the substantial morbidity associated with the illness. The choice of medication should be tailored to the phase of illness in addition to the patient's history of medication response. Furthermore, as large comparative studies have demonstrated few differences in the response to various medications, side effect profiles should be carefully considered when choosing an agent.

Patients are recommended to maintain regular contact with their physician in order to adequately monitor symptoms, treatment response, and adverse events. Common side effects of atypical agents include increased appetite, somnolence, weight gain, motor restlessness, and other extrapyramidal symptoms. Weight gain appears to be a greater problem in youth, as compared to adults, and is associated with subsequent metabolic abnormalities such as diabetes and cardiovascular problems. Recent reports suggest that metformin may be helpful in mitigating these effects in both youth and adult patients, although further study is needed. Baseline and follow-up monitoring is required, including weight, blood pressure, and body mass index, plus laboratory testing of metabolic function, lipids, liver functions, and fasting glucose. Other potential side effects need to be monitored as well, including extrapyramidal symptoms and tardive dyskinesia.

In the acute phase of illness, antipsychotic therapy should be implemented for at least 4 to 6 weeks, using adequate dosages, before judging efficacy. Large medication doses instituted very early in the course of treatment do not necessarily hasten recovery, and may result in excessive doses and increased side effects. A trial of an alternative agent should be undertaken if side effects are not manageable or if no results are apparent after 4 to 6 weeks. For those patients who do not respond adequately to multiple trials of neuroleptics, clozapine should be considered with careful monitoring.

As positive symptoms improve, usually after 4 to 12 weeks of treatment, patients commonly undergo a recuperative phase. They may continue to exhibit confusion, disorganization, and dysphoria, but the severity of their psychotic symptoms and functional impairments tends to diminish. Antipsychotic medication should be maintained during this period to hopefully achieve additional improvements while also reducing the risk of relapse. A gradual dosage reduction may be indicated if high dosages were necessary to control the acute psychotic phase. However, when lowering the dose or changing medications, the patient should be monitored with more frequent visits. Further symptoms may evolve and require treatment using adjunctive medications, although in general it is best to avoid polypharmacy.

During maintenance treatment, physician contact should continue on a regular basis. The goals of pharmacologic treatment in individuals with EOS should be incorporated into other modes of therapy, should be monitored regularly and reviewed with patient and family, and should focus on reducing symptom, improving social and occupational functioning, enhancing quality of life, and reducing risk for relapse.

Some youth may present with treatment refractory or complicated symptom presentations that require the use of adjunctive medications, for example, the use of mood stabilizers or antidepressants to treat concurrent mood episodes. In addition, adjunctive agents are often used to address side effects, for example, benztropine for extrapyramidal side effects or metformin for weight gain and metabolic changes. Although polypharmacy is common in community settings, there are no well-designed studies of this practice for EOS. Medications should be added systematically so that their effectiveness and tolerability can be adequately gauged.

Many patients will likely need to have their medication regimens adjusted over time, given a lack of efficacy, problematic side effects, or noncompliance. A small percentage of remitted patients may not relapse; a trial of medication taper can be considered in youth who have been symptom free for at least 12 months. However, most individuals will require prolonged treatment for ongoing symptoms and for preventing reoccurrence or worsening of the illness.

Psychosocial Interventions

Adjunctive psychosocial interventions are almost always indicated in the treatment of EOS. While EOS is certainly an illness mediated by genetic and neurodevelopmental factors, psychosocial factors often play a powerful role in the expression of the illness course, treatment response, and prognosis. In turn, the illness can wreak havoc on the child's psychosocial world. Psychotherapy as a stand-alone treatment has not proven to be effective for treating schizophrenia. However, adjunctive psychosocial treatments including psychoeducation, behaviorally based family therapy, and cognitive–behavioral therapy (CBT) have been shown to reduce relapse rates and improve positive and negative symptoms in schizophrenic patients.

Psychoeducational therapy is helpful for the patient and his or her family to learn how to cope better with effects of the illness and enhance long-term outcome. Psychoeducation for the patient should include ongoing education about the illness, treatment options, social skills training, relapse prevention, basic life skills training, and problem-solving strategies. Psychoeducation for the family should include information to increase their understanding of their child's illness, treatment options, short- and long-term prognosis, and developing strategies to cope with their child's symptoms and behavioral manifestations of the disorder. Research on adolescents with schizophrenia by Rund and colleagues found that psychoeducational treatment was associated with lower rates of hospitalization and was more cost-effective than standard community treatment.

Family therapies for schizophrenia evolved from research examining the effects of expressed emotion in families on the long-term illness course in schizophrenic patients. Expressed emotion refers to attributes of hostility, overprotectiveness, and/or criticism expressed toward the patient by his or her family members. Relapse rates have been shown to be consistently higher for schizophrenic patients who live in families with high levels of expressed emotion. Therefore, it is not surprising that adjunctive family interventions aimed at educating the family about schizophrenia and the medications used for treating the disorder, improving problem solving, and increasing communication skills have proven to significantly decrease relapse rates.

TABLE 15-3   Treatment Essentials for Early-Onset Schizophrenia (EOS)
• Antipsychotic medications are the frontline treatment for psychosis, with the atypical antipsychotic agents generally considered the drugs of first choice.
• A trial of antipsychotic medication should be implemented for at least 4–6 weeks before any judgment about efficacy can be made. After 4–6 weeks, if significant improvement is not apparent and/or side effects are unmanageable, then a different neuroleptic should be tried.
• Some form of adjunctive psychosocial treatment (e.g., psychoeducation, family therapy, and cognitive–behavioral therapy) is always indicated in the treatment of EOS.
• It is important to educate and collaborate with the child's teachers and school counselors to formulate appropriate expectations, goals, and programming to ensure optimal academic success.
• Other medications, such as antidepressants, mood stabilizers, and/or benzodiazepines, can be used to manage mood and anxiety symptomatology once antipsychotic agents have been given the appropriate time to exhibit effects.

CBT for schizophrenia focuses on challenging and testing key beliefs associated with hallucinations and delusions, teaching problem solving skills, enhancing coping strategies, and increasing medication adherence. In adults, adjunctive CBT has been found to produce large clinical effects on both positive and negative symptoms of schizophrenia. However, there are no published research studies examining the effects of CBT on symptomatic or functional outcomes in patients with EOS. Certainly, the effectiveness of CBT would depend on the developmental level of the patient and whether the patient possesses the metacognitive abilities to "think about one's thinking," which may be beyond what the majority of EOS individuals are capable of during childhood and early adolescence.

Behavioral interventions for weight management may also be indicated in children who gain a significant amount of weight on antipsychotic medications. Traditional behavioral interventions focus on self-monitoring of weight, food intake, and exercise. Unfortunately, research on the effectiveness of behavioral interventions for antipsychotic-induced weight gain is virtually absent. The research literature on nonpsychotic overweight children and adolescents indicates that a comprehensive, multidisciplinary program including a dietician, physical therapist, psychologist, and physician is needed to produce significant weight loss. Clearly, more research on weight management in youths with medication-induced weight gain is greatly needed.

Specialized educational programs and/or vocational training may be indicated for some children or adolescents to address the cognitive and functional deficits associated with the disorder. Some children will require more intensive community support services, including day programs and/or community caseworkers. In more chronic and/or severely ill children, long-term placement in a residential facility may be warranted.

The most important aspects of treatment are summarized in Table 15-3.

Conclusions

EOS is a rare, serious illness associated with significant morbidity, chronicity, and social impairment. Diagnosis of schizophrenia in youth is challenging because of its symptomatic overlap with other serious mental illnesses as well as the developmental factors that can obfuscate the assessment of psychotic symptoms. When EOS is identified accurately, its treatment is likely to be intensive and long lasting in order to facilitate a more positive long-term outcome. Two case vignettes are presented later in the text that document the nature of symptoms, course of treatment, and long-term effects of schizophrenia when it onsets in childhood or adolescence.

CASE VIGNETTES

VIGNETTE 1: JENNIFER, AN ADOLESCENT WITH SCHIZOPHRENIA

Jennifer presented as a 16-year-old girl who had been acting increasingly bizarre at home and at school for the past year. Her parents reported that her grades and school attendance had worsened significantly that year. She was not completing her homework and had been spending excessive amounts of time in the evenings on tarot card and astrology websites trying to predict her future. She had become increasingly oppositional at home and often refused to get out of bed until late afternoon. Her self-care had deteriorated significantly over the past 8 months so that she would shower only once a week at the insistence of her parents. She had become increasingly socially odd and exhibited significant blunting of her affect with sudden periods of inappropriate laughter. Her best friend refused to spend time with Jennifer anymore, because of her behavioral oddities and obsessive interest in the supernatural realm.

During the initial interview, Jennifer complained of seeing ghosts in her house and believed that evil spirits were haunting her. She stated that the devil was trying to kill her when she was asleep and she, therefore, was trying to stay awake at night. Her affect was blunted with virtually no eye contact. She denied any significant symptoms of mania or depression (past or current). Her developmental milestones were slightly delayed, with onset of speech at age 19 months and walking at 16 months. Neuropsychological testing indicated a full-scale IQ within the normal range. There was no documented history of physical, emotional, or sexual abuse. An in-depth physical examination including laboratory tests, an electroencephalograph (EEG), and computed tomography (CT) scan of the head all indicated that she had no significant medical problems. Her family psychiatric history consisted of schizoaffective disorder (maternal grandfather), depression (mother), drug-induced psychosis (paternal uncle), and alcoholism and drug abuse (father and paternal grandfather).

Jennifer was diagnosed with schizophrenia and started on an atypical antipsychotic agent. She also met with a psychologist weekly for support, psychoeducation, and social skills training. Within several months, her hallucinations, delusions, and disorganized thinking were improving. She was attending school on a regular basis and trying to make new friends. Although she had improved, she was still complaining of seeing ghosts at times and continued to exhibit blunted affect with moderate psychomotor retardation. Her concentration at school, ability to complete her homework, and grades had improved, but she remained far below her premorbid level of academic functioning. She participated in an individualized education program at school, which helped her considerably. Jennifer's supportive family environment was a huge asset for her and, ultimately, contributed to her successful completion of high school at age 19. After high school, she continued to live at home with her parents, who supported her financially and were helping her to find appropriate employment.

VIGNETTE 2: TOMMY, A YOUTH WITH VERY EARLY ONSET SCHIZOPHRENIA

Tommy, a 13-year-old boy, was brought in to his physician's office by his mother because of ongoing problems with confused thinking, aggressive behaviors, and refusal to go to school. At age 12 years, Tommy first developed significant problems sleeping because he was terrified that a "bad man" was outside his room trying to kill him and his family. At first, his mother believed he was having nightmares and had perhaps seen a few too many scary movies at his friends' homes. However, over the course of several months, it became apparent that his fear was becoming increasingly excessive and irrational. He often seemed disoriented and confused, and would tape black paper over his windows to keep the "bad man" from spying on him. He described hearing voices (e.g., the "bad man" mumbling threats). He reported that the "bad man" was following him at school and was putting poison in his food. He stopped going to class, and spent a great deal of time in his room, refusing to eat most of his meals.

Tommy's family physician had noted that as a young child, Tommy's developmental milestones were delayed. He had problems with interpersonal relatedness as a toddler, necessitating an earlier referral for a pervasive developmental disorder evaluation. He was diagnosed with an autism spectrum disorder at the age of 5 because of difficulties with interpersonal relatedness, restricted interests, and language delays.

When he first described experiencing auditory hallucinations and paranoid delusions, Tommy was diagnosed with schizophrenia and started on risperidone. The dose was increased over 4 weeks to 6 mg/day. Unfortunately, he experienced some weight gain (15 pounds over 2 months) and exhibited only a very mild improvement in symptoms. Subsequently, he underwent consecutive trials of aripiprazole (up to 30 mg/day) and perphenazine (up to 16 mg/day). However, neither agent adequately addressed his symptoms. In addition, he developed some bradykinesia and rigidity on the perphenazine. At this point, he had not attended school for almost an entire year, and was only marginally functional.

Therefore, his psychiatrist discussed the option of clozapine with the family. His mother was initially concerned over the potential for further weight gain, plus the risk of agranulocytosis. She and Tommy opted to continue the perphenazine. The psychiatrist raised the dose of perphenazine to 20 mg/day and added benztropine 1 mg b.i.d. for extrapyramidal side effects. However, after 1 week Tommy still looked stiff and rigid, and remained distressed and confused. His parents, and Tommy with their urging, decided to undergo a trial of clozapine.

His psychiatrist worked with a local pharmacy and laboratory that managed clozapine monitoring protocols for community mental health centers. She initiated clozapine at 12.5 mg b.i.d. and raised the dose twice per week as tolerated. At the same time she began a slow taper of the perphenazine. After 3 weeks, he was taking 300 mg of clozapine per day, and the perphenazine and benztropine were discontinued. Tommy had blood draws twice per week. The pharmacy confirmed that his blood counts were within the normal range prior to dispensing medication. In addition to blood counts, his physician monitored his weight, glucose levels, and lipids. She also warned Tommy and his family regarding the risk for seizures.

Tommy complained of drowsiness and drooling. However, he was less confused and expressing fewer paranoid concerns. He spent more time out of his room. His psychiatrist raised the clozapine to 400 mg/day, and continued to monitor his blood counts.

After 6 months, Tommy's thinking improved significantly. Although he continued to report some auditory hallucinations, he stated that the voices did not bother him and that he was able to ignore them. He denied being worried about the "bad man," although he still felt that the "bad man" may have been real. He was able to go out of the house on errands with his mom, and expressed a begrudging willingness to start attending school. His mother arranged for a special classroom focused on supportive learning and low stimulus, as part of an individualized education program (IEP). Tommy gained approximately 10 pounds during this time. His mother and psychiatrist worked on dietary programs; although Tommy was resistant to many of the food choices and also refused to exercise. His blood counts remained stable. He continued to have a complete blood count (CBC) checked weekly.

BIBLIOGRAPHY

Addington AM, Gornick MC, Shaw P, et al. Neuregulin 1 (8p12) and childhood-onset schizophrenia: susceptibility haplotypes for diagnosis and brain developmental trajectories. *Mol Psychiatry*. 2007;12(2):195–205.

Álvarez-Jiménez M, Hetrick SE, González-Blanch C, et al. Non-pharmacological management of antipsychotic induced weight gain: systematic review and meta-analysis of randomized controlled trials. *Br J Psychiatry*. 2008;193(2):101–107.

American Academy of Child and Adolescent Psychiatry. Practice parameter for the assessment and treatment of children and adolescents with schizophrenia. PMID: 11434484. *J Am Acad Child Adolesc Psychiatry*. 2001;40(suppl 7):4S–23S.

American Psychiatric Association. *Diagnostic and Statistical Manual of Mental Disorders, Fourth Edition Text Revision (DSM-IV-TR)*. Washington, DC: American Psychiatric Association; 2000.

Carlson GA, Bromet EJ, Sievers S. Phenomenology and outcome of subjects with early- and adult-onset psychotic mania. *Am J Psychiatry*. 2000;157(2):213–219.

Eggers C, Bunk D. The long-term course of childhood-onset schizophrenia: a 42-year followup. *Schizophr Bull*. 1997;23(1):105–117.

Frazier JA, Giedd JN, Hamburger SD, et al. Brain anatomic magnetic resonance imaging in childhood-onset schizophrenia. *Arch Gen Psychiatry*. 1996;53(7):617–624.

Gillberg C. Infantile autism and other childhood psychoses in a Swedish urban region. Epidemiological aspects. *J Child Psychol Psychiatry*. 1984;25(1):35–43.

Gilmore JH, Sikich L, Lieberman JA. Neuroimaging, neurodevelopment, and schizophrenia. *Child Adolesc Psychiatric Clin North Am*. 1997;6(2):325–341.

Goldstein MJ, Miklowitz DJ. The effectiveness of psychoeducational family therapy in the treatment of schizophrenic disorders. *J Marital Fam Ther*. 1995;21(4):361–376.

Gornick MC, Addington AM, Sporn A, et al. Dysbindin (DTNBP1, 6p22.3) is associated with childhood-onset psychosis and endophenotypes measured by the Premorbid Adjustment Scale (PAS). *J Autism Dev Disord*. 2005;35(6):831–838.

Gur RE, Keshavan MS, Lawrie SM. Deconstructing psychosis with human brain imaging. *Schizophr Bull*. 2007;33(4):921–931.

Harrison PJ, Weinberger DR. Schizophrenia genes, gene expression, and neuropathology: on the matter of their convergence. *Mol Psychiatry*. 2005;10(1):40–68.

Kraepelin E. *Dementia praecox and paraphrenia* (trans by RM Barclay of the 8th German Edition of the Textbook of Psychiatry, Vol. III, part ii). Edinburgh: E & S Livingstone; 1919.

Kumra S, Frazier JA, Jacobsen LK, et al. Childhood-onset schizophrenia: A double-blind clozapine-haloperidol comparison. *Arch Gen Psychiatry*. 1996;53(12):1090–1097.

Leff J, Vaughn C. *Expressed Emotion in Families: Its Significance for Mental Illness*. New York, NY: Guilford Press; 1985.

Maziade M, Gingras N, Rodrigue C, et al. Long-term stability of diagnosis and symptom dimensions in a systematic sample of patients with onset of schizophrenia in childhood and early adolescence, I: nosology, sex and age of onset. *Br J Psychiatry*. 1996;169(3):361–370.

McClellan J, Breiger D, McCurry C, et al. Premorbid functioning in early-onset psychotic disorders. *J Am Acad Child Adolesc Psychiatry*. 2003;42(6):666–672.

McClellan J, McCurry C. Early onset psychotic disorders: diagnostic stability and clinical characteristics. *Eur Child Adolesc Psychiatry*. 1999;8(suppl 1):I13–I19.

McClellan JM, Susser E, King MC. Maternal famine, de novo mutations, and schizophrenia. *JAMA*. 2006;296(5):582–584.

Nicolson R, Lenane M, Brookner F, et al. Children and adolescents with psychotic disorder not otherwise specified: a 2- to 8- year follow-up study. *Compr Psychiatry*. 2001;42(4):319–325.

Rapoport JL, Giedd JN, Blumenthal J, et al. Progressive cortical change during adolescence in childhood-onset schizophrenia. A longitudinal magnetic resonance imaging study. *Arch Gen Psychiatry*. 1999;56(7):649–654.

Rector NA, Beck AT. Cognitive behavioral therapy for schizophrenia: an empirical review. *J Nerv Ment Dis*. 2001;189(5):278–287.

Rund BR, Moe L, Sollien T, et al. The Psychosis Project: outcome and cost-effectiveness of a psychoeducational treatment programme for schizophrenic adolescents. *Acta Psychiatr Scand*. 1994;89(3):211–218.

Sikich L, Frazier JA, McClellan J, et al. Double-blind comparison of first- and second-generation antipsychotics in early onset schizophrenia and schizo-affective disorder: findings from the treatment of early-onset schizophrenia spectrum disorders (TEOSS) study. *Am J Psychiatry*. 2008;165(11):1420–1431.

Stone JL, O'Donovan MC, Gurling H, et al. International Schizophrenia Consortium. Rare chromosomal deletions and duplications increase risk of schizophrenia. *Nature*. 2008;455(7210):237–241.

Thomsen PH. Schizophrenia with childhood and adolescent onset: a nationwide register-based study. *Acta Psychiatr Scand*. 1996;94(3):187–193.

Tsuang MT, Stone WS, Faraone SV. Schizophrenia: a review of genetic studies. *Harv Rev Psychiatry*. 1999;7(4):185–207.

Walsh T, McClellan JM, McCarthy SE, et al. Rare structural variants disrupt multiple genes in neurodevelopmental pathways in schizophrenia. *Science*. 2008;320(5875):539–543.

Werry JS, McClellan J, Chard L. Childhood and adolescent schizophrenic, bipolar, and schizoaffective disorders: a clinical and outcome study. *J Am Acad Child Adolesc Psychiatry*. 1991;30(3):457–465.

White T, Cullen K, Rohrer LM, et al. Limbic structures and networks in children and adolescents with schizophrenia. *Schizophr Bull*. 2008;34(1):18–29.

Xu B, Roos JL, Levy S, et al. Strong association of de novo copy number mutations with sporadic schizophrenia. *Nat Genet*. 2008;40(7): 880–885.

SUGGESTED READINGS

American Academy of Child and Adolescent Psychiatry. Practice parameter for the assessment and treatment of children and adolescents with schizophrenia. *J Am Acad Child Adolesc Psychiatry*. 2001;40(suppl 7):4S–23S. (for clinicians who want to know current professional standard for assessment and treatment of schizophrenia in children).

Torrey EF. *Surviving Schizophrenia: A Manual for Families Consumers and Providers*. 5th ed. New York: Harper Collins Publishers, Inc.; 2006. (award-winning basic reference for families).

Mueser KT, Gingerich S. *The Complete Family Guide to Schizophrenia: Helping Your Loved One Get the Most Out of Life*. NY: The Guilford Press; 2006. (a practical, user-friendly resource for families).

Foster M. *Schizophrenia Revealed: From Neurons to Social Interactions*. New York: W.W. Norton and Co; 2003. (for sophisticated families and clinicians seeking information about the neurocognitive aspects of schizophrenia).

Andreasen NC. *Brave New Brain: Conquering Mental Illness in the Era of the Genome*. New York: Oxford University Press; 2001. (information about schizophrenia and other psychiatric illnesses written in a style accessible to families wanting more technical information).

SUGGESTED WEBSITES

A 25-page pamphlet in pdf file on schizophrenia written for families. http://www.nimh.nih.gov/health/publications/schizophrenia/complete-index.shtml

For clinicians interested in having their patients enrolled in an NIMH study on childhood-onset schizophrenia. http://intramural.nimh.nih.gov/chp/cos/

The National Alliance on Mental Illness provides an excellent support network for individuals and families struggling with severe mental illness. http://www.nami.org

NARSAD funds psychiatric research for mental illness such as schizophrenia, bipolar disorder, depression, and anxiety disorders. Their website provides up-to-date research findings and patient and family guides with information about how to cope with these illnesses. http://www.narsad.org

REVIEW QUESTIONS

1. Brain development in EOS differs from typical development in that:
   a. Typical brain development does not involve reductions in cortical brain regions.
   b. Patients with EOS show brain changes that can be used to diagnose illness.
   c. Patients with EOS may show subtle changes, but these do not emerge until late in the course of chronic illness.
   d. Patients with EOS exhibit regional reductions in cortical volumes that are present early in the course of illness.
   e. The regional changes in EOS progress in the reverse pattern compared to typical development.

2. Medication trials in EOS suggest:
   a. Atypical agents are associated with much better response rates than older agents.
   b. Atypical agents are associated with fewer and less severe side effects.
   c. Youth are at less risk for extrapyramidal symptoms of typical agents.
   d. Despite demonstrated efficacy over placebo, the response rates of various antipsychotic agents remains at 50% or lower.
   e. Greater metabolism in children suggests the need for higher doses of medications compared to adults.

3. Which diagnosis should be made when the child's symptoms of schizophrenia have existed for less than 6 months?
   a. Schizoaffective disorder
   b. Schizophreniform disorder
   c. Schizophrenia, brief episode
   d. Psychosis NOS
   e. None of the above

4. Which developmental phenomenon can make it difficult to distinguish true psychotic symptoms in young children?
   a. Developmental delays
   b. Overactive imaginations
   c. Posttraumatic phenomena
   d. Misperceptions of the questions being asked
   e. All of the above

5. Research on the treatment of EOS indicates that:
   a. Atypical psychotic agents are superior to typical agents.
   b. Clozapine is a first-line treatment for EOS.
   c. Antipsychotic therapy should be implemented for at least 4–6 weeks before judging efficacy.
   d. Youth with EOS are less prone to medication-induced weight gain than adults.
   e. All of the above.

Answers: 1-d, 2-d, 3-b, 4-e, 5-c

Autism Spectrum Disorders

Introduction and Background

Autism spectrum disorder (ASD) is the term now commonly used to describe three of the pervasive developmental disorders (PDDs): autistic disorder, Asperger disorder, and pervasive developmental disorder—not otherwise specified (PDD-NOS). Rett disorder and childhood disintegrative disorder (CDD) also fall under the broader PDD umbrella. As the term suggests, ASD describes individuals across a wide range of symptoms, cognitive abilities, and adaptive functioning. A lifelong neurodevelopmental disorder, ASD is characterized by qualitative impairments in social interaction and communication, and the presence of restricted, repetitive, and stereotyped interests and behaviors. Our understanding of this complex disorder has changed dramatically since it was first described by Leo Kanner in 1943 and Hans Asperger in 1944. Research integrating diverse methodologies from the fields of neurobiology, cognitive and developmental neuroscience, developmental psychopathology, and genetics has shed light on the complex pathogenesis of this disorder and its heterogeneous phenotype. This chapter highlights the latest advances in autism research, while also providing useful tools for screening and detection of ASD in primary care settings. Finally, information on evidence-based assessment and treatment approaches and helpful resources for parents and professionals are provided.

Clinical Features and Diagnosis

The cognitive and behavioral deficits commonly seen in individuals with autism are perhaps best understood along a dimension of social communication functioning. However, the *Diagnostic and Statistical Manual*, 4th Edition, Text Revision (DSM-IV-TR) is based on a categorical system, which is less useful for capturing the broader phenotype of a spectrum disorder such as autism.

Diagnostic Criteria and Differential Diagnosis

Autistic Disorder

The diagnostic criteria for autistic disorder, both early onset and regressive types, include a total of six or more symptoms across all three domains of impairment, with at least two symptoms in the domain of reciprocal social interaction, one in communication, and one in restricted, repetitive, and stereotyped interests and behaviors. Additionally, symptoms must be present by age 3 and are not better accounted for by Rett disorder or CDD. The diagnostic symptom list for the ASDs by domain, based on the DSM-IV-TR, is shown in Table 16-1.

Asperger Disorder

Just like autistic disorder, Asperger disorder is characterized by at least two impairments in the domain of reciprocal social interaction and at least one in the domain of restricted, repetitive,

---

TABLE 16-1 Diagnostic Symptoms of Autism Spectrum Disorders by Domain

Social Impairments
- Poor eye contact, lack of facial expression and social gestures
- Failure to develop age-appropriate peer relationships
- Lack of shared interests and enjoyment of achievements
- Lack of social or emotional reciprocity

Communication
- Lack of nonverbal attempts to compensate for verbal impairment
- Inability to sustain conversations if language present
- Awkward, odd, and repetitive language
- Absence of make-believe play and developmentally appropriate social imitation

Restricted and Repetitive Behaviors
- Preoccupation with stereotyped and circumscribed activities
- Repetitive motor movements
- Preoccupation with parts of an object
- Inflexible rituals or routines

---

and stereotyped interests and behaviors, using the symptom list provided in Table 16-1. However, for a diagnosis of Asperger disorder, there must be no early language delays (i.e., single words by age 2, phrases by age 3) and no clinically significant delays in cognitive or adaptive function. Finally, criteria are not met for another specific PDD, including autistic disorder. This means that if a child meets early language milestones on time and has no cognitive delays, but has six or more symptoms across all three domains of functioning, the appropriate diagnosis is autistic disorder, not Asperger disorder (in this case, the diagnosis can be further specified as "high functioning"). That being said, there is little empirical support for a clinically meaningful distinction between high functioning autism (HFA) and Asperger disorder, both in terms of symptom presentation and outcome. Further, the absence of early language delays in Asperger disorder does not imply that language acquisition is normal (e.g., there may be deficits in pragmatic [i.e., social use of] language, or use of overly formal or repetitive and stereotyped language), and as such this distinction remains problematic.

Pervasive Developmental Disorder—Not Otherwise Specified

This diagnosis describes severe and pervasive impairments that do not meet full criteria for a specific PDD, and includes "atypical autism—presentations that do not meet the criteria for autistic disorder because of late age at onset, atypical symptomatology, or subthreshold symptomatology, or all of these." Given this broad definition and the absence of minimum symptom criteria, it is no wonder that in recent years many children with social issues and/or pragmatic communication difficulties have been diagnosed as having a PDD. When considering a diagnosis of PDD-NOS, the clinician should assess for impairments in at least two of the three domains indicated in Table 16-1 to provide evidence of a *pervasive* disorder. Further, given that severe social impairments are a distinguishing feature of ASD, there should be evidence of *marked* impairments in social interest, social motivation, and social relatedness, and not merely deficits in interpersonal skills that are common to a number of disorders, such as attention-deficit hyperactivity disorder (ADHD) and conduct disorder, among others. Figure 16-1 provides an algorithm to guide diagnostic differentiation.

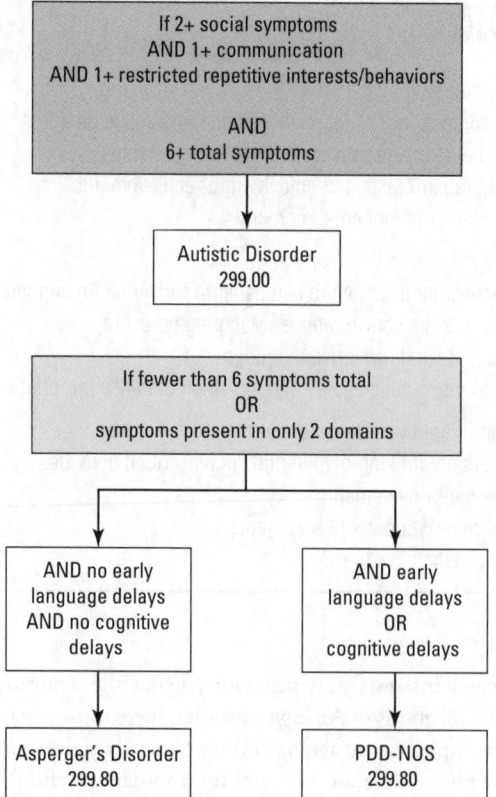

FIGURE 16-1. Diagnostic differentiation: autistic disorder, Asperger disorder, and PDD-NOS.

Other PDDs

Rett disorder and CDD fall under the broader umbrella of the PDDs. In Rett disorder, development in the first 5 months of life is normal, followed by a regression involving deceleration of head growth, loss of previously acquired hand movements and social engagement, the development of stereotypic "hand-wringing" movements, poorly coordinated gait or trunk movements, and severe impairments in language and psychomotor development. CDD is characterized by a period of typical development for the first 2 years of life followed by a regression in language, social or adaptive skills, play, motor skills, and bowel or bladder control. Also present are qualitative impairments in two of the three domains affected in autism. The difference between autism with regression and CDD is that, in autism, the regression typically occurs between 18 and 24 months and, in CDD, the regression occurs *after* 24 months of age.

Symptom Presentation

Every child with autism is unique in terms of number and severity of presenting symptoms. Additionally, symptoms fluctuate across the lifespan.

Social Impairments

Deficits in social attention are primary in ASD. Infants with autism show impairments as early as 8 months of age in *looking at others* and *orienting to name*, as compared to infants with typical and delayed development. A deficit in joint attention—the ability to share attention with another person in regard to an object or event (e.g., pointing to show, following another's eye gaze to an object)—is a core early symptom of autism, present by 12 months of age. Children with autism also show early impairments in motor imitation, social imitative play (e.g., peek-a-boo), and "theory of mind" or perspective-taking abilities.

Communication Impairments

Language development in autism is often (but not always) delayed, with approximately 30% of individuals never acquiring spoken language. Language is also often atypical in children with autism, with unusual prosody and speech patterns (e.g., unusual volume, rhythm, and rate of speech), immediate and/or delayed echolalia (i.e., repetition of words and phrases, often in the same intonation as the speaker), pronoun reversal (e.g., "*you* want a drink" instead of "*I* want a drink"), and deficits in pragmatic or social use of language (e.g., difficulties in reciprocity, pedantic speech, perseveration on particular topics, tangential speech, tendency to interpret speech literally). Symbolic, or pretend, play is also impaired in autism and is associated with the development of both language and social abilities.

Restricted and Stereotyped Behaviors and Interests

These behaviors are often divided into two categories: (1) repetitive, self-stimulatory motor movements, such as hand flapping, finger flicking, toe-walking, and spinning, as well as repetitive, nonfunctional use of objects (e.g., lining up objects, spinning wheels) and (2) more elaborate preoccupations and habits, such as insisting on sameness in routine and schedule, exact ordering of objects, or compulsive-like behaviors (e.g., dressing in a specific order, eating foods in a ritualistic manner, and so on), and intense interests often involving memorization of facts (e.g., antique camera model numbers). It is important for providers to be aware that impairments in this third category are not often present at a very young age in children with autism (i.e., age 2 and younger) and that their absence at this early age does not preclude an ASD diagnosis. Further, while children with typical and delayed development may also engage in ritualistic behaviors, the number, severity, and persistence of these symptoms are distinctive and excessive in children with autism.

Epidemiology

Prevalence

Prevalence rates for the ASDs include 13 per 10,000 for autistic disorder, 2.6 per 10,000 for Asperger disorder, and 21 per 10,000 for PDD-NOS. The estimate for all ASDs (autistic disorder, Asperger disorder, and PDD-NOS collectively) is now close to 1% of all children. There has been much debate in recent years about a possible autism epidemic given the rise in rates of the disorder (now three to four times higher than in the 1970s), which now place it as more common than spina bifida, cancer, and Down syndrome. The increase in rates can be at least partly explained by the broadening definition of autism, changes in DSM nosology from 1980 to present, and the emergence of Asperger disorder as a diagnostic category. Improved identification and use of the diagnosis to qualify for state early intervention programs have also contributed to higher rates of ASD, but environmental factors, although poorly understood, cannot be overlooked.

Demographics

ASDs affect three to four males per female. Females with autism exhibit more severe symptoms, including more severe intellectual disability compared to males with autism. The gender differences found in autism may reflect a higher genetic loading, or increased number of susceptibility alleles, in families with females with autism. Indeed, a genetic study by Schellenberg found unique linkage signals distinguishing families with affected males only versus families with at least one female affected member.

Individuals of all races, ethnicities, and socioeconomic levels are affected by autism. Access to treatment varies and is impacted by racial and ethnic minority status, low education levels, and geographic location. More children with autism are found to have unmet needs for specific health care services as compared to other children with special health care needs.

Etiology and Pathogenesis

There is remarkable heterogeneity within the ASDs—in symptom presentation, course, and response to treatment. This heterogeneity presents a significant challenge to those studying the underlying etiology of these disorders. Only about 10% of cases of autism are associated with known genetic disorders, such as fragile X syndrome; the remaining 90% are idiopathic. While specific causes remain largely unknown, there is substantial evidence for a strong genetic component to autism, with heritability estimates ranging from 91% to 93%.

Genetic Factors

Twin and Family Studies

The concordance rate for monozygotic twins is about 60%; when the broader range of the disorder is included, this rate rises to about 92% for monozygotic twins and 10% for dizygotic twins. The recurrence risk rate for siblings of children with autism is approximately 2% to 8%, compared to a 0.6% general population risk. The rates of autism in second- and third-degree relatives are much lower (0.18% and 0.12%, respectively).

Broader Phenotype

A broader autism phenotype, involving qualitatively similar but milder impairments than those found in autism, has been identified in as many as 25% of siblings and 10% of parents of individuals with autism. Even second- and third-degree relatives have been shown to exhibit broader phenotype impairments. These impairments include social skills deficits, pragmatic language deficits, executive function impairments, deficits in reading comprehension, and higher rates of repetitive and obsessive–compulsive behaviors. Toth and colleagues, and others, have documented broader phenotype impairments (social and communication deficits) in siblings as early as the first 2 years of life.

Candidate Genes

Several regions of interest have been identified, including areas on chromosomes 1p, 2q, 3p, 7q, 15q, and 17q. A region on 7q is thought to be associated with speech and language deficits. Duplications of 15q11–13 are fairly common in affected individuals, occurring in up to 5% of persons with ASD. This region is of particular interest because deletions in this area have been associated with other developmental syndromes, such as Angelman and Prader–Willi syndromes. Among other candidate genes in a growing list are neurexin and neuroligin genes, contactin 4, semaphorin 5A, cadherin genes, *FOXP2*, *RAY1/ST7*, *IMMP2L*, *RELN*, *GABA* receptor and *UBE3A* genes on chromosome 15q11–13, and the oxytocin receptor at 3p25–26.

Epigenetics

Epigenetic regulatory mechanisms have already been implicated in the pathogenesis of Rett syndrome and fragile X syndrome. The reelin gene (*RELN*) is regulated by DNA methylation, which can be modified by both gene (mutation) and environmental factors (prenatal exposures and postnatal experience). Regions on chromosomes 15q and 7q have been found to overlap with regions subject to genomic imprinting and, thus, are likely to confer risk for autism. Epigenetic studies also suggest a central role for GABAergic systems.

Environmental Risk Factors

Associated environmental risk factors that may contribute to autism include low birth weight, maternal education, delays in prenatal care, father's age (younger was associated with risk reduction), and termination of a prior pregnancy. Whether these are liabilities of risk for autism or markers of extant genetic abnormalities remain unknown. Other environmental influences include prenatal exposure to rubella infection, valproic acid, cocaine, and thalidomide.

Two factors that have received a great deal of media attention are the measles, mumps, and rubella (MMR) vaccine, and the ethyl mercury-containing preservative thimerosal that was, until 2001, commonly added to vaccines. Numerous independent investigations have failed to confirm an association between the MMR vaccine or thimerosal exposure or environmental mercury and autism. Aluminum in vaccines has also been studied and does not appear to play a causal role in autism.

Neurobiology of Autism

Brain Volume

Unusual brain growth patterns in children with autism were first reported in 2001 by Courchesne and colleagues. Head circumference in infants with ASD was found to be smaller at birth than that of healthy infants. However, between 6 and 14 months of age, there was an acceleration of head growth such that mean head growth was at the 84th percentile by 6 to 14 months. Further, this increase in head circumference was associated with larger cerebral cortex volumes at 2 to 5 years. Interestingly, at 12 years and older, differences in total brain volume between individuals with autism and typically developing individuals disappear, due to a slight decrease in volume in autism as compared to the increase in volume normally seen at this age.

MRI and fMRI Findings

Frontal lobe development is disrupted in autism, perhaps explaining the deficits in working memory, executive function, and adaptive function seen in individuals with autism. There is also reduced functional connectivity within and between neocortical systems in autism, impacting problem solving, language, working memory, and social cognition. The mirror neuron system, which is active both when imitating and when merely observing others' actions, is also impaired in autism and may contribute to the social–emotional deficits seen in autism.

Face Processing Deficits

Face processing impairments in autism are thought to be the result of fundamental impairments in the neural processing system specialized for faces (i.e., less activation of the fusiform gyrus) combined with fewer early experiences with faces due to decreased social interest and attention. Individuals with autism show abnormalities in how well they process faces, how fast they process faces, and in how they process faces (using features rather than a holistic approach). They also spend less time scanning the eye region and more time looking at mouths, body parts, and objects. Face processing impairments have also been demonstrated in parents and siblings of individuals with autism.

Comorbid Disorders and Behaviors

Intellectual Disability

Forty percent to 55% of individuals with autism also have intellectual disability or mental retardation. Deficits specific to autism include nonverbal communication, imitation, social cognition, play, and emotion recognition. Symptoms common to both autism and mental retardation include motor stereotypies, self-injurious behaviors, and sleep issues.

Seizure Disorders

The epilepsy prevalence rate in individuals with both autism and intellectual disability is 21.5%, as compared to 8% in those with autism alone. The pooled prevalence of epilepsy in females is about 34.5% versus 18.5% in males. Typical age of onset of epilepsy in autism is before 3 years of age or, more frequently, during puberty (11 to 14 years).

Attention-Deficit Hyperactivity Disorder

ADHD is a common initial diagnosis in autism; as many as 31% to 55% of children with autism also meet criteria for ADHD.

Tic Disorders

Roughly 22% of children and adolescents with autism have co-occurring tic disorders, half of those presenting with Tourette syndrome and half with chronic motor tics.

Anxiety and Obsessive–Compulsive Disorder/Phobias

Symptoms of anxiety are so common in autism (both in lower and higher functioning individuals) that they are thought to be part of the disorder. Anxiety in children with ASD tends to be focused on specific things and/or related to changes in routine, novel experiences, and transitions. Over 40% of children with autism are reported to meet diagnostic criteria for a specific phobia, with the most common being needles (shots), crowds, and loud noises. Almost as many (37%) meet criteria for obsessive–compulsive disorder, with half of those exhibiting compulsions involving another person (e.g., parents need to act or respond in a specific way). Also common is the compulsive behavior to repeatedly ask or say something.

Mood Disorders

As many as 30% of individuals with HFA and Asperger disorder also have depressive symptoms. Depression in autism leads to greater withdrawal, noncompliance, and aggressive behaviors. The co-occurrence of bipolar disorder and autism is much less commonly reported in children.

Psychosis

Psychosis in children with autism is also uncommon. The intense preoccupations and circumscribed interests common in autism resemble delusions and thought disorders; therefore, care must be taken when diagnosing these disorders.

Sensory Issues

Many clinicians believe that sensory dysfunction is central to autism. Typical sensitivities include excessive negative reactions to light, sound (e.g., the sound of household appliances), or touch (e.g., certain textures of clothing, objects touching the head), high pain tolerance, and sensory-seeking behaviors (e.g., licking and biting objects, seeking deep pressure by pressing against objects or people, fascination with touching certain textures).

Self-Injurious Behaviors

Self-injurious behaviors are commonly seen both in children with autism and children with intellectual disability, and include biting, head banging, and hair pulling. Self-injurious behaviors are more often seen in younger children, children with more severe symptoms of autism, and children with more severe cognitive and adaptive delays.

Eating and Sleeping Disturbances

Aberrant eating habits are commonly reported (over 90%) by parents of children with autism and fall into three categories: food selectivity, food refusal, and disruptive behaviors at mealtimes.

Sleep difficulties are also noted, including difficulty falling asleep, frequent nocturnal awakening, and waking too early in the morning.

Clinical Course

Early Onset

There appear to be two primary types of clinical onset in autism. With early onset, behavioral symptoms emerge within the first year of life, although these symptoms are not always obvious to parents. Symptoms as early as 8 to 12 months of age include failure to orient to name, lack of pointing and showing, decreased orienting to faces, and less frequent use of babble and words, among others. Of these behaviors, failure to respond to name is most often reported by parents in the first year and is easily assessed within the context of a well baby exam. After a few minutes of interaction, the physician should stand several feet away from (preferably behind) the child and call his or her name. Several attempts should be made with a brief pause in between. Children who do not respond to the first two attempts by turning their head and making eye contact should receive additional follow-up (see the section Assessment).

Regression

The second course of onset, occurring in approximately 30% of cases, is a period of fairly typical development followed by a loss of previously acquired skills typically occurring between 16 and 24 months of age. Losses can occur in social interest and responsiveness, communication, and adaptive skills, although a loss of language skills is almost always reported by parents. No differences in outcomes have been found between children with and without a regression.

Outcomes

Outcomes have improved with earlier diagnosis and treatment. About 50% of individuals with autism have fair to good outcomes based on occupation, friendships, and independent living. Regarding shorter-term outcomes, over 50% of children with autism followed from the age of 2 to 9 years achieved cognitive scores in the average range. The strongest predictors of positive outcomes (i.e., academic and social competence) for individuals with autism include IQ above 50, language (useful speech by the age of 5 years), adaptive functioning, and symptom severity.

Assessment

Early Screening and Diagnosis

The following section provides information on screening and diagnostic tools, as well as an evidence-based approach to assessment of ASDs. See also the American Academy of Pediatrics Clinical Report on Identification and Evaluation of Children with Autism Spectrum Disorders, listed in the Suggested Websites section at the end of this chapter.

Specific Symptoms to Assess

At birth, eye contact is present in typically developing infants and can be assessed at each well baby exam. Babies prefer to look at faces over objects. Engage the infant with talking and smiling; typically developing infants will orient to the face. *By 9 months*, providers can assess not only eye contact (as described above), but also social smiling, response to name, and response to social play (e.g., peek-a-boo). This assessment takes only a minute to complete. Engage the infant with talking and smiling, call the infant by name from several feet away and to the side of the infant, engage in peek-a-boo. Typically developing infants will smile, coo, look at the practitioner, turn when they hear their name, and show enjoyment during games such as peek-a-boo (by smiling and showing increased motor movements). *At 12 months*, most infants are making simple sounds ("ma" and "da"), using simple gestures (waving goodbye), and imitating actions (clap when you clap). By 12 months, most infants will also point to show an object, and follow an adult's point to an object (i.e., joint attention). Again, assessment for these skills takes only a minute or two during an office visit. Engage the infant by calling his or her name, then point to an object across the room and say "look." Play peek-a-boo or other social game (e.g., sing a baby song) and then clap. Wave hello and goodbye to the infant. If a child should fail any of these assessments, providers should obtain additional information from the parent via a clinical interview (to assess whether failure during the office visit is perhaps due to shyness; to determine if the child is showing these behaviors at home and in other settings). Referral to a child development clinic or autism-specific clinic for a more comprehensive evaluation may be warranted. If a child is showing delays in any area, referral to a state Birth-to-Three intervention program is also warranted.

Screening Tools for ASD

For children 16 to 35 months of age. While there are many screening tools available, only the most reliable are included in Table 16-3. The Modified-Checklist for Autism in Toddlers (M-CHAT), a 23-item yes/no parent checklist in the public domain, appears to be most promising for use with children 16 to 35 months of age. The M-CHAT is based on the earlier Checklist for Autism in Toddlers (CHAT), which functions best at capturing classic autistic disorder but not the broader spectrum. Failure of any two critical items or any three items total on the M-CHAT warrants additional assessment (i.e., referral to a specialty clinic). All children should be screened with the M-CHAT starting at 16 months of age. Prior to that time, practitioners should follow the *Act Early* guidelines from the Centers for Disease Control and Prevention, which are available at their website included at the end of this chapter.

For Children 4 Years of Age and Older

The Social Communication Questionnaire (SCQ) is recommended for children 4 years of age and older and is derived from the Autism Diagnostic Interview-Revised (ADI-R), which is used in specialty clinics and in autism research studies. The SCQ is a parent report questionnaire and takes only about 10 minutes to complete. Failure of 15 items or more on the SCQ warrants additional assessment, and possibly referral to a specialty clinic.

Other Tools Used in Specialty Clinics

The Screening Tool for Autism in Two-Year-Olds (STAT) and Pervasive Developmental Disorders Screening Test (PDDST) are designed to be administered by trained clinicians and require more time (20 to 30 minutes) than is often available in primary care settings. The Autism Observation Scale for Infants (AOSI) is designed for infants as young as 6 months; it too, however, requires administration by a trained and reliable clinician and takes about 20 minutes.

Diagnostic Tools

In order to accurately diagnose an ASD, both a detailed history of social, communication, and behavioral development as well as direct observation are necessary. Most autism clinics use the ADI-R and the Autism Diagnostic Observation Schedule (ADOS) to gather this essential information; both require specialized training. The ADI-R provides information on early history as well as low-frequency behaviors that may not be observed during an office visit. The ADOS has four modules and can be used with individuals aged 2 years and older. Instruments used in the assessment of ASDs are summarized in Table 16-2.

Evidence-Based Assessment

A best practice, comprehensive approach to assessing ASDs is typically a combined approach involving a number of professionals: the general practitioner who first screens for autism symptoms, diagnostic assessment by a professional with expertise in ASDs, occupational and speech and language therapists, neuropsychologists, and social workers. This assessment

TABLE 16-2	Screening Instruments and Diagnostic Sensitivity			
	Age	Sensitivity	Specificity	Setting
Screening Instrument				
Checklist for Autism in Toddlers (CHAT)	18+ mo	35%	98%	General practitioner
CHAT Denver Modification	18+ mo	89%	93%	General practitioner
Modified-CHAT (M-CHAT)	16–30 mo	97%	99%	General practitioner
Social Communication Questionnaire (SCQ)	4+ years	85% 75%	75% (PDD vs. non-PDD) 60% (AD vs. PDD)	General practitioner
Screening Tool for Autism in Two-Year-Olds (STAT)	2–3 years	92%	85%	Autism specialist
PDD Screening Test	18–48 mo			Autism specialist
PDDST Stage 1 Stage 2 Stage 3		92% 73% 58%	91% (primary care) 49% (developmental clinics) 60% (autism clinics)	
Autism Observation Scale for Infants (AOSI)	6–18 mo	n/a	n/a	Autism specialist
Diagnostic Instrument				
Autism Diagnostic Interview Revised (ADI-R)	Mental Age of 2+ years	83%–91%[a]	41%–72%[a]	Autism specialist
Autism Diagnostic Observation Schedule (ADOS)	Nonverbal Mental Age of 18+ mo	92%–100%[b]	18%–74%[b]	Autism specialist

[a]Depending on population (i.e., with profound mental retardation; younger than 36 months; mixed group of individuals with autism, PDD-NOS, Asperger disorder, and non-ASD).
[b]Depending on population and whether target diagnosis is autistic disorder, or all three spectrum diagnoses.

should include the following: screening for medical issues, including seizures, sleep difficulties, pica, and sensory-based behaviors that impact day-to-day function; hearing evaluation by an audiologist; screening for psychiatric and behavioral conditions, such as anxiety, depression, and ADHD; assessment of cognitive, language, adaptive, and neuropsychological functioning to inform educational and treatment planning (this can be done in part through state early intervention programs and school districts, and in some cases referral to a neuropsychologist may be warranted); consultation with the school team to inform specialized services and accommodations (often performed by a psychologist or neuropsychologist); occupational therapy evaluation for gross and fine motor impairments and sensory-based behaviors; and assessment of the family system and access to resources (often performed by a psychologist or social worker). The essentials of evidence-based assessment are summarized in Table 16-3.

Treatment

The National Research Council and the Committee on Educational Interventions for Children with Autism recommend a minimum of 25 hours per week of intervention for young children with autism, to include state and school-based programs as well as private and

TABLE 16-3	Essentials of Assessment for Autism Spectrum Disorders

All children should be screened for ASD at well baby exams starting at 16 months of age, and continuing through at least 24 months to capture children who may regress; the Checklist for Autism in Toddlers (M-CHAT) is an excellent instrument for this purpose.

Older children with atypical social relatedness, communication difficulties, and unusual interests and behaviors should also be screened; the Social Communication Questionnaire (SCQ) is appropriate for use with children 4 years and older.

Early symptoms (present by as young as 1 year of age) include not responding to name and reduced eye contact. Assess also for social smiling, pointing and showing objects to others, making simple sounds ("ma" and "da"), and imitating actions (clapping, waving) by 12 months.

A best practices assessment includes screening for medical and genetic disorders, audiological evaluation, screening for behavioral conditions such as ADHD, and assessment of cognitive, language, and adaptive functioning.

Gold standard diagnostic measures include the Autism Diagnostic Interview-Revised (ADI-R) for a detailed developmental history and the Autism Diagnostic Observation Schedule (ADOS) for assessment of social, communication, and behavioral symptoms; both require specialized training.

home-based therapies. Each child with ASD has a unique symptom profile and pattern of strengths and weaknesses, necessitating an individualized treatment approach. That being said, there are a number of specific interventions commonly used for children and adolescents with autism. The essentials of the treatment of children diagnosed with ASDs are summarized in Table 16-4.

TABLE 16-4	Essentials of Treatment for Autism Spectrum Disorders

The National Research Council recommends a minimum of 25 hours per week of intervention services for young children with autism.

Intensive behavioral interventions have the most empirical support and include ABA, Pivotal Response Training (PRT), Incidental Teaching, the Denver Model, TEACCH, Floortime, and Relationship Development Intervention (RDI).

Interventions targeting language and communication are essential as early language skills are a primary predictor of best outcomes for children with autism.

Social skills interventions target the core features of the ASDs and are most effective when they are part of the child's school program; parent involvement has also been shown to be critical for social skills interventions to be most effective.

Special education services addressing academic, speech/language, adaptive, and social skills deficits are critical components of a treatment program; these objectives are achieved through an Individualized Education Plan (IEP) or 504 Plan.

Private therapies addressing communication, motor deficits, and social skills are often warranted.

Pharmacological interventions can be helpful in addressing related behaviors (hyperactivity, irritability, self-injurious behaviors) with cascading effects on core symptoms as well.

Families may qualify for services (e.g., respite, in-home behavioral support) through their state's division of developmental disabilities (DDD) and should be encouraged to apply.

Psychosocial Interventions

Behavioral Interventions

Early, intensive behavioral intervention in autism is associated with higher cognitive scores and a greater likelihood of developing language and being placed in a regular education classroom. A lack of comparative studies precludes recommendation of one behavioral treatment over another, but there are a number of solid approaches.

Applied Behavior Analysis

Applied behavior analysis (ABA) is a therapeutic approach that has been used with children with autism since the 1960s and relies on basic principles of learning and behavior to promote language and social, cognitive, and adaptive functioning; it also has the most empirical support among the various treatments for autism. Intensive (i.e., 25 to 40 hours per week) ABA intervention can lead to normal or near normal functioning for almost 50% of children. A functional analysis of behavior and motivation, followed by clear goals that can be observed and measured daily or weekly, is the backbone of an effective ABA program. These programs are typically conducted at home in a one-to-one format (although the same principles are used in state and school-based intervention programs), can be quite expensive to implement (roughly $25,000 for the first year to cover the cost of a supervisor [generally a PhD level person] and therapists), and are not typically covered by insurance.

Other approaches that employ ABA principles, but capitalize on naturally occurring opportunities for teaching and emphasize child motivation and initiation, include pivotal response training (PRT), incidental teaching, and the Denver model. PRT involves techniques to improve the pivotal behavior of motivation. Originally developed to increase communication and decrease disruptive behaviors, PRT is now used to teach children with autism a variety of skills. A PRT training manual can be found at the Qwest website, listed in the Suggested Websites section at the end of this chapter. Incidental teaching refers to the use of ABA principles in natural, typical settings, such as in daily routines with caregiver and child. This involves structuring goals so that they occur within ongoing, typical activities instead of sitting face to face with the child at a table in a clinical setting. More information can be found at the autism network website. The Denver model combines both ABA techniques and learning-through-play techniques, and can be delivered in any setting and by caregivers, not just professionals. There is detailed information about this model on the UC Davis Mind Institute website.

The TEACCH Method

TEACCH (Treatment and Education of Autistic and related Communication-handicapped CHildren) is an approach most often used by teachers in the classroom, but can also be used by caregivers at home. This approach is based on modifying the environment to support skill acquisition and generalization, as well as independence. Visual and rote memory strengths of children with autism are used to promote less well-developed skills in communication, cognition, and social interaction. This is done by using visual schedules, checklists, and other visual cues (e.g., cards with visual icons) to illustrate daily routines and expectations, as well as to provide predictability, thus easing anxiety, frustration, and disruptive behaviors. More information can be found at Division TEACCH website.

Floortime

Floortime is a developmental, individual differences, relationship-based (DIR) treatment approach that has been used for over 25 years with children with autism, although most of the evidence for its efficacy is anecdotal. This intervention emphasizes following the child's lead and joining the child so that they can be drawn into a shared world. The ultimate goal is for the child to relate and communicate in a reciprocal manner. Three basic abilities are targeted:

establishing closeness, exchanging emotional gestures, and using words or symbols with emotional intent. Like ABA, Floortime can be difficult for families to implement as it is expensive, labor-intensive, and time-consuming. Information on Floortime techniques is available for families at the Floortime website, included at the end of this chapter.

Relationship Development Intervention

Another relationship-based approach that has received much attention recently is Relationship Development Intervention (RDI). This intervention is parent-delivered and involves scaffolding frequent opportunities for the child so they can learn to respond in more flexible ways to novel and challenging situations. Clinicians and parents may find detailed information about the RDI on the RDI website.

Language and Communication Interventions

When behavioral interventions targeting language are implemented prior to age 5, a majority (90%) of children with autism can learn to use verbal communication as a primary method of communication. ABA and other traditional behavioral approaches have been used to target language skills in children with autism. In addition to behavioral approaches, traditional speech and language therapy is an essential component of an intervention program and can augment services the child may be receiving at school, as school-based services are often limited. In addition to traditional techniques, two specialized methods of treatment have been used with success with some children with autism. The first is the PROMPT method (Prompts for Restructuring Oral Muscular Phonetic Targets), a dynamic tactile method of treatment for motor speech disorders based on touch pressure, kinesthetic, and proprioceptive cues. The Prompt Institute website provides families a comprehensive description of their treatment approach. A second approach is the Hanen method, wherein speech and language pathologists educate and coach caregivers on how to foster the child's communication development and make learning to communicate a natural part of everyday life. Several Hanen programs have been developed specifically for children with autism. These programs are outlined on the Hanen website.

Social Skills Interventions

A variety of techniques have been shown to be effective in ameliorating social skills deficits in children with autism, including didactic instruction, role-playing, social stories, social scripts, peer modeling, and video modeling. Social skills interventions capitalize on naturally occurring opportunities. With improved social skills come improvements in other areas, such as communication and behavior. Social skills interventions are most effective when implemented in the school setting and when parents are actively involved. Families are encouraged to seek social skills training opportunities for their child through friendship or social skill groups at school, and through private group therapy programs taught by psychologists, therapists, and speech and language providers.

Special Education Services

The Individuals with Disabilities Education Act (IDEA) ensures services to children with disabilities from birth to age 21. Schools are required to provide fair and unbiased evaluations to determine eligibility for specialized education services, which form the basis of an Individualized Education Program (IEP). The diagnosis of autism alone does not guarantee eligibility. If a child does not qualify for an IEP, another option is to obtain services through Section 504 of the Federal Rehabilitation Act of 1973, which allows for educational accommodations and modifications to help children with autism succeed in school. Accommodations typically include use of individualized visual schedules, checklists, and instructions for multiple-step assignments, designated areas where the child can take a break if feeling overwhelmed, work dividers to eliminate auditory and visual distractions, additional time to complete examinations and assignments, allowing alternate modalities (e.g., oral vs. written), special arrangements for situations likely to cause distress (e.g., fire alarms, assemblies), and behavior modification plans to reinforce appropriate behavior and work completion. Early intervention programs for children from birth to the age of 3 vary widely from state to state. Some involve only limited services (e.g., 1 hour per week of speech and language therapy) while others provide intensive one-on-one behavioral interventions for children with autism. Families should contact their state Family Resource Coordinator to obtain information and to develop an Individualized Family Services Plan (IFSP) for children ages birth to 3.

Occupational/Physical Therapy Services

Occupational and/or physical therapy can address motor deficits, adaptive deficits, and sensory issues. School-based evaluations typically assess motor and adaptive functioning; referral to a private occupational or physical therapist may be warranted for comprehensive evaluation and treatment planning.

State and Federal Resources

Families may also qualify for assistance through their state Department of Developmental Disabilities (DDD) based on diagnosis. Eligibility is often limited to those with the full diagnosis of autistic disorder and/or those with intellectual disability. Services can include in-home behavioral support and respite care. For older individuals, vocational assistance and housing assistance may be available. In addition to DDD services, some families with limited income may qualify for Supplemental Security Income (SSI).

Pharmacological Interventions

Pharmacological treatments for children with autism are typically focused on associated behaviors and symptoms, such as aggression, inattention and hyperactivity, irritability, and mood and anxiety symptoms. While they do not directly target the core symptoms of autism, by treating associated behaviors, pharmacological treatments may allow other interventions (behavioral, educational) to be more successful. Surveys suggest that approximately 30% of children with autism are prescribed at least one psychotropic drug.

Psychostimulants

Studies of methylphenidate indicate highest response rates in children with Asperger disorder and PDD versus autistic disorder, but with less symptom amelioration and more adverse side effects as compared to children without ASD. Currently, studies are in progress to determine the efficacy of amphetamines and nonstimulant agents such as atomoxetine.

Antidepressants

Serotonin reuptake inhibitors (SSRIs) are among the most widely prescribed medications for children diagnosed with ASDs. Anecdotal reports have suggested that SSRIs may be useful in treating repetitive, or what appear to be compulsive, behaviors in children with ASDs. However, King and colleagues' recent randomized controlled study of 149 youths diagnosed with ASDs found that citalopram is ineffective in decreasing such moderate-to-severe repetitive behaviors. There has been some limited data that show that fluoxetine may have positive effects on language, cognition, and social relatedness, and reduce irritability, stereotypic behaviors, and inappropriate speech. However, a multisite placebo-controlled trial targeting repetitive behaviors with fluoxetine was also negative. Other SSRIs have not been well studied in children with ASDs. Overall, based on information available to date, clinicians should be cautious in using SSRIs, particularly because of their propensity to cause increased motor activity, impulsiveness, and sleep disturbance, and should carefully monitor children for their response and progress.

Tricyclic antidepressants, venlafaxine, and bupropion all require further studies, as do the alpha-2 adrenergic agonists.

Antipsychotics

Typical antipsychotics, particularly haloperidol, have been shown to reduce maladaptive behaviors when prescribed at an optimal mean dose of about 1.12 mg/kg/day. Among atypical antipsychotics used to treat self-injurious behaviors, tantrums, and aggression, risperidone has been the most widely studied (even in children as young as 2 years). Risperidone and aripiprazole are approved by the Food and Drug Administration (FDA) to treat irritability and aggression in autism. Despite the dearth of evidence for the use of other atypical antipsychotics, quetiapine and ziprasidone are also widely used to treat ASDs.

Other Medications

Medications used to treat patients with Alzheimer, including donepezil, galantamine, and memantine, have been reported to show some promise in reducing ADHD symptoms and aggression in children with ASD. D-cycloserine is also being studied to target social relatedness and reciprocity. Current pharmacological approaches to children diagnosed with ASDs are summarized in Table 16-5.

Non-Traditional Interventions

Secretin, a gastrointestinal hormone, has been one of the most carefully scrutinized and well-studied treatments for autism following the 1998 report of three children who received intravenous secretin during diagnostic endoscopy and later reported resolution of autism symptoms. Unfortunately, over a dozen subsequent studies failed to confirm a treatment effect.

Despite a lack of empirical evidence, the most popular autism diet is the gluten-free, casein-free (GFCF) diet. Some parents report reduced overactivity, inattention, and sleep problems, while others report no changes in behavior. A Cochrane review of the literature in 2008 concluded that current evidence for the efficacy of this and other diets is poor. The National Institute of Health is currently sponsoring an investigation of the efficacy of a gluten-free diet in the treatment of autism. Probiotics, digestive enzymes, magnesium, cod liver oil, and vitamin supplements (e.g., B6, B12, Super Nu-Thera, dimethylglycine) are also popular alternative interventions used for autism, although empirical evidence is lacking.

Controversial Interventions

There are many other therapies targeted at improving symptoms of autism that families may read about, none of which has empirical support and some of which are dangerous, including chelation, holding therapy, cranial sacral therapy, equestrian therapy, hyperbaric oxygen, and others.

Conclusion

The diagnosis of ASDs is usually made in early childhood based on core deficits in relatedness and communication. Comorbidity with other psychiatric, medical, and developmental disorders may also be evident, both in early childhood and across development. Therefore, assessment is ongoing at each developmental stage and treatment planning is multimodal. The primary interventions focus on educational programs and behavioral interventions. There are now many interventions that help children with ASDs to better approach and achieve developmental expectations. Schools continue to comprise a primary site and source of interventions for these youths. Psychotropic medications may augment educational and psychosocial interventions by ameliorating associated symptoms, decreasing aggression and self-injurious behaviors, and increasing youths' flexibility and, therefore, improve their ability to benefit from various inter-

TABLE 16-5   Pharmacological Interventions

Medication	Target Symptoms	Comments
Stimulants: methylphenidate, dextroamphetamines, amphetamine salts	Hyperactivity	• Effectiveness in decreasing hyperactivity and increasing attention span is variable in youth diagnosed with ASDs • Stimulants may increase agitation and stereotypic behaviors including self-injurious behaviors • Anecdotally, stimulants appear more effective in Asperger disorder than in other ASDs
SSRIs: fluoxetine, sertraline, citalopram, escitalopram, fluvoxamine	Anxiety Perseveration Compulsions Depression Social Isolation	• SSRIs have been popular due to anecdotal reports of effectiveness on behavior, language, cognition, and social relatedness and few adverse effects • A recent randomized controlled study showed citalopram was not effective and increased restlessness, hyperactivity, agitation, and insomnia
Antipsychotics: risperidone, olanzapine, quetiapine, aripiprazole, ziprasidone, haloperidol, thioridazine	Aggression Agitation Irritability Hyperactivity Self-injurious behavior	• Thioridazine and haloperidol have been the most extensively investigated medications for use in ASD • Atypical antipsychotics now comprise the primary medication used for treating behavioral disturbances in ASDs • The complications of severe weight gain, hypertension, hyperlipidemia, and hyperglycemia in the use of atypical antipsychotics warrant caution in the use of atypical antipsychotics with children
Alpha-2a agonists: guanfacine, clonidine	Hyperactivity Aggression Sleep dysregulation	• Anecdotally, alpha-2a agonists may be effective in treating hyperactivity • Clonidine may be useful for sleep dysregulation
Selected anticonvulsants/ mood stabilizers and lithium carbonate	Aggression Self-injurious behaviors	• Also may be useful for cyclical behavior patterns • Need for blood monitoring for lithium, valproate, and carbamazepine limits their use in ASD children without epilepsy
Naltrexone	Self-injurious behaviors	• Naltrexone has been shown to be effective to decrease self-injurious behaviors (not specific to ASD), but usefulness in clinical practice has never been robust • Hepatic monitoring needed
Amantadine	Hyperactivity Irritability Aggression	• Studies suggest amantadine may be effective in treating behavioral disturbances in children diagnosed with ASDs
Melatonin	Sleep dysregulation	• May be effective in treating insomnia in ASD youth

ASD, autism spectrum disorder; SSRI, Serotonin reuptake inhibitor.

ventions. Children with ASDs also experience psychiatric illnesses like mood and anxiety disorders that should be treated. The desperation of families with a child diagnosed with ASD may lead away from evidence-based treatments to unproven and potentially harmful alternative interventions. Clinicians can help to guide families to appropriate interventions throughout the child's development. With appropriate interventions, functioning and quality of life can greatly improve.

CASE VIGNETTES

VIGNETTE 1: TYLER, ASPERGER DISORDER

Tyler is a 15-year-old male who presents with his parents for evaluation of significant symptoms of anxiety and school refusal. Tyler's parents report that he met all developmental milestones on time, although he did show some early problems in motor planning. His parents did not become concerned about Tyler until the second grade, when he began to exhibit extreme anxiety at school, sweating so much his desk would become wet. Academically, Tyler was showing advanced abilities in some areas, such as math. Due to his growing anxiety, his parents placed him in a private school halfway through the second grade year. From second grade to eighth grade he remained at a private school, but constantly struggled with getting homework done. Last year he entered public school, but refused to do homework; by the end of the year he stopped going altogether. In addition to concerns about his education, Tyler's parents note that he has never shown much interest in developing friendships. When the examiner greets Tyler, he looks up briefly and responds with an almost inaudible "hi." During the hour-long assessment, Tyler talks at length about his interests, which include antique watches and mechanisms used in firearms. His descriptions include excessive amounts of detail, particularly involving numbers, such as the weight, cost, and make of the gun safe he wants to buy. His language is more formal than expected for his age, and he shows little interest in participating in a reciprocal exchange, in spite of the examiner's repeated attempts to insert comments or change the topic. Tyler reports having one friend, although his parents confirm that he has spent the entire summer in his room looking up information on watches online. He denies feeling lonely and reports being happy spending time alone. Tyler's parents are very concerned about the widening gap between Tyler's social development and that of his peers, as well as his education and future job prospects. Birth and family history are positive for perinatal problems and an ASD in a paternal family member. Tyler is diagnosed with Asperger disorder and recommendations include an alternative school program (given his age and lack of interest in public school), vocational training, a social skills training intervention, online resources for teens with Asperger, and support group information for his parents.

VIGNETTE 2: ETHAN, EARLY ONSET AUTISM

Ethan is a 4½-year-old male who was referred for an ASD evaluation due to concerns by his speech and language pathologist. Ethan's parents report first concerns about Ethan at 24 months of age due to unusual behaviors, including rituals with food and compulsions around wearing hats. Ethan was about 12 months old when he said his first word, but did not begin using phrases until 4 years of age. Currently, Ethan is reported to have poor eye contact, limited use of gestures such as pointing and waving goodbye, limited pretend play and imitation skills, and limited interest in peers. He does like to show objects to his parents, but less often than other children at that age. Ethan frequently engages in repetitive play, including watching a particular segment of a video over and over, spinning wheels, lining things up, and hoarding objects. Ethan is also ritualistic in how he eats certain foods and compulsive about putting things in an exact order. He is showing both sensory-based behaviors (likes hard pressure, puts his fingers in his ears when hearing everyday sounds) as well as repetitive finger mannerisms. During the assessment, Ethan had difficulty sustaining attention and frequently jumped up to walk around the room, disrupting the assessment. He used short phrases to comment on the materials and to respond to questions, but his articulation was poor and he often used odd intonation (i.e., everything was said with the intonation of a question). He could not sustain a short back-and-forth conversation about pets, and his eye contact was avoidant. He refused to play pretend with a set of toy figures, and rather than participating in routines with the examiner, he preferred to take the toys aside and play by himself. Finally, he rarely initiated interactions, although he could be briefly drawn into interactions initiated by the examiner. Ethan's parents were primarily concerned with his "odd behaviors" and school services. Ethan was diagnosed with autistic disorder and recommendations were made for specialized education services at school delivered by a multidisciplinary team, an ABA home program (although additional resources were provided for parents to learn and deliver this type of intervention themselves due to family financial constraints), private speech and language therapy to augment school services, visual supports to structure his environment at school and at home, medical and genetic follow-up, classroom resources and strategies to help with problems with attention, and resources and reading for Ethan's family, to include support groups and information on applying for benefits through the state Department of Developmental Disabilities. It was also suggested that Ethan be reevaluated in 2 years to assess progress and assist with treatment planning.

BIBLIOGRAPHY

American Psychiatric Association. *Diagnostic and Statistical Manual of Mental Disorders.* 4th ed. Text Revision. Washington, DC: American Psychiatric Association; 2000.

Asperger H. Die 'autistischen psychopathen' im kindesalter. *Archiv für Psychiatrie und Nervenkrankheiten.* 1944;117:76–136. [Translated by Frith U. In: Frith U, ed. *Autism and Asperger Syndrome.* Cambridge: Cambridge University Press; 1991:36–92.]

Courchesne E, Karns CM, Davis HR, et al. Unusual brain growth patterns in early life in patients with autistic disorder: an MRI study. *Neurology.* 2001;57:245–254.

Fombonne E. The changing epidemiology of autism. *J Appl Res Dev Disabil.* 2005;18:281–294.

Kanner L. Autistic disturbances of affective content. *Nerv Child.* 1943;2:217–250.

King BH, Hollander E, Sikich L, et al. Lack of efficacy of citalopram in children with autism spectrum disorders and high levels of repetitive behavior: citaprolam ineffective in children with autism. *Arch Gen Psychiatry.* 2009;66:583–590.

Lord C, Rutter M, LeCouteur A. Autism diagnostic interview-revised: a revised version of a diagnostic interview for caregivers of individuals with possible pervasive developmental disorders. *J Autism Dev Disord.* 1994;24:659–685.

Lord C, Risi S, Lambrecht L, et al. The autism diagnostic observation schedule-generic: a standard measure of social and communication deficits associated with the spectrum of autism. *J Autism Dev Disord.* 2000;30:205–223.

Milward C, Ferriter M, Calver S, et al. Gluten and casein free diets for autistic spectrum disorder. *Cochrane Data Syst Rev.* 2008;(2):CD003498.

National Research Council. *Educating Children with Autism.* Washington, DC: National Academy Press; 2001.

Research Units on Pediatric Psychopharmacology (RUPP) Autism Network. Randomized, controlled, crossover trial of methylphenidate in pervasive developmental disorders with hyperactivity. *Arch Gen Psychiatry.* 2005;62:1266–1274.

Schellenberg GD, Dawson G, Sung YJ, et al. Evidence for multiple loci from a genome scan of autism kindreds. *Mol Psychiatry.* 2006;11:1049–1060.

Toth K, Dawson G, Meltzoff AN, et al. Early social, imitation, play, and language abilities in young non-autistic siblings of children with autism. *J Autism Dev Disord.* 2007;37:145–157.

SUGGESTED READINGS

Michael Powers
Children with Autism: A Parent's Guide
Woodbine Press, (2000) Paperback
(A good reference for parents that includes information about diagnostic criteria, advocacy via the Internet, applied behavior analysis, and Individuals with Disabilities Education Act (IDEA))

Sally Ozonoff, Geraldine Dawson, James McPartland
A Parent's Guide to Asperger Syndrome and High Functioning Autism: How to Meet the Challenges and Help
    Your Child Thrive
Guilford Press (2002) Hardcover
(An informative book for parents with children who have Asperger syndrome or high functioning autism)

Tony Atwood
The Complete Guide Asperger's Sydrome
Jessica Kingsley Publishers (2008) Paperback
(A definitive handbook with information on all aspects of the syndrome for children through adults)

Committee on Educational Interventions for Children with Autism
Educating Children Autism
National Academy Press (2001) Hardcover
(This volume outlines an interdisciplinary approach to education for children with autism spectrum disorders)

Catherine Maurice, Gina Green, Stephen Luce
Behavioral Intervention for Young Children with Autism: A Manual for Parent and Professionals
Pro-Ed (1996) paperback
(Provides a solid information about applied behavioral analysis and other interventions for young children with autism)

Robert Koegel and Lynn Koegel
Teaching Children with Autism, Strategies for Initiating Positive Interactions, and Improving Learning Opportunities
Paul H Brookes Publishing Company (1995)
(More geared for professionals with a good summary of various aspects of treating children with autism)

Michelle Garcia Winner
Inside Out: What Makes a Person with Social Cognitive Deficits Tick
Michelle Garcia Winner (2000) Paperback
(This volume helps anyone develop an understanding of the origins of social dysfunction in children with Asperger
    syndrome and other youths with cognitive deficits)

Jed Baker
The Social Skills Picture Book: Teaching Play, Emotion, and Communication to Children with Autism
Future Horizons (2003) paperback
(A wonderful aid with pictures for therapists and teachers who work with children and adolescents with higher
    functioning autism spectrum disorders)

Temple Grandin
The Way I See It: A Personal Look at Autism and Asperger's
Future Horizons (2008) paperback
(A book filled with personal stories of the inner life of a person with autism and what works best for helping them)

Sandra Harris and Beth Glasberg
Siblings of Children with Autism: A Guide for Families
Woodbine House (2003) paperback
(Provides guidance to parents on sibling issues addresses the many issues that confront brothers or sisters with an
    autistic sibling)

SUGGESTED WEBSITES

AAP Autism Report: American Academy of Pediatrics Clinical Report on Identification and Evaluation of
    Children with Autism Spectrum Disorders, with information for both families and professionals, available at:
    http://www.aap.org/healthtopics/autism.cfm. Accessed October 2, 2009.

Modified-Checklist for Autism in Toddlers: The M-CHAT is a 23-item yes/no parent checklist that can be
    downloaded free along with scoring instructions from the website:
    http://www2.gsu.edu/~psydlr/Diana_L._Robins,_Ph.D..html. Accessed 10/02/09, and from:
    http://www2.gsu.edu/~wwwpsy/faculty/M-CHAT.pdf.

CDC Act Early Guidelines: Basic information regarding developmental guidelines for parents and families
    is available at: http://www.cdc.gov/actearly. Accessed October 2, 2009.

Pivotal Response Training (PRT): Originally developed to increase communication and decrease disruptive
    behaviors, PRT is now used to teach children with autism a variety of skills. A training manual can be found at:
    http://www.users.qwest.net/~tbharris/prt.htm. Accessed October 2, 2009.

Applied Behavioral Analysis (ABA): Incidental teaching refers to the use of ABA principles in natural, typical
    settings, such as in daily routines with caregiver and child. This involves structuring goals so that they occur
    within ongoing, typical activities instead of sitting face to face with the child at a table in a clinical setting.
    More information can be found at: http://www.autismnetwork.org. Accessed October 2, 2009.

The Denver model: The Denver model combines both ABA techniques and learning-through-play techniques, and can be delivered in any setting and by caregivers, not just professionals. For more information see: http://www.ucdmc.ucdavis.edu/edsl/esdm/description.html. Accessed October 2, 2009.

Treatment and Education of Autistic and related Communication-handicapped CHildren (TEACCH): Developed by Eric Schoppler in the 1970s, the TEACCH programs have been helping children with ASD and educating families for many years. More information can be found at Division TEACCH at: http://www.teacch.com/. Accessed October 2, 2009.

Floortime: Developed by Stanley Greenspan, Floortime is a specific technique to follow a child's natural emotions and interests in developing their mastery of social, emotional, and cognitive capacities. For more information see http://www.icdl.com/dirFloortime/overview/index.shtml. Accessed October 2, 2009.

Relationship Development Intervention (RDI): RDI is a relationship-based approach treatment intervention that is parent-delivered. For more information see: http://www.rdiconnect.com/. Accessed October 2, 2009.

Prompts for Restructuring Oral Muscular Phonetic Targets (PROMPT): This method uses prompts for restructuring oral muscular phonetic targets, a dynamic tactile method of treatment for motor speech disorders based on touch pressure, kinesthetic, and proprioceptive cues used in children with autism spectrum disorders. Available at: http://www.promptinstitute.com/. Accessed October 2, 2009.

The Hanen method: The Hanen method is for promoting communication skills in child with communication disorders and autism spectrum disorders. Several Hanen programs have been developed specifically for children with autism. Available at: http://www.hanen.org. Accessed October 2, 2009.

Supplemental Security Income (SSI): In addition to DDD services, some families with limited income may qualify for SSI. For more information see: http://www.ssa.gov/pgm/links_ssi.htm.

REVIEW QUESTIONS

1. What is the best screening tool for children under age 3 years in primary care settings?
   a. Autism Diagnostic Observation Schedule (ADOS)
   b. Children's Autism Rating Scale (CARS)
   c. Autism Observation Scale for Infants (AOSI)
   d. Modified Checklist for Autism in Toddlers (M-CHAT)
   e. Autism Behavior Checklist (ABC)

2. Which psychiatric diagnosis in **NOT** commonly seen in children with Autism Spectrum Disorders?
   a. Schizophrenia
   b. Intellectual disability
   c. Attention deficit hyperactivity disorder
   d. Seizure disorders
   e. Anxiety disorders

3. Core interventions for children with autism spectrum disorders include all of the following **EXCEPT:**
   a. Psychodynamic psychotherapy
   b. Speech and language therapies
   c. Behavior modification
   d. Social skills training

4. What behaviors can be directly assessed within the context of a well child visit?
   a. Imitation
   b. Vocalizing simple sounds
   c. Response to name
   d. Eye contact
   e. All of the above

5. What are the earliest (12 months and younger) emerging behavioral symptom(s) of autism?
   a. Lack of response to name
   b. Lack of eye contact
   c. Lack of smiling
   d. b and c
   e. a and b

Answers: 1-d, 2-a, 3-a, 4-e, 5-e

CHAPTER

17

David Breiger, Ph.D.
and Jenise Jensen, Ph.D.

Learning Disabilities

Introduction and Background

Reports of individuals who acquired a sudden inability to read, write, or perform mathematical calculations after some type of neurological insult have been published since the 17th century. However, it was a description by Dr. W. Pringle Morgan in 1896 of a 14-year-old boy named Percy that led to the hypothesis that learning difficulties were due to a specific congenital or developmental disorder. Dr. Morgan's report of Percy's difficulty with learning to read, despite his overall normal intellect and intact visual and mental calculation skills, led another doctor, James Hinshelwood, MD, to conclude that this difficulty was due to problems with the visual memory system for words. The term "congenital word blindness" was coined in the early 1900s to describe this condition and represents the beginning of the research in the field of learning disabilities (LDs).

Later modifications to Hinshelwood's theory resulted in the hypothesis that the inability to learn to read was due to problems with left–right orientation and strephosymbolia, or twisted word imagery, that was caused by a lack of cerebral dominance. Therefore, it was reasoned that deficits in the visual system resulted in seeing letters backwards ("b" for "d") or transposing letters in words ("was" for "saw"). Until as recently as 30 years ago, this was one of the leading theories about the causes of developmental reading problems.

Another important point in the history of understanding childhood LDs was the 1918 flu pandemic. Many children who survived demonstrated attention, perceptual-motor, learning, and behavior problems despite having normal physical and neurological examinations. Because these difficulties could not be readily attributed to mental retardation or other forms of social or emotional disturbance, the term "minimal brain damage" was used to indicate that these learning and attention problems were due to some congenital factor intrinsic to the child. Further research and debate resulted in the term "minimal brain dysfunction" to reflect that a specific brain insult was not required to cause these problems. Attempts to identify neurological soft signs that might be diagnostic and predictive of which children would develop learning problems were also prominent throughout this period, to no avail.

It was not until the last 40 years that the official terms "learning disability" and "learning disorder" came into popular use. Dr. Samuel Kirk, a psychologist and special educator, first coined the term *specific learning disability* in 1963 to describe a group of children who had disorders of development in language, speech, reading, and associated communication skills that were not due to either sensory handicaps or mental retardation. The following chapter provides a summary of the current understanding of LDs, including their clinical features and course, prevalence, and etiological factors. Issues of assessment, identification, and treatment of LDs will also be discussed. The majority of this chapter will be primarily targeted at reading disabilities (RDs) as it has been the most researched, and hence is the best understood, of the LDs.

The Individuals with Disabilities Education Act (IDEA)

The term Learning Disorders is used in the *Diagnostic and Statistical Manual of Mental Disorders*, Fourth Edition, Text Revision (DSM-IV-TR) to refer to a group of disorders that are characterized by learning problems resulting in an individual's measured academic achievement falling substantially below the level expected given the person's chronological age, educational level, and intellectual ability. The three primary LD diagnoses defined by the DSM-IV-TR are Reading Disorder, Mathematics Disorder, and Disorder of Written Language. The DSM-IV-TR also allows for the diagnosis of Learning Disorder Not Otherwise Specified (LD-NOS) to account for learning problems that do meet criteria for any specific LD.

The terms *learning disorder* and *learning disability* have largely been interchangeable in both the educational and psychiatric literature since the federal government officially adopted Kirk's term "specific learning disability" in 1975 with the passage of Public Law 94-142. This federal law mandated schools to provide publicly funded special education and related services to students whose disabilities adversely affected their educational performance. PL 94-142 is currently named the Individuals with Disabilities Education Act (IDEA). The IDEA governs how states and public agencies provide early intervention, special education, and related services to more than 6.5 million eligible infants, toddlers, children, and adolescents with disabilities across the United States. Children from birth to 2 years of age with disabilities and their families receive early intervention services under IDEA Part C. Children and adolescents (ages 3 to 21) receive special education and related services under IDEA Part B.

The IDEA defines the term "Specific Learning Disability" as: "A disorder in one or more of the basic psychological processes involved in understanding or in using language, spoken or written, that may manifest itself in an imperfect ability to listen, speak, read, write, spell, or to do mathematical calculations, including conditions such as perceptual disabilities, brain injury, minimal brain dysfunction, dyslexia, and developmental aphasia." This term does not include a learning problem that is primarily the result of visual, hearing, or motor disabilities, of mental retardation, of emotional disturbance, or of environmental, cultural, or economic disadvantage.

IDEA was reauthorized in 2004. A number of noteworthy changes were incorporated including the following: alignment of IDEA with "No Child Left Behind"; emphasis on "Adequate Yearly Progress" (AYP); a mandate that Individual Education Plans (IEPs) must have measurable goals; increased certification standards for Special Education teachers; and requirement that parents receive quarterly reports on goal attainment. In addition, children who are homeless and disabled need to be identified, evaluated if necessary, and provided with IEPs.

Although IDEA provides a federal definition of specific LDs, states and local school districts have flexibility in how they identify which students meet criteria for special education services. The majority of school districts have traditionally used a discrepancy model to identify students with learning problems substantial enough to qualify for special education services under the classification of Specific Learning Disability. This formula requires a statistically significant difference of at least 1.5 to 2 standard deviations between assessed academic achievement and cognitive ability in order to qualify for special education. This type of identification system relies on *categorical* definitions of LD. However, there is also a debate that LDs, like many other medical and psychological disorders, may actually fall on a *continuum* and that a dimensional or spectrum model may be more appropriate. This type of identification system would allow children who would have otherwise been characterized as "poor readers," but not learning disabled, to receive needed services. For example, a student whose overall cognitive ability was measured in the "low average" range (standard score of 85) and single word reading skills were in the "below average" range (standard score of 70) would not necessarily be identified as LD and receive services. This is because the student's reading ability, while low, is often interpreted as being commensurate with his or her inherent ability using the traditional discrepancy model.

The latest revisions of the IDEA beginning in 2004 included an alternative to using the achievement–aptitude discrepancy formula to identify children with an LD. The revision prohibited requiring a severe discrepancy (while still allowing the use of the information) and allowed school districts to use Response to Intervention (RTI) as part of the evaluation process. RTI is the practice of providing high-quality instruction and interventions matched to student need, monitoring progress frequently to make decisions about changes in instruction or goals, and applying child response data to important educational decisions.

The implementation of RTI can be described as follows:

1. Students are provided "effective instruction" by their teacher(s).
2. Students' progress is frequently monitored.
3. Students who do not make progress then receive either different instruction or more of the same instruction.
4. Progress continues to be monitored.
5. Students who continue to not make progress either qualify for special education, or qualify for a special education evaluation.

Conceptually, RTI holds great promise for improving educational experience for children with LDs. However, effective implementation of RTI is fraught with difficulties. Readers interested in the strengths and weaknesses of RTI can find more information in the Suggested Readings section at the end of the chapter.

Reading Disability

Clinical Features

A reading disability (RD), also known as dyslexia, is characterized by the presence of deficits in an individual's reading achievement despite having average intelligence and educational opportunities. However, considerable research has demonstrated that single word reading (decoding) is not strongly related to global measures of intellectual functioning. Current diagnostic criteria in the DSM-IV-TR as well as the achievement–aptitude model do not reflect the overwhelming consensus of researchers in the field of dyslexia. Research in the past 20 years has demonstrated that dyslexia is related to deficits in processing the basic sounds that make up language, a skill that is referred to as *phonological awareness*. Specifically, these children demonstrate an isolated weakness with phonological processing that results in difficulty with decoding or being able to "sound out" words, although higher order cognitive skills of thinking, reasoning, and understanding abstract concepts are intact and possibly advanced.

In order to become an effective reader, a child must first be able to hear and identify the individual sounds in a spoken word. These are called *phonemes* and are the basic building blocks of language. For example, the word "mat" is comprised of three phonemes: "mmm," "aah," and "tuh." Phonological processing allows one to identify, understand, store, and retrieve each of these sounds so that they can be put together to form a word or *morpheme*. This process occurs automatically in spoken language through a process called *coarticulation* where individual phonemes are rapidly compressed or blended together to produce speech that is understandable and not taxing on the memory system. Hence, the spoken word "mat" is perceived as one single sound, rather than the three separate phonemes that it actually contains.

In reading and writing, these individual phonemes are mapped onto letters that share the same structural sound properties. For example, the letter "B" makes the /b/ or "buh" sound. This process is termed the *alphabetic principle*. Reading requires that an individual be able to *decode* words by simultaneously segmenting each letter into its representative sound, retain these sounds in memory, and then blend them together to form a word. Effective reading also requires that an individual become fluent in this skill so that attentional and cognitive resources can be used for the purpose of recalling previous words and sentences in a paragraph in order to obtain meaning.

The core weakness of dyslexia lies in developing an awareness that spoken and written words are made up of phonemes. Hence, children with reading problems have difficulty recognizing that words are made up of much smaller segments representing individual sounds. These problems are then compounded further by the process of reading, which requires that a child learn that these sounds are tied to squiggly lines on paper called letters. Finally, a child must then understand that when these letters are put together to form words, they represent the same number and sequence of sounds that are heard in a spoken word. Children must first develop phonemic awareness in order to become effective readers and learn how to decode and decipher words into their representative phonemes.

Although children with dyslexia can be taught phonological awareness skills, many continue to have difficulty with the automatization of this process that allows them to read fluently, or in a quick, smooth, and accurate manner. Effective readers are able to identify individual words with a little to no effort, and thus, are able to devote the majority of their cognitive resources to comprehension. Poor fluency can have an immense effect on comprehension when an individual is pressured by time or has a large volume of written material to understand and integrate. This is because so much energy must be dedicated to decoding text with few reserves left over for understanding critical pieces of information, recalling previously read material, and drawing inferences from prior knowledge. It is also important to note that because higher order cognitive skills are intact in dyslexic individuals, comprehension can be largely unaffected when they are allowed to read at their own pace or they are able to use visual cues to help them derive meaning from the text.

Many dyslexic individuals also have considerable difficulties with rote memorization and rapid word retrieval which is also thought to be related to poorly developed phonemic awareness. This is often the most frustrating paradox of dyslexia since the inability to quickly find *the* correct word is often misinterpreted as the person being slow or below average intellectually when the converse is actually true. Many individuals with dyslexia have been shown to have strong receptive vocabulary, grammar and syntactic skills, but have difficulty retrieving words on demand due to the inability to use the phonemic properties of the word to assist with quick and easy access from long-term memory. In fact, sound-based slips of the tongue often are not indicative of poor understanding of the word's meaning, but rather of confusion regarding the word's sounds (e.g., saying the word "intrepid" for "interrupted"). This is also one of the more persisting symptoms of dyslexia, as adults who develop adequate reading skills will continue to demonstrate difficulties with rapid and fluent word retrieval and will have speech characterized by long pauses, fillers ("um"), and nonspecific language ("that thing").

Epidemiology

RD is the most common form of LD, accounting for 50% to 80% of all diagnosed LDs. Prevalence in the DSM-IV-TR is estimated at 3% to 10% of the population with a ratio of males to females of 3 to 4:1. However, other studies suggest that the prevalence rate is actually closer to 17% to 20% with a much more equal rate between boys and girls. The lower prevalence rate and bias toward males cited in previous studies are likely due to the manner in which subjects were identified for these studies. The majority of these samples relied on children who were clinic-referred or already qualified for special education services. Because boys are more likely to display disruptive behavior in the classroom when confronted with academic challenges, whereas girls tend to display quietly inattentive behavior, boys are more often referred for evaluation. In fact, longitudinal studies that have obtained a representative sample of all young children entering school have found that the rate of RD is much higher than previously indicated, as well as much more equal between females and males. It is also interesting that recent research has begun to question a previously held notion that dyslexia only occurs in individuals who speak alphabetic languages, and not in individuals who speak logographic languages such as Chinese.

Clinical Course

Previous theories about LDs posited that they represented a developmental lag that could be outgrown or effectively treated with a short-term "booster" of intervention that would allow a child to catch up. It is now understood that LDs can be persistent over time, although the manner in which the specific symptom is exhibited can vary. In fact, nearly 75% of children classified as RD in the third grade continue to demonstrate reading problems in the ninth grade. Specifically, adults who were identified as having an RD as children often continue to demonstrate difficulties with decoding unfamiliar words, spelling, and fluency. Reading can continue to be frustrating for adolescents and adults whose comprehension often depends upon a laborious, time-consuming process of relatively slowed word retrieval. This is especially true for those bright individuals whose academic or vocational ambitions require a considerable amount of reading.

Many children with RD exhibit a reluctance to attend school, moodiness, self-derogatory comments about their ability, and disruptive behavior due to boredom, frustration, and/or shame. In fact, school dropout rates for children and adolescents with LD are estimated to be as high as nearly 40%, resulting in major problems with employment as adults. Other profound lifelong psychosocial correlates of dyslexia include self-perceptions of lower intellectual ability, more generalized psychological distress, and less social mobility.

The term *Matthew effects* has been used to characterize the accumulated disadvantage of not being able to fluently read. Third grade has been identified as the turning point in school where instruction models switch from "learning to read" to "reading to learn." Unfortunately, if children have not learned adequate decoding and fluency skills by this age, the achievement gap between them and their peers in all academic areas begins to widen. Longitudinal studies of children who did not receive early and intense intervention have demonstrated that these students continue to lag behind their peers throughout high school in many academic areas, but especially in those areas that require a great deal of reading.

Etiology and Pathogenesis

RD has been shown to be both familial and genetic with a nearly 80% concordance rate reported in monozygotic (MZ) twins in comparison to less than 50% concordance rate in dizygotic (DZ) twins and other siblings. Furthermore, if one family member is affected, the rates for other members are much higher than that in the general population. For example, the rates of reading problems in children of dyslexic parents have been found to be as high as 30% to 60%. Parents of children with RD are also more likely to have reading problems (25% to 60%), with a higher risk for fathers (46%) than mothers (33%). Finally, linkage studies suggest a major role for chromosomes 6 and 15, with additional potential markers on chromosomes 1 and 2.

Structural and functional neuroimaging studies have demonstrated differences in brain structure and activation for children and adults with RD compared to matched normal controls. Structural studies have revealed possible differences in the left-hemispheric regions that support language in individuals with RD, most notably in the areas of the planum temporale, insular cortex, and corpus callosum. The most consistent findings have demonstrated that skilled readers generally demonstrate an asymmetry of the planum temporale favoring the left side, whereas individuals with dyslexia demonstrate a lack of, or reversed, asymmetry.

Functional neuroimaging studies have also supported left-hemispheric differences between individuals with and without RD, notably in the basal temporal, temporoparietal, and inferior frontal regions. Specifically, increased activation in the angular gyrus, Wernicke's area, and basal temporal areas within the left temporoparietal region has been shown on word-recognition tasks

TABLE 17-1   Differential Diagnoses for All Learning Disabilities
• Vision or hearing problems • Mental retardation • Psychological or mental health problems • Environmental or cultural factors • Medical disorders including seizures, sleep disorders, genetic disorders

in skilled readers. In contrast, adults and children with RD exhibit increased activation in the anterior portions of the brain, as well as a reversed pattern of hemispheric activation in the right temporoparietal region, on these tasks.

Although there is strong evidence that RD is a genetic and neurobiological disorder, the effect of the environment cannot be ignored. Parents who have reading problems often have fewer books in the home and are less likely to read to their children or to model reading as a preferred and rewarding activity. Furthermore, it is becoming clearer what the effect of inadequate instruction has on brain development. Neuroimaging studies suggest that intervention aimed directly at addressing the core phonological deficit of RD produces changes in brain activation that more closely resemble nondisabled readers. Recent work has also demonstrated neural plasticity in typically developing readers in response to reading interventions. For these reasons, it is clear that both neurobiological and environmental factors interact to produce the phenotype that is currently defined as dyslexia.

Differential Diagnoses and Common Comorbidities

The most common differential diagnoses for all LDs are summarized in Table 17-1. These include ruling out sensory problems related to vision or hearing difficulties and mental retardation. The DSM-IV-TR and special education definitions also specify that inadequate educational opportunities, poor motivation, and significant emotional problems must be ruled out as well. However, it is important to note that the mere presence of these factors does not rule out the diagnosis of LD. Instead, their presence can contribute to and interact with a comorbid learning disability, making a differential diagnosis quite difficult. Finally, methods of assessment and interpretation of testing results should be sensitive to an individual's ethnic or cultural background, as well as a child's current proficiency in developing a second language, to avoid possibly mislabeling a child as LD or mentally retarded.

LDs, including RD, often occur in association with general medical conditions, such as very low birth weight, prematurity, lead poisoning, fetal alcohol syndrome, and fragile X syndrome. However, the presence of these disabilities does not necessarily indicate learning problems, and many individuals with LD do not have such a history.

The most common comorbidities with RD are primarily related to emotional and behavioral disturbances, as summarized in Table 17-2. Attention-Deficit/Hyperactivity Disorder (ADHD) is the most frequently reported comorbidity with RD in both epidemiological and clinical studies, regardless of whether individuals are selected for reading problems or for ADHD. Between 15% and 26% of individuals with dyslexia also meet criteria for ADHD, whereas 25% to 40% of individuals with ADHD have reading difficulties. Furthermore, the core deficits in language and phonological processing specific to dyslexia have been shown to be independent of a comorbid diagnosis of ADHD.

RD can also take a high toll on children's psychological health. Emotional or physical symptoms (e.g., anxiety, depression, stomach aches, reluctance to go to school) are common in children and adolescents with RD, with studies indicating that 14% to 32% of RD children

TABLE 17-2	Common Comorbidities for All Learning Disabilities

- Other learning disabilities
- Developmental or acquired language disorders
- Attention-deficit/hyperactivity disorder (ADHD)
- Disruptive behavior disorders
- Mood disorders
- Anxiety disorders
- Environmental or cultural factors
- Medical disorders including seizures, sleep disorders, genetic disorders

experience depressive moods and feelings of lack of control and low self-efficacy. Twin studies have supported higher rates of all internalizing and externalizing disorders in individuals with RD. Gender differences have also been found with a stronger association toward externalizing symptoms for boys and internalizing symptoms for girls with reading difficulties.

Assessment

The essentials of assessment for RD are summarized in Table 17-3 and explicated here. Children with normal reading processes spontaneously begin to identify and segment the sounds or phonemes in words around the ages of 4 to 6 years. For example, children at these ages are particularly attuned to and take pleasure in rhymes and can begin to group words by their initial and ending sounds. This has been shown to be a critically important skill for learning to read and, hence, difficulties in this area can be very predictive markers for reading problems. Early assessment of dyslexia usually focuses on three areas that are related to phonological processing: (1) *phonemic awareness* or the ability to identify phonemes and manipulate words by removing and replacing sounds; (2) *rapid automatic naming* or the ability to quickly and efficiently retrieve phonologic information from long-term memory; and (3) *phonologic working memory* or the ability to temporarily store bits of verbal information.

The first area of assessment, *phonemic awareness*, can be measured in several ways, including sound comparison, segmentation, blending, and manipulation of phonemes in words. Sound comparison involves asking a child to decide which words are alike based on their initial, ending, or middle sounds. For example: "Which word begins with the same sound as pan: tub, pig, or can?" Segmentation can be measured by asking a child to either report how many sounds are in a word or to pronounce the sounds he hears. For example: "How many sounds are there in the word cat?" "Three" or "kuh" "aaa" "tuh." Alternatively, asking a child what sounds "kuh" "aaa" and "tuh" makes requires him to blend these phonemes together to form a word. Finally, the most advanced phonemic awareness skill involves having a child add, move around, or delete sounds from one word in order to form another word. For example: "What word do you get if you take the /l/ sound away from the word *slide*?" It is important to note that most children have mastered the majority of these skills by the end of first grade.

The second area, *rapid automatic naming*, is assessed by having a child name as quickly as he or she can an array of stimuli arranged in rows on a card. Because the purpose of the task is to assess how efficiently a child can retrieve information (rather than measure the child's vocabulary), the stimuli used are usually very familiar items such as letters, numbers, colors, or objects. Finally, *phonologic working memory* is a critical skill when learning to read as sounding out a word is a complex process that requires decoding letters into their sounds, storing these sounds in memory while decoding the remaining letters of a word, and then blending these sounds to form a word. Assessment of phonologic working memory usually involves having a child repeat strings of

TABLE 17-3   Assessment Essentials for Reading Disorder

Domain	Commonly Administered Measures (List is Not Exhaustive)
Rule out sensory problems	Thorough screening of hearing and vision
Cognitive ability	
To obtain understanding of cognitive strengths and weaknesses and qualify for special education	Wechsler Intelligence Scale for Children (WISC-IV)[a] Wechsler Adult Intelligence Scale (WAIS-IV)[a] Stanford-Binet (SB-V)[a]
Assessment of early language development	
Difficulties with rhyming Poor articulation and pronunciation Word finding problems Poor knowledge of letter names	Developmental history Parent interview Observation Ask child to name capital and lower-case letters Identify corresponding letter sounds
Areas of diagnostic assessment	
Family history Phonemic awareness	Parent interview Comprehensive Test of Phonological Processing (CTOPP)[a]
Single-word decoding of real and nonsense words	Woodcock Johnson (WJ-III) Tests of Achievementa[a] Letter-Word Identification subtest Word Attack subtest
Rapid automatic naming	CTOPP[a]
Reading fluency (oral and silent reading speed and accuracy)	Gray Oral Reading Test (GORT)[a]
Reading comprehension	Reading Comprehension subtests from the WJ-III Tests of Achievement[a] and/or the Wechsler Individual Achievement Test (WIAT-III)[a]
Other assessment areas for differential diagnosis, comorbidity, and attention problems	
Attention and concentration	Parent/teacher interview and rating scales Conners' Continuous Performance Test (CPT)[a]
Receptive and expressive vocabulary	Peabody Picture Vocabulary Test (PPVT-4)[a] Expressive One-Word Picture Vocabulary Test (EOWPVT)[a] WISC-IV[a] Vocabulary subtest
Verbal fluency	NEPSY 2[a] Word Generation subtest
Listening comprehension	WIAT III[a] Listening Comprehension subtest
Understanding of print conventions	Process Assessment of the Learner (PAL): Test Battery for Reading and Writing[a]
Problems with mood, anxiety, behavior problems, and/or self-esteem	Behavior Assessment Scale for Children (BASC-2) Achenbach Child Behavior Checklist (CBCL)[a]

[a]Indicates measure is standardized.

TABLE 17-4	Early Warning Signs of Reading Disability

- Early warning sings of reading disorder by the end of kindergarten:
  - Delay in developing speech
  - Difficulties with articulation or pronunciation
  - Takes little enjoyment in hearing and repeating nursery rhymes
  - Difficulty with rhyming
  - Difficulty naming all upper and lower-case letters
- Early warning signs of reading disorder by 1st grade:
  - Difficulty segmenting words and grouping them by their initial, ending, and middle phonemes
  - Difficulty naming letter sounds
  - Difficulty counting number of sounds in small words
- Expressive language seems to lag behind receptive language

random numbers, letters, or words. Table 17-4 lists several early warning signs for clinicians and parents to be aware of in children who may exhibit RD.

Another important area of assessment in young children is the knowledge of letter names and letter sounds. Developmentally, it is expected that children who are exposed to letter concepts will begin to show an interest in and ability to identify letters and their corresponding sounds by preschool with proficiency by early first grade. Difficulties with naming letters and identifying their corresponding sounds by this age should warrant a referral for further evaluation. A commonly held notion that writing poorly formed or backwards letters represents a core symptom of dyslexia also deserves comment. It is now recognized that the base rate of this difficulty in young children is fairly high. Whereas children without dyslexia seem to outgrow this difficulty by second grade, many children with dyslexia continue to demonstrate such problems. Contrary to previous beliefs, the cause of this problem is not due to "seeing" letters backwards. Rather, these problems can again be attributed to poor phonological processing skills that make it very difficult and cumbersome for a child to tie letters with their corresponding sounds.

Three additional areas are generally targeted for assessment when evaluating for RDs in school-aged children: (1) single word reading; (2) reading fluency; and (3) reading comprehension. Assessment of *single word reading* is fairly simple and involves having a child read aloud lists of real words, as well as phonetically regular nonsensical words. Nonsense words are a particularly important measure of phonological decoding as many children with dyslexia initially try to learn to read by memorizing the letter groupings of real words. *Reading fluency* is a measure of an individual's speed and accuracy in reading. It is measured by timing how quickly and smoothly a child can read a list of single words, a group of sentences, or multiple paragraphs on a page without errors. Reading fluency is generally assessed through oral reading, although assessment of silent reading fluency can be important with older students or adults. *Reading comprehension* is measured by having an individual read a paragraph, story, or piece of text and then asking him questions about what they read. Although appearing to be a fairly straightforward concept, comprehension can be affected by many task variables. These include differences in passage length and response format (free recall vs. multiple choice), timed versus untimed reading of material, presence of other forms of contextual information (pictures, graphs, etc.), and an individual's knowledge of the material.

The role of assessing a child's cognitive or intellectual ability continues to this day to remain central to both educational and psychiatric diagnostic systems for LDs. This harkens back to the originally proposed notion that problems with learning to read represent an *unexpected* difficulty that is not consistent with a child's innate cognitive ability. This hypothesis was based on research demonstrating a high correlation between cognitive ability and reading achievement in normal readers. However, current research on the role of phonological processing with reading problems has demonstrated that overall cognitive ability and achievement are not highly correlated in individuals with dyslexia. In fact, IQ tests are poor predictors of both later reading problems and response to treatment. Furthermore, the disturbing paradox with using IQ tests to diagnose or qualify a child with reading problems can be that many dyslexic children do not present with a significant enough discrepancy between their aptitude and achievement in the early grades to qualify for services. It is not until they have "failed" reading for several consecutive grades that their gap becomes wide enough to meet diagnostic or educational criteria, which can be too late to prevent subsequent academic and behavioral problems. For this reason, IQ tests are frequently not recommended in the assessment of early identification of reading problems, although understanding a child's overall cognitive ability can be useful to help inform other treatment goals. This difficulty further underscores the aforementioned controversy of using a discrepancy model rather than a continuum model in identifying children with RD, or any LD.

Treatment

Early identification and intervention are essential for optimal prevention of further learning, emotional, and behavioral problems. Developing fluent reading skills requires the old adage of "practice, practice, practice." Thus, the older a child is before a diagnosis is made, the greater the gap between him and his peers. The essential pieces of an effective intervention include intense and high-quality instruction of sufficient duration.

Specifically, Shaywitz suggests that a child receive systematic and direct instruction in increasing phonemic awareness (noticing, identifying, and manipulating the sounds of language), as well as phonics (how written letters and letter groups represent the sounds of spoken language). Improving a child's ability to decode or sound out words, blend sounds together to form words, recognize words by sight, spelling skills, and reading comprehension strategies is critical. Recent research has indicated that effective interventions for reading problems entail frequent instruction (between 30 and 60 minutes a day, 4 to 5 days a week) delivered in a one-to-one, or at most, a three-to-one setting. Other core elements to an effective reading program include an emphasis on letter identification, vocabulary development, the ability to recall and retell sentences and stories, and practice in writing words and sentences with an emphasis on vocabulary development and planning and organization of written material.

To facilitate reading fluency and comprehension, children with RD should be provided with materials that they are able to read easily, with an error rate of no more than 10%. It is further recommended that children receive practice in identifying key facts from written material to assist with developing an understanding of the structure of sentences, paragraphs, and stories and being able to extract important concepts from reading material.

Several comprehensive reading programs are available that utilize a direct instruction approach with a systematic and integrated format that teaches phonetic skills in a structured and comprehensive manner. These include DISTAR (The Direct Instructional System for Teaching Arithmetic and Reading), Reading Mastery, Open Court Reading, Success for All, and the REACH System to name a few. However, it is important to emphasize that no single program is sufficient to meet all instructional reading needs, nor a panacea for addressing all reading-related problems. Furthermore, the quality of instruction with teachers or tutors who are well-trained in the technology of teaching reading cannot be ignored as a critical part of any intervention.

Despite developing adequate decoding and reading skills, many older children and adolescents with dyslexia continue to demonstrate problems with fluency. These difficulties can represent a considerable impediment to their being able to access challenging learning opportunities and warrant academic accommodations. These may include providing extra time and/or alternate formats for tests (e.g., oral), quiet environment for test taking, computer assistance, books on tape or CD-ROM, and recording lectures.

Three additional recommended interventions for a child with RD deserve mention. First, because of the impact reading problems can have on a child's self-confidence, it is critically important to focus on providing positive experiences that emphasize his strengths, provide him with enjoyment, and an opportunity to shine in his own way. Second, medications have not been beneficial for remediating reading or learning problems per se, but can be useful in addressing comorbid attention problems. Finally, several interventions that have not received empirical support for remediating reading problems, but nonetheless continue to be promoted, should be noted. These include treatment methods aimed at simultaneously stimulating several modes of sensory input to develop better "learning patterns," early motor training, improving eye–hand coordination, eye exercises, tinted lenses, biofeedback, and special diets.

Mathematics Disability

Mathematical computation deficits in individuals with LDs have been less frequently reported historically, but have been noted for as long as RDs. Overall, educators, clinicians, and researchers have devoted less time to understanding mathematics disabilities (MDs) than RDs. This may be due to the central role that reading plays in academics and in vocational success.

Definitional issues in the area of arithmetic disabilities, such as RDs, are currently an area of considerable difficulty. Consistent standards or inclusion/exclusion rules to determine the presence of an LD in math do not exist, although several general terms are in common use, such as developmental arithmetic disability, specific math disability, as well as dyscalculia. As in RD, the assumptions that underlie these terms are intact (normally developed) language, reading, and writing skills. Although deficits in math commonly occur with other LDs, it is possible for difficulties with math computation to occur in isolation. The relationship between language and reading problems with learning mathematical concepts is unclear. However, significant difficulty with reading comprehension can interfere with a child's successful completion of arithmetic problems involving reading, for example, story problems. It can also interfere with being able to obtain information from textbooks.

Clinical Features

Competence in the area of math involves mastering *basic number skills, counting,* and *arithmetic. Basic number skills* involve learning the English number words and the correct sequence of numbers, for example, 1, 2, 3. The quantities associated with the number words and numbers must be learned, for example, 2 and two are symbols that indicate a group of any 2 things. In addition, children must learn to translate numbers from one form to another, for example, " twenty two" into "22." Several other skills must be mastered including an understanding that numbers can be decomposed into smaller numbers or combined to make larger numbers. The most challenging feature of the number system is that it is based upon a base-10 structure and it is necessary to understand this in order to master other domains in arithmetic. Research suggests that children with MD do not have a basic inability in the ability to understand or learn basic number skills.

Learning to count in order, for example, "one, two, three" is mastered by most children. Learning the concepts/rules that allow for effective and accurate counting are critical skills to develop. These basic rules include: one-to-one correspondence, stable order, cardinality, abstraction, and order-irrelevance (items do not have to be adjacent to be counted). Research findings indicate that children with math disabilities in 1st and 2nd grade understand the concepts of one-to-one correspondence, stable order, and cardinality as well as children without LD. However, many children with MD experience difficulty on tasks that require an understanding of the order irrelevance principle, that is, items do not have to be adjacent to be counted.

TABLE 17-5	Frequently Exhibited Problems in Children with Math Disabilities

- Concentration
  - Difficulty maintaining attention to steps needed for problem solving
  - Difficulty sustaining attention/concentration to instruction
- Memory/retrieval
  - Unable to retain mathematical facts
  - Difficulty counting from within a sequence
  - Forgets steps in algorithm
  - Performs poorly on review lessons
  - Difficulty telling time
  - Difficulty solving multistep word problems
- Visual–perceptual/visual–motor
  - Loses place on page
  - Difficulty keeping numbers aligned, writing straight across page
  - Difficulty with directional aspects, for example, up–down, left–right
  - Difficulty using number line

Many children with math disabilities recall fewer basic *arithmetic* facts, such as 5 + 5 = 10, and are slower retrieving the facts they do know. This pattern appears to be chronic and not one that is "outgrown." Children with MD use immature problem-solving procedures, or strategies that are more commonly used by younger typically learning children. For example, when solving the problem 5 + 4 the immature approach would be to hold up nine fingers and begin counting from one. The more mature approach would be to begin with 5 and then add on the smaller number, for example, six, seven, eight, nine. Although a sizable number of children with MD are able to catch up to their peers by the middle of elementary school, a subset of children demonstrates persisting difficulties in counting procedures throughout elementary school and sometimes later. Table 17-5 summarizes problems frequently exhibited by children with arithmetic disabilities.

Core Processes

Recent research has identified two problem areas that are found in children with arithmetic disabilities: basic math processes and procedural difficulties. The first problem area of basic math processes impacts a child's ability to learn mathematical concepts, represent concepts, and retrieve math facts. Difficulties with these processes will be expressed as slow computation speed, as well as inaccurate or inconsistent computations. Some children will use counting because they are unable to quickly or with minimal effort retrieve a math fact. The second problem type involves difficulty with mastering the procedural aspects of math. This will appear as difficulties with counting.

The underlying processes for both of the problem areas described above seem to be related to working memory and executive function skills. Poor working memory skills are defined as difficulties with temporarily storing and manipulating information in order to solve a cognitive task. Executive function skills utilized in math include strategy knowledge and the ability to use working memory efficiently. Both functions are related to math disabilities.

Children with dual-diagnoses of RD and MD are more impaired on language-related tasks than children with only single word decoding deficits. These children have difficulty with all aspects of math, for example, learning math facts, retaining and easily retrieving math facts. Neuropsychological studies have attempted to subtype LDs based on different patterns of performance related to patterns of academic achievement. For example, groups of children with low achievement in arithmetic relative to reading and spelling demonstrate low scores on visual–perceptual and visual–spatial measures. In contrast, their performance on measures of auditory-verbal measures was higher relative to children with low achievement in reading and spelling.

Epidemiology

The prevalence of MDs has been estimated to be 5% to 6% of school-aged children. No consistent evidence of gender differences in math achievement has been found and little is known of the developmental course. It does appear that a significant number of children with identified MDs in elementary school will continue to meet the diagnostic criteria for the disability several years later. Like RD, MDs appear to be chronic and persist through school. Little is known about the development and course of children with deficits only in math and not reading.

Etiology and Pathogenesis

MDs have been found to be more common in some families. One study found the prevalence in parents and siblings to be between 40% and 66%. Other studies have also found substantial shared variance between RD and MD. It is important to note that approximately 40% to 60% of individuals with a disability in one area will also have a disability in another, for example, RD.

Studies of either brain structure or brain function have not been carried out on children with MD. Research in adults has suggested that calculation involves the inferior prefrontal cortex in the left hemisphere as well as the angular gyrus. These areas are also involved in language.

Differential Diagnoses and Common Comorbidities

RD is very common in children with MDs. Specifically, 50% or more of children with MD will also experience difficulty learning to read. Table 17-2 summarizes additional common comorbidities. Furthermore, it is not uncommon that children with MD have difficulties on tasks requiring visual–perceptual and visual–motor integration.

Assessment

Although MD can occur in isolation it is much more common to find it together with a RD. The approach to assessment should include measures to rule out a reading disorder in addition to understanding the child's math competence. In elementary school-aged children, the evaluation should include measures of computation skill as well as computational accuracy. In addition, assessment of arithmetic concepts should be included, for example, time, measurement, as well as working memory. Unfortunately, school districts vary significantly with regards to the math curriculum they adopt. In addition, districts and states frequently change curriculum at least several times in a student's life. This makes evaluation of math skills very difficult as national norms may not reflect the local curriculum.

Treatment

Much less is known about effective remediation approaches to MD as compared to RD. This is due in large part because little is known about the nature and course of MD. Math and DISTAR Arithmetic Program have been shown to increase computational and math problem-solving skills using approaches such as teacher modeling, strategy training, direct instruction, and cooperative learning groups. A number of other validated instructional techniques have also been documented for children with MD, including: (1) providing demonstration, modeling, and feedback; (2) increasing fluency; (3) using concrete–abstract teaching sequence; (4) setting goals; (5) combining demonstration with permanent model; (6) using verbalization while solving problems; (7) teaching strategies for computation and problem solving; and (8) using computerized instruction.

Disorder of Written Language

No current definition of disorders of written expression clearly articulates the variety of component processes necessary for adequate writing skills. Written expression is linked and likely dependent upon oral expression skills. In addition, written expression performance will not exceed reading competence in most children. However, written expression is also related to basic skills such as handwriting and spelling, as well as executive functions, such as planning, self-monitoring, organizing, and perspective taking. In general, selective difficulties with psychomotor skills or spelling are not considered to be disorders of written expression.

Clinical Features and Core Processes

Written expression is a complex activity that involves a host of cognitive and executive functions, as well as the automatization of lower level skills. Cognitive and executive functions needed include expressive vocabulary skills, general world knowledge, and planning/organizational skills. Lower level skills include the production of letters and spelling, as well as understanding rules of grammar. Additionally, other factors that can impact writing skills include motivation, speed of processing, sustained attention, and interest in and knowledge of a topic. In summary, it appears that difficulties with writing can include problems with handwriting, spelling, or the ability to express ideas through text, all of which have different underlying subcomponents. Spelling is related to phonological analysis, knowledge of letter–sound correspondence, and single word reading. Handwriting is related to fine motor skills, motor planning, and rapid retrieval of symbols. Finally, written expression is related to executive functioning, including working memory and language skills.

Epidemiology

Most children with LDs have difficulty with at least one aspect of writing, for example, handwriting, spelling, content or form. Epidemiological data is lacking regarding the prevalence of disorders of written language. However, given the rate of developmental language disorders and RD, deficits in written language likely affect at least 15% to 25% of school-aged children.

Etiology and Pathogenesis

The number of skills necessary for the development of writing makes it likely that a large number of etiologies are possible and interact with each other. These include biological, genetic, psychosocial, and environmental (including instructional variables) causes. Difficulties with language-related skills (e.g., phonological analysis, rapid retrieval), executive functioning (e.g., working memory), visual–spatial skills, and motor systems could each impede the development of writing skills. Component skills related to writing such as spelling and reading has been found to have a significant heritability although their specificity with regards to writing is unclear.

There is limited information regarding the causes, course, prognosis, and treatment of disorders of written language. The distinction between children who demonstrate differences with motor versus idea generation may be an important clinical and research goal. Specifically, children with expressive writing difficulties that are not primarily due to language-based disorders may have different etiological causes compared to children with language problems.

Differential Diagnoses and Common Comorbidities

Children with RD will invariably have difficulty with written expression as well. Common problems may involve any aspect of writing, including spelling, sentence structure, grammar, fluency, and clarity of ideas. Please see Table 17-2 for a list of common comorbidities for disorders of written expression as well. Furthermore, it is important to evaluate for the presence of visual–motor and language disorders.

Assessment

Intuitively, an individual's written expression skills will seldom exceed their reading skills—otherwise they would be unable to read what they write! First it will be important to evaluate for the presence of a RD. It will be important to evaluate the visual–motor skills of the student to evaluate the possibility that motor difficulties are not the primary cause. If it is, then the diagnosis of dyspraxia is likely. Evaluation for a disorder of written expression will include knowledge of the alphabet, spelling, punctuation, and grammar. In addition, evaluation of oral expressive skills is necessary as written expression is a reflection of oral expression abilities. Measures of writing fluency are also helpful.

Treatment

There are a number of intervention components that have been shown to improve the writing of children with LDs. These include: (1) consistently using a basic framework of planning, writing, and revision; (2) direct instruction of the critical steps in the writing process; (3) providing consistent feedback regarding the child's writing; and (4) providing early intervention. When planning what to write, it is helpful if teachers use techniques such as semantic maps to help a child respond to questions such as "Who am I writing for?" "Why am I writing?," "What do I know?," "How do I group my ideas?," and "How will I organize my ideas?" Providing feedback of already written material is often directed at aspects of writing such as organization, punctuation, and interpretation.

Conclusions

LDs are common and when undetected and untreated cause significant morbidity and distress to the child and family. Research has revealed that LDs do not represent a lag; that is, there is no "catching up" that occurs later in childhood. However, there is good support for early screening and detection of children at risk for RDs because early intervention has been shown to be effective in improving a child's ability. In addition, if beginner readers are taught using materials that develop skills identified as core processes in reading (e.g., phonemic awareness, knowledge of phonics) the incidence of RD is significantly reduced. The latest revision of the IDEA has important implications for future detection and treatment of LDs in the nation's schools. Most importantly, school districts can now identify children at risk for the development of a learning disability and provide interventions prior to the student qualifying for special education. Hopefully, this will lead to fewer children developing LDs and experiencing success in school and adulthood.

CASE VIGNETTES

VIGNETTE 1: 9 YEAR OLD GIRL WITH A READING DISORDER

Sue is a 9-year-old who is in the third grade. She is brought to the pediatrician's office by her parents due to concerns regarding her behavior at home and school. Specifically, her parents scheduled the appointment because Sue has demonstrated an increased difficulty with her homework completion, incomplete assignments, and below average reading scores on school-administered tests. Her teacher reports that she is often off-task in school, and fails to complete her assignments in the allotted time.

Sue's developmental history is unremarkable. The family history is notable for difficulty in learning to read by Sue's father, who reports he is a poor speller and does not read book length material for pleasure, although he did graduate from college. Sue was described as having difficulty finding the right word but seemed to understand a great deal. She mispronounced many words and often left off the beginning or ends of words. Upon further questioning, her parents report that Sue was not interested in Dr. Seuss type books as a preschooler, did not seem to enjoy word play or rhyming, and did not learn the letters of the alphabet until the summer after kindergarten. They remarked that she was different from her older sister who was a good student. Sue's parents became concerned with her reading development in kindergarten. They reported that she was given some extra reading help at the end of first grade, which continued through second grade. Sue was good at artwork and could spend hours on intricate drawings or puzzles. Her current third-grade teacher has raised concerns regarding Sue's attention and activity level, as well as poor performance on reading tasks.

The pediatrician referred Sue for a neuropsychological evaluation. The results indicated that Sue had well-developed cognitive skills, but that her single word reading was slow and her accuracy was below average. Reading comprehension and written math calculations were average. Spelling and writing skills were low to below average. Sue performed below average across a number of tasks that assess skills shown to be important in the development of reading. In particular, she exhibited deficits in the area of phonemic awareness and phonemic analysis (e.g., the ability to deal explicitly and segmentally with sound units smaller than the syllable) and rapid naming. For example, she had difficulty when asked to read nonsense words (made up words that can be pronounced, e.g., dop). In addition, she was able to only accurately read 50% of words at the third-grade level. She did not demonstrate a pattern of difficulty on tasks involving speed of processing, sustained effort, inhibition, or planning. Behavioral questionnaires completed by parents and teachers highlighted concerns with learning, homework completion, and completing academic work involving reading and writing.

Discussion

Sue demonstrated several disruptive behaviors that could be suggestive of an attentional or behavioral disturbance, including hesitation and anxiety when called on to read aloud, off-task or inattentive behaviors, poor sustained effort with school assignments and homework, non-compliance, and anger directed at her parents regarding her school performance. Although ADHD, emotional disturbance, or parent–child problems are appropriate differential diagnoses in this case, further evaluation revealed that Sue's difficulties with reading were the cause of these other problems. Specifically, her early history of difficulty with precursors to phonological analysis (e.g., rhyming), the father's history of early reading, and spelling problems are very important. Results from her neuropsychological testing indicated that she had difficulty with reading single words, decoding nonsense and unfamiliar words, as well as poor fluency and spelling. Her reading comprehension, in contrast, was superior to her decoding skills when there were no time limits. Moreover, the use of standardized behavior questionnaires did not reveal a pattern of significant or pervasive inattention, impulsivity, or overactivity. Taken together these do not support a diagnosis of ADHD.

The recommendations from the evaluation included reading interventions that are empirically validated, and would include sustained and systematic instruction (approximately 30 minutes a day, 4 days a week) with an emphasis on: (1) *phonemic analysis*—detection of sounds that comprise words; (2) *synthetic phonics*—production of sounds that comprise letters and practice in blending; and (3) *reading fluency*—additional practice in reading. Information regarding effective reading programs was provided as well as a number of helpful websites including: The National Reading Panel. It was recommended that the results of the evaluation be shared with Sue's school in order to start the eligibility process for special education support. In addition, a number of accommodations under Section 504 of the American with Disabilities Act were provided, including extra time to complete assignments, reduced amount of material to read, preparation before being called on in class, access to recorded materials when possible, as well use of an optical character reader when possible for assignments. Sue began in special education and received remediation using an empirically supported reading program. In addition, her parents had her work with a tutor for 6 months. Her reading accuracy and fluency improved and she was exited from special education the following school year.

VIGNETTE 2: 12 YEAR OLD BOY WITH ADHD AND A READING DISORDER

Joe is a 12-year-old who is in the sixth grade and the first year of middle school. He was brought to the pediatrician's office by his parents due to concerns regarding his behavior at home and school. Specifically, his parents scheduled the appointment because Joe has been unable to complete his homework on a regular basis in his academic classes and has become disruptive in class. Family history is remarkable for Joe's dad indicating he was an underachiever who frequently was off-task in elementary school and had notes sent home detailing his disruptive behavior in class. Joe's developmental history is remarkable for increased activity while a toddler and frequent accidents including a broken wrist. He experienced difficulty throughout elementary school keeping up in all subjects and focusing his attention throughout the school day. Joe would improve with additional support provided at home and by teachers. Joe is very social and athletically skilled. His performance on statewide examinations varied, but he failed some sections which necessitated extra assistance. At home, Joe is described as disorganized and impulsive. Joe's parents think he needs more supervision than other children of his age but also think that he just needs some extra time to catch up with his peers.

The pediatrician referred them for a neuropsychological evaluation. The results indicated that Joe had average cognitive skills; however, he demonstrated significant impulsive behavior during the assessment as well as being easily distracted. Assessment of academic achievement revealed below average single word reading, below average reading comprehension, low to below average math computation skills, due in part to careless errors, and writing characterized by punctuation and grammatical errors. Neuropsychological assessment revealed deficits in phonological awareness, sustained attention, impulsive responding, and decreased vigilance. In addition, on measures of certain aspects of executive functioning, including organization, planning, and working memory Joe's performance was below age expected levels. Learning and recall, as well as visual–perceptual skills were age appropriate.

Behavioral questionnaires completed by parents and teachers highlighted clinically significant elevations in the areas of attention, overactivity, learning, homework completion, and completing academic work involving reading and writing.

Discussion

Joe demonstrated several disruptive behaviors that are consistent with an attentional disturbance, including clowning around when called on to read aloud, off-task or inattentive behaviors, overactivity, poor sustained effort with school assignments and homework, noncompliance, and anger directed at his parents regarding his school performance. In this case, difficulties with a number of aspects of attention, executive functions as well as deficits in phonological awareness and reading indicate that Joe meets the diagnostic criteria for both ADHD and a RD. Joe's past behavior at home and school is also consistent with a long-standing difficulty in both areas. The increase in the "challenge level" at middle school (e.g., multiple teachers, schedule that varies) exceeded Joe's coping skills and resulted in his presenting complaints.

The recommendations from the evaluation included qualification for special education with specially designed instruction for reading (likely to occur in a resource room) and accommodations under Section 504 of the Rehabilitation Act of the Americans with Disabilities Act. Accommodations included extra time to complete reading and written work, copies of notes provided, use of optical character reading software and organization reminders. In addition, a number of behavioral supports were developed to help with sustained attention and work completion in the classroom. It was recommended that a medication trial be considered and that Joe's parents work with a psychologist to develop supportive strategies at home for work completion and behavior problems.

BIBLIOGRAPHY

Aylward EH, Richards TL, Berninger VW, et al. Instructional treatment associated with changes in brain activation in children with dyslexia. *Neurology*. 2003;61:212–219.

Denckla MB, Cutting LE. History and significance of rapid automatized naming. *Ann Dyslexia*. 1999;49:29–42.

Deutsch GK, Dougherty RF, Bammer R, et al. Children's reading performance is correlated with white matter structure measured by diffusion tensor imaging. *Cortex*. 2005;41:354–363.

Fuchs L, Powell S, Seethaler P, et al. Remediating number combination and word problem deficits among students with mathematics difficulties: a randomized control trial. *J Educ Psychol*. 2009;101(3):561–576.

Gertsten R, Baker S. *Teaching Expressive Writing to Students with Learning Disabilities: A Meta Analysis*. Eugene, OR: University of Oregon; 1999.

Hatcher, P. Phonological awareness and reading intervention. In: Snowling MJ, Stackhouse J, eds. *Dyslexia, Speech and Language: A Practitioner's Handbook*. 2nd ed. London: Whurr; 2006:167–197.

Hatcher PJ, Hulme C, Miles JNV, et al. Efficacy of small group reading intervention for beginning readers with reading-delay: a randomized controlled trial. *J Child Psychol Psychiatry*. 2006;47:820–827.

Kaufmann L, Nuerk HC. Numerical development: current issues and future perspectives. *Psychol Sci*. 2005;47(1):142–170.

Kaufmann L, Nuerk HC. Interference effects in a numerical Stroop paradigm in 9- to 12-year-old children with ADHD-C. *Child Neuropsychol*. 2006;12(3):223–243.

Kronenberg WG, Dunn DW. Learning disorders. *Neurol Clin N Am*. 2003;21:941—952.

Passolunghi MC, Marzocchi GM, Fiorillo F. Selective effect of inhibition of literal or numerical irrelevant information in children with Attention Deficit Hyperactivity Disorder (ADHD) or Arithmetic Learning Disorder (ALD). *Dev Neuropsychol*. 2005;28(3):731–753.

Phinney E, Pennington BF, Olson R, et al. Brain structure correlates of component reading processes: implications for reading disability. *Cortex*. 2007;43(6):777–791.

Puolakanaho A, Ahonen T, Aro M, et al. Very early phonological and language skills: estimating individual risk of reading disability. *J Child Psychol Psychiatry*. 2007;48:922–931.

Reynolds C, Fletcher-Janzen E, eds. *Neuropsychological Perspectives on Learning Disabilities in the Era of RTI: Recommendations for Diagnosis and Intervention*. Hoboken, NJ: Wiley; 2008.

Richards T, Berninger V, Winn W, et al. Functional MRI activation in children with and without dyslexia during pseudoword aural repeat and visual decode: before and after treatment. *Neuropsychology*. 2007;21(6):732–741.

Snowling MJ, Muter V, Carroll JM. Children at family risk of dyslexia: a follow-up in adolescence. *J Child Psychol Psychiatry*. 2007;48:609–618.

Snowling MJ. Specific disorders and broader phenotypes: the case of dyslexia. *Q J Exp Psychol*. 2008;61:142–156.

Stuebing KK, Fletcher JM, LeDoux JM, et al. Validity of IQ discrepancy classification of reading disabilities: a meta-analysis. *Am Edu Res J*. 2002;39:465–518.

Temple E, Deutsch GK, Poldrack RA, et al. Neural deficits in children with dyslexia ameliorated by behavioral remediation: evidence from functional MRI. *Proc Natl Acad Sci USA*. 2003;100:2860–2865.

Vellutino FR, Fletcher JM, Snowling MJ, et al. Specific reading disability (dyslexia): what have we learned in the past four decades? *J Child Psychol Psychiatry*. 2004;45(1):2–40.

Willcutt EG, Pennington, BF. Psychiatric comorbidity in children and adolescents with reading disability. *J Child Psychol Psychiatry*. 2000;41:1039–1048.

Wilson AJ, Dehaene S. Number sense and developmental dyscalculia. In: Coch D, Dawson G, Fischer K, eds. *Human Behavior, Learning, and the Developing Brain: Atypical Development*. New York, NY: Guilford Press; 2007:212–238.

Yin WG, Weekes BS. Dyslexia in Chinese: clues from cognitive neuropsychology. *Annals Dyslexia*. 2003;53:255–279.

SUGGESTED READINGS AND RESOURCES

General Resources

Neuropsychological Perspectives on Learning Disabilities in the Era of RTI: Recommendations for Diagnosis and Intervention, 2008. This paper describes "Response to Intervention" (RTI), a provision under IDEA for improving educational experience for children with learning disabilities, as well as its difficulties in implementation.

Pennington BF. *Diagnosing Learning Disorders: A Neuropsychological Framework*—Second Edition. New York: Guilford Press, 2009.

Rayner K, Foorman BR, Perfetti CA, Pesetsky D, Seidenberg MS. How psychological science informs the teaching of reading. *Psychological Science in the Public Interest* 2:31–74, 2001.

Shaywitz SE. *Overcoming Dyslexia: A New and Complete Science-Based Program for Reading Problems at Any Level.* New York: Knopf, 2003.

Reading Intervention Materials

Phonological Awareness Training for Reading, by Joseph Torgesen & Brian Bryant. PRO-ED Publishing, 8700 Shoal Creek Blvd, Austin, TX 78757-6897. Phone (512) 451-3246, $129 kit.

Phonemic Awareness in Young Children: A Classroom Curriculum, by Adams, Foorman, Lundberg & Beeler. Brooks Publishing Co., P.O. Box 10624, Baltimore, MD 21285-0624. Phone (800) 638-3775, $22.95.

Earobics, by Jan Wasowicz. Cognitive Concepts, Inc.,1123 Emerson Street, Suite 202, Evanston, IL 60201. Phone 847-328-8099 or 888-328-8199.

Homework/Study Skills

"Seven Steps To Homework Success: A Family Guide For Solving Common Homework Problems" by S. S. Zentall

"How to Do Homework Without Throwing Up" by Trevor Romain, Elizabeth Verdick

"Ending The Homework Hassle" by John Rosemond

"Homework Without Tears" by Lee Canter

"Thinking Organized for Parents and Children: Helping Kids Get Organized for Home, School and Play" by Rhona M. Gordon

Learning Disabilities

"Nonverbal Learning Disabilities at Home: A Parent's Guide" by Pamela Tanguay, by Byron P. Rourke

"Learning Outside the Lines: Two Ivy League Students with Learning Disabilities and ADHD Give You the Tools for Academic Success and Educational Revolution" by Jonathan Mooney and David Cole

Math Resources

"Math on Call: A Mathematics Handbook" by Andrew Kaplan, Carol Debold, Susan Rogalski, & Pat Bourdreau.

"Do the Math: Secrets, Lies, and Algebra" by Wendy Lichtman.

SUGGESTED WEBSITES

The website related to IDEA and special education is: http://idea.ed.gov/explore/home

The LD online website is: http://www.ldonline.org

The Core Knowledge website is: http://www.coreknowledge.org/

The Recording for the Blind and Dyslexic website is: http://www.rfbd.org/applications.htm

The All Kinds of Minds Website is: http://www.allkindsofminds.org/

The National Institutes of Health Learning Disabilities Website is: http://www.ninds.nih.gov/disorders/learningdisabilities/learningdisabilities.htm

The National Reading Panel website is: http://www.nationalreadingpanel.org/.

REVIEW QUESTIONS

1. Which of the following is not considered to be a specific learning disability:
   a. Reading disability
   b. Disorder of written expression
   c. Intellectual disability
   d. Mathematics disorder

2. Response to Intervention (RTI) refers to:
   a. Practice of providing high-quality instruction
   b. Using interventions matched to student need
   c. Monitoring progress frequently to make decisions about changes in instruction or goals
   d. Applying child response data to important educational decisions
   e. All of the above

3. A core deficit identified in dyslexia is:
   a. Phonics
   b. Rhyming
   c. Vocabulary
   d. Phonemic awareness

4. The most common comorbidity of Reading Disability is:
   a. Anxiety
   b. ADHD
   c. ODD
   d. Intellectual disability

5. The course of learning disabilities is best described as:
   a. A lag with a catch up in high school
   b. A constant decline in skills
   c. A chronic course with improvement following appropriate intervention
   d. Variable, depending upon timing and type of intervention
   e. c and d

6. Children may qualify for special education as a learning disabled student if:
   a. Their IQs are above 100
   b. They have a medical diagnosis
   c. Their achievement is discrepant from their IQ
   d. Their achievement is below grade expected levels
   e. c and d

Answers: 1-c, 2-e, 3-d, 4-b, 5-e, 6-e

CHAPTER **18**

Mary Margaret Gleason, MD, FAAP,
and Chia Granda, MD

Early Childhood Mental Health in Clinical Practice

Introduction

The field of infant mental health (IMH) focuses on promoting mental health in infants, toddlers, preschoolers, and their families. This multidisciplinary field strives to support emotional and behavioral development and reduce current suffering through prevention for very young children at risk for developing mental health problems and early intervention for those with clinically significant mental health problems. This chapter will describe the principles of IMH practice, assessment strategies, diagnoses, and treatment.

History and Principles of Infant Mental Health

The field of IMH developed from collaboration among developmental psychologists, pediatricians, child psychiatrists, occupational therapists, and other early childhood specialists. The field gained momentum in the 1960s, when John Bowlby presented a theory of parent–child attachment relationships and Mary Ainsworth began to test the theories in real-world settings. Since then, the field of IMH has focused on the mental health of very young children in the real-world contexts that influence their mental health, including two primary contexts: parent–child relationships and development.

The parent–child relationship begins prenatally and includes multiple components. An early component of this relationship, bonding, is the parents' emotional connection to the child that develops in the perinatal period. Although it is clear that the parents' emotional ties to their infants continue to evolve beyond the child's first moments, early interactions and experience may influence the developing relationship. The attachment relationship is a central component of the parent–child relationship and presents with discernable developmental stages in the first few years of life. Attachment relationships are defined by the infant's behaviors toward the parents. In the first two months, infants show preferences to their mothers; they look at their mother's face, and turn to her voice or her smell preferentially. The second major stage of development in the parent–child relationship occurs in months 2 to 7, when infants' social repertoire blossoms. They continue to respond preferentially to parents, but will interact socially with most people and can elicit comfort in a nondiscriminated way from strangers. At 7 to 9 months of age, infants first demonstrate focused attachment behaviors toward their primary caregivers. That is, they preferentially seek proximity to and comfort from their primary caregivers during times of distress. This important developmental shift is accompanied by new distress with separation from a parent and anxiety with strangers.

Parents' consistent and predictable comfort, nurturance, and protection of an infant provide a foundation for healthy emotional development and physical safety. When an attachment relationship is healthy or "secure," an infant can elicit comfort effectively from the parent in times of distress. Conversely, when a child has not experienced a caregiver as a reliable protector, the child may not seek proximity to or comfort from the caregiver, or may show a pattern of resistance to comfort, such as an inability to calm, or may even actively turn away from the parents' comfort. Longitudinal studies by Weinfield and colleagues demonstrate that secure attachment relationships in infancy, toddlerhood, and preschool ages predict social, emotional, and relationship competence and overall mental health in childhood, which can predict well-being into adulthood.

Although attachment relationships are defined by behaviors, the way that a parent and a child think of each other (the "internal representation" or "working model") is thought to strongly influence the relationship. These parental representations are influenced not only by the experiences with the infant but also by the parents' experiences in other intimate or caregiving relationships. In 1975, Fraiberg characterized these past relationships as "Ghosts in the nursery" when they negatively influence the parents' view of the child. In 2003, Lieberman and Amaya-Jackson reminded us that these relationships may also have positive influences and serve as "Angels" in the nursery. An example of "ghosts" could be a mother who has experienced abuse within intimate relationships. These past relationships may shape her view of herself as unlovable, and she may experience her infant's crying as a confirmation of that belief and as a criticism of her parenting. Thus, understanding parents' past experiences is crucial for understanding a parent–child relationship and a child's current experiences.

A child also contributes to the developing parent–child relationship in many ways, including temperament. Temperament is the early and stable pattern of emotional reactivity that appears to modulate the interaction between the child and his or her environment. Fox's research describes the behavioral presentation of temperament as an approach-withdrawal dichotomy that is apparent at birth. These emotional reactions become more complex (e.g., manifestations of joy vs. interest) with development, specifically with associations with prefrontal cortex and corpus callosum development in the first few years of life. Neuroanatomically, patterns of emotional reactivity correlate with asymmetric activation of and interactions between the left and right prefrontal cortices. These biologically related patterns of emotional reactivity can be influenced by early childhood experiences—including treatment—although they are often moderately stable over time and treatment does not change the biologic correlates. Since the early 1990s, Davidson and others have examined the propensity of children with behaviorally inhibited temperament to develop psychopathology. Although fewer than one third of children with behavioral inhibition develop social anxiety, their risk is two to three times that of nonbehaviorally inhibited children. These temperamental patterns of approach and withdrawal behaviors can influence the child's future developmental trajectories and form part of the child's contribution to the parent–child relationship.

Rapid development in the first years of life is another major context of early childhood mental health practice. The first years of life are the period of most rapid growth, especially in the central nervous system (CNS). By age 4, a child's brain is 90% of adult size. Early childhood brain development is characterized by extraordinarily high rates of synaptogenesis, myelinization, and neuronal pruning. Adverse and positive environmental factors influence the CNS development. For example, both lead and maternal depression exposure are

TABLE 18-1	Other Contexts of Infant and Early Childhood Mental Health
Marital/partner relationships and family support	Quality of marital/partner relationships can protect or increase risks in early childhood mental health Family supports (parent groups, religious community, and social services) enhance child mental health
Parental psychopathology and medical illnesses	Impacts intrauterine environment, family environment, and genotype/genetic risk for disorder
Physical health and attributes	Health problems impact (1) type of care needed and (2) perceived vulnerability Congenital anomalies may trigger parental impulse to protect, blame, or avoid infant, impacting developing relationship Physical similarities with other family members may be associated with attributing the infant with someone else's characteristics and influencing the way in which the parent interacts with infant
Socioeconomic factors	Number of social risk factors (not specific factors) predicts adverse child outcomes Financial resources are often associated with additional access to community support, safe child-focused activities, and time to interact with child
Cultural expectations	Culture defines beliefs about quality parenting behaviors and traditions (e.g., acceptable discipline approaches; developmental expectations regarding behavior, and toilet training) Cultural norms define expectations about the roles of family members, including roles of extended family in child care

associated with measurable CNS impairment. In addition, important studies by Nelson and colleagues in 2007 and Dozier and colleagues in 2006 demonstrate that nonbiologic interventions focused on enhancing the caregiving environment for high-risked children can improve CNS functioning, including substantial increases in IQ and normalization of electroencephalogram (EEG) patterns and cortisol patterns. The rapidity of early development across domains means that early childhood mental health intervention targets a dynamic process rather than a static system and enhances the potential for affecting important changes early in life. The practice of IMH views a child within many other contexts as well, as young children's mental health may be influenced by a range of family, community, and societal factors. Table 18-1 presents the impact of other contexts of infant and young child mental health. Table 18-2 summarizes the essentials of healthy infant and early childhood mental health development.

TABLE 18-2	Essential Principles of Infant and Early Mental Health
Infant mental health is synonymous with healthy social and emotional development.
The parent–child relationship, which includes the parent and child behaviors and the parent's internal representations of the child, is a central factor in infant mental health.
The rapidity of early childhood development means that early intervention has the potential to make substantive changes in the developing central nervous system even in high-risk children.
Many intrinsic and extrinsic factors influence infant's development including biologic, genetic, and constitutional makeup; the caregiver's relationship; family; culture; and socioeconomic status.

Applying IMH Principles: Universal Interventions

The principles of IMH can be applied in all settings where infants are seen including primary care settings; early intervention settings; Women, Infants, and Children (WIC) nutrition offices; child care settings; as well as specialty IMH programs, and any setting where children and their families receive services. In this section, we present opportunities for universal interventions intended to promote IMH by meeting the needs of young children and by supporting parents in the challenging task of caregiving.

Create a Family-Friendly Environment

Providers can convey to a family that children are valued by creating a physical space that welcomes young children and providing a child-safe environment, child-size furniture, and activities for children while parents are occupied, and private space for breast-feeding. Parents who feel valued and respected are more likely to treat their child in a nurturing and sensitive manner. For some parents, a family-friendly office staff member may be the first to model this type of interaction.

Promote Early Childhood Mental Health by Discussing and Screening for Mental Health Problems Universally

Universal systematic screening with validated measures in primary care settings may facilitate discussions about mental health, reduce the perceived stigma of mental health, and facilitate early identification of children with mental health needs. A number of valid, psychometrically strong measures can be used in clinical practice settings or child care settings to identify young children in need of mental health. Screening for maternal mental health is also a way of communicating that parenting is valued and may increase identification of parents in need of referrals and treatment. Table 18-3 presents some common instruments used to screen for mental health problems in young children.

Parent-report measures represent the parents' perception of the child's behaviors or emotional patterns and can be influenced to some degree by parental depression, distress, or concern about how the responses will be used. Thus, positive screens may represent child psychopathology, or parental distress, or a combination, but nearly always reflect a clinical situation in need of

TABLE 18-3	Selected Screens for Identifying Children in Need of Further Assessment	
Measure	**Ages (months)**	**Characteristics**
Ages and Stages Questionnaire: Social Emotional (Squires et al., 2002)	1–60	Different measures for each age range Strong psychometric properties 10–15 minutes to complete, 2–3 minutes to score
Brief Infant Toddler Social Emotional Assessment (Briggs-Gowan & Carter, 2002)	18–36	Identifies problems and strengths Strong psychometric properties including predictive validity 7–10 minutes to complete, 5 minutes to score
Early Childhood Screening Assessment (Gleason, Dickstein, & Zeanah, 2010)	24–60	36 items focused on child emotional and behavioral symptoms Four items focused on parent mental distress and depression
US PHTF Depression Screener (Olson et al., 2006)	Adult	Parental depression Two questions to identify parental depression

attention. Negative screens reflect a lower risk of mental health problems and may offer an opportunity for anticipatory guidance and positive reinforcement for parenting skills. No single measure should be considered a diagnostic tool. The results of a screen should be considered in the context of clinician observations, reports from other adults including child care providers, and clinician knowledge of other risk factors. Structured developmental screening using a validated measure is recommended by the American Academy of Pediatrics, as noted in the "Suggested Readings" section of this chapter.

Applying the Principles: Assessments of Infants and Young Children

Ideally, an early childhood mental health team includes or has access to child and adolescent psychiatrists, psychologists, social workers, developmental–behavioral pediatricians, other developmental specialists, and case managers. They generally collaborate with speech and language pathologists, occupational and physical therapists, primary care providers, and pediatric specialists such as geneticists and neurologists.

Making a Referral

Parents may have misconceptions about the meaning of an early childhood mental health referral. It is not uncommon for parents to be concerned that the referral reflects criticism of their parenting capacity, that the child is permanently disordered, or that a referral may result in losing custody of their child. Addressing these misconceptions early may facilitate the referral and assessment process. Referring clinicians can help parents understand the goals of the referral and what to expect in the assessment process and what they know about the specific approach used by the specialty provider. It can be helpful to use the words the mother has used to describe her concerns. If the parent described concerns about "fits," the referring clinician can talk about how the specialty provider will help understand the "fits." Often, statements like "She can help understand what is going on with your child's feelings and help your child learn to organize her feelings and behaviors" or "His job is to help your child be as happy and successful as possible and to help you and your child have chances to enjoy each other" can help to clarify the role of the early childhood mental health evaluation.

Infant and Early Childhood Assessment

Assessments occur over the course of multiple visits, with multiple informants and multiple approaches to information gathering that allow the provider to integrate a three-dimensional view of the child. The assessment includes time alone with the parents to discuss sensitive information such as pregnancy planning, family history, and family violence histories and time with both the parents and the child in the room to observe behavior and interactions informally. With older children, the time with everyone in the room allows the clinician to help reframe the presenting complaint from blaming or negative words to behavioral descriptions. For example, a clinician may reframe "he's so bad" to "it sounds like he has a hard time sitting still in school." Such an intervention can help engage the child in the process and reduce the child's negative experiences.

An important focus of an IMH assessment is attention both to the information the parents provide and to the way they provide it (narrative qualities). These qualities reflect the parent's internal representation of the child and may be heard in the degree to which the parent's discussion of the child includes a balance of both positive and negative characteristics, whether it is shaped or distorted by the parent's other intimate relationships or experiences, the overall tone the parent uses to discuss the child, and the degree to which the narrative holds together as a cohesive picture of the child. An example of distortion is a mother whose child experienced an arm injury due to a birth trauma and who was unable to talk about the child in any way without connecting the discussion to the traumatic birth events. Her narrative demonstrated that she saw her child through the lens of a traumatic event that shaped and distorted the picture. A strong body of literature led by groundbreaking work by Benoid, Parker, and Zeanah in 1997 documents the association between narrative qualities—even prenatally—and the quality of the attachment relationship and the child's later mental health outcomes.

Taking the History

The major components of an IMH history are similar to the categories of history elicited about older children. In IMH assessments, parents and other adults provide most of the history of present illness. Clinicians primarily use observational and interactive approaches to elicit information directly from the child. This is especially true with infant assessments, in which most of the assessment focuses on the history provided and on the parent–infant relationship, which will be the path through which intervention addresses the presenting problem. Although infant and preschool assessments often differ in the content of the presenting complaint and the proportion of time spent on *DSM*-specific symptoms, the major components are similar.

The clinician focuses on the parent's primary concern, using open-ended questions and probes to understand who is concerned, what specifically has been observed, how adults respond to the concerning symptoms, how the problem resolves, the meaning that the caregivers attribute to the behavior, and how they have been coping with the challenge of the symptom. A complete history of the presenting concern and review of systems informs the differential diagnosis. In infants, the review of symptoms focuses heavily on regulatory processes (soothability, feeding, sleeping patterns, and sensory issues) and less on the typical domains of older children. Review of symptoms in toddlers and preschoolers include attention both to regulatory processes and to the traditional psychiatric domains like mood, anxiety, behavioral regulation, and social skill development.

A few items in the standard psychiatric history for very young children warrant further explanation as they may serve different purposes than a typical mental health history. The history should include the preconception period including pregnancy history, intention to become pregnant, or fertility treatments. If a mother did not plan or want to be pregnant, it can be useful to understand what influenced her decision (or nondecision) to have the child, and whether she changed her mind during the pregnancy. Early events including becoming pregnant unexpectedly, a history of fertility treatment, domestic violence, medical problems, the absence of supportive relationships, and major life events during the pregnancy all can influence how a parent thinks about and reacts to a very young child and can influence the developing relationship with a child. For example, a mother with a history of multiple pregnancy losses may view her infant as especially vulnerable even after birth and continue to monitor and protect the infant as if the world actively threatens the baby. She may present with excessive sleep deprivation because she sets an alarm clock every hour to check that her 15-month-old is breathing. Additionally, it is useful to ask about the transition to the role of parent. Understanding the parent's view of the new role and the degree to which she feels supported by her partner, extended family, and other supports helps the clinician gauge the context of her concerns and opportunities for enhancing support. A mother who is isolated and unsupported is at higher-than-usual risk for developing postpartum depression or experiencing parenting and her infant as burdensome.

It is important to take a developmental history as well, with attention to motor milestones, language development, self-care skills like toilet training, as well as social development. Standardized measures such as the Ages and Stages Questionnaire can be useful adjuncts to this history in developmental risk categories. Medical issues most relevant to an IMH evaluation are any CNS processes such as seizures or head trauma, pregnancy or perinatal events, failure to thrive, and in older children, pica. Generally, it is prudent to review the primary care records to avoid unnecessary duplication of lead levels or other blood tests. Any chronic illness or frightening medical event may influence the degree of vulnerability a parent sees in a child as well as increase child anxiety, and thus is important in the infant and early childhood mental health context.

Family psychiatric history provides information about possible genetic loading, and also about a child's and a parent's caregiving experiences. Parental psychiatric disorders may affect how a parent attends to the child's needs, the consistency of caregiving style, their patience with the child, affective tone toward the child, and punishment styles. Research shows that maternal depression occurs at rates of 20% to 30% in the preschool years and is associated with a range of biologic and psychological adverse child outcomes including EEG asymmetry, low developmental quotient, abnormal catecholamine excretion, and emotional, behavioral, and social problems. Thus, depression and comorbid conditions must be identified and addressed as part of an IMH assessment. When parents have a history of depression or any other psychiatric disorder, clinicians explore how their symptoms impact parenting. For example, a question such as "Sometimes people get frustrated or upset with their children more easily than they want to. Does that happen to you?" may give a parent permission to describe the impact of depression on parenting.

Drawing a genogram allows clinicians to understand family relationships, and the parents' own caregiving experiences, and to identify supportive or abusive caregiving relationships. The genogram allows the clinician to begin to identify the "ghosts" and "angels" in the nursery and helps identify genetic factors that may influence the child's clinical presentation.

In the social history, the clinician focuses on contexts of the child's experiences including cultural beliefs about child development, safety of home environment, and the people involved in the child's caregiving, with a goal of identifying protective and risk factors. Sameroff and Fiese research reminds us that no specific single risk factor is determinative; the number of social risk factors predicts a child's outcome. Understanding the community, cultural, and household contexts in which a child is developing informs a biopsychosocial assessment and identifies targets for nonclinical interventions.

Observations

A clinician can create opportunities for multiple types of observations during the assessment. Informal observations in the waiting room and while taking a history can be quite valuable in revealing the child's and dyad's typical patterns including how a child interacts with the clinician for the first time. Table 18-4 provides a structure for describing observations in an IMH setting. Although IMH mental status examinations share domains with those for older patients, a few differences warrant attention. First, appearance is especially important in an IMH assessment. Size for age provides information about the child's nutrition or medical status. A clinician also observes whether a patient has stigmata of genetic syndromes. The most commonly seen dysmorphic features include unusual placement or shape of the ears, presence of epicanthal folds, unusual shape of the nose and nasal bridge, philtrum, and the presence of micrognathia, although a clinician should be aware of any congenital dysmorphism. Evidence of "baby bottle carries" may suggest a low level of parental supervision while feeding, and excessive occipital alopecia may suggest that the baby spends significant time on his or her back. A child's developmental level in the domains of language, fine and gross motor skills, and school readiness in older children are part of the mental status evaluation. If any developmental concerns are raised during the mental health assessment, the child should be referred for formal testing by a developmental specialist. Most of the observations of a child can be done during play, which is the primary communication tool for young children and informs a clinician's understanding of the child's thought process and thought content.

During the early childhood mental health assessment, the clinician attends to the patterns of the parent–child interactions. The first opportunity for these observations is the waiting

TABLE 18-4	Essential Observations in Infant and Early Childhood Assessment
Appearance	Size (height and weight for age), dress and hygiene, maturity compared to age, dysmorphia and congenital anomalies, bruises or other marks, degree of occipital alopecia in infants, dentition (e.g., baby bottle caries)
Observed reaction to new situation	Initial reaction to setting and to strangers (e.g., fearful, clingy, indiscriminate friendliness) and rate of adaptation to the setting
Parent–child interactions	Pattern of interactions including proximity seeking, eye contact, joy sharing, child's tone in interactions, parental engagement with child, responsiveness to child's needs, enthusiasm, and parent tone; child use of parent after brief separation (eye contact, approach, and ability to be soothed)
Relatedness	Physical contact with caregiver, eye contact, interactive style, level of verbal engagement, play engagement, and turn taking in older children
Development	
Motor muscle tone and strength	Gross motor coordination, fine motor coordination
Speech/language	Vocalization and speech production; receptive language; expressive language; volume, rate, and prosody in verbal children
Cognition	Use information from all above areas, especially play, language use, symbolic functioning, and problem-solving, school readiness skills
Developmentally specific mental status observations	
Infants: self-regulation	Predominant state and rage of states observed during session, patterns of transition, sensory regulation, unusual behaviors, activity level, attention span, frustration tolerance, aggression
Infants: affect and mood	Modes of expression (facial, verbal, body tone and positioning), range of expressed emotions, duration of emotional state, intensity of expressed emotions Self-reported mood in preschoolers
Toddlers, preschoolers: behavior	Activity level, impulsivity, ability to follow directions, stereotypies, responses to limit setting
Toddlers, preschoolers: mood	How they identify their mood; can be facilitated by drawing pictures of happy, sad, mad, and scared, checking that the child can identify these feelings accurately and then asking them to identify their own mood
Toddlers, preschoolers: thought process	Ability to maintain attention at developmental level Degree and quality of organization of play and (when developmentally applicable) speech
Toddlers/preschoolers: thought content	Predominant themes in play and speech (with attention to aggression, sexual play, caregiving themes)

room, when the clinician can observe how the child responds to the presence of a stranger (the clinician) and the degree to which the child references the parent to check about the safety of the stranger. Throughout the observation, the clinician attends to the child's interactions with the parent, including patterns of proximity seeking, comfort seeking, and social referencing. Disturbances of these behaviors may represent a wide differential including relationship disturbances, temperamental patterns (extremes of approach or withdrawal behaviors), and pervasive developmental disorders. During the evaluation, and especially during mild stressors, the clinician notes the affective tone of the interactions (e.g., warm, joyful, harsh, wary, or fearful), the way the infant or child uses the parents for comfort and to help them regulate their emotions, the parent's ability to anticipate the child's needs, limit setting and the child's response to the limits, and comfort level playing together/interacting. Formal, structured observations such as those used in Crowell's procedure provide information about how the dyad plays together, copes with limit setting, and negotiates easy and difficult puzzle tasks, and how the child uses the parent for comfort after a separation. In healthy dyads, a child will seek out the parent who anticipated the potential for distress and offers comfort, and the child will soothe quickly. In other situations, the clinician may note that the child approaches the clinician for comfort, that the parent did not recognize the child's need and does not offer comfort or is dismissive of the child ("he's too big to cry about that"), or that despite reasonable efforts to calm the child, the child cannot organize his or her feelings. Each of these findings would suggest important difficulties in the parent–child relationship or the child's emotional regulation.

Diagnosis

In 2006, Egger and Arnold reported that approximately 10% of preschoolers exhibit patterns of symptoms that meet criteria for a severe, impairing psychiatric disorder, with generalized anxiety disorder and oppositional defiant disorder tied for most prevalent at over 6%. A small but increasing literature supports the validity of the use of the use of the *Diagnostic and Statistical Manual, Fourth Edition (DSM-IV)* with preschoolers, primarily regarding major depressive disorder, post traumatic stress disorder, and attention deficit hyperactivity disorder (ADHD) diagnoses, respectively in preschoolers. These disorders tend to persist over time and can be distinguished from each other and from developmentally normative behaviors by observation, symptom report, and in the cases of MDD and PTSD, biologic markers. In short, preschool disorders are neither phases nor normal development. Clinicians may find that the *Diagnostic Criteria: Zero to Three (Revised) (DC:0–3R)* is a clinically useful tool as a developmentally sensitive alternative to the *DSM-IV*. It provides a standardized approach to diagnosis in infants, toddlers, and preschoolers and includes structured ways to report parent–child interaction patterns. Table 18-5 provides a crosswalk between *DC:0–3R* and common *DSM-IV* diagnoses.

TABLE 18-5 Crosswalk between *DSM* and *DC:0–3R* Diagnoses	
DSM-IV	*DC:0–3R*
Attention-deficit hyperactivity disorder	Regulatory disorder of sensory processing: sensory seeking/impulsive or hypo-/underresponsive
Oppositional defiant disorder	Regulatory disorder of sensory processing: negative/defiant
Generalized anxiety disorder	Generalized anxiety disorder
Reactive attachment disorder	Deprivation maltreatment disorder
Posttraumatic stress disorder Acute stress disorder	Posttraumatic stress disorder
Major depressive disorder	Type I major depression
Feeding disorder of infancy	Feeding behavior disorder Feeding behavior disorder of caregiver infant reciprocity Infantile anorexia

TABLE 18-6 Essentials of Infant and Early Childhood Assessment
Nonspecialty settings provide opportunities for observations and universal screening
A warm, consistent, and nurturing environment is critical to for assessment and treatment
Parents' content and narrative qualities in the history inform the assessment process
Multiple visits using multiple assessment modalities and multiple reporters are necessary in this age group
History includes attention to usual components of history plus details of pre- and perinatal events, development, attention to regulatory and attachment behaviors, and family history of psychiatric disorders and caregiving strengths or challenges
Observations include developmentally specific factors including size, dysmorphic features, behavioral regulation, organization of behavioral and emotional responses, ability to respond to parental support and parent–child interactions, and qualities of play
Careful application of diagnostic criteria may facilitate communication and treatment planning

Although historically controversial, using standard diagnostic nosologies enhances communication among providers, helps children access services, allows for billing for IMH services, and informs treatment planning. It is important that clinicians and parents understand the limits of these diagnoses in predicting the longitudinal courses, especially for those disorders with the most limited data, such as anxiety disorders or bipolar disorder.

Formulation in IMH should be organized in the same way as for older children using the biopsychosocial model. A clinician considers all of the information obtained in the assessment, including biologic factors (medical problems, possible or known genetic factors, and a child's developmental status), parent and child psychological factors (how the parent perceives the child and himself/herself, the child's self-regulatory patterns, and the use of parents and other caregivers as part of the regulatory approach), and family and child social factors (especially exposure to violence, maltreatment, and limited access to resources). Depending on the clinical situation, the formulation may focus primarily on the child's own intrinsic biologic or psychological patterns, on the parent–child relationship, or on exposure to social risk factors. Sometimes, the assessment will identify the need for clinical attention to developmental issues or basic needs such as housing or food. Most importantly, the formulation must provide an understanding of the child and family at a point along a developmental trajectory, rather than a static assessment unlikely to change. Table 18-6 summarizes the essentials of assessment during infancy and early childhood.

Infant Mental Health Treatment Approaches

Non-IMH providers play an important role in promoting infant and early childhood mental health by providing anticipatory guidance to parents about social-emotional development and helping address challenges of normal variations of regulation like sleep difficulties and picky eating. Many clinical interactions provide opportunities for providers to observe dyadic interactions and identify strengths ("Wow! He really calmed down when you hugged him after the shots. He feels safe when he's close to you.") or opportunities ("I see him looking right at you now after the shots. I wonder if he might calm down if you held him."). Such brief interventions may help families toward healthy developmental trajectories and/or identify emerging problems that may benefit from early interventions. Basic information about positive reinforcement and safe discipline strategies can also be applied in non-IMH settings. Clinicians can also guide parents toward resources with reliable information about young

TABLE 18-7	**Essentials of Infant and Early Childhood Mental Health Treatment**
Nonspecialty settings can create family-friendly environment with useful psychoeducation regarding infant mental health that promotes infant and early childhood mental health in a universal intervention	
Evidence supports the use of relationship-focused psychotherapies that can target internal experiences/perceptions and/or behaviors in the parent and/or child	
Successful therapy includes use of play as a primary modality for interacting with toddlers and preschoolers	
Psychopharmacologic treatment of very young children has limited empirical support and some known risks, although may be an appropriate adjunctive treatment in severe cases	

children, as noted in the "Suggested Readings" and "Suggested Websites" sections at the end of this chapter.

A growing evidence base supports the efficacy of early childhood mental health interventions. Most focus on parent–child relationships and intervene at the caregiver level, with the expectation that changes in caregiver behaviors or perception of the child's behaviors will impact the child's experience and ultimately improve the child's mental health status. Because caregivers usually seek treatment for their child rather than for themselves or the dyad, it is essential that clinicians ensure that parents do not experience the parent focus as an unspoken criticism. It can be useful to be explicit, using phrases like "You are the most important person in the child's life and using you as part of the therapy is the most powerful way we can help." As children get older and develop more language and cognitive capacity, the potential for child-focused therapy increases. Treatment is usually multimodal and should include attention to basic needs including housing, food, safety, and educational and legal advocacy.

The following sections present specific forms of evidence-based treatments for early childhood disorders or risk conditions, which are summarized in Table 18-7.

Attachment-based Therapy

Dyadic or parent–child therapies based on attachment theory focus on strengthening disordered infant–parent relationships. They primarily target the parent's internal representations of the child and parent behaviors with the child in order to change the child's experiences in the parent–child relationship, increase emotional regulation capacity, and enhance their sense of safety. Treatment for infants always includes dyadic therapy and may also include individual treatment for the parent. Dyadic therapy includes a strong emphasis on developing a strong, respectful, and nurturing therapeutic alliance with the parent. One evidence-based attachment-based therapy, Infant and Child Parent Psychotherapy developed by Alicia Lieberman, explicitly focuses on creating a "corrective attachment relationship" with the caregiver, developing an understanding of the influence of past caregiving relationships on the parent–child relationship and building upon existing strengths. This intervention has demonstrated strong and persistent decreases in traumatic stress symptoms in young children who have experienced trauma and improvements in their mothers' mental health symptoms. A number of other attachment-based therapies have been shown to be effective in increasing parenting sensitivity, increasing rates of secure attachment status, and reducing rates of later psychopathology in at-risk infants.

Parent-Management Training

A number of evidence-based treatment approaches use parent-management training to address behavioral problems, primarily in older toddlers and preschoolers. These programs, including Eyberg's Parent–Child Interaction Therapy and Webster-Stratton's Incredible Years Series, target the child's behavior by changing parent behavior. Both use psychoeducation and provide opportunities for parents to practice positive discipline. The Parent–Child Interaction Therapy includes two primary components—the first in which parents practice the "PRIDE" skills (*p*raise, *r*eflection, *i*mitation, *d*escription, *e*nthusiasm) and the second in which parents learn to structure a safe discipline plan and to follow through when a child does not obey instructions. With parent-management training, child behavior problems decrease with the treatments and the improvement is sustained over years.

Cognitive–Behavioral Therapy

For preschoolers, cognitive–behavioral therapy (CBT) has also been used to treat trauma-exposed children. CBT for young children includes a focus on learning anxiety-management strategies such as progressive muscle relaxation, diaphragmatic breathing, and guided imagery, as well as graduated exposure to a narrative of the traumatic event. CBT for preschoolers also includes attention to parents' symptoms and their responses to the trauma and to the treatment. In 1997, Cohen and Mannarino reported that young children could participate effectively in CBT and the treatment was associated with a persistent decrease in trauma-related, internalizing, and externalizing symptoms in sexually abused children 2 to 7 years old.

Play Therapy

Virtually all therapy for young children includes some element of play. In play therapy, the play becomes the vehicle for change. Play therapy is founded upon the understanding that children use play to express their internal experiences and that they may be able to resolve internal distress or conflicts through play. Play therapy does not lend itself to randomized controlled trials and limited data exist. However, nondirected, unstructured play therapy provides a child a safe space and a relationship with a positive, nurturing adult. Structured play therapy for trauma-exposed children provides opportunities to understand the trauma and integrate the memories and experience of the trauma into a cohesive narrative rather than an intrusive set of unprocessed images and sensations.

Medications

Rates of prescriptions for very young children have increased in the last 20 years to approximately 3 to 9 per 1000 children, according to Zito and colleagues' 2006 research. Despite this trend, most children with a psychiatric disorder do not receive any form of treatment, including medication. The current state of the literature highlights the need for caution when considering medications in very young children because of the limited knowledge related to short-term efficacy and safety and long-term effects on development.

Preschool and psychopharmacology experts have provided some general principles to guide the consideration of psychopharmacologic intervention, as noted in Table 18-8. First, psychotherapy should be the first-line treatment for preschoolers with psychiatric disorders, as the risks are lower and the empirical support is often equal to or stronger than that for medications. Because of the lack of systematic research, psychopharmacologic therapy is not recommended for children under 36 months. When considering medications, clinicians should have a clear plan for monitoring treatment effects and adverse effects using structured symptom-specific measures. At the beginning of treatment, clinicians should discuss a plan to discontinue the medication after a period of successful treatment (e.g., 6–9 months) to allow a reassessment of the child's clinical status. Lastly, given the limits of evidence regarding safety for single medications, concomitant use of more than one medication should be a rare occurrence and more than one medication should not be started at the same time.

Comprehensive treatment recommendations are beyond the scope of this chapter but are available in a Gleason and colleagues' 2007 review and guidelines. In every case, prescribers should consider the degree of certainty of the diagnosis, the level of impairment associated with the disorder, the relative strength of evidence for psychotherapy compared with psychopharmacotherapy, and the risk of adverse effects when developing a treatment plan. There may be

	TABLE 18-8 Preschool Disorders and Pharmacologic Treatments*			
Disorder	FDA Indication for Preschoolers	RCTs of Psychotherapy	RCTs of Psychopharmacology	Other Medications with Published Data in Preschoolers (Level of Evidence, Sample Size)
ADHD	D-Amphetamine Clonidine	Yes—parent-management training (Sonuga-Barke et al., 2001)	Yes—methylphenidate: large, multisite RCT (Greenhill et al., 2006), 10 smaller studies	Atomoxetine: open trial, FDA > 6 y.o. (Kratochvil et al., 2007) Guanfacine: open trial, FDA no pediatric indications (Hunt, 1995) Clonidine: chart review, (Prince et al., 1996)
Aggression	None	Yes—parent-management training, multiple studies (Eyberg et al., 1988; Webster-Stratton et al., 1997)	None	Risperidone: case series, FDA no aggression indication if no PDD (Cesena et al. 2002) Risperidone: retrospective chart review, FDA no aggression indication if no PDD (Staller, 2007)
Anxiety (GAD, SAD, selective mutism, PTSD, OCD)	Hydroxyzine	CBT for sexually abused preschoolers (Cohen & Mannarino, 1997)	None	Clonidine: open trial for PTSD + aggression, FDA no anxiety indication (Harmon & Riggs, 1999) Fluoxetine: case reports, FDA OCD > 7 y.o. (Wright et al., 1995; Avci et al., 1988; Celik et al., 2007) Sertraline: case series, FDA OCD > 6 y.o. (Oner and Oner, 2008)
Autism/PDD	Risperidone (> 5 y.o.)		Risperidone: minimal difference vs. placebo on core symptoms, (Luby et al., 2006); (2–9 y.o.) (Nagaraj et al., 2006)	Risperidone: case series, FDA > 5 to treat aggression and irritability (Masi et al., 2003)

(continued)

331

TABLE 18-8 Preschool Disorders and Pharmacologic Treatments* (continued)

Disorder	FDA Indication for Preschoolers	RCTs of Psychotherapy	RCTs of Psychopharmacology	Other Medications with Published Data in Preschoolers (Level of Evidence, Sample Size)
Bipolar disorder	None	None		Risperidone: open trial, $n = 16$, FDA > 10 y.o. (Biederman et al., 2005) Valproate: retrospective chart review, $n = 9$, FDA no bipolar indication (Mota-Castillo et al., 2001)
Major depressive disorder	None	None	None	None
Reactive attachment disorder	None	Placement in foster care reduces rates of RAD for institutionalized children (Zeanah et al., 2009)	None	None

*Positive effects unless otherwise noted.

FDA, Food and Drug Administration; RCT, randomized clinical trial; PDD, pervasive developmental disorder; GAD, generalized anxiety disorder; SAD, separation anxiety disorder; PTSD, posttraumatic stress disorder; OCD, obsessive–compulsive disorder; CBT, cognitive–behavioral therapy; RAD, reactive attachment disorder.

patients for whom supportive therapy and attention to basic needs may be the treatment plan with the highest likelihood of success and lowest risk of adverse effects.

There are limited data to guide dosing strategies in very young children except with methylphenidate, as described later in the text. In general, using the lowest possible dose (one fourth of a tablet of the smallest dose) is recommended with a slow upward titration, recognizing young children may be especially susceptible to adverse effects. There are also limited data to guide laboratory and other safety monitoring, so generally, guidelines like the *Practice Parameters* for older children developed by the American Academy of Child and Adolescent Psychiatry in 2009.

Only two medications have been tested in randomized controlled trials: methylphenidate for ADHD and risperidone for aggression and irritability in children with autism. The 2006 Preschool ADHD Treatment Study (PATS) by Greenhill and colleagues is a landmark, placebo-controlled, multisite trial of methylphenidate for preschoolers with ADHD. The research group reported that methylphenidate was superior to placebo in treating symptoms of ADHD by parent and teacher report. Children's individual optimal dose ranged from 7.5 to 30 mg divided three times per day, but was not associated with weight. Compared with studies in older children, the PATS demonstrated a smaller effect size (only 21% achieved full remission), higher rate of adverse effects, and slower clearance of methylphenidate. Thus, this study both highlights the potential benefits of methylphenidate as an effective treatment for preschool ADHD and reminds us of the limits of extrapolating results from other age groups to preschoolers. Because of the level of evidence supporting methylphenidate compared to other medications for preschool ADHD, it is recommended as the first-line treatment for therapy-resistant ADHD in this age group, using doses in the PATS. Although no studies have examined the safety or efficacy of long-acting formulations of methylphenidate, these have logistical advantages and may be used after it is clear the patient can tolerate the immediate-release stimulant. For children who fail trials of methylphenidate, reassessment of the diagnosis and the adequacy of the psychotherapy is warranted. If the diagnosis appears accurate and psychotherapy appropriate, amphetamine formulations such as mixed amphetamine salts or D-amphetamine may be a reasonable next step. As shown in Table 18-8, limited data guide approaches beyond stimulants and warrants discussion with colleagues, especially physicians with training or experience working with very young children.

There are no randomized controlled trials of psychopharmacologic interventions for preschoolers with disruptive behavior disorders. This contrasts dramatically with the strong evidence demonstrating the efficacy and effectiveness of parent-management training, such as the Parent–Child Interaction Therapy and the Incredible Years Series. Thus, medication to treat preschool disruptive behavior disorders is rarely indicated except when dangerous aggression is prominent and environmental and behavioral interventions have failed to reduce these risks. Pharmacologic treatment of comorbid ADHD with disruptive behavior disorders is appropriate and should occur before consideration of medication specifically to target disruptive behaviors. Of medications with data supporting their use for disruptive behavior disorders in older children, risperidone has the most data related to safety and is approved for use in children as young as 5 years for aggression related to pervasive developmental disorders. Reported doses in preschoolers range from 0.25 to 3.0 mg/day. Adverse effects of risperidone in preschoolers can be significant. Extraordinary weight gain (15 kg in one case report), sedation, and elevated prolactin levels have all been reported. Children on these medications should have regular monitoring of growth parameters and laboratory screening including fasting glucose and lipid panels as well as prolactin. Like other medications, risperidone should not be continued if a child experiences significant adverse events.

Although anxiety disorders are common in preschoolers, there are no systematic studies of psychopharmacologic interventions for preschoolers with anxiety disorders. On the other hand, preschoolers are able to participate in CBT, which is an effective treatment for preschool posttraumatic symptoms and the first-line treatment for anxiety disorders in older children. Thus, CBT is the first-line treatment for preschoolers with anxiety disorders. Adverse effects of selective serotonin reuptake inhibitors (SSRIs) in children under 7 have been reported to be higher than in older children, with nearly 20% discontinuing the medication because of adverse effects and over half experiencing behavioral activation. Based on the balance of risks, benefits, and alternatives, SSRIs should be used with caution and in collaboration with a mental health professional.

Pharmacologic intervention for preschool mood disorders is a complex topic beyond the scope of this chapter. No studies have examined the treatment of the well-validated disorder of major depression in preschoolers, and researchers who work with this population rarely use medications to treat this disorder. Dyadic and/or play therapy seems to be effective, sometimes in conjunction with parental treatment, for preschool depression. On the other hand, a number of reports have described pharmacologic treatment of bipolar disorder, a disorder whose diagnostic criteria continue to be controversial in this age group. None of the reports employed systematic approaches to diagnosis. Thus, it is difficult to generalize from these reports, which largely used atypical antipsychotic agents and mood stabilizers.

There are neither empirical nor theoretical reasons to consider psychopharmacologic interventions for preschoolers with reactive attachment disorder. This disorder should be addressed by providing a safe caregiving environment. Children who have experienced pathogenic caregiving may be at risk for other disorders, which may warrant therapy or, in some cases, medications. Assessment of these children with multiple risk factors and high rates of comorbidity is complex and should be done by a clinician with experience working with very young children.

Because of the shortage of child psychiatrists, primary care providers play an active role in the treatment of very young children with severe mental health problems. This role is optimally done in collaboration rather than in isolation. Although clinicians may feel pressure to "do something" when children present with extreme mental health problems and intense parental distress, the importance of a reasonable assessment, diagnosis, and formulation cannot be underestimated. Nonmental health prescribing clinicians are encouraged to follow as many of the steps of the assessment described earlier in the text as possible before considering medication for a young child. Minimally, before prescribing, clinicians should assess recent stressors or family events, use history and observation to inform biopsychosocial diagnostic formulation, obtain collateral information from other adult caregivers, reconsider the treatment plan if the child does not meet criteria for a diagnosis, and consider a broad range of nonpharmacologic interventions. Psychopharmacologic treatment without these steps may prevent identification of and intervention for important etiologic factors such as maltreatment, developmental delays/learning disorders, and parental psychopathology. Additionally, quick use of a prescription may create an expectation that the problem is likely to be resolved with medication alone, a belief that the PATS study suggests may be unrealistic. Suggested readings and websites for clinicians treating young children are included at the end of this chapter.

Conclusions

IMH is a multidisciplinary specialty that considers the emotional well-being of young children within the contexts of their caregiving relationships, family, development, and community factors. Assessment of very young children with mental health problems is a multidisciplinary and multimodal process. A number of psychotherapeutic modalities are effective in reducing mental health problems of very young children, but may not be accessible to all children or clinicians. Psychopharmacologic interventions may be effective as an adjunct treatment for very young children, but have a higher risk of adverse effects, and further study is necessary to understand long-term effects.

CASE VIGNETTES

VIGNETTE 1: POSTPARTUM DEPRESSION AND INFANT MENTAL HEALTH

Ethan is 6 weeks old. He and his parents have recently moved to a new town and have no family or friends in the area. His father, Peter, works long hours, and his mother, Jane, is home alone with him during the day. His mother has been extremely tired and tearful throughout the day, and has been avoiding answering her telephone. When Ethan begins crying in his crib, his mother sighs but does not approach him and sometimes turns up the TV to block out Ethan's cries. When his crying persists, she often cries as well. When she feeds him, she holds him facing out and they make little eye contact. Her obstetrician diagnosed her with depression and started an SSRI, which she did not take because she was worried it would make her too sleepy. Ethan's pediatrician was concerned because he made little eye contact or vocalizations, and referred the dyad to an IMH specialist and the Part C Early Intervention Program, which had an IMH specialist on the team. The therapist initiated Infant Parent Psychotherapy and together they explored Jane's interpretation of Ethan's crying as a sign of her failure as a mother. The sessions focused on developmentally appropriate expectations and on identifying the outside influences that were shaping how she thought about Ethan, supporting their social engagement, providing a supportive relationship with her, and developing strategies to enlist Ethan's father as a critical part of the caregiving team. Additionally, the therapist encouraged Jane to discuss her concerns about the medication with her physician. She began to identify Ethan's cues as his only way of communicating with her rather than condemnation, and both she and the therapist noted that Ethan made increased positive bids for attention and stronger eye contact.

VIGNETTE 2: AGGRESSION IN A PRESCHOOLER WHO HAS BEEN EXPOSED TO DOMESTIC VIOLENCE

Jessica was a 3-year-10-month-old girl referred for behavioral difficulties at school and at home, including hitting other children, throwing toys, and yelling, often when the home or classroom was already loud, and appeared hyperactive, impulsive, and fidgety. Her mother, Susan, also reported that she had developed nightmares, was afraid of being around men, and became distressed with parades and television shows that portrayed arguments. During free play in the assessment, Jessica used the father figure doll to hit the mother figure over and over. Further history revealed she had witnessed her mother's boyfriend assault her mother shortly before the behavioral difficulties began. Her mother had not seen him since, but continued to be frightened as well. In addition to Jessica's mother receiving a referral to legal aid services, Jessica and her mother participated in CBT focused on PTSD, learned relaxation techniques, and began a graduate course of exposure to triggers. Behavioral difficulties at school and at home resolved quickly, and her anxiety symptoms also decreased.

VIGNETTE 3: POLYPHARMACY IN A PRESCHOOLER

Kaleb is a 3-year-4-month-old boy referred for evaluation from his primary care provider for consultation regarding medications. Kaleb's mother reported that he was experiencing impulsivity, irritability, sleep problems, and severe aggression toward his infant brother. He had been diagnosed with bipolar disorder by a local adult psychiatrist at age 2 year 4 months and started on zyprexa, fluoxetine, clonidine, and lisdexamphetamine. With each medication, he seemed to have a response for a few weeks and the symptoms resolved. Full evaluation revealed a 60-pound boy who had severe expressive speech delay but evident social skills, notable impulsivity, and some provocative aggressive behaviors, usually in response to his mother yelling loudly and harshly at him, which she did repeatedly during the evaluation. She reported untreated symptoms of moderate depression and said she had been diagnosed with borderline personality disorder. Formal diagnosis was deferred because of the unknown effects of the medications on his underlying disorder. He was diagnosed provisionally with ADHD, expressive speech delay, and Rule out oppositional defiant disorder, Rule out sleep disorder, and Rule out mood disorder NOS. He was referred to the school department for more extensive IQ testing and for speech therapy. Monitoring labs revealed triglyceride and cholesterol levels in the borderline range for his age, and BMI was well above the 95 percentile for his age. Pharmacotherapy focused on weaning him off the medications: first the atypical antipsychotic agent and then the SSRI and the alpha agonist. He continued to demonstrate hyperactivity and severe impulsivity on and off the lisdexamphetamine, which was discontinued. He did well in a child care setting and at home on 30 mg of intermediate duration methylphenidate per day. Psychotherapy focused on Parent–Child Interaction Therapy. His mother was initially reluctant to participate, but after developing a trusting relationship with the therapist, enjoyed the positive reinforcement she received in the therapy and the changes she saw in his behavior, which became more organized, less provocative, and less aggressive. Follow-up labs were within the normal range, and he maintained a stable weight.

BIBLIOGRAHY

Amaya-Jackson L, Ziv Y, Greenberg MT, eds. *Enhancing Early Attachment: Theory, Research and Intervention.* New York: Guilford Press; 2003:100–123.

American Academy of Child and Adolescent Psychiatry. Practice parameter on the use of psychotropic medication in children and adolescents. *J Am Acad Child Adolesc Psychiatry.* 2009;48(9):961–973. Available at: http://www.aacap.org/cs/root/publication_store/practice_parameters_and_guidelines.

American Academy of Pediatrics. Developmental surveillance and screening of infants and young children. *Pediatrics.* 2001;108:192–195.

American Psychiatric Association. *Diagnostic and Statistical Manual of Mental Disorders, Fourth Edition, Text Revision (DSM-IV-TR).* Washington, DC: American Psychiatric Association; 2000.

Avci A, Diler RS, Tamam L. Fluoxetine treatment in a 2.5-year-old girl. *J Am Acad Child Adolesc Psychiatry.* 1988;37(9):901–902.

Bakermans-Kranenburg MJ, van Ijzendoorn MH, Juffer F. Less is more: meta-analyses of sensitivity and attachment interventions in early childhood. *Psychol Bull.* 2003;129(2):195–215.

Benoit D, Parker KCH, Zeanah CH. Mothers' representations of their infants assessed prenatally: stability and association with infants' attachment classifications. *J Child Psychol Psychiatry.* 1997;38(3):307–313.

Biederman J, Mick E, Hammerness P, et al. Open-label, 8-week trial of olanzapine and risperidone for the treatment of bipolar disorder in preschool-age children. *Biol Psychiatry.* 2005;58(7):589–594.

Briggs-Gowan MJ, Carter AS. *Brief Infant Toddler Social Emotional Assessment (BITSEA) Manual Version 2.0.* New Haven, CT: Yale University; 2002.

Carter A, Briggs-Gowan MJ, Davis NO. Assessment of young children's social-emotional development and psychopathology: recent advances and recommendations for practice. *J Child Psychol Psychiatry.* 2004;45(1):109–134.

Celik G, Diler RS, Thiroglu AY, et al. Fluoxetine in posttraumatic eating disorder in two-year-old twins. *J Child Adolesc Psychopharmacol.* 2007;17(2):233–236.

Cesena M, Gonzalez-Heydrich J, Szigethy E, et al. A case series of eight aggressive young children treated with risperidone. *J Child Adolesc Psychopharmacol.* 2002;12:337–345.

Cohen JA, Mannarino AP. A treatment study for sexually abused preschool children: outcome during one year follow-up. *J Am Acad Child Adolesc Psychiatry.* 1997;36(9):1228–1235.

Crowell JA. Assessment of attachment security in a clinical setting: observations of parents and children. *J Dev Behav Pediatr.* 2003;24(3):199–204.

Davidson RJ, Jackson DC, Larson CL, et al. Approach-withdrawal and cerebral asymmetry: emotional expression and brain physiology. *J Pers Soc Psychol.* 1990;58(2):330–341.

Dozier M, Manni M, Gordon M. Foster children's diurnal production of cortisol: an exploratory study. *Child Maltreat.* 2006;11(2):189–197.

Egger HL, Angold A. Common emotional and behavioral disorders in preschool children: presentation, nosology, and epidemiology. *J Child Psychol Psychiatry.* 2006;47(3–4):313–337.

Eyberg SM. Parent-child interaction therapy: integration of traditional and behavioral concerns. *Child Fam Behav Ther.* 1988;10:33–46.

Field T, Diego M. Maternal depression effects on infant frontal EEG asymmetry. *Int J Neurosci.* 2008;118(8):1081–1088.

Fox NA, Henderson HA, Marshall PJ, et al. Behavioral inhibition: linking biology and behavior within a developmental framework. *Annu Rev Psychol.* 2005;56:235–261.

Fraiberg S, Adelson E, Shapiro V. Ghosts in the nursery: a psychoanalytic approach to the problems of impaired infant-mother relationships. *J Am Acad Child Adolesc Psychiatry.* 1975;14:387–421.

Gaensbauer TJ. Psychotherapeutic treatment of traumatized infants and toddlers: a case report. *Clin Child Psychol Psychiatry.* 2000;5(3):373–385.

Gleason MM, Egger HL, Emslie GJ, et al. Psychopharmacological treatment for very young children: contexts and guidelines. *J Am Acad Child Adolesc Psychiatry.* 2007;46(12):1532–1572.

Gleason MM, Zeanah CH, Dickstein S. Recognizing young children in need of mental health assessment: Development and preliminary validity of the Early Childhood Screening Assessment. *Infant Ment Health J.* 2010;33:353–357.

Greenhill L, Kollins S, Abikoff H, et al. Efficacy and safety of immediate-release methylphenidate treatment for preschoolers with ADHD. *J Am Acad Child Adolesc Psychiatry.* 2006;45(11):1284–1293.

Harmon RJ, Riggs PD. Clonidine for posttraumatic stress disorder in preschool children. *J Am Acad Child Adolesc Psychiatry.* 1999;35(9):1247–1249.

Hunt RD, Arnsten AF, Asbell MD. An open trial of guanfacine in the treatment of attention-deficit hyperactivity disorder. *J Am Acad Child Adolesc Psychiatry.* 1995;34(1):50–54.

Kratochvil CJ, Vaughan BS, Mayfield-Jorgensen ML, et al. A pilot study of atomoxetine in young children with attention-deficit/hyperactivity disorder. *J Child Adolesc Psychopharmacol.* 2007;17(2):175–185.

Lahey BB, Pelham WE, Stein MA, et al. Validity of DSM-IV attention-deficit/hyperactivity disorder for younger children. *J Am Acad Child Adolesc Psychiatry.* 1998;37(7):695–702.

Lieberman AF, Amaya-Jackson L. Reciprocal influences of attachment and trauma: using a dual lens in the assessment and treatment of infants, toddlers, and preschoolers, in enhancing early attachment: theory, research and intervention. In: Berlin L, ed. New York: Guilford Press; 2003:100–123.

Lieberman AF, Ippen CG, Van Horn PJ. Child-parent psychotherapy: 6 month follow-up of a randomized controlled trial. *J Am Acad Child Adolesc Psychiatry.* 2006;45:913–918.

Luby JL, Heffelfinger A, Mrakotsky C, et al. Preschool major depressive disorder: preliminary validation for developmentally modified DSM-IV criteria. *J Am Acad Child Adolesc Psychiatry.* 2002;41:928–937.

Luby JL, Mrakotsky C, Statelets MM, et al. Risperidone in preschool children with autistic spectrum disorders: an investigation of safety and efficacy. *J Child Adolesc Psychopharmacol.* 2006;16(5):575–587.

Masi G, Cosenza A, Mucci M. A 3-year naturalistic study of 53 preschool children with pervasive developmental disorders treated with risperidone. *J Clin Psychiatry.* 2003;64(9):1039–1047.

Mota-Castillo M, Torruella A, Engels B, et al. Valproate in very young children: an open case series with a brief follow-up. *J Affect Disord.* 2001;67:193–197.

Merrell K. *Preschool Kindergarten Behavior Scale: Test Manual.* Brandon, VT: Clinical Psychology Publishing; 1994.

Nagaraj R, Singhi P, Malhi P. Risperidone in children with autism: randomized, placebo-controlled, double-blind study. *J Child Neurol.* 2006;21(6):450–455.

Nelson CA, Zeanah CH, Fox NA, et al. Cognitive recovery in socially deprived young children: the Bucharest early intervention project. *Science.* 2007;38(5858):1937–1940.

Olson AL, Dietrich AJ, Prazar G, et al. Brief maternal depression screening at well-child visits. *Pediatrics.* 2006;118(1):207–216.

Oner O, Oner P. Psychopharmacology of pediatric obsessive-compulsive disorder: three case reports. *J Psychopharmacol.* 2008;22(7):809–811.

Prince JB, Wilens TE, Biederman J, et al. Clonidine for sleep disturbances associated with attention-deficit hyperactivity disorder: a systematic chart review of 62 cases. *J Am Acad Child Adolesc Psychiatry.* 1996;35(5):599–605.

Sameroff AJ, Fiese BH. Models of development and developmental risk. In: Zeanah CH, ed. *Handbook of Infant Mental Health.* New York: Guilford Press; 2000:3–19.

Scheeringa MS, Peebles CD, Cook CA, et al. Toward establishing procedural, criterion, and discriminant validity for PTSD in early childhood. *J Am Acad Child Adolesc Psychiatry.* 2001;40(1):52–60.

Scheeringa MS, Salloum A, Arnberger RA, et al. Feasibility and effectiveness of cognitive-behavioral therapy for posttraumatic stress disorder in preschool children: two case reports. *J Trauma Stress.* 2007;20(4):631–636.

Seifer R, Dickstein S, Sameroff A, et al. Infant mental health and variability of parental depressive symptoms. *J Am Acad Child Adolesc Psychiatry*. 2001;40(12):1375–1382.

Sonuga-Barke EJS, Daley D, Thompson M, et al. Parent-based therapies for preschool attention-deficit/hyperactivity disorder: a randomized controlled trial with a community sample. *J Am Acad Child Adolesc Psychiatry*. 2001;40(4):402–408.

Squires J, Bricker D, Twombly E. *Ages and Stages Questionnaires: Social-Emotional*. Baltimore, MD: Paul H Brookes Publishing Co; 2002.

Staller J. Psychopharmacologic treatment of aggressive preschoolers: a chart review. *J Neuropsychopharmacol Biol Psychiatry*. 2007;31:131–135.

Webster-Stratton C, Hammond M. Treating children with early-onset conduct problems: a comparison of child and parent training interventions. *J Consult Clin Psychol*. 1997;35(1):93–109.

Weinfield N, Whaley G, Egeland B. Continuity, discontinuity, and coherence in attachment from infancy to late adolescence: sequelae of organization and disorganization. *Attach Hum Dev*. 2004;6(1):73–97.

Wright HH, Cuccaro ML, Leonhardt TV, et al. Case study: fluoxetine in the multimodal treatment of a preschool child with selective mutism. *J Am Acad Child Adolesc Psychiatry*. 1995;34(7):857–862.

Zeanah CH, Benoit D, Hirschberg L, et al. Mothers' representations of their infants are concordant with infant attachment classifications. *Dev Issues Psychiatry Psychol*. 1994;1:9–18.

Zeanah CH, Boris NW, Larrieu JA. Infant development and developmental risk: a review of the past 10 years. *J Am Acad Child Adolesc Psychiatry*. 1997;36(2):165–176.

Zeanah CH, Egger HL, Smyke AS, et al. Institutional rearing and psychiatric disorders in Romanian preschool children. *Am J Psychiatry*. 2009;166:777–785.

Zero to Three Diagnostic Classification Task Force. *Diagnostic Classification of Mental Health and Development Disorders of Infancy and Early Childhood: DC:0–3R*. Washington, DC: Zero to Three Press; 2005.

Zito JM, Tobi H, Lolkje TW, et al. Antidepressant prevalence for youths: a multi-national comparison. *Pharmacoepidemiol Drug Saf*. 2006;15(11):793–798.

SUGGESTED READINGS

Barkley, RA. *Defiant Children: A Clinician's Manual for Assessment and Parent Training*. 2nd ed. New York: The Guilford Press; 1997.

Brazelton TB. *Touchpoints (0–3 and 3–6)*. Cambridge, MA: DaCapo Press; 2005.

Greene RW. *The Explosive Child*. 2nd ed. New York: Harper Collins; 2001.

Lieberman A. *Emotional Life of the Child*. New York: The Free Press; 1993.

Lieberman A, Horn P. *Psychotherapy for Infants and Young Children: Repairing the Effects of Stress and Trauma on Early Attachment*. New York: Guilford Press; 2008.

Webster-Stratton C. *The Incredible Years. A Trouble-Shooting Guide for Parents of Children Aged 3–8*. Toronto, Ont.: The Umbrella Press; 2005.

Zeanah CH. *Handbook of Infant Mental Health*. 3rd ed. New York: Guilford Press; 2009.

Zero to Three. *Diagnostic Classification: 0–3R*. Washington, DC: Zero to Three; 2008.

SUGGESTED WEBSITES

www.circleofsecurity.org (includes links to valuable attachment literature and parent-friendly descriptions of the parent–child relationship)

www.PCIT.org (Parent–Child Interaction Therapy)

http://www.incredibleyears.com/ resources (handouts on elements of positive parenting including praise and play)

www.waimh.org (World Association of Infant Mental Health with links to local affiliates including practicing infant mental health specialists)

www.zerotothree.org (parent information about basic parenting skills and support)

www.circleofsecurity.org (parent handouts about the emotional needs of young children)

REVIEW QUESTIONS

1. IMH is best described as:
   a. A subspecialty in psychiatry focusing on the first year of life
   b. A multidisciplinary field focusing on promoting mental health in infants, toddlers, preschoolers, and their families
   c. Babies on analysts' couches
   d. Mental health specialty not involving physicians

2. What of the following factors impact very young children's mental health status?
   a. Child's developmental status
   b. Parental experiences of caregiving or intimate relationships
   c. Community violence
   d. Temperament
   e. All of the above

3. Which of the following is a hallmark of infant and early childhood mental health assessments?
   a. Focus on how parents may have created the child's problems
   b. Multimodal assessments using a team approach and multiple appointments
   c. Assessment of the child alone for the majority of the assessment
   d. Able to be done without meeting the child

4. Which of the following diagnoses are the most prevalent among preschoolers?
   a. GAD and ODD
   b. ADHD and bipolar disorder
   c. PDD and MR
   d. MDD

5. Which of the following are form(s) of evidence-based treatments for early childhood disorders or risk conditions?
   a. Attachment-based therapy
   b. Parent-management therapy
   c. Cognitive–behavioral therapy
   d. All of the above

6. Which of the following medication statements is supported by demonstrated efficacy in a randomized clinical trial?
   a. Guanfacine is an effective sleep agent for preschool sleep disorders.
   b. Haldol is an appropriate first-line medication for treating preschool psychosis.
   c. Risperidone is effective and safe as a treatment for aggression in typically developing preschoolers.
   d. Methylphenidate is superior to placebo in treating ADHD symptoms.
   e. Fluoxetine is recommended as first-line treatment for preschool PTSD.

7. Which of the following medications have FDA approval for use in children under 5 for psychiatric conditions?
   a. Risperidone
   b. Methylphenidate
   c. D-Amphetamine
   d. Fluoxetine

Answers: 1-b, 2-e, 3-b, 4-c, 5-d, 6-d, 7-a

Fetal Alcohol Spectrum Disorders

Introduction and Background

A large and still growing body of animal and human literature has described the long-term effects of maternal alcohol use during pregnancy on offspring outcome. Alcohol is a neurobehavioral teratogen, a substance that affects fetal growth and brain development. In group studies, alcohol's teratogenic effects have been most clearly evident on children's outcomes when use was heavy, but more subtle effects have also been seen with the moderate alcohol exposure characteristic of social drinking. Importantly, no clear threshold of "safe drinking" has been identified.

This body of research has shaped public policy, and gestational alcohol use is now seen as a global public health problem. For example, in 1981 and again in 2005, the United States (US) Surgeon General issued a statement warning women who are pregnant and women who may become pregnant to abstain from alcohol use during pregnancy. Over the past three decades, there has been growing attention on the hazards of drinking during pregnancy in countries around the world. There have been public health education campaigns and extensive media coverage, and warning labels have been posted at sites of alcohol purchase. Governmental task forces and workgroups have been formed to develop a coordinated public health response. Professional organizations have developed position statements and guidelines, and there are ongoing preservice and continuing education offerings for professionals in many disciplines. Collaborative international research efforts on drinking during pregnancy are underway, yet much remains to be done to address this major public health concern.

It was not until the late 1960s and early 1970s when French and then US physicians identified a birth defect called "fetal alcohol syndrome" (FAS). Professionals then began to take notice of a medical condition evident in newborn children prenatally exposed to alcohol. In 2004, clinicians, researchers, policymakers, and families in the United States reached a consensus that there is a wider spectrum of the effects of prenatal alcohol exposure beyond FAS, and reached an agreement on appropriate terminology. The umbrella term fetal alcohol spectrum disorders (FASD) is now used to refer to individuals who have FAS *and* to those who have other alcohol-related neurodevelopmental disabilities.

Over about the past decade, investigators in the field have begun to produce diagnostic guidelines—and to start designing and testing FASD prevention approaches and intervention strategies tailored to the needs of individuals with FASD and their families. Unfortunately, despite advancements in the field, organized prevention efforts are not yet common. Also, many individuals with FASD are still not recognized and do not receive proper diagnosis or treatment, and so miss the chance for help to lessen potentially deleterious life outcomes. Yet the public health problem of prenatal alcohol effects can be addressed in an important way if medical and mental health professionals become knowledgeable about FASD, learn to screen families, and move them toward essential diagnosis and treatment, and carry out much-needed FASD prevention activities.

Diagnostic Considerations and Clinical Features

Diagnostic Considerations

Currently accepted essentials of diagnosis are presented in Table 19-1. Medical and mental health professionals can screen for FASD. Diagnosis is ideally made by medical professionals working with an interdisciplinary team, because test data and psychosocial information indicating central nervous system (CNS) damage/dysfunction are central to the diagnosis.

The most obvious manifestation of the developmental effects of prenatal alcohol exposure is the full FAS. FAS is a permanent birth defect syndrome known to be caused by maternal alcohol consumption during pregnancy. FAS can be recognized by a pattern of characteristic dysmorphic facial features, smooth philtrum, thin upper lip, short palpebral fissure lengths (Fig. 19-1), pre- or postnatal growth deficiency, and a variable manifestation of CNS damage/dysfunction. Diagnostic researcher Astley maintains that the specificity of the FAS facial phenotype to prenatal alcohol exposure supports a clinical judgment that the cognitive and behavioral dysfunction observed among individuals with FAS is due, at least in part, to brain damage caused by a teratogen. Studies by the Centers for Disease Control and Prevention show FAS rates ranging from 0.2 to 1.5 cases per 1000 live births, comparable to other common developmental disabilities such as Down syndrome or spina bifida.

TABLE 19-1	Essentials of Diagnosis for Fetal Alcohol Spectrum Disorders to Inform Diagnostic Screening

Diagnostic Terms (ARBD not included)
- **FAS:** All diagnostic criteria must be met. It is possible to have a diagnosis of FAS without evidence of confirmed prenatal alcohol exposure if growth and <u>all</u> characteristic facial features are present.
- **Partial FAS:** All diagnostic criteria must be met, though the full expression of the characteristic facial features does not have to be present OR significant growth impairment may not be present. There must be evidence of confirmed prenatal alcohol exposure.
- **ARND:** For a diagnosis of ARND, there must be confirmed prenatal alcohol exposure. There is no requirement for growth deficiency or expression of the characteristic facial features. However, there <u>must</u> be evidence of central nervous system dysfunction across multiple functional domains. *Note that several diagnostic systems use terms other than 'ARND' to describe conditions on the wider fetal alcohol spectrum.*

Diagnostic Criteria
- Evidence of confirmed prenatal use of alcohol
- Evidence of growth deficiency (prenatal and/or postnatal) not explained by significant postnatal environmental influences
- Expression of three characteristic facial features:
  - Small palpebral fissures
  - Smooth philtrum (groove above the upper lip)
  - Thin upper lip
- Central nervous system (CNS) impairment as evidenced by structural and/or functional deficiencies (i.e., including but not limited to: microcephaly, seizures, and/or evidence of delays in cognition/learning, language, motor skills, executive functioning, social skills/adaptive function. When children are young, it is more difficult to obtain the testing evidence necessary to completely document CNS impairment.)

Note: Different diagnostic systems have defined cutoffs and evidence of CNS impairment in very different ways. See text for discussion of FASD diagnosis.

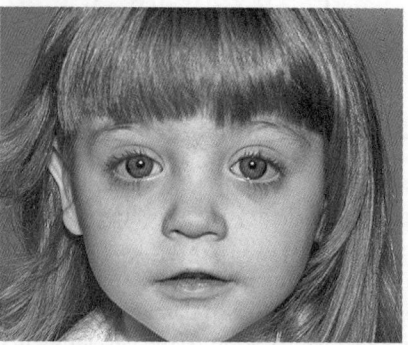

FIGURE 19-1. Facial features characteristic of fetal alcohol syndrome. (© 2009 University of Washington. With permission, Susan Astley, PhD.)

Prenatal alcohol exposure, however, is also known to cause a wider spectrum of adverse functional outcomes, whether or not the characteristic facial features occur. Over the years, clinicians and researchers have given a variety of labels to those who lack some or all of the physical features of FAS, but still have neurobehavioral deficits presumed to be related to prenatal alcohol exposure. Labels include descriptive terms such as the outdated term "fetal alcohol effects" (FAE), which should no longer be used in clinical or research settings. To label conditions across the spectrum, the Institute of Medicine (IOM) recommended other terms for diagnostic purposes, which are described below. Alcohol-related conditions resulting from prenatal alcohol not meeting the criteria for FAS are believed to occur about three times as often as does FAS, and some have estimated the rates of the full range of FASD to be as high as 9 or 10 per 1000 live births.

Initially, diagnostic emphasis was placed on physical findings, including growth deficiency and the cluster of minor facial anomalies characteristic of the fetal effects of alcohol. But in 2000, researchers Streissguth and O'Malley argued that diagnosis based on facial features is problematic, especially because the FAS face arises from prenatal exposure occurring during only a very short period of vulnerability, and so is quite tied to the timing of prenatal alcohol exposure. In 2005, Chudley and colleagues stated that "in the wide array of FASDs, facial dysmorphology is often absent and, in the final analysis, has little importance compared with the impact of prenatal alcohol exposure on brain function" (p. 56). More recently, then, there has been increasing diagnostic emphasis on the neurobehavioral deficits presumed to be related to prenatal alcohol exposure, as these are of greater functional significance than the physical features—and are highly associated with caregiver stress, and may be present even when characteristic physical features are not. There has also been a research emphasis on trying to identify a "behavioral phenotype" of FASD, or characteristic profile of learning and behavioral deficits. This line of research is relatively new and challenging. To date, no commonly accepted behavioral phenotype has been described, but increasing evidence reviewed by the researcher Kodituwakku notes generalized deficits in processing complex information.

Diagnostic systems for clinical and epidemiologic settings are under intensive development because of efforts to make diagnosis more accessible and reliable across settings. In 1996, the IOM in the United States defined five conditions along the spectrum with categories of: (1) FAS with confirmed prenatal alcohol exposure; (2) FAS without confirmed prenatal alcohol exposure; (3) partial FAS; (4) alcohol-related neurodevelopmental disorder (ARND); and (5) alcohol-related birth defects (ARBD). The IOM made recommendations that research data be gathered to allow refinement and validation of diagnostic system(s). Since then, national guidelines for diagnosis have been and are now being developed around the world.

Presently, national guidelines for diagnosis of the full FAS exist in the United States, but various systems also exist for diagnosing the full spectrum of FASD in the United States, Canada, and other countries. These various diagnostic systems are being used to define samples in much of the research now accumulating in the field of FASD. Consensus has not yet been reached on a single diagnostic system, although there are many areas of agreement between the systems in common use. Work to clarify diagnostic systems and understanding conditions across the fetal alcohol spectrum is of great importance. It is of clinical, epidemiologic, and research interest to generate accurate diagnoses of individuals, and also to reliably differentiate between meaningful subgroups on the fetal alcohol spectrum. At present, clinicians recognizing only the characteristic facial features of FAS may indeed identify individuals with the full syndrome, but miss the much larger number of individuals (such as those with ARND or partial FAS) actually showing debilitating CNS effects of prenatal alcohol, but not any or all of the facial features.

Clinical Features

Individuals diagnosed with FASD show neurobehavioral deficits across a number of developmental domains, with no "behavioral phenotype" identified at this point in time. In this medical condition, difficulties can occur in cognition and executive function, attention, learning and memory, speech and language, visual–spatial skills, fine and gross motor skills, and/or adaptive behavior. These difficulties impact how the affected individual functions in all life settings, including home activities, school performance, how they get along with peers, and success in employment. Families, researchers, and clinicians believe that neurodevelopmental difficulties are the basis for the behavior and lifestyle problems often seen among those with FASD—and that what are actually difficulties in learning, memory, or behavioral regulation, or a generalized deficit in processing complex information, may often be misinterpreted as oppositional, stubborn, noncompliant, or even antisocial behavior. While there is some research evidence to support these speculations, further studies are needed to draw a firm conclusion. But few would argue that it is the difficulties with behavior that often lead families to seek professional support for their alcohol-affected child, teen, or adult.

Because of the variable way in which alcohol exposure impacts fetal development and causes CNS damage and dysfunction, no two individuals with FASD are alike in clinical features, although they share common areas of likely deficit. These clinical features persist over time, changing their "look" somewhat as individuals grow and mature. It should be noted that children born prenatally alcohol-exposed often have other prenatal exposures, such as to cigarettes or street drugs, and most have some degree of postnatal environmental risk. While animal and longitudinal study of children with moderate levels of alcohol exposure do clearly show that alcohol is a neurobehavioral teratogen, there are certainly other factors associated with adverse developmental outcomes. But prenatal alcohol exposure is a central concern, and FASD is a descriptive and diagnostic term that captures a crucial aspect of the clinical and educational presentation of an affected individual. FASD has some prognostic value, definite implications for treatment and, importantly, may suggest that FASD prevention is needed.

Behavior Problems, Social Skills Deficits, and Psychiatric Conditions

Because individuals with FASD often have challenging behavior, although this may actually arise from underlying neurodevelopmental difficulties, maladaptive behavior is discussed first. While not all individuals with FASD show maladaptive behavior, many children with FASD demonstrate behavior problems and psychiatric disorders, such as attention deficits, depressive and other internalizing disorders, oppositional defiant behavior and conduct disorders, and specific phobias, when compared to typically developing peers. This high prevalence of behavioral difficulties and psychiatric conditions continues into adolescence and adulthood among those with heavy prenatal alcohol exposure. Social skills deficits are common among children diagnosed with FASD based on both parent and teacher report. Social skills deficits can include important areas of relationship development such as cooperation, initiation of conversations, making friends, and responding appropriately to conflict situations, all contributing to poor social behavior across multiple settings. Other specific social and behavioral deficits in children with FASD include poor understanding of consequences, temper tantrums and angry outbursts, unpredictable behavior, noncompliance, and difficulty regulating behavior. Other psychosocial difficulties include a higher risk of legal difficulties, alcohol and drug abuse, and other maladaptive behaviors, compared to typically developing peers.

Psychiatric and behavior problems occur in individuals across the spectrum of FASD, and not just among those diagnosed with FAS. These problems persist across time, and appear at a greater rate than would be expected based on the presence of cognitive deficits or environmental factors. Individuals with conditions on the wider fetal alcohol spectrum may actually have more debilitating behavior and lifestyle problems than those with the full FAS, perhaps because their problems go unrecognized or are inappropriately treated. These social and behavioral deficits affect an individual's function in all life settings, and likely arise in a large part from underlying global or complex neurobehavioral deficits resulting from the teratogenic effects of prenatal alcohol exposure. Because the effects of prenatal alcohol exposure are contingent upon multiple maternal and fetus factors, and on dosage patterns, damage to the developing fetus can be widespread and diffuse. The impact on CNS structure and function is variable from person to person, making treatment quite complex and necessarily individualized.

There is no clear consensus about how FASD is acknowledged in current psychiatric or medical diagnostic coding schemes. Some consider FASD a medical condition that modifies the presentation of other psychiatric conditions. Some advocate other strategies for denoting that prenatal alcohol exposure, or clinical effects like FASD, as part of how a child's situation is conceptualized. There is a specific code in the current medical coding system (ICD-9-CM: 760.71) used for general medical conditions that is utilized *both* for the full "FAS" and for "toxic effects of alcohol," and there are other codes that might be used depending on a clinician's case formulation. But the wider fetal alcohol spectrum and the lifelong aspect of this disorder are not adequately dealt with in psychiatric, medical, educational, or legal/judicial/correctional systems.

Adaptive Behavior

Accumulating research has shown that children prenatally exposed to alcohol, including both those with FAS and those falling within the wider fetal alcohol spectrum, often have significant adaptive function deficits in areas such as socialization, communication, and daily living skills. These youth show lower performance than might be expected from overall cognitive level, but it should be noted that lower adaptive functioning does not appear specific to more severe prenatal alcohol exposure. Interestingly, comparison of adaptive function between children with FASD and other clinically referred populations has not revealed differences in level of adaptive skills in infancy to early childhood. But they do tend to demonstrate arrested development of social adaptive functioning after the age of 4 to 6 years when compared to peers. Furthermore, difficulties with adaptive behavior do seem highly associated with caregiver stress and with executive function deficits.

Cognition and "Executive Functions"

Among the most commonly recognized difficulties for children diagnosed with FASD are deficits in intellectual status, although a wide range of intellectual abilities, ranging from the above average to well below average, occur.

Early on, alcohol-affected children may show developmental delays. Recent work suggests that over half of such children may show marked developmental delay in the first three years of life, including those later diagnosed with FAS or partial FAS. Yet as many as one-fourth of these children may show developmental profiles well within normal limits. Among older individuals, cognitive deficits may appear as difficulty understanding abstract concepts and a concrete learning style, poor reasoning skills, or as real-life problems such as poor understanding of time-sensitive tasks and behavior that appears "immature" or younger than expected for their chronological age. A strong correlation has been found between the degree of morphological damage of facial features and cognitive abilities, as assessed by standardized measures, at least among those with the full FAS; this is not true of those without characteristic facial features, and this point is still controversial. For most individuals with FASD, performance on standardized cognitive assessments remains consistent over time, and does not decline with age. Yet although many individuals with FASD may have cognitive skills broadly within the average range, over time the presence of secondary disabilities, such as mental health problems, may mean they do not function at their actual intellectual level, because they are not able to effectively problem solve and process complex information.

Individuals diagnosed with FASD may also show problems with "executive functions." Specific executive function impairments found in this population may include difficulty with planning ahead, cognitive inflexibility, inability to multitask, and problems in generalizing information from one situation to another. Executive function deficits may manifest themselves in real-life behavior problems such as acting without thinking about consequences or in struggling to plan a sequence of activities or actions.

Attention

Attention deficits have often been cited as a hallmark feature of FASD, perhaps affecting over 60% of children diagnosed with FASD. There may be some specificity in the types of attention deficits, with difficulties in attentional control rather than with global attention deficits. Attention deficits likely impact daily functioning at school and at home. It is thought that attention deficits can be linked to underlying deficits in working memory or to the greater cognitive effort required to respond accurately to attentional demands. A large body of research has noted that these attention deficits manifest themselves independently of cognitive deficits and persist over time.

Language

Prenatal alcohol exposure appears to affect verbal functioning. Individuals with FASD are reported to have difficulty with language learning, verbal fluency, naming, word comprehension, phonological working memory, grammatical and semantic abilities, and pragmatics. Deficits in receptive and expressive language skills impact individuals with FASD across multiple life settings, and contribute to difficulty using language to reason and analyze, and to interpret verbal and nonverbal cues. Importantly, deficits in language skills may often be overlooked or misunderstood earlier in life because many children with FASD can appear very "chatty" and seem to have age-appropriate language, although this may be less true as individuals with FASD grow older, and especially as they try to communicate effectively with peers. An interesting line of research has been tracking problems in higher-level "integrative" language abilities, like the ability to tell cohesive and coherent narratives, which may be a particular problem for those with FASD.

Problems in Learning, Memory, Visual–Spatial Skills, and Fine Motor Performance

Individuals with FASD show difficulties in learning and memory. For example, briefly put, deficits can be seen on measures of verbal fluency, efficient encoding of various kinds of information and, more generally, in working memory. On verbal memory tasks, intrusion errors and perseverative errors are common, and individuals with FASD often experience cognitive interference. Processing speed, or difficulties in balancing the trade-off between accuracy and speed, are seen. Difficulties are also seen in visual motor integration. Visual–perceptual tasks that require integration of local and global information also appear affected, although it is possible that this may reflect a function of overall intellectual functioning, which is required to efficiently integrate visual–perceptual stimuli. In addition, in the area of motor skills, both fine and gross motor deficits have been found, particularly difficulties in fine motor precision and speed, steadiness, and dynamic movement, and in overall balance.

Academic Achievement and School Performance

Problems in school performance may have many sources, such as deficits in short and long-term memory, cause-and-effect reasoning, difficulty appreciating time or sequencing of events, visual–spatial deficits, or problems with skills such as number processing or phonological processing. As a consequence, individuals affected by prenatal alcohol exposure may show specific academic deficits in areas of reading, writing, and especially, mathematics. School performance may also be affected by problems with adaptive function and maladaptive behavior. Children and adolescents with FASD may appear unmotivated or unorganized, though this may actually arise from underlying difficulties in learning. The situation can become worse, and school performance increasingly affected, when problems go unrecognized, misdiagnosed, or inappropriately treated.

Etiology and Prevention Efforts

There is a great deal of individual variation in CNS dysfunction among those affected by maternal drinking, which is thought to arise from the wide natural variability in the dose, pattern, and timing of prenatal alcohol exposure. This highly variable exposure means there is great variability in which developing brain structures are affected. Highly variable prenatal alcohol exposure is coupled with variability in maternal factors, such as a woman's age or nutrition during pregnancy, which also affects fetal development. Differences in genetic factors also contribute to the variable effects of prenatal alcohol exposure, because of biologically based differences in metabolism and sensitivity to alcohol of the parent and fetus. Given the multiple and diverse factors determining the fetal effects of maternal alcohol consumption during pregnancy, it makes sense that a broad spectrum of individually variable learning and behavior disabilities would be found. This remarkable individual variation means that comprehensive diagnosis and individualized intervention are required.

Maternal age and the degree of alcoholism appear to moderate the effects of prenatal exposure in school-aged offspring, with greater effects seen among those born to older women and heavier drinkers. It is speculated that the natural aging process and additional strain on the body of chronic alcoholism cause physical changes in the body related to absorption/elimination of alcohol, the viability of the reproduction system, and reduction of available nutrients for the fetus. But it is quite possible for younger women to have children with FASD. On an individual basis, the impact of drinking during pregnancy is not predictable.

Indeed, no safe amount of alcohol use during pregnancy has been recognized. The public health message from the US Centers for Disease Control and Prevention, for example, recommends that women who are planning to become pregnant, at-risk for pregnancy, or who are pregnant abstain from drinking alcohol. Prevention is important, and can be accomplished by individual providers aware of FASD and the effects of prenatal alcohol exposure reaching out to their patients, or by more formal prevention programs.

A number of successful prevention efforts to reduce the risk of alcohol-affected pregnancies have been developed, and public health plans have been proposed in the United States and other countries. Prevention efforts range widely. There are "universal" public health education efforts, including warning signs at alcohol points of purchase or public service announcements.

There are "selected" interventions for women already pregnant, such as alcohol counseling at centers providing low-income maternal/child health care or counseling by obstetricians. There are also "indicated" interventions for women who have already had one alcohol-affected pregnancy, such as long-term paraprofessional support programs for women with serious chemical dependency problems. There is intense and widespread interest in recent, effective, scientifically validated FASD prevention programs that include preconception counseling or brief interventions to reduce the use of alcohol among women at-risk for pregnancy, or already pregnant, that use a multimethod approach combining cognitive behavioral techniques, education, and motivational enhancement.

FASD prevention efforts remain sorely needed. Recent studies in the United States have found that roughly 50% of women of childbearing age report using alcohol within the previous month and, of these, 13% met criteria for heavy drinkers, while an additional 12% report binge drinking which is particularly harmful for the fetus. Health care and mental health professionals who work with children, or with teens and older women of childbearing age, should carefully consider their role in FASD prevention efforts. Within their own agency's guidelines, it is suggested they develop practice policies for how to counsel clients, or the parents of child clients, about alcohol use and pregnancy. Further policy consideration is needed to address the important fact that alcohol use by a partner or spouse can be highly related to a woman's own alcohol use during pregnancy.

Clinical Course

Because FASD is a lifelong medical condition, the clinical course is chronic but manifests differently across the life span. The clinical course may well differ in surprising ways for those with the full FAS versus those with conditions on the wider fetal alcohol spectrum.

It is important to note that when FASD is being considered, questions must first be asked about prenatal alcohol exposure, by both families and professionals, even if these questions are somewhat uncomfortable. Simply put, if questions are not asked about alcohol exposure during pregnancy, and/or records not reviewed for evidence of alcohol exposure, FASD will be missed. Professionals in health care and mental health need training on how to inquire about drinking during pregnancy in a supportive, nonjudgmental way, and training on how to connect families with FASD diagnosis and, if needed, substance abuse treatment for parents or adult clients.

The clinical course of this condition can be discussed in terms of the defining features of FASD: facial dysmorphology, growth, and CNS damage/dysfunction. Facial dysmorphology may exist beginning at birth, become more apparent to observers during the childhood years, and grow less apparent to observers with the changes of puberty. But observers must learn to be aware of the characteristic facial features, how to assess them, and their importance. Growth is not always a defining characteristic of FASD, but prenatal or postnatal growth impairment can occur. If a young child is found to have even mild growth impairment in the presence of prenatal alcohol exposure, this can signal the need to examine facial dysmorphology and ascertain whether there is additional evidence of developmental, learning, or behavior problems.

There is a complex clinical course of "primary disabilities" in CNS dysfunction and learning arising from teratogenic alcohol effects. At any age, small head circumference can signal the possibility of alcohol-related CNS damage, as can the presence of sensorineural hearing loss, seizure activity, or clinical findings on magnetic resonance imaging (MRI). But these "hard signs" of neurological impairment are not a necessary feature of FASD, nor are they specific to this medical condition. Interestingly, it appears that only about half of young children prenatally exposed to alcohol show marked developmental delay in the first 3 years of life, including those later diagnosed with FAS or partial FAS. But learning problems can emerge later.

In the school years, problems in CNS dysfunction can manifest in any combination of the developmental domains discussed in the Clinical Features section, or as global cognitive delays.

The clinical course of this condition can also be discussed in terms of "secondary disabilities" or real-life problems in lifestyle and daily function. Because of the wide range of individually variable developmental deficits found among those with FASD, there will be differences in the manifestation and severity of real-life secondary disabilities. But some surprising data exist suggesting that real-life difficulties are *less* common among those with FAS than in those with conditions on the broader fetal alcohol spectrum who do not show facial dysmorphology.

A pioneering evaluation of a large clinical sample of individuals with FASD carried out by researcher Streissguth and her team was reported in 2004. This study revealed a high prevalence of adverse lifestyle outcomes over the life span. This early study has limitations, as it focuses on a nonrepresentative clinical sample without a comparison group and the sample was diagnosed before many community interventions were available. Nevertheless, this study is informative by revealing the high rate of secondary disabilities found among individuals diagnosed with FASD, with little difference in rates of males and females. Of the 415 individuals in this study, 80% were not raised by their biological mothers. Examining secondary disabilities, 60% of this group experienced a variety of disrupted school experiences, such as being expelled, dropping out, difficulty completing school work, poor peer relations, and being disruptive in class. In addition, 14% of the children and 60% of the adolescents and adults were reported to have some type of trouble with the law. Moreover, 35% of those over 12 years of age were reported to have substance abuse problems. A wide spectrum of inappropriate sexual behaviors, ranging from minor to major issues, were also reported to be an adverse life outcome in 39% of children and 48% of adolescents diagnosed with FASD over 12 years of age.

Follow-up research describing the clinical course of FASD has also been carried out in other countries. In Sweden, children with FAS followed into early to midadolescence demonstrated continuing problems such as learning disabilities, attention deficits, motor control problems and, in some cases, severe intellectual deficits. In Germany, follow-up research suggests that for most individuals with FASD intellectual functioning does not change over time and psychiatric disorders persist. Moreover, while age-specific psychiatric disorders, such as enuresis or eating difficulties decreased after preschool, the extent of behavioral difficulties remained relatively constant over time because new problems emerged. For example, difficulties with social relationships and attention emerged in the school years. Sleep problems were important over time. Further follow-up research into young adulthood demonstrated persistence or evolution into more impairment of many of the difficulties seen in childhood and adolescence, including attentional problems, intellectual disability, dependent living, poor occupational opportunities, and behavioral problems.

Assessment of FASD

An initial work-up is always indicated and is helpful in determining appropriate interventions. The usual task of an individual medical or mental health professional is to screen for FASD and appropriately refer to a diagnostic clinic. Typically, an assessment for FASD is accomplished by an expert multidisciplinary team of professionals knowledgeable about FASD and experienced in evaluating communication, fine and gross motor skills, cognitive ability, learning, memory, processing, and general development. A multidisciplinary approach is necessary because of the broad array of disabilities seen in this population. However, FASD diagnostic clinics are not always available, although this network is growing, so referral can be made to child guidance centers or other neurodevelopmental clinics. Table 19-2 gives the essentials of an FASD work-up.

TABLE 19-2 **Essentials of Assessment for Fetal Alcohol Spectrum Disorders**

- Early detection and diagnosis of at-risk individuals to ensure early intervention.
- Screening in any health care, social service, or treatment system in which an individual with FASD may be found.
- Determine alcohol use during pregnancy including frequency, amount, and type.
- Evaluate growth of the affected individual for impairment during the prenatal and/or postnatal period that is not fully explained by genetic and/or significant postnatal environmental influences.
- Specialist evaluation of facial morphology for small palpebral fissures, smooth philtrum, and thin upper lip. Facial dysmorphology is characteristic only of FAS. An individual may be affected by prenatal alcohol exposure and not show these facial features.
- Monitor developmental progress for delays or deficits related to central nervous system (CNS) dysfunction, as per formal testing evidence or confirmed caregiver report of difficulties in development.
- Query for postnatal environmental influences that significantly affect growth or CNS dysfunction of the affected individual.
- Refer patient to an appropriate developmental clinic to be evaluated for FASD and treatment options.
- Refer patient for evaluation and treatment of co-occurring mental health disorders.
- Follow-up on progress of diagnostic evaluation and treatment. Help promote continuity of care.
- Assess caregiver needs.

The first step is to determine alcohol use during pregnancy including frequency, amount, and type. Asking questions about alcohol use requires some training and practice. All highly exposed individuals should be referred for further evaluation, even if they were also exposed to other drugs. To put alcohol exposure in perspective, clinicians should also query about postnatal environmental influences that could affect growth or CNS dysfunction of the affected individual. However, the postnatal environment should not completely explain problems of the exposed individual. Next, evaluate growth for impairment either during the prenatal and/or postnatal period that is not fully explained by genetic and/or postnatal environmental influences. Examination of the facies for dysmorphology will help to establish the full syndrome of FAS. These features include small palpebral fissures, smooth philtrum, and thin upper lip. This evaluation requires specialized training which is available online. Facial dysmorphology is characteristic only of FAS, and absence of this does not preclude other conditions on the fetal alcohol spectrum. An individual may be quite affected by prenatal alcohol exposure and not show facial dysmorphology. Therefore, individuals exposed to alcohol before birth who also have learning or behavior problems should be referred even if there is no dysmorphology.

As the exposed individual develops, monitoring is crucial to measure progress and detect delays or deficits related to CNS dysfunction. Any testing results or caregiver report of difficulties in any of the following domains should be examined: executive function; cognitive/learning/memory; language; fine motor; gross motor; problems in behavior/social skills; attention; visual–spatial skills; adaptive behavior; or academic performance. Exposed individuals who have suggestions of deficits should be referred to an appropriate developmental clinic to be evaluated for FASD and treatment options. It is important to recognize that a diagnosis of FASD does not rule out other co-occurring disorders, such as attention-deficit hyperactivity disorder. Thus, part of the result of a developmental assessment may be to reveal other problems in need of treatment. It is important to realize that assessment for alcohol-exposed individuals is ongoing throughout development. Thus, follow-up on the progress of evaluations and recommended treatments is crucial to the individual's welfare and to help promote continuity of care. What is often most important in a work-up of FASD is support for the caregiver and provision of resources and supports on the local and national level.

A final comment on neuroimaging is warranted, as a role for neuroimaging in the evaluation of FASD is not yet established, but emerging. Research advances in MRI, MRS, fMRI coupled with neuropsychological testing have clarified that not all individuals with identifiable CNS effects of prenatal alcohol exposure display the facial features of FAS. Preliminary neuroimaging data with small samples suggest that selected brain structures and neuronal arrays may be implicated, but the teratogenic effects of alcohol on fetal development are complicated. Excellent research reviews are available and listed in the references. In research so far, there do seem to be brain structures more susceptible to alcohol's teratogenic effects, such as the cerebellum, basal ganglia, corpus callosum, and frontal lobes—but much more study is needed. There are clearly dramatic individual differences in how affected individuals manifest CNS damage/dysfunction related to prenatal alcohol exposure. New understanding will emerge as researchers attempt to define meaningful subgroups across the full fetal alcohol spectrum, and provide convincing evidence of the characteristics of FASD through data on alcohol-related differences in CNS morphology, neurochemistry, neurological function, and neurodevelopmental performance. What is clear now is that no matter what their facial features, those children clinically identified with FASD do show evidence of impairment using neuroimaging technology, so that even individuals with ARND can show measurable changes in brain structure, function, and neurochemistry. Although neuroimaging research is a promising addition to the field, the implications for clinical practice are not yet clear.

Treatment

Early diagnosis is critical to early intervention, but neurodevelopmental and psychological evaluations at successive developmental stages are also important to document strengths and weaknesses, to refine the treatment plan, and to monitor progress over the long term.

Prompted by caregiver advocacy and legislative action, governmental agencies joined together in the formation of the National Task Force on FAS and FAE, among other efforts. In 2009, this task force produced a federal-level "call to action" for more research and public policy to provide treatment for those with FASD and their caregivers. There are many treatment suggestions (Table 19-3). Data support the importance of early diagnosis and interven-

---

TABLE 19-3 Essentials of Treatment for Fetal Alcohol Spectrum Disorders

- Individualized, multidisciplinary services across systems, appropriate for the disability, including as needed: early intervention; special education; medical care; mental health care; psychopharmacotherapy; speech-language therapy; occupational therapy; vocational training; recreational activities; social skills/teen groups; substance use education/treatment; sexuality education; mentoring programs; legal, correctional and judicial assistance; and FASD prevention.
- Individualized family and caregiver support across systems, including as needed: parent training in behavior management, advocating for child's needs, neurodevelopmental disabilities, and long-term planning; respite care; referral to parent and sibling support groups; referral to federal and state financial supports.
- Neurodevelopmental/psychological evaluations at successive developmental stages to document strengths and weaknesses, and to plan and monitor treatment.
- Collaboration among service providers for affected individual and the family, and planning for continuity of care.
- Long-term planning for the individual and caregivers.

tion for children prenatally affected by alcohol, and the field of early intervention has begun to deal with this issue. But there is a clear need to provide multimodal, effective services to families of individuals with FASD, from early childhood through adulthood. This need is a growing and significant public health concern. Ensuring that diagnosis is accessible, and then understanding and delivering appropriate treatment approaches, is essential for professionals not only in health care, mental health, and social services—but also for those in the educational, juvenile justice, legal, drug treatment, vocational rehabilitation, adult day care, and adult correctional systems. Professionals in all these settings are already serving individuals with FASD, even if this medical condition is currently unrecognized as part of a client's or patient's diagnostic profile.

Even when appropriately diagnosed, it is sometimes difficult for individuals with FASD to be recognized as eligible for services they actually need. Often service systems, such as special education or funding through state departments of developmental disabilities, have simple cutoffs, such as low IQ or the presence of physical disabilities, which may not adequately define those with FASD. For instance, individuals with FASD may have "scattered" cognitive profiles (e.g., IQ within the average range but evidence of complex learning disabilities), and not show global delays. They may also show "higher-order" language problems which compromise their school learning and social skills, but pass the tests of vocabulary and grammar generally used to permit access to services. The overarching issue is that individuals with FASD may not meet eligibility for services but still appear to have serious or odd behavior problems, and have underlying learning deficits that go unrecognized and untreated.

A wide range of services is needed for this population. A "care network," including services that differ over the life span, is needed for individuals with FASD. In general, to address the complex needs of this population, what is required are multimodal, multisystem interventions. Effective communication between service providers and planning for the continuity of care are of the utmost importance. In the past decade there has been considerable progress in thinking about psychosocial interventions for children and families impacted by FASD. There are several new publications discussing "state-of-the-art" thinking in planning for effective intervention, as discussed briefly below and listed in the recommended references.

Parent Education and Support

Both informal parent support, and more formal parent education (typically using parent groups) have growing momentum as an important part of the continuum of FASD intervention. Informal parent support has been identified as a powerful predictor of positive outcome in the broader developmental disabilities literature. Parent support/advocacy groups, often initiated and run by the parents themselves, play a role in providing emotional support and validation, instilling hope for the future, problem solving difficult behaviors and life situations, gaining practical assistance such as babysitting and community resources, providing a platform for services (such as social skills groups, summer camps, and recreational opportunities), and increasing social support.

Parent Education and Behavioral Consultation

Natural history research indicates that important correlates of positive outcome among those with FASD include descriptors of a nurturant, stable, appropriately stimulating environment during middle childhood, absence of victimization or traumatic experiences, not living with a parent involved in substance abuse, and availability of appropriate social services. Appropriate caregiving for children with FASD, especially the many who have challenging behavior, can be a daunting task. An intervention that includes supportive behavioral consultation and advocacy training, provided by a specialist in neurodevelopmental disabilities and positive behavior support approaches who collaborates with a parent/guardian, has data to support its efficacy. Researcher Carmichael Olson and her team describe the Families Moving Forward (FMF) Program, a caregiver-focused behavioral consultation intervention which uses specific treatment processes useful when the affected individual has neurological impairment. The FMF intervention has so far been found to be efficacious in helping birth, adoptive, and foster parents raising preschool and school-aged children with FASD improve feelings of parenting effectiveness, increase parental self-care, report their family needs have been met, and report reduced disruptive child behavior. Other parenting approaches have also been tested, including behavioral parent training, with some positive results. There are also "key worker" programs in countries such as Canada that provide advocates to assist parents once an FASD diagnosis has been rendered, which show high rates of parent satisfaction.

Early Intervention

Like most developmental disabilities, early recognition of prenatal alcohol exposure and identification of FASD is imperative for appropriate provision of health care, education, and social services that promote well-being. Early identification of this medical condition (before age 6 years) is an important correlate of many positive life outcomes among those with FASD. Early identification allows the family to plan for appropriate intervention and advocacy. Early intervention may be more successful when family support is paired with direct intervention using effective teaching methods. Interventions targeting readiness to learn, or teaching specific skills such as math and handwriting, studies by Coles, Kable, and colleagues, have shown good results with children with FASD and their families. As the field of FASD intervention grows and develops, there will likely be interest in effective strategies used in early childhood mental health such as enhancing parent–child attachment, teaching realistic developmental expectations, and parenting strategies more generally useful for children with developmental disabilities. There will likely also be interest in interventions that address other areas of impairment, such as motor training, sensory-integration deficits, and the ongoing and notable problems individuals with FASD have in sleep.

Social Skills Groups

Deficits in the area of social skills have been a core feature of children diagnosed with FASD. Research and practice have taken two approaches to remediating social skills deficits: (1) direct skills instruction; and (2) creating social space, such as teen groups, retreats, and conferences for children and teens with FASD. Children's friendship groups, such as those carefully studied by O'Connor and her colleagues that explicitly teach and provide practice on specific social skills with parent assistance, have good data to support their efficacy in improving friendship skills in a sustained manner. Other groups that focus on improving behavioral self-regulation have been tested with some positive results, and have very promising anecdotal support.

Educational Testing and Support

For those with prenatal alcohol exposure, diagnostic facilities are not always available, careful learning evaluation may not always be done, and misdiagnosis of emotional disturbance or conduct problems rather than the medical condition of FASD may occur. Thus, school-aged children with FASD do not always receive necessary or appropriate educational services. Moreover, even when children with FASD are diagnosed appropriately, recognized to have learning problems, and given adequate testing to explain their unique cognitive and learning profile, school systems may not know how to deal with students who show a scattered profile of deficits across multiple developmental domains. To improve school performance, comprehensive assessment, scaffolded instruction of skills, functional behavioral assessment, effective instructional strategies, and positive communication between family and school can help to appropriately accommodate students diagnosed with FASD. Supportive services, including occupational therapy and speech-language therapy, can be especially helpful for those with FASD who have sensory processing, motor, and higher-level language impairment.

Psychopharmacology

Given the many behavioral problems and psychiatric conditions found among these children, it is not surprising that psychopharmacology treatment has been widely used. What is surprising is the scarcity of data on the frequency of use and efficacy of different medication regimens. Children with FASD are frequently prescribed multiple medications, including psychoactive medications, that are taken simultaneously. Most psychoactive medication use with children is generally still off-label. At present, available treatment guidelines advise prescribing professionals to have specialized training in psychiatry-specific knowledge about FASD, and pediatric experience if prescribing for children. The principles of "start low, go slow," with careful and close monitoring of medication treatment (including objective data collection) are advised. More research in this area is sorely needed.

Other Services

There are other services needed by individuals with FASD and their families, given the life span nature of this developmental disability. Respite care is important, from infancy through adolescence. Specialized consultation by those knowledgeable about FASD is required within multiple systems, including the educational system, juvenile justice, and adult correctional systems, legal and judicial systems, and social services. Mentoring and advocacy programs are needed for adolescents and young adults with FASD. Supportive living and work situations must be created for adults with FASD, as well as specialized parent–child assistance programs for adults with FASD who have become parents.

Conclusions

Alcohol is a potent neurobehavioral teratogen, and prenatal exposure to alcohol can have wide-ranging, individually variable consequences on development that last lifelong. Individuals affected by alcohol in utero have diagnosable medical conditions, grouped together under the umbrella term of FASD. The most significant impact among those with FASD comes from their neurodevelopmental disabilities, which affect learning, behavior, daily function—and quality of life for affected individuals and their families. The majority of those affected by FASD still go unrecognized and are often inappropriately served. This means it is essential for medical and mental health professionals to become aware of FASD, and then to screen for this condition, refer possibly affected individuals for diagnosis, and respond with appropriate treatments. Assessment should occur as early as possible, with diagnosis by an interdisciplinary team that can create a multimodal treatment plan. The treatment plan must change as the affected individual grows older, and provide a "care network" which will likely reach into health and mental health care, education, social services, vocational training, and even into the substance use, legal, judicial, and correctional systems. Providing formal and informal support and advocacy training for caregivers and families is also crucial. FASD is a significant public health problem that is preventable, and research is defining effective prevention methods. It is vital for medical and mental health professionals to act to prevent FASD, finding methods that fit with their discipline, agency guidelines, and personal decisions.

CASE VIGNETTES

VIGNETTE 1: A CHILD WITH FETAL ALCOHOL SYNDROME

Grace is a small, lively, cheerful child of mixed ethnicity who was born exposed to alcohol and cigarettes, and also to brief illicit drug use. Early on, there were developmental concerns and Grace received early intervention because she was "drug-exposed." Intervention stopped when she was just 3 years old and her family moved to a rural area, but at that time she was doing well. When Grace was 4 years old, though, she was tantrumming and her new doctor noticed unusual facial features she had seen in articles on FAS. A review of medical records confirmed Grace had been alcohol-exposed in a pattern that fit with medical literature placing the fetus at "high risk" because the hospital worker had written that Grace's birth mother had been a heavy drinker throughout pregnancy. Records further noted that because Grace's birth mother was very willing to receive services, Grace was sent home. But even though her mother struggled to do well, records noted that Grace was later removed because of neglect and placed in the child welfare system.

Over the years, Grace's foster family had become her legal guardians. They provided a stable, structured home with clear routines. The family moved to a ranch, which suited Grace well. Once Grace's doctor pointed out the possibility of FAS, the doctor and her family located an FASD diagnostic clinic which required them to drive to another state to be seen. By the time of Grace's clinic visit, she had just celebrated her 6th birthday, been purposefully started late in kindergarten, and her school was awaiting the outcome of the diagnostic visit.

At the FASD diagnostic clinic, the physician did standardized measurements, finding that Grace had a "severe" level of expression of facial features compared to norms. A record review showed persistent growth impairment. The multidisciplinary team found small head size and evidence in speech, occupational therapy, and psychology testing that showed complex learning disabilities. The team felt Grace met criteria for a diagnosis of FAS. The clinic gave information on FAS to the family, who then went online to learn all they could. They talked to Grace's school psychologist, who helped them get Grace qualified for special education as developmentally delayed, and referred them to a family counselor to process their surprise and grief about the diagnosis.

As Grace grew older, her doctor saw her regularly, eventually giving an additional diagnosis of ADHD. The doctor monitored stimulants and sleep medication, though medication was not that effective. As Grace progressed through school, her eligibility classification changed from Developmentally Delayed to Other Health Impaired. The occupational therapist consulted with her teacher to set up the classroom so Grace could best learn and behave. Her parents enrolled her in swimming and 4-H, and joined an FASD parent support listserve to get ideas from other parents.

Near the end of 3rd grade, Grace was making academic progress but her rate of achievement was starting to slow even in special education. School testing showed borderline IQ with real variability in aspects of learning (with some skills in the average range). Grace was understood at school to be active and distractible, but that did not bother her teachers who found her likable. When faced with something hard at school, Grace always kept trying (which her teachers appreciated), but she was disorganized and did not check her work. What did bother her teachers was that Grace acted out in odd, random ways at school. She also had trouble explaining things, and when there was trouble and she was asked what happened, Grace gave a disorganized explanation without needed details.

To a mental health provider, Grace's parents lovingly described their now almost 10-year-old daughter as sometimes cooperative and helpful, but also as very distractible, active, impulsive—

with many tantrums, odd behaviors, and problems communicating. They said adults liked her, but were saddened because Grace really had no friends of her own age. Her behavior was an increasing challenge, especially at home. The mental health provider looked into available treatments, found information about FASD intervention and received some specialized training, then worked closely with the family for over a year with good success. The family enrolled Grace in a social skills group even though this meant a long drive for them. Of importance, the mental health provider helped the family begin to come to terms with the fact that Grace would need lifelong assistance.

VIGNETTE 2: A CHILD WITH ALCOHOL-RELATED NEURODEVELOPMENTAL DISORDER

Andrew is a boy whose mother and father both had a history of substance use, including alcohol use. His mother had no prenatal care. Yet Andrew was born full term, without growth or medical concerns, and with no dysmorphology. His parents tried hard to raise him but, as a toddler, Andrew was moved to several foster homes. While living in one foster home, Andrew was referred by his doctor for developmental screening because of difficulty focusing and "problems with hitting." Testing showed intact developmental skills, except in language, but Andrew was still considered "at-risk" due to distractible and active behavior, and was described as being "a handful" during the evaluation. Early intervention was recommended to support adaptive behavior and language development. Unfortunately, intervention was not started, and not considered again until after Andrew had moved to his adoptive home at age 4½ years and showed continuing troublesome behaviors.

Around the time Andrew began 2nd grade, his adoptive placement was quite firm and he had transferred to a new health care provider who was doing ongoing medical care. This provider was very concerned about Andrew's adoptive parents' report of their son's ongoing problems in the presence of known prenatal alcohol exposure. He referred Andrew for an FASD diagnostic work-up. Clinic evaluators found Andrew to have a condition called "alcohol-related neurodevelopmental disorder" (ARND). Their testing showed IQ within normal limits, but also distractibility, poor adaptive behavior, sensory sensitivities, some memory difficulties, and higher-level language deficits (even though Andrew was now very talkative and had a good vocabulary). With advocacy, clinic results allowed Andrew to qualify for speech-language therapy and resource room support. His family had to seek outside occupational therapy services because the school could not justify providing these services. Although Andrew benefited from learning support at school, behavior was still an issue at school and at home.

As he moved through elementary school, Andrew continued to have behavior problems, changing schools once when his problems with peers became too great. His grades slipped lower, but school interventions were for challenging behavior rather than learning issues. Home life was difficult, with Andrew often refusing to do what his parents asked him to do. Andrew had also been acting out in the community and had one minor legal infraction which worried his parents greatly. Andrew's parents decided to enroll him in counseling. He was diagnosed with oppositional defiant disorder, although the usual interventions did not seem to help him or his parents. His counselor felt he lacked "insight" into his problems.

As time went on, Andrew's parents and health care providers talked about various plans to address learning and behavioral problems related to ARND. Finally, Andrew was referred for psychological testing and classroom observation by a specialist in neurodevelopmental disabilities because of the chance that Andrew's learning issues were partly responsible for his behavior problems. Testing showed that Andrew had clear memory deficits, slow and inaccurate information processing, and specific learning disabilities. He had real trouble in the classroom when instructions were presented quickly and spoken (and not written). Observations revealed when Andrew did not understand, he would just act out.

Test results and advocacy finally resulted in additional learning supports at school. In addition, his mental health provider learned about FASD interventions, and changed the approach she was using with Andrew. She began to use more concrete, "role-playing" techniques to address self-regulation and rule-following with Andrew. But she mostly focused on separate behavioral consultation with Andrew's parents, which research so far has found efficacious for FASD. With the additional support, Andrew's learning and behavior improved. He found one best friend, who had also struggled with learning problems. He started more often following school and home rules. Everyone was happy with his progress, although seriously thinking ahead about what to do when he reached middle school.

Andrew had a condition on the fetal alcohol spectrum that was certainly not a mild problem. It was not until the adults around Andrew "reframed" his behavior problems as partly due to underlying learning issues that he was given the type of interventions he needed to progress. Andrew certainly had early risk factors, but these did not explain all his issues or point toward the most effective interventions. Knowledge of his condition of ARND, along with other diagnosable conditions and a full understanding of his learning problems, proved to be important in finding treatments to help life be more successful for Andrew.

ACKNOWLEDGMENT

This work was supported in part by a grant from the Centers for Disease Control and Prevention, U01DD00038, "Transitioning Science-Based FASD Intervention to the Community," awarded to Heather Carmichael Olson, Principal Investigator. The authors also acknowledge the support of the Seattle Children's Hospital Research Institute, Seattle, Washington.

REFERENCES

Aronson M, Hagberg B. Neuropsychological disorder in children exposed to alcohol during pregnancy: a follow-up study of 24 children to alcoholic mothers in Goteburg, Sweden. *Alcohol Clin Exp Res.* 1998;22(2):321–324.

Astley S. *Diagnostic Guide for Fetal Alcohol Spectrum Disorders: The 4-Digit Diagnostic Code.* 3rd ed. Seattle: University of Washington; 2004.

Astley SJ, Aylward E, Olson HC, et al. Functional magnetic resonance imaging outcomes from a comprehensive magnetic resonance study of children with fetal alcohol spectrum disorders. *J Neurodevel Dis.* 2009;1:61–80.

Astley SJ, Olson HC, Kerns K, et al. Neuropsychological and behavioral outcomes from a comprehensive magnetic resonance study of children with fetal alcohol spectrum disorders. *Can J Clin Pharm.* 2009;16(1):e178–e201.

Bertrand J, Floyd LL, Weber MK. Guidelines for identifying and referring persons with fetal alcohol syndrome. *MMWR Recomm Rep.* 2005;54(RR-11):1–14.

Chudley AE, Conry J, Cook JL, et al. Public health agency of Canada's national advisory committee on fetal alcohol spectrum disorders. Fetal alcohol spectrum disorder: Canadian guidelines for diagnosis. *Can Med Assoc J.* 2005; 172(5):S1–S21.

Fryer SL, McGee CL, Matt GE, et al. Evaluation of psychopathological conditions in children with heavy prenatal alcohol exposure. *Pediatrics.* 2007;119(3):733–741.

Interventions for Children with FASD Research Consortium (ICFRC). Interventions for children with fetal alcohol spectrum disorders (FASDs): overview of findings for five innovative research projects. *Res Del Disabil.* 2009;30(5):986–1006.

Jacobson SW, Jacobson JL, Sokol RJ, et al. Maternal age, alcohol abuse history, and quality of parenting as moderators of the effects of prenatal alcohol exposure on 7.5-year intellectual functioning. *Alcohol Clin Exp Res.* 2004;28(11):1732–1745.

Jones KJ, Smith DW. Recognition of the fetal alcohol syndrome in early infancy. *Lancet.* 1973;302(7836): 999–1001.

Kalberg WO, Buckley D. FASD: what types of intervention and rehabilitation are useful? *Neurosci Biobehav Rev.* 2007;31(2):278–285.

Kodituwakku PW. Defining the behavioral phenotype in children with fetal alcohol spectrum disorders: a review. *Neurosci Biobehav Rev.* 2007;31(2):192–201.

Mattson SN, Calarco KE, Lang AR. Focused and shifted attention in children with heavy prenatal alcohol exposure. *Neuropsychology.* 2006;20(3):361–369.

Mattson SN, Riley EP, Delis DC, et al. Neuropsychological comparison of alcohol exposed children with or without physical features of fetal alcohol syndrome. *Neuropsychology.* 1998;12(1):146–153.

Mattson SN, Schoenfeld AM, Riley EP. Teratogenic effects of alcohol on brain and behavior. *Alcohol Res Health.* 2001;25(3):185–199.

May P, Gossage J. Estimating the prevalence of fetal alcohol syndrome: a summary. *Alcohol Res Health.* 2001;25(3):159–167.

Miller D. Students with fetal alcohol syndrome. *Teaching Exceptional Children.* 2006;38(4):12–18.

National Task Force on Fetal Alcohol Syndrome and Fetal Alcohol Effect Post Exposure Writing Group. *A Call to Action: Advancing Essential Services and Research on Fetal Alcohol Spectrum Disorders—A Report of the National FAS Task Force on Fetal Alcohol Syndrome and Fetal Alcohol Effect.* Atlanta, GA: Centers for Disease Control and Prevention; 2009.

O'Connor M, Frankel F, Paley B, et al. A controlled social skills training for children with fetal alcohol spectrum disorders. *J Consult Clin Psychol.* 2006;74(4):639–648.

Olson, HC. The current state of FASD intervention: an overview to spark debate and new ideas. *Iceberg Newsletter.* 2006;16(4). http://fasiceberg.org/newsletters/Vol16Num4_Nov2006.htm#currentstate. Accessed February 5, 2009.

Olson HC, Jirikowic T, Kartin D, et al. Responding to the challenges of early intervention for fetal alcohol spectrum disorders. *Infants Young Child.* 2007;20(2):162–179.

Olson HC, Oti R, Gelo J, et al. Family matters: fetal alcohol spectrum disorders and the family. *Dev Disabil Res Rev.* 2009;15(3):235–249.

Paley B, O'Connor MJ. Intervention for individuals with fetal alcohol spectrum disorders: treatment approaches and case management. *Dev Disabil Res Rev.* 2009;15(3):258–267.

Riley EP, McGee CL. Fetal alcohol spectrum disorders: an overview with emphasis on changes in brain and behavior. *Exp Biol Med.* 2005;230(6):357–365.

Schonfeld AM, Paley B, Frankel F, et al. Executive functioning predicts social skills following prenatal alcohol exposure. *Child Neuropsychol.* 2006;12(6):439–452.

Spadoni AD, McGee CL, Fryer SL, et al. Neuroimaging and fetal alcohol spectrum disorders. *Neurosci Biobehav Rev.* 2007;31(2):239–245.

Spohr HL, Willms J, Steinhausen HC. Fetal alcohol spectrum disorders in young adulthood. *J Pediatr.* 2007; 150(2):175–179.

Steinhausen HC, Spohr HL. Long-term outcome of children with fetal alcohol syndrome: psychopathology, behavior, and intelligence. *Alcohol Clin Exp Res.* 1998;22(2):334–338.

Steinhausen HC, Willms J, Spohr HL. Correlates of psychopathology and intelligence in children with fetal alcohol syndrome. *J Child Psychol Psychiatr.* 1994;35(2):323–331.

Streissguth AP, Bookstein FL, Barr HM, et al. Risk factors for adverse life outcomes in fetal alcohol syndrome and fetal alcohol effects. *J Dev Behav Pediatr.* 2004;25(4):228–238.

Streissguth AP, O'Malley K. Neuropsychiatric implications and long-term consequences of fetal alcohol spectrum disorders. *Semin Clin Neuropsychiatry.* 2000;5(3):177–190.

Stratton K., Howe C, Battagliam F. Institute of Medicine (U.S.). Division of Biobehavioral Sciences and Mental Disorders. Committee to Study Fetal Alcohol Syndrome. *Fetal Alcohol Syndrome: Diagnosis, Epidemiology, Prevention and Treatment.* Washington DC: National Academy Press; 1996.

Thomas SE, Kelly SJ, Mattson SN, et al. Comparison of social abilities of children with fetal alcohol syndrome to those of children with similar IQ scores and normal controls. *Alcohol Clin Exp Res.* 1998;22(2):528–533.

Whaley SE, O'Connor MJ, Gunderson B. Comparison of the adaptive functioning of children prenatally exposed to alcohol to a nonexposed clinical sample. *Alcohol Clin Exp Res.* 2001;25(7):1018–1024.

SUGGESTED READINGS

1. Fetal Alcohol Syndrome: A Guide for Families and Communities
   Author: Ann Streissguth
   Publisher: Paul H. Brookes Publishing Company, 1997
   (This classic, still current book is for parents, educators, and health professionals seeking to understand the medical and social implications of children and adults with FASD.)
   Paperback 306 pages
2. Special Issue: Fetal Alcohol Spectrum Disorders. Dev Disabil Res Rev. 2009 Volume 15. (This issue provides an overview of the research advances on fetal alcohol spectrum disorders.)

3. Fantastic Antone Succeeds: Experiences in Educating Children with Fetal Alcohol Syndrome
   Editors: Judith Kleinfeld and Siobhan Wescott
   Publisher: University of Alaska Press, 1993
   (This timeless book presents personal stories and advice to parents, teachers, and families providing education to children with FASD.)
   Paperback 372 pages

4. Fantastic Antone Grows Up: Adolescents and Adults with Fetal Alcohol Syndrome
   Editors: Judith Kleinfeld, Siobhan Wescott, and Barbara Morse
   Publisher: University of Alaska Press, 2000
   (This easily readable book presents information that is still very current on the challenging transition to adolescence and adulthood for those with fetal alcohol syndrome, from the perspective of young people with FASD, their parents, teachers, and mental health professionals.)
   Paperback 425 pages

5. Prenatal Alcohol Use and Fetal Alcohol Spectrum Disorders: Historical and Future Perspectives
   Editors: Susan Adubato & Deborah E. Cohen
   Publisher: Bentham Science: Bentham e-Books, in press
   (This electronic book provides a state-of-the-art overview of the impact of prenatal alcohol use on the development of affected individuals and their families, and on society. Chapters provide a historical overview, discussion of the prevalence of maternal drinking and efforts toward prevention, information on diagnosis, and characteristics of the clinical conditions of FASD, and a variety of chapters that discuss intervention research and innovative treatment ideas from infancy through adulthood.)

6. Storm Riders
   Author: Craig Lesley
   Publisher: Picador USA, 2001
   (This beautifully written novel portrays the struggle of a father raising an adopted son who has been diagnosed with FAS.)
   Paperback 352 pages

7. A Call to Action: Advancing Essential Services and Research on Fetal Alcohol Spectrum Disorders—A Report of the National FAS Task Force on Fetal Alcohol Syndrome and Fetal Alcohol Effect.
   Authors: National Task Force on Fetal Alcohol Syndrome and Fetal Alcohol Effect Post Exposure Writing Group.
   Publisher: Centers for Disease Control and Prevention, 2009
   (This useful booklet presents the latest information on FASD and recommendations for public policy and services that communities should build to respond to this under-recognized medical condition.)
   Paperback, 30 pages

RECOMMENDED ONLINE RESOURCES

- The National Organization on Fetal Alcohol Syndrome can be found at: http://www.nofas.org/ *This is a national FASD nonprofit organization that is committed to primary prevention, advocacy, and support. NOFAS has international affiliations, as well as US state affiliate organizations.*

- The Fetal Alcohol Syndrome Diagnostic and Prevention Network (FAS DPN), based at the University of Washington, can be found at: http://depts.washington.edu/fasdpn/ *The FAS DPN website provides access to the manual for the 4-Digit Diagnostic Code. This diagnostic system can be learned by providers to assess the characteristic facial features of fetal alcohol syndrome, and to diagnose conditions across the fetal alcohol spectrum. The FAS DPN website also provides information on FASD, access to research literature, and links to other important websites on FASD.*

- The Iceberg newsletter website can be found at: www.fasiceberg.org/ *This is a quarterly international educational newsletter on FASD (Fetal Alcohol Spectrum Disorders) from FASIS, a parent/professional partnership. "Because the problems we readily see are only the tip of the iceberg."*

- The Centers for Disease Control and Prevention, Office of Fetal Alcohol Spectrum Disorders, can be found at: http://www.cdc.gov/ncbddd/fasd/index.html. *This is a US Department of Health and Human Services website, offering information, prevention toolkits, and curriculum guides for families and providers, with the aim of enhancing public health. This is the specific FASD website.*

- The Substance Abuse & Mental Health Services Administration, FASD Center for Excellence can be found at: http://www.fasdcenter.samhsa.gov/ *The Center was created by a federal initiative "…devoted to preventing and treating FASD." The Center provides training and technical information, and the website presents comprehensive information on prenatal alcohol exposure and FASD, research, resources, and more.*

- The National Institute on Alcohol Abuse and Alcoholism can be found at: http://www.niaaa.nih.gov/. *NIAAA is an organization providing national research leadership in an effort to reduce alcohol related problems.*

- The Research Society on Alcoholism, Fetal Alcohol Spectrum Disorders Study Group, can be found at: http://www.rsoa.org/fas.html *This is a society of professionals dedicated to fully understanding FAS and FASD, and improve the lives of all individuals living with alcohol related disabilities.*

REVIEW QUESTIONS

1. One of your patients is a newly adopted toddler with suspected exposure before birth to alcohol and other drugs. A physical examination reveals some mild to moderate facial dysmorphology and delayed growth, and, from your brief interaction, you suspect the child also has mild cognitive and language delays. How do you proceed?
   a. Consult with a colleague familiar with FASD.
   b. Conduct a thorough evaluation of medical history, including the extent of alcohol and drug use during pregnancy.
   c. Inform the family of your concern about FASD and provide them with information about the condition.
   d. Refer the family to a clinic specializing in diagnosis and treatment for FASD, or a clinic that specialized in neurodevelopmental disabilities, for evaluation and treatment recommendations.
   e. All of the above.

2. Which of the following statements is TRUE?
   a. The US Surgeon General issued a statement warning women who are pregnant and women who may become pregnant to abstain from alcohol use during the final trimester of pregnancy.
   b. The problems of individuals with the full fetal alcohol syndrome (FAS) are worse than those with conditions on the wider fetal alcohol spectrum (often called alcohol-related neurodevelopmental disorder, or ARND).
   c. FAS is far less common than Down Syndrome or spina bifida.
   d. There has been increasing emphasis in diagnosis on the neurobehavioral deficits presumed to be related to prenatal alcohol exposure, because these are related to caregiver stress and to the affected individual's day-to-day function.
   e. None of the above is true.

3. You are contacted by a foster parent who has been referred to you by her foster child's school. This seventh grader has been diagnosed with the full FAS, and has experienced several disrupted home placements because of volatile behavior. The school reports that this middle school student has learning problems and a "scattered" cognitive profile despite an average IQ. She also appears to have delays in social language use. She has very few friends, and wants her parents to give her more time to do things on her own. The family and school would like recommendations from you about appropriate next steps. What recommendations are necessary to support this preadolescent?
   a. This girl will automatically receive social services because of her FAS diagnosis, so you can simply refer to the Division of Developmental Disabilities in your state.
   b. Refer the family to a resource that can conduct neurodevelopmental or psychoeducational testing to provide the family and school with a learning profile of individual strengths and weaknesses, and create an accommodation plan at school and structured social skills instruction even though she has average IQ.
   c. This girl needs insight into her behavior, so she should be referred to a counselor who can provide talk therapy and come to terms with the disruption she experienced earlier in life.
   d. Counsel the family to give this girl more independence, and a chance to participate in social activities such as school dances and team sports so she can find a group of same-aged friends.

4. Which of the following statements is FALSE?
    a. There is no "behavioral phenotype," or characteristic set of clinical features in behavior, identified at this point in time for FASD.
    b. It is usually behavioral difficulties that lead families to seek professional support for their alcohol-affected child, teenager, or adult.
    c. It is unusual for individuals with FASD to have co-occurring psychiatric conditions.
    d. There is a clear consensus for how to code FASD in current medical, psychiatric, and educational coding schemes.
    e. Answers c and d are both FALSE.

5. Which of the following statements are TRUE?
    a. Individuals with conditions on the fetal alcohol spectrum typically have IQ in the range of intellectual deficiency.
    b. Attention deficits are very often seen in those with FASD.
    c. Younger women cannot have children with FASD.
    d. Health and mental health professionals rarely have a role to play in the prevention of FASD.
    e. All the above statements are TRUE.

Answers: 1-e, 2-d, 3-b, 4-e, 5-b

CHAPTER 20

Elizabeth Super, MD
and Kyle P. Johnson, MD

Pediatric Sleep Problems

Introduction and Background

While pediatric sleep disorders have long been recognized by parents and pediatricians, systematic study has only recently been applied. Nineteenth and early twentieth century clinicians were primarily interested in sleep-related breathing problems. Some of the earliest descriptions of pediatric sleep disorders are in the literary works of Charles Dickens, most famously the depiction of Joe in the *Pickwick Papers* published in 1836. Joe was an obese boy who was always excessively sleepy. He snored loudly and likely had right-sided heart failure as a result of severe obstructive sleep apnea (OSA). In 1892, William Osler described childhood OSA in his classic textbook, *The Principles and Practice of Medicine*. Over 60 years passed before there was further study, linking OSA to adenotonsillar hypertrophy and cardiac failure.

In the second half of the twentieth century, as adult sleep medicine was developing into a medical science, systematic study of children and adolescents started at Stanford University under the direction of Dr. Mary Carskadon. For 10 years beginning from 1976, Dr. Carskadon and her colleagues ran the Stanford Summer Sleep Camp. Basically, the same cohort of preadolescents and adolescents returned each summer allowing for the systematic collection of data. This information provided the first objective description of pediatric sleep and how it changes with development. During the same time span, other pioneers in the field such as Dr. Richard Ferber and Dr. Thomas Anders concentrated on sleep in infants, toddlers, and school children.

More recently, studies have documented the deleterious effect of persistent sleep disturbance on various areas of functioning in children and adolescents. Sleep loss in adolescents is associated with excessive daytime sleepiness, depressed mood, and poor school performance. OSA can result in serious sequelae such as failure to thrive and cor pulmonale as well as neurocognitive deficits such as learning problems and disruptive behavior. In young children who are at particular risk for adenotonsillar hypertrophy, these neurocognitive deficits present similarly to attention-deficit/hyperactivity disorder (ADHD). Treatment for OSA often improves daytime functioning and school performance.

Increasingly, sleep is being investigated in special pediatric populations. For example, it has been discovered that the majority of children with autism spectrum disorders experience insomnia. Patients with Down Syndrome, Prader Willi, and those with cleft palates are at increased risk for OSA. Treatment can improve their daytime functioning and ability to learn.

Review of Normal Sleep in Children and Adolescents

In simple behavioral terms, sleep is a reversible state of perceptual disengagement from and unresponsiveness to the environment, typically occurring while lying down, quiet with closed eyes. Although the exact purpose of sleep still eludes investigation, we do know that it is necessary for healthy functioning as persistent disturbance causes psychological and sometimes physical impairments.

TABLE 20-1	Average Sleep Needs Over Development
Age	**Duration of Sleep Over 24 Hours**
Newborn	16–20
Infant (0–1 year)	14
Toddler (1–3 years)	12
Preschooler (3–5 years)	11–12
School Age (6–12 years)	10–11
Adolescent (>12 years)	9
Young Adult (19–22 years)	8–8.5

There are two states within sleep, nonrapid eye movement sleep (NREM) and rapid eye movement sleep (REM), which are distinct from one another as well as from wakefulness based on a myriad of physiological parameters. According to the American Academy of Sleep Medicine Manual for the Scoring of Sleep and Associated Events, NREM sleep is divided into three stages (N1, N2, and N3) which correspond to the depth of sleep. Stage N3 is also referred to as slow-wave sleep or delta sleep. Fragmented mental activity occurs in NREM and bodily movement is possible. REM sleep is defined by electroencephalogram (EEG) activation, muscle atonia, and periodic bursts of REMs. Mental activity is more continuous in REM sleep and is associated with dreaming. In adults, approximately 20% of sleep is REM sleep and 80% is NREM, and these stages alternate in 90–120 minute cycles. Sleep changes over the course of development with the most pronounced changes occurring in the first 5 years of life, as outlined in Table 20-1.

At birth, normal full-term newborns spend 16 to 20 hours out of 24 hours asleep. As any new parent knows, sleep in the first month of life is not consolidated at night, instead occurs in 3 to 4 hour cycles throughout a 24-hour period of time. After the first month, the infant starts adapting to the light–dark cycle and regularly recurring time cues. By 6 months of age, most infants have a continuous sleep period of 6 hours during the night. At 1 year, the infant is sleeping 14 to 15 hours per day with the majority of sleep occurring at night and two naps during the day. In the second year, sleep decreases to about 12 hours and the morning nap usually ceases. The afternoon nap tends to drop out by 4 to 5 years of age. Infants spend more time in REM sleep compared with adults and actually enter sleep through REM, a phenomenon considered pathologic in adults. REM and NREM cycles are of 50 to 60 minutes in infants and young children and progressively increase until adult cycle lengths are reached in adolescence.

School-aged children demonstrate excellent sleep as evidenced by high sleep efficiencies and considerable daytime alertness compared to other age groups. Sleep efficiency is the ratio of total sleep time to time in bed expressed as a percentage. Problems with sleep or daytime alertness at this age is reason for concern. School-aged children need 9.5 to 11 hours of sleep typically, usually consolidated at night. Adolescents' sleep requirements do not decrease significantly, if at all, compared with school-aged children. However, they tend to delay preferred sleep times, going to bed on school nights an average of an hour later than school-aged children. Teenagers tend to have lower levels of alertness during the day, particularly during the morning and early afternoon hours. This appears to be a normal part of development since the level of daytime sleepiness correlates more with pubertal development (Tanner Stages) than age when adequate amounts of sleep are ensured. Adolescents also have more irregular sleep patterns than the school-aged child, delaying sleep onset even longer on weekend nights and then sleeping later the next morning.

Epidemiology

Sleep problems in children and adolescents are very common. Population studies of toddlers demonstrate bedtime settling or frequent-awakening problems occurring at most nights or every night at rates of 20% to 25%. Once these sleep problems are established in toddlers, they tend to persist into early childhood at rates ranging from 25% to 84% over a 3-year period. The prevalence of parent-reported sleep problems in school-aged children is 11% to 37%. OSA occurs in approximately 2% of the pediatric population. Narcolepsy, which occurs in 1/2000 people, usually onsets during adolescence. Many patients with restless legs syndrome (RLS) experience the onset of symptoms in childhood, with an estimated prevalence of 2%. Delayed sleep phase syndrome (DSPS) affects approximately 5% to 10% of adolescents.

Insufficient sleep and irregular sleep patterns are particularly common in adolescents with the majority of students getting inadequate sleep during school nights. Children with developmental and neurological disabilities are at high risk for severe sleep disturbances. Up to 80% of children with mental retardation, Down syndrome, brain damage, and blindness suffer with clinically significant sleep disorders. The prevalence rates of sleep problems in children who have autism range from 44% to 83%. Sleep disturbance is often comorbid with psychiatric disorders including depression, anxiety, trauma-related pathology, and disruptive behavior disorders. Thus, sleep problems are common, but probably inadequately considered or evaluated, in clinical practice.

Sleep Disorder Syndromes

Overview and General Issues

Sleep disorders in children and adolescents differ from those occurring in adults. Some sleep disorders are specific to childhood while others occur across the developmental spectrum but may have different presentations and etiologies in children and adolescents. In pediatric sleep medicine, the parents are often the ones to complain, not the child, making parental perception an important part of the picture. Often the complaint is more consistent with a problem rather than a true disorder. What is defined as a sleep problem will vary from family to family and culture to culture. Therefore, pediatric sleep disturbances need to be considered within the specific psychosocial context of the child being assessed. In fact, pediatric insomnia has recently been defined with family considerations in mind. A consensus paper on the subject in 2006 by Mindell and colleagues defined pediatric insomnia as follows: "Repeated difficulty with sleep initiation, duration, consolidation, or quality that occurs despite age-appropriate time and opportunity for sleep and results in daytime functional impairment for the child and/or family."

Sleep problems have a bidirectional relationship with many child and adolescent psychiatric disorders, particularly ADHD, anxiety disorders, and depression. Insomnia is a criterion symptom for depression and many of the anxiety disorders experienced in childhood. Conversely, chronic insomnia and sleep deprivation place children at increased risk to suffer with these conditions. Although insomnia is not a criterion symptom of ADHD, a large percentage of children with ADHD have sleep problems including initial insomnia, RLS, and OSA. Clinical and experimental research shows that sleep deprivation can result in ADHD-type symptoms and behaviors.

Sleep disorders are classified into four major categories in the *Diagnostic and Statistical Manual*, Fourth Edition (*DSM-IV*): Primary Sleep Disorders; Sleep Disorder Due to a Medical Condition; Sleep Disorder Due to Another Mental Disorder; and Substance-Induced Sleep Disorder. These *DSM-IV* categories appropriately describe sleep disorders in adults, but are inadequate for categorizing sleep disorders in children. Instead, it is easier to conceptualize pediatric sleep problems in three broad categories: sleeplessness; excessive daytime sleepiness; and disturbed behavior during sleep. Some of the more common pediatric sleep disorders are summarized in Table 20-2 and discussed below.

TABLE 20-2   Common Pediatric Sleep Disorders

Category		Typical Age	Prevalence	Symptoms/Signs	Evaluation	Interventions
Excessive daytime sleepiness	OSA	3- to 8-year olds and adolescents	1–2% of children	Habitual snoring, noisy breathing, pauses in breathing, nocturnal sweating, mouth breathing	Full PSG is gold standard; limited channel cardiopulmonary study; home oximetry	Adenotonsillectomy; CPAP/BIPAP
Excessive daytime sleepiness	DSPS	Adolescents	5–10% of adolescents	Delayed sleep onset (usually after midnight) with difficulty awakening in a.m.; sleep very late on weekends; normal sleep quality	Detailed sleep history; sleep diaries; actigraphy	Chronotherapy; behavioral interventions; light therapy; motivational counseling; potentially melatonin
Excessive daytime sleepiness	Narcolepsy	Adolescents	1/2000	Cataplexy, hypnogogic hallucinations, sleep paralysis, sleep attacks	PSG and MSLT	Modafinil or stimulants for EDS; SSRI's or TCAs for cataplexy; scheduled naps
Disturbed sleep behaviors	Sleep terrors	Toddlers and school-aged children	3%	Occur in first third of the night; autonomic arousal with tachycardia, tachypnea, sweating; inconsolable screaming; amnesia for event	Detailed sleep history with attention to timing of episodes; family history of parasomia; video taping	Reassurance of parents; avoid sleep deprivation; benzodiazepines for severe cases
Disturbed sleep behaviors	Sleep walking	4- to 8-year-olds	15–40% have one episode; 3–4% have weekly/monthly episodes	Usually occur 1–2 hours after sleep onset; walks for a few minutes up to one-half hour; confusion; incoherence; difficult to awaken; amnesia for event	Detailed sleep history; video taping; family history	Reassurance of parents; safety measures (lock outside doors and windows; alarm on bedroom door); benzodiazepines for severe cases

Sleeplessness	Sleep-onset association disorder	Infants and toddlers	25–50% of 6- to 12-month-olds; 15–20% of 1- to 3-year-olds	Frequent signaling of parents after nightwakings; initiation of sleep requires parental involvement; inappropriate sleep associations (falls asleep in parent's arms)	Detailed sleep history with attention to reinforcing behaviors of parents; charting of sleep associations; sleep diaries; video taping	Behavioral interventions (put to bed awake but sleepy); parental guidance regarding bedtime routines and sleep scheduling, education on graduated extinction.
Sleeplessness	Restless legs syndrome	School age and adolescents	2%	Uncomfortable sensation in legs; urge to move legas at time of rest, relieved with movement	Clinical history, family history, at times PSG appropriate to evaluate for overlapping periodic limb movement disorder	Avoidance of caffeine Iron replacement if low Dopamine agonists

OSA, obstructive sleep apnea; CPAP, continuous positive airway pressure; DSPS, delayed sleep phase syndrome; PSG, polysomnogram; MSLT, multiple sleep latency test; EDS, excessive daytime sleepiness; SSRI, selective serotonin reuptake inhibitor; TCA, tricyclic antidepressant.

Sleeplessness

Sleeplessness is a broad category which can be broken down into three basic types: problems settling and initiating sleep; frequent awakenings during the night; and awakening too early in the morning. These particular forms can occur in isolation or combination. It is important to determine the specific type of sleeplessness as etiologies will differ and, subsequently, so will treatment. In addition, potential causes of sleeplessness change according to the age of the child or adolescent.

Infants and toddlers often experience problems with settling and frequent awakenings. Potential medical causes (such as colic, middle ear disease or gastroesophageal reflux) need to be considered, although are rarely the problem for persistent nightly awakenings. In addition, it is quite uncommon for pain to be the cause of frequent awakenings in children. If pain were the cause of the awakenings, the child would not be able to return to sleep after being held or fed. Difficult temperaments can also manifest as sleeplessness. Behavioral issues are often the cause, specifically inappropriate sleep associations, clinically described as "sleep-onset association disorder." Sleep-onset is a learned behavior and, therefore, is assisted or inhibited by certain environmental stimuli. If a child learns to fall asleep at bedtime in the mother's arms, it will be difficult for the child to initiate sleep independently during a nighttime awakening. These children will signal care providers to aid in the transition back to sleep.

Family expectations can play a part in "sleeplessness" in toddlers. Often, parents expect a child to sleep more than is biologically necessary. When total sleep time is added up, including daytime naps, expected sleep is excessive leading to a decrease in homeostatic sleep drive. A sleep diary can help determine this cause.

According to the 2007 International Classification of Sleep Disorders, behavioral insomnia of childhood is divided into sleep-onset association type or limit-setting type. Inadequate limit-setting and sleep routines are often the culprits especially in overwhelmed or chaotic families. Sleep-onset association insomnia is characterized by an extended process of falling asleep that requires special conditions which are highly problematic or demanding for caregivers. In the absence of the associated conditions, sleep onset is significantly delayed or sleep is otherwise disrupted. Nighttime awakenings required caregiver intervention to return to sleep. In limit-setting insomnia, the child has difficulty initiating or maintaining sleep, refuses to go to bed at an appropriate time or refuses to return to bed after a nighttime awakening. The caregiver demonstrates insufficient and/or inappropriate limit setting to establish appropriate sleeping behavior in the child.

School-aged children (5 to 12 years) have the best sleep efficiency of any age group, so sleeplessness is concerning when it happens. Psychiatric disorders such as anxiety and depression become more common at these ages as well as circadian rhythm disturbances. Children can develop into either "larks" or "owls" based on their tendency to advance or delay their sleep schedules. The intrinsic, biologically driven sleep/wake rhythms may be in conflict with parental and societal expectations leading to a perception of sleeplessness, particularly problems falling asleep or arising either too late or early in the morning. If these children are allowed to sleep their own schedule, they sleep soundly and are rested during waking hours. Behavioral sleep disorders continue to be prevalent in this age group.

More recently, RLS has been described in children. Manifestations of RLS include uncomfortable sensations in the legs associated with urges to move the legs and motor restlessness. Patients may describe the sensation as "crazy legs, creepy-crawlies" or "growing pains." These symptoms are experienced during times of rest and relaxation particularly in the evening and night when one is recumbent. The uncomfortable feeling is relieved when the legs are moved. RLS tends to cause sleep-onset problems as the behaviors that relieve symptoms (movement) are likely to interfere with sleep onset. In a large population-based survey, criteria for definite RLS were met by approximately 2% of 8- to 17-year-olds. RLS is thought to be an autosomal dominant condition and, therefore, shows strong familial trends. Reduced iron stores appear to play a role in children and adults with RLS. Synthesis of iron is the rate-limiting step of dopamine synthesis and metabolism. Thus, it is compelling to consider that iron deficiency plays a role in other central nervous system dopamine-related conditions like ADHD. In this population-based study, there was approximately 35% comorbidity of self-reported ADHD and RLS. Further work has found that children with RLS and ADHD tend to have lower ferritin levels than children with ADHD alone, and tend to be more severely affected by ADHD.

Adolescents experience sleeplessness for reasons similar to those described for school-aged children. In addition, substances such as caffeine and illicit drugs can disrupt sleep. Social and academic pressures may cause worry and anxiety and, subsequently, sleep disturbance. Other psychiatric disorders to consider in teens are bipolar disorder and psychotic illnesses such as schizophrenia, both of which can cause sleeplessness. DSPS is a circadian rhythm disturbance often manifesting at puberty. Adolescents with this problem have sleep-onset insomnia and excessive daytime sleepiness during the first half of the day.

Excessive Daytime Sleepiness (EDS)

Sleepiness differs from tiredness. Tiredness is similar in nature to fatigue, lethargy, or exhaustion and typically has a medical cause such as depression or endocrine dysfunction. Sleepiness describes an actual urge to fall asleep which tiredness does not entail, although the two conditions can simultaneously exist. Daytime sleepiness in children and adolescents has long been ignored, only recently supported by systematic research. Sleepiness can range from mild to severe and can present differently depending on age. Preschoolers and school-aged children usually do not manifest the behavioral signs seen in adolescents and adults, that is, difficulty in initiating or sustaining motor activity, droopy eyelids, or head nodding. Instead, they often present paradoxically with hyperactivity, increased impulsivity and aggressiveness, as well as impaired concentration and irritability.

EDS is often unrecognized in children because it presents similarly to other conditions such as learning disabilities or ADHD. A standard way to objectively measure daytime sleepiness is the Multiple Sleep Latency Test (MSLT). The patient is asked to try to take a nap on four or five separate occasions separated by 2 hours during the day. The time it takes to fall asleep (sleep latency) is recorded as well as sleep stages, most importantly sleep-onset REM periods. Research using the MSLT has demonstrated that school-aged children tend to be very alert during the day (longer sleep latencies during MSLT) compared with adolescents.

There are multiple causes for EDS in the pediatric population with leading causes differing among age groups. The most frequently encountered etiologies will be reviewed here. The reader is referred to pediatric sleep medicine textbooks listed in the suggested readings for a more detailed discussion.

Obstructive Sleep Apnea (OSA)

It has been estimated that 2% of children from infancy through adolescence have some degree of sleep-related upper airway obstruction. Prevalence rates have been variable due to varying definitions. In 2002, the American Academy of Pediatrics published a Technical Report on the Diagnosis and Management of Childhood Obstructive Sleep Apnea Syndrome in *Pediatrics*, that reviewed articles from 1966 to 2000 reporting a prevalence from 0.7% to 13%. Children between the ages of 3 and 8 years are most commonly afflicted with OSA due to higher rates of the main etiology, adenotonsillar hypertrophy. Adolescents who are obese or have craniofacial abnormalities are also at risk.

Snoring is a major symptom of OSA. Approximately 10% of children habitually (almost every night) snore to some degree, with about 20% of this group meeting criteria for OSA when formally studied in a sleep laboratory. Since snoring alone does not predict OSA, other risk factors need to be considered in determining who undergoes a formal sleep study. Other symptoms of OSA include witnessed apnea, snoring or gasping for breath while asleep, excessive sweating, restlessness, and unusual extension of the neck during sleep. Daytime functioning is often affected and includes sleepiness, mood instability, and poor attention and concentration with associated poor school performance. Findings suggestive of OSA on physical examination are enlarged tonsils, deviated nasal septum, large tongue, abnormal palate or uvula, and craniofacial abnormalities such as midface hypoplasia or micrognathia. Obesity is not a common risk factor for OSA in children, as compared to adolescents and adults, although obesity does increase the risk if present.

When these symptoms and signs are present, further evaluation is indicated by someone familiar with pediatric OSA. Specialists in this area include sleep medicine clinicians, pediatric otolaryngologists, and pulmonologists. A sleep study may be needed, preferably an overnight, full-channel polysomnogram (PSG). A PSG is the gold-standard for assessing OSA in children and adults. It measures electrical activity in the brain and movements of eyes allowing staging of sleep. The PSG also measures airflow, effort of breathing, oxygen saturation, and often levels of carbon dioxide. Once OSA is diagnosed, appropriate treatment is highly successful.

Narcolepsy

Narcolepsy is a neurological syndrome that afflicts about 1 in 2000 persons. Multiple case series indicate that approximately 50% onset before 15 years of age. Its chief symptoms, apart from daytime sleepiness, are cataplexy (sudden loss of muscle tone induced by strong emotions) and daytime sleep attacks. Other symptoms include sleep paralysis (inability to move although fully conscious during the onset of sleep or while waking) and hypnagogic hallucinations (dream-like auditory or visual hallucinations at the onset of sleep). These symptoms arise when REM sleep intrudes into waking periods. The diagnosis is confirmed with a PSG and MSLT. The time it takes to fall asleep (sleep latency) is measured and sleep stages are determined. An average sleep latency of less than 8 minutes and the presence of REM sleep in two or more naps are diagnostic of narcolepsy.

Narcolepsy has a strong genetic component, although the pattern of hereditary transmission is not yet known. In recent research, it has been linked to decreased numbers of the neurons in the hypothalamus that produce a neuropeptide called hypocretin (also known as orexin). An autoimmune etiology has been proposed.

Insufficient Sleep

Inadequate amount of sleep is the most common cause of EDS particularly in adolescents. In young children, parents may underestimate the amount of sleep needed by a child of a certain age. Adolescents face other impediments to getting adequate sleep. As noted previously, adolescents delay their sleep schedule by an average of 1 hour over the course of puberty while overall sleep needs remain essentially the same as for latency-aged children. Coupling this biologically driven delay in sleep-onset with earlier school schedules in high school and increasing social, occupational, and academic demands leads to chronic sleep deprivation and EDS. Although most adolescents need approximately 9 hours of sleep, surveys indicate that during the school week, average sleep times are closer to 7.5 hours. Only 15% of adolescents sleep as long as eight and half hours on school nights, and 26% say they usually sleep six and a half hours or less. Teenagers generally compensate on weekends by sleeping nearly 2 hours longer. This "catch-up" sleep is a normal response in adolescents not getting enough sleep during the week.

Circadian Rhythm Disorders

Disorders of circadian rhythms may take the form of delayed sleep phase syndrome (DSPS) or irregular sleep–wake schedules. Children with blindness are particularly at risk for irregular sleep–wake cycles. Blind children and adolescents may be unable to consistently consolidate sleep at night due to underlying circadian rhythm pathology. Research demonstrates that many blind youths and adults, especially those with no light perception, have circadian rhythms that progressively drift later and later over time or "free-run." Free-running rhythms lead to episodes of insomnia and EDS when the endogenous rhythm for sleep is out of phase with preferred nighttime sleep schedules.

DSPS is most common among adolescents due to the normal delay in circadian rhythms which occurs with puberty. This is a disorder defined by society, as sleep quality and quantity is normal if the patient is left to sleep his/her own schedule. Adolescents with DSPS have a delay in sleep onset of at least 3 to 4 hours compared with adolescents with normal sleep patterns. This syndrome should be suspected if EDS resolves when the patient is allowed to sleep on his/her own biologically driven schedule, for example, 2 am until 12 noon. Adolescents with DSPS are at risk of developing poor sleep habits, such as using the bed for other purposes besides sleep.

Patients with DSPS have severe sleep deprivation which impairs academic and social functioning. DSPS may be an unrecognized cause of behavior that looks like adolescent delinquency or depression. Patients may miss many days of school, causing grades to slip because of their inability to wake in the morning, often causing conflict with parents. They may drop out of sports because of the inability to attend morning practices and avoid social events during daytime because of their sleep schedule. The cycle is worsened by their peers who are also up in the late evenings socializing on the internet or phone.

Disturbed Sleep Behaviors (Parasomnias)

Parasomnias are recurrent, undesirable physiological or mental phenomena which occur during sleep such as autonomic arousal, skeletal muscle activity, emotions, thoughts and images. The etiology is thought to be a state dissociation involving aspects of sleep impinging on wake, essentially getting caught between the two states. Children are at particular risk given developmental differences in sleep architecture, namely greater amounts of slow-wave sleep compared with adults.

Parasomnias can be primary sleep phenomena or secondary to medical or psychiatric disorders and may develop out of different sleep states (REM vs. NREM). The most concerning potential medical cause is nocturnal seizures. Although an EEG is not routinely ordered in the work-up of a parasomnia, this procedure should be considered when the problem is refractory or associated with atypical features. EEG telemetry is often needed to capture an event.

The most common parasomnias seen in clinical practice are the arousal disorders, including sleep terrors, confusional arousals, and sleep walking. These disorders arise out of NREM slow-wave sleep and, therefore, occur typically in the first third of the night. They tend to run in families. Children with arousal disorders will have amnesia for the events. Sleep terrors are usually the most disturbing to parents because the child experiences autonomic arousal and appears terrified. Sleep terrors occur most frequently in 4 to 12 year olds and usually disappear by adolescence. The event typically lasts 3 to 5 minutes and may recur during the night. Sleep walking is prevalent, occurring in as many as 20% of children. Usual onset is between the ages of 4 and 6 years and events typically last 5 to 15 minutes. Sleep walking can potentially be dangerous if a child falls down the stairs or wanders outside. Confusional arousals are more common in infants and toddlers and typically last longer than sleep terrors with less autonomic arousal. Arousal disorders can be precipitated by sleep deprivation, stress, or medical illnesses.

Nightmares are another common form of parasomnia. Nightmares are dream phenomena arising out of REM sleep. They are differentiated from sleep terrors in that they tend to occur in the second half of the night when REM sleep is frequent. Another differentiating feature is that the child recalls the perceptual phenomena in dreams.

Rhythmic movement disorder is a stereotyped parasomnia characterized by purposeless, repetitive movements such as head banging and body rocking. These behaviors occur during the sleep–wake transition either at initial sleep onset or after arousal from sleep. These movements occur in normal infants and young children, typically beginning by 6 months of age and remitting by 5 years of age. Persistence into adolescence is unusual unless there are comorbid developmental disabilities such as mental retardation or autism. Reassurance and safety precautions (extra padding for head banging) are the treatments of choice.

Assessment

Initial work-up for a sleep complaint in a child or adolescent should include a detailed history of sleep including sleep schedule and environment, unusual behaviors during sleep, and sleep-related breathing problems. The clinician must also assess daytime alertness by questioning the patient, parents, and possibly collateral sources such as teachers. Medical, developmental, and psychiatric histories are instrumental in considering differential diagnoses. Family sleep, medical, and psychiatric histories are important in assessing risk factors for certain conditions that run in families such as depression and RLS. The differential diagnosis of pediatric sleep disorders is listed in Table 20-3.

A tailored physical exam is also needed especially in assessing risk factors for OSA such as micrognathia (small jaw), enlarged tonsils, deviated nasal septum, and abnormal palate and uvula. Weight and height measurements are important for assessing obesity, another risk factor

TABLE 20-3 Differential Diagnosis of Sleep Problems	
Medical	**Substances/Medications**
Allergies/eczema	Alcohol
Asthma	Antiepileptic drugs
Gastroesophageal reflux disease	Antidepressants
Migraine headaches	Antipsychotics
Neuromuscular disorders	Lithium
Arnold–Chiari malformation	Stimulants
Chronic renal failure	Opiods
Seizure disorders	Hypnotic agents
Ear infections	Corticosteroids
Diabetes mellitus	Caffeine
Pain syndromes	Nicotine
Iron deficiency anemia	Theophylline
Hyperthyroidism	**Psychosocial**
Hypothyroidism	Abuse
Psychiatric	Chaotic home life
Anxiety disorders	TV/computer in bedroom
Mood disorders	Parental sleep disorder
Disruptive behavior disorders	Inappropriate sleep-onset associations
Posttraumatic stress disorder	Marital conflict
Pervasive developmental disorder	New infant in home
Psychotic disorders	
Substance-use disorders	
Reactive attachment disorder	
Obsessive compulsive disorder	

for OSA. Assessing mental status is important given the possibility of psychiatric conditions. Laboratory tests should be ordered on a case-by-case basis, depending on the condition suspected. OSA is common in hypothyroidism, so thyroid function testing may be indicated in patients with hypothyroid symptoms or signs. Given the association between iron deficiency and RLS, obtaining iron indices, particularly ferritin levels, in patients with a clinical history consistent with RLS is appropriate. Drug screening should be considered in adolescents with EDS.

Questionnaires have a role in screening for specific sleep disorders. The Pediatric Sleep Questionnaire (PSQ) can be used to screen for pediatric sleep problems particularly sleep-related breathing disorders and sleepiness. It is a reliable measure validated by polysomnography. The Children's Sleep Habits Questionnaire (CSHQ) is a useful screening instrument for school-aged children. The CSHQ gives both a total score and eight subscale scores, reflecting the important sleep domains of the major behavioral and medical sleep disorders in this age group. There is also a role for scales that measure depression and anxiety.

A pediatric sleep specialist may use other assessment tools including an actigraph which is worn on a patient's wrist for several weeks. The actigraph measures movement and correlates this with sleep/wake, allowing for objective assessment of sleep schedules over time. As mentioned previously, sleep studies are indicated for assessing medical causes of sleep disturbances such as OSA, periodic limb movement disorder, and narcolepsy.

Referral to a pediatric sleep specialist is warranted when underlying sleep disrupters are suspected such as sleep apnea or periodic limb movements. Consultation with a pediatric sleep specialist is also indicated for the evaluation and management of children with EDS, RLS, or treatment-refractory parasomnias. The essentials of assessment of pediatric sleep disorders are summarized in Table 20-4.

Treatment

Education of patient and family is the first step in treatment. In some cases, this may be the only treatment necessary, that is, when parents have inflated sleep expectations of children. Parents can be referred to various sources for education. Improving sleep hygiene is important

---

TABLE 20-4   Essentials of Evaluation for Pediatric Sleep Disorders

- Must consider sleep disorders in the differential diagnosis when evaluating children and adolescents with cognitive, emotional, and behavioral problems
- Screen all children and adolescents for OSA by asking parents about snoring, apnea, and labored breathing
- When assessing excessively sleepy youth, ask screening questions for narcolepsy, for example, cataplexy, sleep paralysis, and hypnagogic hallucinations
- Carefully assess sleep schedules and sleep amounts on weekdays, weekends, and school holidays. Consider use of a sleep diary
- Remember that insufficient sleep is the most common cause of EDS
- Assess bedtime routines and sleep-onset associations especially in younger children with behaviorally based sleep disorders
- Conduct a physical exam particularly assessing risk factors for OSA such as craniofacial anomalies, tonsillar size, septal deviation of the nose

OSA, obstructive sleep apnea; EDS, excessive daytime sleepiness.

in almost every case and may be the only treatment needed in behavioral sleep disorders or insufficient sleep syndrome. Parents should be counseled on age-appropriate sleep times. A relaxing and enjoyable 20 to 30 minute bedtime routine is paramount. This should be continued in adolescents. The television should be removed from the bedroom. Television, video games, and computer use should be discontinued at least 30 minutes prior to bedtime to avoid additional light exposure and stimulation close to bedtime. Dinner and exercise should be completed an hour prior to bedtime. The child should be placed in a dark, quiet, and cool environment.

Cognitive behavioral interventions are helpful in many pediatric sleep disorders. Sleep restriction, stimulus control (using the bed for sleep only), and relaxation techniques are particularly useful especially in treating insomnia.

School interventions may be needed in certain situations. In correcting circadian rhythm disorders such as DSPS, it may be necessary to alter individual school start times at least temporarily. EDS associated with narcolepsy can be treated with scheduled daytime naps at school.

Treatment of OSA varies depending on etiology. In younger children, primarily ages 3 to 8, enlarged tonsils and adenoids are usually the culprits. Referral to a surgeon for adenotonsillectomy is the treatment of choice in this group of patients with OSA. Older patients, especially those with comorbid obesity, are candidates for continuous positive airway pressure (CPAP), which entails using a mask and positive air pressure to keep the airway open during sleep. Rare patients with craniofacial abnormalities and OSA may need maxillofacial surgery. Oral appliances are used to expand the airway during sleep in certain cases.

Influencing circadian rhythms has a role in pediatric sleep medicine. Melatonin has been used in totally blind adults to entrain the free-running rhythm to the 24-hour environmental cycle, and research is underway to replicate this in children and adolescents. Melatonin also has been used successfully in treating irregular sleep–wake schedules in neurologically compromised patients. Melatonin appears to be generally well tolerated in this population although there are concerns for increasing seizure frequency in patients with epilepsy. DSPS can also be treated with a melatonin dose at bedtime. When recommending melatonin, one needs to keep in mind that it is not approved for sleep by the Federal Drug Administration (FDA), but instead is a nutritional supplement. There is a theoretical risk of exogenous melatonin impacting pubertal onset (postponing onset). Light therapy is also helpful in circadian rhythm disorders such as DSPS. The timing of light exposure is crucial. Light must be given in the morning after waking up in order to provide a corrective phase advance in DSPS. Depending on the season, natural light exposure can suffice, but often, especially in the winter at higher latitudes, artificial light is needed. Broad-spectrum light boxes which provide 2,500 to 10,000 lux of nonultraviolet light are preferred. Light exposure of 30 minutes is often enough in the morning.

There is minimal research data on the pharmacologic treatment of pediatric sleep disturbances even though these problems are common and impairing. Despite the paucity of research, medications are frequently recommended and prescribed. A survey of primary care pediatricians showed that 75% of practitioners had recommended nonprescription medications and 50% had prescribed a sleep medication. These medications were prescribed most often for acute pain, travel, and children with special needs (autism, ADHD, and mental retardation). Antihistamines were the most commonly recommended nonprescription medications followed by melatonin. Alpha-agonists such as clonidine were the most frequently prescribed medications. Other medications often prescribed include choral hydrate, benzodiazepines, tricyclic antidepressants, and trazodone. A more recent survey of child and adolescent psychiatrists reveals that prescription or nonprescription medications are frequently used to manage insomnia in the following disorders: primary insomnia, depression, bipolar disorder, anxiety, posttraumatic stress disorder (PTSD), DSPS, ADHD, autism spectrum disorder, chronic pain, oppositional disorder, and mental retardation/developmental delay.

Diphenhydramine, which is available over the counter, is the most popular antihistamine used to facilitate sleep in children. Although this commonly used medicine will shorten sleep latency, it often causes significant side effects such as dry mouth and morning sedation. Chloral hydrate is frequently used for sedation around procedures, but there are safety and tolerability concerns regarding its long-term use. The active metabolite of choral hydrate, trichoroethanol, has a long half-life leading to next-day sedation especially in infants and young children.

Melatonin is frequently recommended for the treatment of insomnia particularly sleep-onset insomnia. Although melatonin is a nutritional supplement and not a licensed drug (at least in the United States), there are more placebo-controlled trials using it to treat pediatric insomnia than licensed drugs. Melatonin has been found effective in treating insomnia in typically developing children, children with ADHD, and children with autism spectrum disorders.

Benzodiazepines have a role in treating severe parasomnias as they tend to decrease deep, slow-wave sleep. Clonazepam is the most frequently used and can be effective in very small doses (0.125 to 0.5 mg at bedtime). Trazodone, mirtazipine, and less commonly tricyclic antidepressants are used for insomnia associated with psychiatric disturbances such as depression and anxiety disorders. Trazodone, in particular, seems to be fairly well tolerated in the long term, at least anecdotally. Clonidine, an alpha2-adrenergic receptor agonist, has been prescribed for sleep disturbances associated with ADHD, PTSD, and neurological impairment. The potential risks far outweigh the benefits when considering use of an antipsychotic to treat insomnia not associated with psychosis.

The nonbenzodiazepine benzodiazepine receptor agonists include zolpidem and zaleplon. Zolpidem is available in an immediate-release formulation and a controlled-release formulation. These medications are FDA-approved for the treatment of insomnia in adults only. Although the FDA-approved indication is for short-term insomnia, these medicines are often used for long term in adults with chronic, severe insomnia. Eszopiclone is a racemic isomer of zopiclone, a sedative–hypnotic used for many years in Europe. Although the precise mechanism of action is not known, eszopiclone is suspected to work similarly to zolpidem and zaleplon. Zolpidem, zaleplon, and eszopiclone differ primarily in their half-lives. Zolpidem and zaleplon have very short half-lives, making them much less likely to cause daytime sedation. In comparison, eszopiclone has a longer half-life, but not so long as to cause next-day sedation. Eszopiclone is particularly helpful for sleep-maintenance insomnia. Although there is little to no published research on the use of these newer hypnotics in the treatment of pediatric insomnia, there is a role for their "off-label" use in certain cases of severe insomnia.

Ramelteon is a potent FDA-approved melatonin agonist used for the treatment of initial insomnia in adults. According to product labeling, reproductive development may be affected in adolescents or children taking ramelteon given the potential effect on the endocrine system. Ramelteon should not be prescribed to patients taking fluvoxamine since fluvoxamine is a major inhibitor of CYP1A2.

Sedative–hypnotics can cause significant side effects. In March 2007, the FDA requested that all manufacturers of sedative–hypnotic medications change their product labeling to include the risks of severe allergic reactions and complex sleep-related behaviors including sleep-driving sleep-eating. Children and adolescents may be particularly at risk for hypnagogic hallucinations if these medicines are dosed too early prior to bedtime.

There is more support for the use of medications to treat children and adolescents with narcolepsy. The treatment of narcolepsy is complicated and best left to a sleep specialist at least during the initiation phase. EDS can be treated with modafinil, a novel alerting agent, or stimulants such as methylphenidate. Cataplexy is treated with REM-suppressing medications such as protriptyline, fluoxetine, and venlafaxine. Sodium oxybate, also known as gamma

TABLE 20-5	Essentials of Treatment for Pediatric Sleep Disorders

- Refer suspected cases of OSAS and narcolepsy to a sleep center for further assessment with PSG and/or MSLT.
- The treatment of choice for OSAS is adenotonsillectomy. CPAP can be used if surgery is not possible or if OSAS persists after adenotonsillectomy.
- A follow-up polysomnogram should be done in any child continuing to have OSAS symptoms after adenotonsillectomy.
- Initiation of pharmacologic treatment of narcolepsy is best left to a sleep specialist or neurologist with experience in managing narcolepsy patients. Alerting medications such as modafinil and stimulants are useful for EDS; TCA's and SSRI's are helpful for cataplexy.
- DSPS is common and can be readily treated with chronotherapy, light therapy, and potentially melatonin as long as the patient is motivated.
- Educate parents and the youth on sleep needs and hygiene and refer them to appropriate sources of information (see Suggested Readings).
- Treat parasomnias with reassurance and safety measures, using benzodiazepines sparingly for severe, potentially dangerous cases.
- Behavioral interventions are the treatment of choice for young children with bedtime struggles and frequent awakenings. Resist using medications unless the child is neurodevelopmentally compromised and unresponsive to behavioral treatments.

OSAS, obstructive sleep apnea syndrome; PSG, polysomnography; MSLT, multiple sleep latency test; CPAP, continuous positive airway pressure; EDS, excessive daytime sleepiness; TCA, tricyclic antidepressant; SSRI, selective serotonin reuptake inhibitor; DSPS, delayed sleep phase syndrome.

hydroxybutyrate (GHB), is FDA-approved for the treatment of cataplexy and narcolepsy and EDS in patients older than 16, but due to its abuse potential (the "date rape drug"), it should be judiciously used with close monitoring.

If symptoms of RLS result in prolonged sleep onset or severe leg discomfort, treatment is indicated, but best under the guidance of a sleep physician. Caffeine, alcohol, and antihistamines are known to exacerbate RLS and should be avoided. Antidepressants, particularly the serotonin reuptake inhibitors, can also exacerbate RLS. Bupropion, however, does not cause RLS symptoms and is the preferred antidepressant to use when clinical depression is comorbid with RLS. Iron indices should be obtained since RLS can be exacerbated by iron deficiency even in the absence of anemia. A 2007 treatment survey given to members of the American Academy of Sleep Medicine Pediatric Section indicated that iron is the first-line treatment in children with RLS. The dopamine agonists, ropinerole or pramipexole, are FDA-approved for the treatment of RLS in adults. There are case reports of these medications being helpful in youth with RLS. Other treatment options include benzodiazepines, clonidine, gabapentin, and opiates. A summary of treatment essentials for pediatric sleep disorders is presented in Table 20-5.

Conclusions

In conclusion, pediatric sleep disorders are common and disabling. The majority of pediatric sleep disorders are behavioral in origin but medical conditions such as OSA and RLS must be considered in the differential diagnosis. One should consider sleep disorders when assessing a child or adolescent with psychiatric complaints since sleepiness often manifests as neurobehavioral problems. Most pediatric sleep disorders can be managed by primary care physicians, but some conditions may require consultation with a pediatric sleep specialist especially if sleep laboratory tests are needed.

CASE VIGNETTES

VIGNETTE 1: SCHOOL-AGED BOY WITH SLEEPINESS

Tommy was a 7-year-old boy referred to the sleep clinic for concerns regarding both excessive daytime sleepiness and hyperactivity. Although Tommy had not seen his pediatrician for many years due to loss of health insurance, he had a recent well child check at which his parents reported worsening of his loud snoring, which had been occurring nightly since age two. Often he would stop breathing briefly in his sleep, which his parents attributed to his asthma. He would breathe primarily through his mouth both night and day. He would often wake with a dry mouth and occasional headaches. In bed he was very restless and would drench the sheets with sweat. Adding to his parent's concern, he was incredibly difficult to wake in the morning. Often it would take his mother 2 hours to get him out of bed, resulting in 10 days of missed school. He had trouble with enuresis and currently his parents have to wake him twice nightly to use the bathroom, otherwise he will wet the bed.

His second-grade teacher has witnessed him napping during class several times. His grades have fallen since last year. Tommy reports that often his legs feel jumpy, and that he has to move them, sometimes while trying to get to sleep and in the afternoons. Past medical history is significant for asthma.

His father snores nightly with pauses in his breathing, but has had no evaluation. His father believes he has restless legs syndrome, but his symptoms are mild.

Physical exam reveals an obese child (BMI greater than 95%) with a large neck. His tonsils were enlarged with a large overbite. A 16-channel overnight polysomnogram was preformed with the mother present for the study. Objective evidence from this sleep study supported the diagnosis of OSA. The child averaged three obstructive apneas and five hypopneas (partial airflow limitation) per hour of sleep. These events occurred primarily in REM sleep. Sleep efficiency was low for his age and cyclic oxygen desaturations and arousals were noted in REM sleep.

On recommendation of the sleep specialist, the child was referred to a pediatric otolaryngologist who performed an adenotonsillectomy. After recovery from the procedure there was resolution of snoring and witnessed apnea. Tommy no longer had morning struggles, and stopped missing school. His grades and attention improved. His parents are monitoring for symptoms of restless legs syndrome by keeping a diary of growing pains and urge to move his legs close to bedtime. In addition, his parents were encouraged to increase his activity and improve his eating habits to achieve a more healthy weight. They were told that although his sleep apnea had resolved with surgery, he remains at risk for recurrent obstructive sleep apnea in adolescence especially if significant weight is gained.

VIGNETTE 2: TODDLER WITH MULTIPLE NIGHT AWAKENINGS

Sydney is a 2-year-old healthy female referred to the sleep clinic by her pediatrician after six months of intense bedtime struggles. As an only child, Sydney has been rocked to sleep since birth. This never presented problems for parents, as they enjoyed the bedtime interaction. She has been unable to fall asleep at night and at naps without the presence of her mother rocking her to sleep. For the last year, Sydney had 1–3 awakenings per night, but was able to be rocked back to sleep quickly by her mother, not causing much family disruption.

Things worsened tremendously 6 months ago with the birth of her brother and the start of daycare. Sydney falls asleep easily at bedtime if she is rocked, but has had up to ten awakenings every night, yelling for her parents. Often the awakenings have disturbed her baby brother. She has not been able to nap at daycare. There have been no new illnesses. Growth and development have been normal. In fact, Sydney is an incredibly bright girl that often challenges her parents with her stubbornness.

A detailed sleep history was obtained by the sleep specialist. Bedtime routines, nap routines, bedroom environment, history of snoring, labored breathing, sleeping in strange positions, history of parasomnias, symptoms of daytime sleepiness were assessed. The remainder of the sleep history was normal, except for Sydney's need to be rocked to sleep and increased perceived daytime tiredness by parents.

The sleep specialist diagnosed Sydney with behavioral insomnia of childhood, sleep-onset association type. During the physiologically normal 3 to 5 awakenings in the middle of the night, Syndey is unable to fall back asleep without the presence of her mother, causing disrupted sleep and daytime consequences. There was no indication on history of sleep disordered breathing or movement disorder during sleep and thus a polysomnogram was not indicated.

Education was given to Sydney's parents regarding the normalcy of her nighttime awakenings. Her mother was interested in helping Sydney to learn self-soothing skills which would assist her in returning to sleep after a natural awakening. Parents were very motivated to change and embarked on a behavioral treatment program.

A timeline was implemented with agreed upon goals by both parents. A fun and soothing bedtime routine was recommended. The end of the routine would be to place Sydney in the crib drowsy but awake. Use of a transitional object was recommended.

Focus on bedtime sleep initiation without rocking was prioritized. If Sydney was unable to fall asleep and was crying for her mother, her mother would go into Sydney's room to briefly check on her. Her mother felt that she could listen to Sydney crying for 6 minutes without responding. After six minutes she was to go into her room and calmly say, "I love you, time to go to sleep." She would repeat this checking routine until Sydney was asleep. Parents were warned that the behavior may worsen prior to improving (extinction burst). Parents were counseled to continue middle of the night rocking to sleep until Sydney was able to fall asleep easily on her own at bedtime. Sydney was rewarded in the morning with stickers if she was able to sleep through the night.

After a 2-week follow-up, Sydney was doing much better. It took 3 days of up to 2 hours of crying for Sydney to fall asleep on her own without her mother rocking her. Her signaling for parents diminished to once per night. Parents felt her daytime behavior was much improved with less tantrums. They were encouraged to continue the bedtime routine and to not respond to nighttime awakenings. Upon follow-up after 1 month, Sydney was falling asleep on her own with no signaling for parents during the night. Parents continued to use a sticker chart and positive praise. Sydney takes her stuffed bear to daycare with her to help her fall asleep. They are hopeful that they will be able to implement more healthy sleep habits with their 3-month-old son.

BIBLIOGRAPHY

American Academy of Sleep Medicine. *ICSD-2—The International Classification of Sleep Disorders, 2nd ed.: Diagnostic and Coding Manual.* Westchester, IL: American Academy of Sleep Medicine; 2007.

American Academy of Pediatrics, Section on Pediatric Pulmonology, Subcommittee on Obstructive Sleep Apnea Syndrome. Technical Report: Diagnosis and Management of Childhood Obstructive Sleep Apnea Syndrome. *Pediatrics.* 2002;109:e69–e69. See http://pediatrics.aappublications.org/cgi/content/abstract/109/4/e69

Carskadon MA. *Adolescent Sleep Patterns: Biological, Social, and Psychological Influences.* Cambridge: Cambridge University Press; 2002.

Chervin RD, Hedger K, Dillon JE, et al. Pediatric sleep questionnaire (PSQ): validity and reliability of scales for sleep-disordered breathing, snoring, sleepiness, and behavioral problems. *Sleep Med.* 2000;1:21–32.

Garcia J, Rosen G, Mahowald M. Circadian rhythms and circadian rhythm disorders in children and adolescents. *Semin Pediatr Neurol.* 2001;8:229–240.

Garstang J, Wallis M. Randomized controlled trial of melatonin for children with autistic spectrum disorders and sleep problems. *Child: Care, Health Dev.* 2006;32(5):585–589.

Gaylor EE, Goodlin-Jones BL, Anders TF. Classification of young children's sleep problems: a pilot study. *J Am Acad Child Adolesc Psychiatry.* 2001;40:61–67.

Guilleminault C, Pelayo R. Narcolepsy in children: a practical guide to its diagnosis, treatment and follow-up. *Pediatr Drugs.* 2000;2:1–9.

Halbower AC, Ishman SL, McGinley BM. Childhood obstructive sleep-disordered breathing: a clinical update and discussion of technological innovations and challenges. *Chest.* 2007;132:2030–2041.

Ivanenko A, Tauman R, Gozal D. Modafinil in the treatment of excessive daytime sleepiness in children. *Sleep Med.* 2003;4:579–582.

Jan JE, Wasdell MB, Reiter RJ, et al. Melatonin therapy of pediatric sleep disorders: recent advances, why it works, who are the candidates and how to treat. *Curr Pediatr Rev.* 2007;3:214–224.

Johnson KP, Malow BA. Sleep in children with autism spectrum disorders. *Curr Neurology Neurosci Rep.* 2008;8:155–161.

Konofal E, Arnulf I, Lecendreux M, et al. Ropinirole in a child with attention-deficit hyperactivity disorder and restless legs syndrome. *Pediatr Neurol.* 2005;32:350–351.

Konofal E, Cortese S, Marchand M, et al. Impact of restless legs syndrome and iron deficiency on attention-deficit/hyperactivity disorder in children. *Sleep Med.* 2007;8(7–8):711–715.

Kuhn BR, Elliott AJ. Treatment efficacy in behavioral pediatric sleep medicine. *J Psychosomatic Res.* 2003;54:587–597.

Mindell JA, Emslie G, Blumer J, et al. Pharmacologic management of insomnia in children and adolescents: consensus statement. *Pediatrics.* 2006;117:e1223–e1232.

Mindell JA, Owens JA. *A Clinical Guide to Pediatric Sleep: Diagnosis and Management of Sleep Problems.* Philadelphia, PA: Lippincott Williams & Wilkins; 2003.

Mitchell, RB. Adenotonsillectomy for obstructive sleep apnea in children: outcome evaluated by pre- and postoperative polysomnography. *Laryngoscope.* 2007;117:1844–1854.

Murali H, Kotagal S. Off-label treatment of severe childhood narcolepsy-cataplexy with sodium oxybate. *Sleep.* 2006;29:1025–1029.

O'Brien LM, Holbrook CR, Mervis CB, et al. Sleep and neurobehavioral characteristics of 5- to 7-year-old children with parentally reported symptoms of attention-deficit/hyperactivity disorder. *Pediatrics.* 2003;111:554–563.

Owens JA, Rosen CL, Mindell JA. Medication use in the treatment of pediatric insomnia: results of a survey of community-based pediatricians. *Pediatrics.* 2003; 111:e628–e635.

Owens JA, Spirito A, McGuinn M. The Children's Sleep Habits Questionnaire (CSHQ): psychometric properties of a survey instrument for school-aged children. *Sleep.* 2000;23:1043–1051.

Picchietti DL, Allen RP. Restless legs syndrome: prevalence and impact in children and adolescents—The peds rest study. *Pediatrics.* 2007;120:253–266.

Reed MD, Findling RL. Overview of current management of sleep disturbances in children: pharmacotherapy. *Current Ther Res: Clin Exper.* 2002;63:B18–B37.

Rosen CL, Owens JA, Mindell JA, et al. Use of pharmacotherapy for insomnia in children and adolescents: a national survey of child psychiatrists. *Sleep.* 2005;28 (abstract supplement):A79–79. Available at http://www.journalsleep.org/PDF/AbstractBook2005.pdf

Sheldon SH, Ferber R, Kryger MH. *Principles and Practice of Pediatric Sleep Medicine.* Elsevier Saunders; Philadelphia, PA; 2005.

Smits MG, van Stel HF, van der Heijden K, et al. Melatonin improves health status and sleep in children with idiopathic chronic sleep-onset insomnia: a randomized placebo-controlled trial. *J Am Acad Child Adolesc Psychiatry.* 2003;42:1286–1293.

Szeinberg A, Borodkin K, Dagan Y. Melatonin treatment in adolescents with delayed sleep phase syndrome. *Clin Pediatrics.* 2006;45:809–818.

Weiss MD, Wasdell MB, Bomben MM, et al. Sleep hygiene and melatonin treatment for children and adolescents with ADHD and initial insomnia. *J Am Acad Child Adolesc Psychiatry.* 2006;45:512–519.

Wills L, Garcia J. Parasomnias: epidemiology and management. *CNS Drugs.* 2002;16:803–810.

Wolfson AR, Carskadon MA. Sleep schedules and daytime functioning in adolescents. *Child Dev.* 1998;69:875–887.

SUGGESTED READINGS

Sleeping Through the Night, Revised Edition: How Infants, Toddlers, and Their Parents Can Get a Good Night's Sleep
Author: Jodi A. Mindell, PhD
Publisher: Collins Living, 2005

Solve Your Child's Sleep Problems: New, Revised, and Expanded Edition
Author: Richard Ferber, MD
Publisher: Fireside, 2006

Take Charge of Your Child's Sleep: The All-in-One Resource for Solving Sleep Problems in Kids and Teens
Authors: Judith A. Owens, MD, and Jodi A.Mindell, PhD
Publisher: Da Capo Press, 2005

A Clinical Guide to Pediatric Sleep: Diagnosis and Management of Sleep Problems, Second Edition
Authors: Jodi A. Mindell, PhD, and Judith A. Owens, MD
Publisher: Lippincott Williams & Wilkins, 2010
(Practical review of pediatric sleep disorders for clinicians. Includes online access to excellent handouts and
    questionnaires).

Clinician's Guide to Pediatric Sleep Disorders
Editors: Mark Richardson, Norman Friedman
Publisher: Informa Healthcare, 2007

Sleep and Psychiatric Disorders in Children and Adolescents
Editor: Anna Ivanenko, MD
Publisher: Informa Healthcare, 2008

SUGGESTED WEBSITES

http://www.sleepfoundation.org/ Home of the National Sleep Foundation. Excellent resource for parents and clinicians.
http://www.sleepforkids.org/ Specific pediatric content from the National Sleep Foundation directed at parents,
    teachers and kids.
http://www.sleepeducation.com/ Content from the American Academy of Sleep Medicine for patients.

REVIEW QUESTIONS

1. In school age children obstructive sleep apnea is MOST often manifested by
    a. Daytime sleepiness
    b. Hyperactivity, often overlapping with symptoms of ADHD
    c. Morning struggles with difficulties waking from sleep
    d. Both B and C

2. Delayed sleep phase syndrome in teenagers:
    a. Diagnosis requires an overnight polysomnogram
    b. Is often mistaken for depression or adolescent delinquency causing conflicts at
        home and school
    c. Excessive daytime sleepiness resolves if patient is allowed to sleep preferred schedule
    d. Rarely occurs in the general population
    e. Both B and C

3. Signs and symptoms of obstructive sleep apnea in children include all of the following except:
    a. Snoring, pauses of breathing during sleep
    b. Excessive sweating during sleep
    c. Wheezing at night
    d. Enuresis
    e. Morning headaches

4. Restless leg syndrome in children:
    a. Needs a polysomnogram for diagnosis
    b. Often has a strong family history

   c. Can cause occasional fevers
   d. Is exacerbated by sugary foods

5. The most common cause of excessive daytime sleepiness in adolescents is:
   a. Obstructive sleep apnea
   b. Narcolepsy
   c. Inadequate amounts of sleep
   d. Delayed sleep phase syndrome

Answers: 1-d, 2-e, 3-c, 4-b, 5-c

CHAPTER

21

Kelly Schloredt, PhD,
Cynthia Flynn, PhD,
Brent Collett, PhD,
and Kathleen Myers, MD, MPH, MS

Suicidality and Youth: Identification, Treatment, and Prevention

Introduction

Adolescents face many developmental challenges academically, socially, and within their families. The large majority of youth handle this developmental period without major difficulty. However, this is also the time when rates of depression and suicide begin to increase. Youth suicidality has become a public health concern. Whether suicidal youth are encountered in the office with depressed mood and passive suicidal ideation or in the emergency department (ED) after an attempt, clinicians are faced with difficult decisions regarding their care. Not only must clinicians decipher when to recommend hospitalization, but they must also determine how best to facilitate outpatient treatment and, in some cases, figure out how to manage recurrent suicide attempts and begin to ameliorate the social chaos that often surrounds suicidal youth. These decisions are taxing under the best circumstances for even the most experienced clinicians. All too often, however, clinicians find themselves with limited time, limited training in mental health in general, and/or limited experience with youth.

This chapter reviews the salient features of child and adolescent suicidality that primary care physicians, general psychiatrists, and other primary clinicians must consider as they are the front-line clinicians encountering youth at risk. Emphasis is on delineating an approach to the assessment of suicidality and disposition of suicidal youth from the primary clinician's office to other services. The literature on the management and treatment of suicidal youth is reviewed.

Classification of Suicidal Behaviors and Methods

Historically, there has been some debate as to how best to define and classify a range of behaviors on the suicide spectrum. Some authors draw parallels between suicide and self-injury enacted without the intent to die, referring to these nonlethal behaviors as "parasuicide" or "suicidal gestures." Understanding these phenomena is important, as a subset of youth use self-injury to manage negative affect and communicate their distress to significant others, and studies estimate that 50% to 75% of teens who engage in nonsuicidal self-injurious behavior have also made at least one prior suicide attempt. These issues are complex and the subject of much investigation. In the current chapter, suicidality includes *preoccupations and overt behaviors enacted with the intent to cause one's own death*. Although the intent to die is an essential element of this definition, it is important to note that children and developmentally delayed youth may not have a mature concept of the finality of death or an accurate assessment of the lethality of their behavior. If youth expect that their behavior will bring about death, then that behavior should be considered a suicidal act, even if of low lethality. The main "differential" will be self-injurious and high-risk behaviors without the intent to die. Such nonlethal behaviors are a concern in that they cause suffering and have an association with suicidality, but require different interventions.

Youth with emerging personality disturbance, highly dysregulated affect, and dissociative features often engage in self-injurious behaviors, such as cutting or burning, in an effort to manage negative affect and communicate distress to others without an intent to die. They may report a sense of relief upon such injury or may acknowledge that they wanted to "get back at" a significant other for a perceived transgression. Self-injurious behaviors without suicidal intent are more likely to be repetitive, with multiple injuries over relatively short periods of time.

High-risk behaviors such as reckless driving, frequent accidents, and running in front of vehicles must be differentiated from suicide attempts. There is some suggestion that suicidal individuals engage in endangering behavior, even at a very young age. Youth with disruptive behavior disorders put themselves in harm's way, either without consideration of the consequences or with the assumption that nothing bad will happen to them, such as driving fast, provoking police, or binging on drugs or alcohol. Open-ended questioning about such youth's assumptions regarding their intent and the expected outcome of their behavior helps to differentiate suicide from reckless behavior.

Epidemiology of Youth Suicidality

Rates of Suicidality

Suicidal ideation and nonlethal attempts are a major concern for youth at all ages. In the Methods for the Epidemiology of Child and Adolescent Mental Disorders (MECA) study of 9- to 17-year-olds, 5.2% of youth reported suicidal ideation and 3.3% reported having attempted suicide. Data from the 2007 Youth Risk Behavior Surveillance—United States report show that in the 12 months prior to the survey, 14.5% of youth had seriously considered suicide, 11.3% of youth had made a plan about how they would attempt suicide, and 6.9% had made one or more attempts—2% of which required treatment. Across studies, annual rates of suicide attempts range from 1.7% to 8.3%, and rates of suicide attempt over the lifetime range from 7% to 9.7%.

Overall, each year in the United States, 2 million adolescents attempt suicide, but only 25% ever come to medical attention, suggesting that many of these youths are missed by current systems of care. The risk of recurrent suicide attempts is high. Among youth hospitalized for suicidality, 18% attempt to kill themselves again within 6 months of discharge and 42% reattempt within 44 months. Similarly, in community samples of youth with prior suicide attempts, 25% will reattempt suicide within 3 months after an initial attempt. Finally, postmortem data suggest that 10% to 46% of youths who eventually complete suicide had prior suicidal behaviors.

Over the past several years, data collected by the Centers for Disease Control and Prevention (CDC) show that suicide has accounted for the death of nearly 2000 youth (ages 5 to 19) each year. While these data show that the rates of suicide climbed steadily through 1988, peaking at a rate of 4.36 per 100,000, this number decreased by 35% and reached a low of 2.83 per 100,000 in 2003. Since then, however, youth suicide rates in 2004 and 2005 were higher by 12.4% and 7.8%, respectively, and there has been concern that the rate may again be on the rise in the United States. While it is difficult to know the reasons, one hypothesis has been that the decreased use of antidepressants following the black box warning from the Federal Drug Administration (FDA) in 2004 left depressed youth untreated. This issue of how antidepressants both treat depression and precipitate de novo suicidality continues to be debated and investigated.

Overall, these findings indicate that suicidality is a recurrent phenomenon and increases in severity over time and with age. These findings further suggest the importance of talking with all youth about previous suicidality. This is of utmost importance as such a history may not be known to caregivers who generally tend to be unaware of their children's subjective distress.

Methods

Data from the CDC show that the use of firearms, suffocation (mostly hanging), and poisoning have been the three most common methods by which youth commit suicide. Since the early 1990s, however, there have been some changing trends in youth suicide methods. More specifically, between 1992 and 2001, rates of youth suicide by firearm and poisoning decreased, while that by suffocation increased. Although firearms continue to be the most predominant method of suicide for older adolescents (15 to 19 years), suffocation has eclipsed firearms as the predominant method of suicide among younger adolescents (10 to 14 years).

Firearms are the most lethal method of suicide attempt, being 200 times more likely to result in death than other methods, and currently account for approximately 46% of completed youth suicides. Youth in rural areas, where guns are readily available, are particularly vulnerable. The proportion of suicide victims who have detectable blood alcohol levels has also risen dramatically. Youth who use firearms to kill themselves are more likely to have been drinking than those who choose other methods. Thus, alcohol combined with access to firearms comprises a highly dangerous situation that differentiates completed suicides from serious suicide attempts.

Suffocation, mostly hanging, accounts for 39% of the suicides by youth 10 to 24 years old. Children, in particular, are much more likely to use suffocation. Poisoning is the third most common method of youth suicide, accounting for about 8% of completed suicides. Many families are not aware of the dangers of many medications, particularly common analgesics, such as acetaminophen and aspirin, which are often purchased in bulk through warehouse stores. Youth, then, may have easy access to large quantities of lethal medicines that are innocently stored in the family medicine cabinet and that often prove lethal when used in a suicide attempt. Likewise, youth who are allowed to take their medications without supervision have easy access to means by which to attempt suicide. Generally, the method chosen varies by sex, age, and opportunity. Girls favor poisonings, while boys and older attempters choose more lethal means, such as firearms and suffocation. Also, a suicide attempt by unusual methods and medically serious attempts are predictive of further suicide attempts, as well as of eventual completed suicide.

Etiology and Risk Factors

The etiology of youth suicide is unknown. It appears that there are several pathways to this outcome and that a multitude of risks may play a role leading to this tragedy. Risk factors appear to be cumulative; that is, the number of risk factors, as well as the severity and acuity of individual risks, is important in predicting suicide. Common risk factors are outlined in Table 21-1.

Demographics

Age

Youth suicide rates increase with age. According to the CDC, suicide is rare among children (0.01 per 100,000 between the ages 5 and 9), but increases dramatically during the preadolescent and adolescent years (1.3 per 100,000 in youth between the ages of 10 and 14, and 7.67 per 100,000 in teens between 15 and 19 years). There are two predominant theories for this rise with age. First, it has been suggested that the lower rate of suicide among preadolescents is due to their cognitive immaturity and inability to successfully plan and execute a lethal suicide attempt, despite a desire to do so. A second explanation centers on increasing risk factors in adolescence, such as psychiatric and substance-use disorders, which

TABLE 21-1	Essential Risk Factors for Suicidality

- **History of suicidality (past attempts predict future suicidality)**
- **Lethality of suicide attempt/medical compromise (intent)**
- **Access to means (decreased time to consider options)**
  - Firearms, especially in rural areas
  - Other highly lethal means
  - Inadequate supervision
- **Demographics**
  - Age
  - Race/ethnicity
  - Sexual orientation
  - Religion
- **Psychopathology (fuels suicidality)**
  - Major depression
  - Bipolar disorder, depressed or manic phase
  - Psychosis
  - Substance abuse, especially alcohol
  - Conduct disorder, especially impulsive/aggressive
- **Personality traits and individual risks (act on suicidal thoughts)**
  - Impulsivity
  - Anger/hostility/aggressiveness
  - Attributional style
  - Hopelessness
  - Cognitive inflexibility (black and white thinking)
  - Interpersonal problem-solving

- **Environmental stressors**
  - Child maltreatment
  - Family dysfunction/poor parent–child communication
    - Parental suicidality
    - Parental mood disorders
    - Parental substance abuse
    - Family conflict and communication
  - Interpersonal problems/loss events
    - Loss events: parents, peers, romantic, prestige
  - Acute stressors
    - Disciplinary crises
    - Legal involvement
    - Incarceration
    - Academic difficulties

Note: Risk factors are cumulative in predicting suicide. Severity of risk factors is important in predicting suicide, especially severe acute stressors.

independently increase the risk of suicide. It is likely that both of these issues contribute to the rise of suicide with age.

Gender

It is estimated that in the average US high school classroom, approximately 1 male and 2 females have attempted suicide within the past year. It has long been established that while females are more likely to attempt suicide, males are more likely to succeed. More specifically, between 1.5% and 10.1% of females make a suicide attempt in their lifetime, compared to 1.3% to 3.8% of males. However, boys are about four times more likely to die by suicide. In fact, the increased rate of adolescent suicides from the 1950s to the 1990s predominantly reflected boys' choice of more lethal methods and girls' choice of nonlethal methods. For both males and females, a prior suicide attempt is predictive of later completed suicide. While a previous suicide attempt is the most potent predictor of eventual suicide for boys, the most potent risk factor for girls is depression followed by a previous suicide attempt.

Race and Ethnicity

Data from the CDC Web-based Injury Statistics Query and Reporting System (WISQARS) database show that while completed suicide in children between the ages of 5 and 9 is rare across all racial groups, differences begin to emerge among youth aged 10 to 14 and 15 to 19 years. Between 1999 and 2005, suicide in 10- to 14-years-olds was most prevalent among American Indian/Alaska natives, followed by White youth, Black youth, and Asian/Pacific Islander youth. In 15- to 19-year-olds, racial differences in suicide rates are much more pronounced. Among males 15 to 19 years old, American Indians have the highest rate (26.64 per 100,000), followed by Whites (13.48 per 100,000), Blacks (7.80 per 100,000), and Asian/Pacific Islanders (6.75 per 100,000). In females, the racial trends are similar, but less dramatic, for both American Indians (9.40 per 100,000) and Whites (3.00 per 100,000). Suicide among Asian/Pacific Islander females between the ages of 15 and 19 (2.76 per 100,000) is somewhat more common than in Black females (1.38 per 100,000). These data are not well understood. Although there is great variability among Native American and Alaska Native tribes, rates appear highest within tribes that have experienced erosion of traditional culture and that have high rates of delinquency, alcoholism, and family disorganization. As African American suicide victims tend to be from families of upper socioeconomic status (SES), it has been hypothesized that greater educational and employment achievement has led to identification with the majority White culture, along with the erosion of some traditional protective values. Although the overall rates of suicide are lower among Hispanic youth, suicide is, nevertheless, the third leading cause of death, and appears to be growing, with firearms, suffocation, and poisoning being the most common methods. More specifically, Hispanics in grades 9 to 12, particularly females, report more hopelessness, sadness, and suicidal ideation and attempts than non-Hispanic White and non-Hispanic Black youth. Hypothesized risk factors for this group include mental illness, substance use, acculturative stress, family issues, and low SES.

Sexual Orientation

The rate of completed suicide for gay, lesbian, and bisexual youth is comparable to heterosexual youth. It should be noted, however, that these youth are thought to be more than twice as likely to attempt suicide than their heterosexual peers. Their heightened risk for depression and suicide is hypothesized to result from the additional stress of managing the stigma of "coming out" and developing an identity as a gay man or lesbian woman.

Religion

Religion seems to have a protective effect and reduces the risk for suicidality. This may be due to religious proscriptions against suicide, community involvement, and other beneficial effects of spirituality. However, the precise mechanism is difficult to establish, as religion is often confounded with reductions in other risks, such as substance abuse and parental divorce, precluding firm conclusions.

Psychopathology

As noted earlier in the text, most suicidal youth have a major psychiatric disorder regardless of the severity of suicidality. Risk for suicide is estimated to increase 35-fold in the face of psychiatric disorder and, with each psychiatric comorbidity, the likelihood of a suicide attempt increases by nearly 250%. It has been suggested that most psychiatric disorders are associated with an increased risk of suicide attempts, although the nature of this association changes during the course of development. For example, an association between suicide and some disorders (e.g., major depression, substance-use disorders, and attention-deficit hyperactivity disorder [ADHD]) becomes more robust as youth move into young adulthood, while the association with other disorders (e.g., conduct disorder and panic disorder) is attenuated.

As major depression and other depressive disorders are most commonly associated with suicidality in youth, there has been some suggestion that suicidality may represent a severe variant of depression rather than a separate construct. In general, any form of psychopathology that is associated with high levels of emotional reactivity and low levels of inhibition, and interferes with self-regulation, judgment, and perception, confers risk for suicide in youth. In addition to depressive disorders, examples would include behavioral disorders, substance-use disorders, psychosis, and borderline personality disorder. Conduct disorder, in particular, places youth at risk due to impulsivity, low threshold for violent behavior, and poor judgment that accompanies this disorder. Additionally, youth with conduct disorder face recurrent stressors in the form of disciplinary crises, legal difficulties, peer problems, and social alienation. It can also be speculated that youth with conduct disorders may be more likely to use drugs and alcohol and may more readily have access to lethal weapons by virtue of the company they tend to keep.

While psychopathology places youth at increased risk for suicide, it should be noted that there are instances of suicide in which the behavior appeared to come "out of the blue" and a psychological autopsy does not reveal any significant psychopathology.

Personal Skills/Resources Deficits

To varying degrees, personal skills and resources, such as problem-solving ability and social effectiveness, can mitigate risk, whereas skills deficits and lack of personal resources, such as impulsivity, anger, aggressiveness, cognitive inflexibility, attributional style, hopelessness, and poor interpersonal problem-solving, have been found to be related to suicidality. In general, these factors are less well understood in youth than in adults, but data exist. *Impulsive* youth are at increased risk as they do not think through the repercussions of their behavior. They may hastily engage in high-risk behaviors, failing to recognize the consequences of their actions.

The association of suicidal behaviors with elevated levels of anger, hostility, and aggression supports the role of abnormal serotonergic function. *Attributional style* refers to individual's approach to explaining life events. A negative attributional style is characterized by a tendency to attribute negative events as due to factors that are internal, stable, and global. This pattern has been associated with depression, as well as suicidality. *Hopelessness* is related to attributional style, and refers to pessimism about the future. Although hopelessness has been associated with suicide, in youth it is unclear whether hopelessness provides a unique role in predicting suicide. Youth who are hopeless, however, also often struggle with *cognitive inflexibility* and struggle with "black and white" thinking. The inability to see the shades of gray in a situation can lead suicidal youth to believe that their current situation and psychological pain will never improve, and as such, can lend itself to hasty decision-making in the face of high levels of stress and agitation. *Poor interpersonal problem-solving* is also commonly observed among suicidal youth who appear to generate fewer approaches to problems. These deficits discriminate suicidal youth from their peers even after controlling for depression. Such deficits likely prevent these youth from accessing social supports from peers during times of stress. These deficits in personal skills or resources can be considered liabilities that are expressed during times of stress when a youth's coping resources are tested, rather than considered the primary force driving suicidality.

Environmental Stressors

Debate continues over the relative importance of psychosocial stressors in explaining suicidal behavior. Overall, there appears to be a unique role for selective life stressors, such as child maltreatment, family dysfunction, and poor parent–child communication, interpersonal problems and losses, school problems, and legal or disciplinary crises, in accounting for suicidal behavior. The relative contribution of these stressors may even be comparable to that of primary psychopathology. In particular, legal and disciplinary crises provide additional predictive value in the assessment of suicide risk after controlling for the presence of psychiatric disorders.

Maltreatment, both sexual and physical, is associated with the development of depression and suicidality. Sexual abuse appears to be especially prevalent among suicide attempters, and increases the risk of repeated suicide attempts up to eightfold, independently of associated factors such as depression or the contextual factors under which the abuse occurred. Physical abuse also contributes to repeated attempts. A 17-year longitudinal study found that maladaptive parenting and maltreatment lead to profound interpersonal difficulties in middle adolescence. In turn, these difficulties mediate the association between maladaptive parenting and suicidality in later adolescence. Youth experiencing such adverse experiences may have difficulties in developing skills that are essential for maintaining healthy relationships with both adults and peers when under stress. Perhaps such adverse experiences also account for the tendency of suicidal youths to engage in other risky behaviors.

Even in the absence of overt maltreatment, family dysfunction, and poor parent–child communication have consistently been identified as salient factors for young suicide attempters and completers. Specific risks include lack of an intact family, depressed mothers, fathers with legal difficulties, and a family history of suicidal behavior. In addition, families of suicidal youth have been described as less supportive, with more conflict and poor communication. Children in such families may also lack supervision. Likewise, suicidal adolescents have described their families as experiencing difficulties in adapting to change, problem-solving, and being prone to crises, with ineffective communication and more power struggles. Although some suicidal teens perceive their families as emotionally disengaged, others perceive them as enmeshed.

Another family issue relates to the risk conferred by a family history of suicidality. However, it is difficult to disentangle the relative contributions of genetic mechanisms from social factors associated with having a psychiatrically ill parent. Overall, studies suggest that suicidality is heritable and runs in families. Postmortem studies with adults have suggested a role for decreased functioning of central serotonin.

Interpersonal problems with peers have long been identified as precipitants to suicidal behaviors. In particular, conflicts with and separations from a romantic relationship play an important role as precipitants to both attempted and completed suicide. More generalized social alienation also appears to pose substantial risk. Such youngsters may give the impression of "drifting," without affiliation with a school, community, or work institution. Comment is needed regarding ecological precipitants to suicidality. Studies of suicide "contagion" among high school students suggest that students with current major depression or past depression and suicidality may be the most likely to become suicidal subsequent to a peer's suicide, regardless of the closeness of the relationship to the suicide victim. Furthermore, students who are close friends of a suicide victim may become suicidal at a lower threshold of psychopathology.

Finally, the directionality of risks and suicidality is not always clear. Stressors leading to suicidality may be normative outcomes of uncontrollable events, such as a death in the family. Alternatively, such stressors may ensue from the underlying mental disorder, for example, legal crises for conduct-disordered youth. The important issue is that the youth with a mental disorder may face greater numbers of stressful events, or may perceive such events as more stressful.

Assessment

The importance of the front-line clinician in assessing and preventing suicide is suggested by three factors. First, only a minority of suicidal youth will access mental health treatment and, of those who are referred for such care, many may not receive effective treatments or may drop out of treatment prematurely only to resurface during crises. Second, many suicidal youth seek medical attention for factors unrelated to suicidality in the months prior to an attempt. Third, front-line clinicians usually have contact with a child and family members over a prolonged period and can, therefore, monitor behavioral and environmental changes that may suggest a youth is at risk. The essential aspects of assessment of suicidal youth lie with the interview.

Interviewing about Suicidality

A critical part of any assessment of suicidality includes an interview with the youth and a care-giver. Caregivers usually are able to report a history of depression or disruptive behaviors, but may not be aware of their child's suicidality or even of prior attempts. Caregivers may not be aware that a child has been depressed. In addition, youth can reveal sources of stress that their parents are unaware of or are reluctant to report themselves, such as abuse, domestic violence, or parental psychopathology. Thus, it is critical to conduct an interview with the youth alone.

Interviewing the Youth

Clinicians may be hesitant to initiate a candid interview about suicidality due to fears that they will encourage or increase suicidal ideation or behavior. To the contrary, it can be helpful to provide a safe environment to discuss these feelings with an adult who can assist in accessing resources for help. It is important to conduct the interview matter-of-factly while communi-cating confidence that help can be obtained. Promises of confidentiality should be avoided. Youth can be reassured that some details may be kept confidential; however, they should be aware that some information may need to be shared with their parents/caregivers and other providers in order to provide for their safety. In general, information directly related to risk for suicidal behavior and appropriate supervision and treatment will need to be shared.

When interviewing youth, questions should be posed in a developmentally appropriate manner that assesses the severity of ideation, intent, and plan. It is most effective to begin with broad, open-ended questions (e.g., "It sounds like you have been feeling really sad lately, how bad has it gotten?") and then follow-up with probes to assess specific risk factors for suicidal behavior, such as thoughts about death and dying, frequency and intensity of suicidal ideation, level of intent to harm one's self, and whether or not the child has developed a plan for how to commit suicide or has made any prior attempts. Attention should be given to the specificity, lethality, and anticipated outcomes that the child associates with a suicide attempt. It is also important to ask about associated risks such as current stressors, level of agitation, perceptions of social support, and reasons for living and dying. Inquiry about a child's reasons for *not* com-mitting suicide can reveal potential protective factors. For some, these reasons may include re-ligious proscriptions, fear of pain, knowledge of the emotional pain inflicted on loved ones, or awareness of missing an event in life. These steps may provide a brief therapeutic intervention by making suicide seem a less viable "solution" to life's problems, and by instilling hope.

Interviewing the Parent(s)

Parents may be better reporters of their child's externalizing behaviors and can clarify the child's impulsivity and judgment. Young children, in particular, often have difficulty reporting the course of their symptoms and identifying the relationship between precipitants and the onset of their suicidality. An interview with parents also serves a preventive role, as clinicians can provide information regarding risks for parents to monitor and review proactive steps such as limiting access to means for suicide and providing supervision. Interviewing other adults, such as teachers and counselors, also can elucidate precipitants as well as sources of monitoring.

In sum, the clinician should ascertain the nature, intensity, and frequency of suicidal thoughts, seriousness of intent, plans for committing suicide, history of prior attempts, and level of lethality of past attempts and current plans. This information should be accompanied by assessment of current stressors and perceptions of reasons not to engage in suicidal behav-ior. Assessment for underlying psychopathology should focus on mood lability and emotional dysregulation, inappropriate affect, cognitive distortions, lack of insight and poor judgment, impulsivity, and substance use. Caregivers and other adults should be accessed for contextual information and their assessment of the child's mental health status. If a youth is expressing feelings of being stressed, hopeless, agitated, and/or lacking support, this can add to their risk for suicidal behavior. If a child or an adolescent expresses suicidal ideation, he or she should be monitored while other evaluation and triage are undertaken.

Adjunctive Approaches

Paper-and-pencil rating scales are an efficient method for gathering information about risk factors, past suicidal behavior, and current ideation. Some youth may be more forthcoming in revealing their level of suicidality on a rating scale than in personal interview. Rating scales can provide a comparison to normative levels of symptoms and thoughts about death and dying. They can also be useful for tracking changes in suicidal target symptoms during treatment. Scales assessing both suicidality and depression are most helpful. Suicidality is commonly assessed with the Columbia Suicide Screen (CSS) and depression by the Moods and Feelings Questionnaire (MFQ), both of which are in the public domain. However, rating scales have limitations. Neither these scales comprise stand-alone assessments of suicidality nor are they able to predict suicidal behavior, and some youth may provide more accurate information when interviewed than on a paper-and-pencil measure. Clinicians should consider them supplementary to the clinical interview process. More information is provided in Chapter 3 "Rating Scales."

Approach to Triage

Despite accumulating data regarding the risk factors for suicidality in youth, suicide prediction remains elusive. In part because suicidality has a heterogeneous etiology, no single factor is pathognomonic for suicide. There are numerous potential risk factors, none of which is individually necessary or sufficient. It can be challenging for the clinician to differentiate youth truly at risk from those who can be safely maintained at home. Evaluation of the interplay between the various risk and protective factors offers the best prediction of outcome. Organizing these factors into a few dimensions can be helpful to optimize assessment and triage of suicidal children and adolescents. The following four dimensions should be considered: (1) underlying psychopathology, (2) personal skills and/or deficits, (3) environmental stressors, and (4) access to means. Essential factors relevant to these four dimensions are summarized in Table 21-2.

Psychopathology is present in most suicidal youth. However, mental health problems may not have been previously identified. Depression is associated with suicidality, but is not a necessary factor and is not always present in suicidal youth. Other underlying mental health problems such as impulsiveness, rapid mood shifts, and/or thought disturbances reduce the ability to resist suicidal impulses and to generate healthier options. Substance use contributes to risk by decreasing inhibitions for suicidal behavior. Clinicians should routinely screen for mental health problems and substance use so as to provide referral for further assessment and treatment. Follow-up is advised to ensure that patients do follow such recommendations.

Personal skills/resources and/or deficits may attenuate or exacerbate a child's risk and should be considered in conjunction with the presence or absence of underlying psychopathology and environmental factors. The presence of coping, problem-solving, and social skills can create options not available to children or adolescents with deficits in these areas. Social supports in the form of understanding and helpful caregivers and/or positive peer support can provide resources that can ameliorate risk. For example, a child with strong religious beliefs or a close family might better endure personal loss. However, a child who lacks the interpersonal skills needed to access social support during times of distress would be considered at greater risk than a child who has such skills. A depressed adolescent with perfectionistic traits might suffer loss of prestige poorly. A child who is feeling hopeless may drop out of treatment. Depressed youth who turn to alcohol rather than social supports has exacerbated their risk for suicidal behavior. In addition, it is important to be aware that skill deficits and the presence of psychopathology can lead some individuals to behave in a manner that may generate stressors. For example, mood lability combined

TABLE 21-2	Essential Assessment of Suicidality

Underlying psychopathology
- Determining a youth's psychopathology and its severity is critical; especially look for disturbances in mood, thinking, or impulsivity, *regardless of specific diagnosis*.
- The interview of the youth is the critical element in determining suicidality. The *youth should be interviewed separately from the parents* with developmentally appropriate questions related to depression, substance abuse, physical or sexual abuse, and self-harm.

Personal skills
- Can youth form an alliance to report suicidal impulses and maintain safety?
- Youth's personal attributes such as commitment to others, investment in activities, and past resilience in adversity help to determine the severity of risk, as well as disposition to *less restrictive* intervention.
- Youth's personal deficits, such as self-reproach, hopelessness, alienation, inflexibility, and perceived lack of options, help to determine disposition *to more restrictive* interventions.

Environmental stressors
- Are there recent stressors at home, in school, in the community, and with peers that are beyond the youth's ability to tolerate?
- *Parents should be interviewed separately from the youth* to clarify issues at home, particularly domestic violence, parental problems, and communication.
- How aberrant are the communications between youth and parent?

Access to means
- *Both the youth and parents* should be queried about access to lethal means of harm in the home, especially firearms and their proximity to ammunition.
- The parents should be queried about access to alcohol in the home.
- Parents' ability to supervise youth physically and emotionally should be ascertained if youth is to be sent home.

with impulsivity and poor interpersonal skills can result in behavior toward peers or family that will perpetuate and increase environmental stressors and increasing risk.

Environmental stressors are sometimes given undue causal weight for suicidal behavior; that is, a stressful event is thought to have caused a suicide. Obviously, no single event will elicit the same response from all people. Nonetheless, it is vital to gather information regarding both the objective presence of environmental stressors and the individual's subjective perception of stress. For example, youth with a history of maltreatment may have an exaggerated response to parental discipline, and youth sensitive to peer rejection may feel unable to cope with typical social challenges. In addition, a child's perceived efficacy to cope can vary dependent on other factors such as social support and the ability to tolerate emotional distress. For example, youth in the juvenile justice system may fear prolonged incarceration and turn to suicide as a quick "solution" to escape psychological distress. Finally, response to the suicide of relevant others can make suicidal behavior seem like a viable, or even glamorous, option.

Access to means for suicide is an important variable in the prediction of risk for suicidal behavior. Access decreases the effectiveness of mitigating factors as it provides immediate and potentially lethal action on a suicidal urge. Restricting access to means can create a delay between an urge and an opportunity to act, thus allowing personal skills, social resources, and treatment interventions time to work. Both children and their parents should be queried about access to means, especially firearms. Restriction of access will necessitate increased monitoring of the child as well as removal of means from the child's milieu. This can be difficult. Parents may assume that routine safety measures, such as locking firearms or storing ammunition and guns separately, will ensure safety. This is not the case. Children frequently have greater awareness of how to access these weapons than their parents realize. Many means of suicide, for example, over-the-counter medications, can be overlooked or difficult to remove, given their daily usage. The clinician should assist families in problem-solving how to decrease access to means and provide safety in the home. Psychoeducation regarding the interplay among risk factors can give frightened caregivers some sense of efficacy in being able to alter the risk for their child.

Safety Contracts

When a youth endorses suicidal ideation or a past attempt, common practice has been to obtain a safety or "no-harm contract," in which the patient promises to (1) refrain from hurting himself or herself and (2) notify a therapist, parent, or other appropriate adult if he or she feels suicidal again. A contract can identify potential future precipitants and a sequence of alternatives that the youth can employ for future crises. It can also provide a change in focus from distress to optimism. The process of defining the terms of the "no-harm contract" can help the clinician to better understand the youth's desire to live or die, and his or her strengths and weaknesses, and inform appropriate disposition. For example, a youth refusing to contract may then be referred for hospitalization. However, there is a danger that a "no-harm contract" will create a false sense of security. The youth might not be in a mental state to understand the contract, or may agree to a contract with no actual intent to follow through, or may agree but later, in a moment of distress, resort to suicidal behavior anyway. There is no scientific evidence that "no-harm contract" is effective at preventing suicidal behavior. If it is used, both family and clinician must know not to relax their vigilance just because a contract has been signed. Ultimately, the assumed benefits of a "no-harm contract" can all be obtained, and enhanced, by a frank and compassionate interview that includes assessment of precipitants, psychoeducation, help for feelings of distress, crisis prevention planning, increased supervision and restriction of access to means, and appropriate disposition. Finally, the "no-harm contract" provides no legal protection. Careful clinical assessment and disposition are the cornerstones to preventing suicide.

Disposition: Psychiatric Hospitalization versus Outpatient Treatment

Deciding on a disposition can be challenging. Clinicians usually prefer to "err on the side of caution," a reasonable practice given the consequences of failing to identify and appropriately triage a youth at risk. However, this practice can sometimes lead to "false positives" and can pose difficulties depending on the availability of resources. Thus, the goal is to identify the disposition that has the highest likelihood of preventing the patient from engaging in suicidal behavior while maintaining him or her in the least restrictive setting possible.

The four dimensions assessed during the interview should be helpful in determining disposition. Disposition can be elucidated by thinking of each dimension as a variable contributing to the overall risk. First, consider the severity of the underlying psychopathology, as well as the characteristics of the presenting suicidality and history of prior attempts. Second, consider the youth's personal skills and resources for coping with strong affect. Third, consider the presence/absence of environmental stressors. Lastly, take into account access to means for completing suicide, the likelihood of appropriate levels of supervision, and the availability of community resources. Using this approach, if risk outweighs protective factors, a more restrictive disposition is indicated. If the severity of suicidality is mild and protective factors are high, a less restrictive disposition is possible. Some cases will be clear. For example, a depressed and/or substance-abusing youth presenting with ideation and a recent suicide attempt will require hospitalization. At the other end of the spectrum, a child experiencing mild suicidal ideation with no intent or plan and no newly emerging disorder who has an established mental health treatment team can be referred back to that team after notification to caregivers and providers.

Of course, there are multiple scenarios between these two extremes. The restrictiveness of the disposition should vary from less to more restrictive as risk increases in proportion to protective

TABLE 21-3	Triage of Suicidal Youth in Outpatient Settings

- **Suicide attempt**
  - Hospitalize
  - Emergency room, or other emergent evaluation, if psychiatric bed not readily available or if patient does not agree to hospitalization

- **Suicidal ideation with plan or suicidal ideation with highly lethal thoughts**
  - Urgent outpatient psychiatric assessment, if interim safety can be ensured
  - Parents must agree to supervise adequately and to secure lethal means of self-harm in home while awaiting urgent outpatient assessment
  - Emergent evaluation, if interim safety cannot be ensured

- **Suicidal ideation without plan**
  - Routine psychiatric assessment, if within reasonable time, and if parental supervision is adequate, and if removal of means of self-harm is ensured
  - Urgent psychiatric assessment, if due to exacerbated psychiatric disorder, or if routine appointment not readily available, or if parent cannot adequately supervise or secure means of self-harm

Note: "Emergent" is defined as that day, as soon as possible; "urgent" evaluation is defined variably as within 48–72 hours; "reasonable time" and "routine" refer to within 3 weeks but also according to the family's ability to safely supervise in interim.

factors. A minimal algorithm for assistance in determining disposition from the outpatient office is provided in Table 21-3. Finally, many youth will have to be sent home while awaiting outpatient services. Discharge can be considered if the clinician is satisfied that adequate supervision will be available and that the adults have disposed of potentially lethal means. Good assessment with full knowledge of risks and protective factors is vital to appropriate disposition. If this is not possible for whatever reason, "erring on the side of caution" can allow time for further assessment in a safe setting.

Treatment and Other Interventions

Overall Interventions

Treatment will be part of any disposition for the suicidal youth. Historically, treatment has focused on the underlying psychopathology. While this is appropriate, it also is advisable to directly treat the youth's suicidality. The clinician first encountering the suicidal youth can provide some useful initial interventions. The front-line clinician should work from some general principles to establish a helping relationship and begin the therapeutic process. Most suicide attempters and their families benefit from straightforward interventions determined by the youth's mental status and family circumstances. Some such interventions that are easily implemented in the clinician's office are summarized in Table 21-4. Note that these in-office interventions are educational, directive, and almost prescriptive, recognizing the family's need for a professional to assure them that something can be done and to jumpstart the process.

There have been few empirical studies of treatments for suicidality in youth. In general, treatment addresses risk factors on the aforementioned four levels: treating underlying psychiatric illnesses, ameliorating social and problem-solving deficits, family psychoeducation and conflict resolution to address environmental stressors, and decreased access to lethal means (Table 21-5). Also, because of the need to respond to a suicidal crisis, treatment should be provided within a continuum of care that includes resources for inpatient, short- and long-term

TABLE 21-4	Essential In-Office Interventions

- Be aware of one's own ability and limitations in predicting youth's behavior, forming a therapeutic bond, and eliciting family's compliance with recommendations.
- Be aware that suicidality tends to be recurrent; therefore, establish rapport for the longer term and plan for future triage and/or other referrals or interventions; have an "emergency" plan established.
- Considering the risk for suicide completion, educate youth and parents about the nature of suicidality in young people, particularly its relationship to psychiatric disturbance and the need for treatment of such disturbance
- Considering the response of suicidal youth to parental difficulties and family dysfunction, educate parents about the need for minimizing harmful family environments; encourage parents to get help for themselves, if indicated.
- Offer hope through relationship with youth, encouragement, and noting youth's success with past distress.
- Educate youth and parents about the disinhibiting effects of alcohol and drugs particularly on judgment. Actively advise against the use of such substances.
- Obtain parental commitment to secure firearms and other means of harm.
- Obtain parental commitment to provide appropriate supervision.
- Obtain parental commitment to obtain mental health care for youth.
- Determine that appointment for mental health care has been made, and kept.
- Consider pharmacotherapy especially if ongoing mental health care is delayed; especially relevant for rapid mood swings or psychosis.

outpatient, and emergency interventions, as well as respite care and/or in-home stabilization when possible.

Treatment of Underlying Psychiatric Illness

Treatments vary depending on the underlying psychopathology, as covered in the relevant chapters in this text, particularly major depressive disorder, substance-use disorders, and conduct disorder. Treatments often include both pharmacologic and psychotherapeutic components. Thus, suicidal youth may be treated by multiple providers. The team may include the primary care provider, a child psychiatrist, a mental health clinician, a family therapist, and/or a care coordinator particularly for youth treated in the public mental health sector. There are advantages to an interdisciplinary approach as multiple clinicians can provide a higher level of

TABLE 21-5	Treatment Essentials for Suicidal Youth

- Identification and development of a continuum of interventions, including use of emergency room, crisis services, inpatient unit, outpatient services, "wrap around" services, and respite care
- Development of a treatment team that includes various providers, including primary care provider, primary mental health clinician, child and adolescent psychiatrist, school counselor, and other clinicians as needed and available
- Active diagnosis and aggressive treatment of psychiatric illness
- Individual therapies emphasizing the development of problem-solving skills and impulse control; cognitive–behavioral therapies; dialectal behavior therapy
- Development of family and community resources; emphasize community supports for youth with compromised parents or from unsupportive homes
- Family interventions emphasizing the development of nonviolent conflict resolution skills
- "Harm reduction" through modifications of stressful life obligations such as school schedule

monitoring and address multiple dimensions of the problem concurrently. They may also share the stress of caring for these youth who may experience multiple life crises. A collaborative treatment plan should include all team members, as well as the youth and family.

A few comments are warranted regarding pharmacologic treatment of underlying depressive disorders, particularly with the selective serotonin reuptake inhibitors (SSRIs). Several studies over the past several years suggest that the SSRIs can precipitate suicidal impulses leading the FDA to mandate "black box" labeling of all antidepressants. This issue is complex. It appears that 3% to 4% of youth treated with SSRIs compared with 1% to 2% of placebo-treated youth develop new-onset suicidal thinking. However, subsequent work reported that many medication-naïve youth treated with psychotherapy alone also developed new-onset suicidality. It should be emphasized that in these studies suicidality referred to suicidal ideation; none of the youth completed suicide. Furthermore, following the black box warning, studies with adults found that antidepressant prescriptions decreased by 18 to 20%, and rates of completed suicide quickly increased which was attributed to a decrease in the effective treatment of depression. Such a relationship has not been explored with youth. However, the Treatment for Adolescent Depression Study (TADS) has documented the efficacy of fluoxetine in treating depressed and suicidal youth, particularly in combination with cognitive–behavioral therapy (CBT). An important finding in the TADS study was that CBT appeared to protect against suicidality in the youth randomized to combined treatment with both an antidepressant and CBT. These findings strongly support the need for suicidal depressed youth to receive psychotherapy, not just pharmacologic treatment. Therefore, the clinician must be aware of both the potential benefits and the risks of treating youth with antidepressants. Furthermore, benefits and risks must consider youth's frequent noncompliance with treatment. All these factors continue to fuel the debate regarding the best practices with depressed and suicidal youth. The best approach is to discuss these issues with youths and their families, obtain their consent, and closely monitor progress and complications including suicidality. Preferably, youth should be engaged in a course of CBT or another psychotherapy as combined treatment both enhances treatment outcome and decreases the risk of suicidality.

Remediation of Social and Problem-Solving Deficits

Suicidal youth tend to have difficulty in problem-solving, especially generating alternatives to suicide as a means to solve their life problems. Thus, evidence-based treatments focus on practical skills such as improving problem-solving and teaching social skills especially for youth who are at risk for dropping out of school. Core components of such programs include regular monitoring of mood, school behaviors, and drug use as well as skills training in four areas: self-esteem enhancement, decision-making, personal control (anger, depression, and stress management), and interpersonal communication. Other programs include key elements of peer group and teacher support, monitoring, and skills training, generally over short-term group or individual sessions. Some programs also involve family interventions (family support, meeting family goals, and addressing family distress/conflict). Such programs have found success in decreasing suicide risk behaviors and distress with the most efficacious components being reinforcing personal skills such as increased personal control and problem-solving.

One psychotherapy that has been developed, primarily by Marsha Linehan at the University of Washington for recurrently suicidal adults, specifically to help patients with suicidal and self-harming behaviors to improve their skills at self-management is dialectical behavior therapy (DBT). DBT addresses the core deficits in suicidal patients, such as underlying illness, psychoeducation and conflict resolution to contain potential catalysts, amelioration of social and problem-solving deficits, and decreased access to means of suicide. DBT has been successfully adapted for adolescents. In brief, DBT is a structured psychotherapy that incorporates features of CBT with philosophies and strategies related to Eastern practices, such as "radical acceptance" and "mindfulness." The basic hypothesis is that suicidal patients show a core deficit in emotion regulation. Interventions are utilized to address a hierarchy of therapeutic needs including reduction in suicidal and self-injurious behaviors, reduction in behaviors that interfere with therapy, enhancement of quality of life and reasons for living, and building inter-personal skills. Skill building is included to improve the patient's ability to identify and regulate emotion, to increase coping skills, and to improve interpersonal effectiveness. Mindfulness assists patients in emotion regulation by reducing rumination about past events and reducing spi-raling anticipatory anxiety. Acquisition of these skills increases individual's ability to cope with triggering situations and to manage their emotional response, thus reducing impulsive respond-ing. DBT is an intensive, multimodal, and team-based approach, including individual therapy and group therapy to facilitate skills training. There is also recognition of the high demand that these patients place on clinicians, and consultation groups are used to reduce therapist burnout. An evidence base with adolescents is being established. Some other therapies have adapted com-ponents of DBT into their curricula.

Another new therapy is cognitive–behavioral therapy for suicide prevention (CBT-SP). CBT-SP is a manual-based therapy that works to prevent further suicidality by adolescents who have attempted suicide. It is based on a stress-diathesis model of suicidality and incorporates principles of DBT, CBT, and targeted therapies for suicidal youths with depression. It focuses on developing skills that will enable the adolescent to refrain from further suicidal behavior by using more effective means of coping when faced with stressors that trigger suicidal crises. There are acute and continuation phases, each lasting about 12 sessions. The parents are involved to help their child to develop suicide risk reduction strategies. CBT-SP does not aim to address all of the youth's problems, and recognizes the need for further treatment after resolution of the suicidality. Formal randomized trials are still needed to determine efficacy.

Another protocol for suicide assessment and treatment is being developed by Jobes and colleagues, which specifically addresses suicidality during individual psychotherapy. The effec-tiveness of this approach has been validated in adult populations. Early findings with adolescents suggest that regularly assessing environmental stressors, suicidal ideation, intent, degree of psy-chological pain and hopelessness, as well as reasons for living or dying can be informative and can provide important targets for therapeutic intervention.

Family Psychoeducation and Conflict Resolution

Adolescent suicide attempts occur most frequently during the late afternoon/evening between school and bedtime, a time that may be unstructured and/or unsupervised. When social sup-port is increased, suicide risk behaviors, and even depression, decrease. Focused awareness and supervision are especially important after precipitants such as family fights and increased par-ent–child discord, as these are common precipitants for suicidal behaviors, especially among girls. Increased supervision is an immediate and effective intervention to recommend in any clinician's office, particularly for at-risk youth whose parents are motivated to make changes.

Similarly, this is a good time to recommend lowering conflict in the home. "Expressed emotion" is a well-researched construct that may be applicable for suicidal youth, as it is for depressed and psychotic youth. Expressed emotion refers to high rates of negative emotion, criticism, blaming, and discounting one another in families. This has been shown to nega-tively affect recovery for depressed and psychotic youth, which in turn results in relapse and higher levels of care. Intensification of suicidal impulses may also be expected. Thus, another recommendation that can be made is for families to reduce conflict in the home. Increasing structure is helpful in accomplishing this goal, reducing the need for frequent negotiation of house rules. If this appears challenging, follow-up with a family therapist may be indicated.

Despite the advisability of psychotherapeutic services for suicidal youth, some families encounter obstacles to heeding this advice. They may be willing to make other changes though, for example, increased supervision or reduced family conflict, if the home environment is linked to the youth's welfare. In addition, the triaging clinician can plan an opportunity to check in, and possibly problem-solve, with families about progress in establishing these services.

Means Restriction

Restricting access to easy means is a very effective ecological intervention in prevention of completed suicide. As noted earlier in the text, the most common means of suicide among young people is firearms, particularly among impulsive youth, or those abusing alcohol or drugs. There has been increasing effort to educate the public in general, and parents of at-risk youth in particular, about the danger of having firearms in the home. The American Academy of Pediatrics has sponsored a campaign to inform pediatricians as part of routine practice to ask about firearms in the home and to educate families about firearm safety. At a minimum, routine safety measures and appropriate storage of firearms should be recommended, that is, suggesting locking firearms, storing weapons unloaded, and keeping guns and ammunition in separate locations. For acutely suicidal youth, recommending storage of weapons outside of the home is warranted. However, families show low compliance with such a recommendation, even when they are compliant with other safety recommendations. Education should include a variety of firearm storage options that are directed specifically at the parent who is the primary gun owner. Other recommendations might focus on removing toxic substances and knives and other instruments for cutting. Removal of alcohol may also decrease risk. It may not be possible for families to remove all potentially dangerous means for suicide; thus, it is vital to also stress the importance of increased parental supervision and monitoring.

Conclusion

Suicide among young people is a serious problem of growing concern for both children and adolescents. Even suicidal behaviors without completion confer great morbidity and interfere with the quality of young people's lives. Suicidality is a complex, multifaceted, and multidetermined problem with roots at the neurobiologic, psychodynamic, family, and societal levels. While these multiple sources of difficulty may seem overwhelming, they also provide multiple points for intervention. The outpatient clinician may provide the first intervention point by identifying suicidality, appropriately triaging the youth to services, participating in the youth's care as part of a treatment team, and providing a safe haven when things go awry.

Treatment is multifaceted, often with a team of clinicians. Creating a unified and collaborative plan with the child and their family is important. Treatment may evolve through different stages depending on the acuity and recurrence of suicidality, moving from more restrictive and intensive interventions to customary outpatient care as safety allows. Treatment generally combines psychotherapy and pharmacotherapy geared to the underlying psychopathology, remediating problem-solving deficits, building interpersonal skills, and containing family dysfunction. An evidence base is building for assessment and treatment directly targeting suicidal urges and behavior.

CASE VIGNETTES

VIGNETTE 1: A 17 YEAR OLD MALE WITH CHRONIC AND ACUTE RISKS FOR SUICIDALITY

As a pediatrician, you have cared for Jeremy since birth. He is a 17-year-old Caucasian male who has historically struggled with issues of ADHD and impulsivity, but has managed without medication since approximately 13 years of age. Today he presents to you for his annual sports physical. In talking with him during the examination, he seems less gregarious than he was in previous years and, in fact, appears somewhat withdrawn and hopeless. You discuss the fact that he is going into his senior year in high school, and he shares some concerns regarding his future, including whether his grades are high enough to meet eligibility requirements to play football in his senior year, as well as whether they are high enough to get into the college of his choice. He notes that he had a particularly rough junior year with regard to his grades, social relationships, and stressors at home. In talking with him further, he noted that his parents are in the process of divorcing and that he has had significant conflict with both of them. Suspecting that he may be depressed, you query him with regard to symptoms. At this time, he admits to symptoms of increased sadness and irritability, anhedonia, hypersomnia, increased appetite, poor concentration, and feelings of worthlessness. You directly ask him about feelings of suicidality, and he responds with a vague "kind of." As you query him further, he notes that he has had significant periods of feeling as though life were not worth living. He denies having made any suicide attempts, but reveals that he has been drinking heavily with some of his friends as a way to "forget my pain" and notes that on a couple of occasions he has taken "several" Tylenol PM in an effort to "just sleep." Concerned, you query him about a number of other issues. In the process you learn that his girlfriend recently broke up with him, his father has firearms in the home, and his parents are so absorbed in their divorce proceedings that they are, from Jeremy's perspective, unaware of how miserable he feels. Although Jeremy denies having a current plan, he notes that he has thought of various methods on several occasions. Today he notes that he feels "safe," but highlights that his mood can shift rapidly in the face of a "bad day." You note his multiple risks for suicidality and together with Jeremy, inform his parents of his status. You collaborate with other clinicians to further evaluate and treat his ADHD, depression, and substance abuse.

VIGNETTE 2: A 13 YEAR OLD TRAUMATIZED GIRL PRESENTING WITH SELF-INJURY

Sarah is a 13-year-old African American girl who is new to your care. She returns to your office today at the request of her adoptive mother, who learned that Sarah has been cutting on upper thigh. Her mother perceives this as a bid for attention, and is hoping that you can talk to her about the consequences of cutting, saying, "maybe if she hears it from you, she'll listen." Sarah has a tumultuous psychosocial history, including sexual abuse and neglect, which resulted in her placement in foster care at age 7 years. After a few changes in placement, she came to live with her parents when she was 11 and was later legally adopted. Sarah has been seen by multiple mental health providers over the years, with previous diagnoses including oppositional defiant disorder (ODD), posttraumatic stress disorder (PTSD), and mood disorder not otherwise specified. Her psychiatric care has been fragmented due to her multiple changes in placement and poor compliance on Sarah's part (e.g., refusing to talk to her counselor). Information about her family psychiatric history is limited, though her biologic mother had an unspecified mood disorder and her biologic father was incarcerated. Sarah is not taking any psychiatric medications, nor is she participating in psychotherapy. When you initially meet with Sarah and her mother, she looks at the floor and responds to questions with little more than a shrug of her shoulders. You ask her mother to step out of the room, and Sarah becomes more engaged. She acknowledges feeling sad and anxious, with prominent sleep disturbance, boredom, and irritability. Sarah reports that she had consensual sex with a male peer about a month ago, and he has "not even talked to [her] since then." Several peers found out and have been making rude comments when they pass her in the hall at school. Sarah began cutting on herself 3 weeks ago, and has made six to eight cuts that are superficial but still readily apparent on her leg. When asked about her plans for the future, Sarah replies "I don't know." She is unsure whether she will be able to improve her grades, does not have any plans for extracurricular or other activities, and is not at all sure what to do about her problems at school. Although she denies suicide attempts and is clear that her cutting was not an attempt to kill herself, Sarah acknowledges thinking about death every other day or daily, has considered ways that she could kill herself (overdose or cutting her wrists), has found medications in the home that she believes would be lethal (her mother's prescription sleep medication), and has thought about times when her parents would be unlikely to find her. Sarah fantasizes about the guilt that her peers would feel if she were gone. When you ask whether she thinks she'll be ok if she goes home, Sarah replies, "I don't know" and begins to cry. You note Sarah's chronic stresses and self-injury and enroll her in a DBT program at a local agency.

BIBLIOGRAPHY

Brent DA. Risk factors for adolescent suicide and suicidal behavior: mental and substance abuse disorders, family environmental factors, and life stress. *Suicide Life Threat Behav.* 1995;25:52–63.

Brent D, Baugher M, Birmaher B, et al. Compliance with recommendations to remove firearms in families participating in a clinical trial for adolescent depression. *J Am Acad Child Adolesc Psychiatry.* 2000;39: 1220–1225.

Brent D, Bridge J, Johnson B, et al. Suicidal behavior runs in families: a controlled family study of adolescent suicide victims. *Arch Gen Psychiatry.* 1996;53:1145–1152.

Brown J, Cohen P, Johnson JG, et al. Childhood abuse and neglect: specificity of effects on adolescent and young adult depression and suicidality. *J Am Acad Child Adolesc Psychiatry.* 1999;38:1490–1496.

Centers for Disease Control and Prevention. Youth risk behavior surveillance – United States, 2007. *MMWR Morb Mortal Wkly Rep.* 2008;57(SS04):1–131.

Centers for Disease Control and Prevention (CDC). Web-based Injury Statistics Query and Reporting System (WISQARS) [Online]. National Center for Injury Prevention and Control, CDC (producer); 2009. Available at: www.cdc.gov/injury/wisqars/index.html. Accessed January 31, 2009.

Department of Health and Human Services. Mental health and mental disorders: objectives for improving health, Part B. *Healthy People 2010.* 2003;18:1–33.

Evans E, Hawton K, Rodham K, et al. The prevalence of suicidal phenomena in adolescents: a systematic review of population-based studies. *Suicide Life Threat Behav.* 2005;36:239–250.

Gould MS, Greenberg T, Velting DM, et al. Youth suicide risk and preventive interventions: a review of the past 10 years. *J Am Acad Child Adolesc Psychiatry.* 2003;42:386–405.

Gould MS, Marrocco FA, Hoagwood K, et al. Service use by at-risk youths after school-based suicide screening. *J Am Acad Child Adolesc Psychiatry.* 2009;48(12):1193–1201.

Jobes, DA. *Managing Suicidal Risk: A Collaborative Approach.* New York: The Guilford Press; 2006.

Johnson JG, Cohen P, Gould MS, et al. Childhood adversities, interpersonal difficulties, and risk for suicide attempts during late adolescence and early adulthood. *Arch Gen Psychiatry.* 2002;59:741–749.

King RA, Schwab-Stone M, Flisher AJ. Psychosocial and risk behavior correlates of youth suicide attempts and suicidal ideation. *J Am Acad Child Adolesc Psychiatry.* 2001;40:837–846.

Lewinsohn PM, Rohde P, Seeley JR. Adolescent suicidal ideation and attempts: prevalence, risk factors, and clinical implications. *Clin Psychol Sci Pract.* 1996;3:25–46.

Mann J, Brent DA, Arango V. The neurobiology and genetics of suicide and attempted suicide: a focus on the serotonergic system. *Neuropsychopharmacology.* 2001;24:467–477.

Miller AL, Rathus JH, Linehan MM. *Dialectical Behavior Therapy with Suicidal Adolescents.* New York: The Guilford Press; 2007.

Nemeroff CB, Kalali A, Keller MB, et al. Impact of publicity concerning pediatric suicidality data on physician practice patterns in the United States. *Arch Gen Psychiatry.* 2007;64:466–472.

Olfson M, Shaffer D, Marcus SC, et al. Relationship between antidepressant medication treatment and suicide in adolescents. *Arch Gen Psychiatry.* 2003;60:978–982.

Richardson LP, DiGiuseppe D, Christakis DA, et al. Quality of care for medicaid youth treated with antidepressant therapy. *Arch Gen Psychiatry* 2004;61:475–480.

Rotheram-Borus MJ, Piacentini J, Cantwell C, et al. The 18-month impact of an emergency room intervention for adolescent female suicide attempters. *J Consult Clin Psychol.* 2000;68:1081–1093.

Shaffer D, Craft L. Methods of adolescent suicide prevention. *J Clin Psychiatry.* 1999;60:70–74.

Shaffer D, Scott M, Wilcox H, et al. The Columbia Suicide Screen: validity and reliability of a screen for youth suicide and depression. *J Am Acad Child Adolesc Psychiatry.* 2004;43:71–79. Available at: http://www.teenscreen.org. Accessed April 2010.

Sorenson SB, Rutter CM. Transgenerational patterns of suicide attempt. *J Consult Clin Psychol.* 1991;59:861–866.

Sorenson SB, Shen H. Youth suicide trends in California: an examination of immigrant and ethnic group risk. *Suicide Life Threat Behav.* 1996;26:143–154.

Stanley B, Brown G, Brent DA, et al. Cognitive-behavioral therapy for suicide prevention (CBT-SP): treatment model, feasibility, and acceptability. *J Am Acad Child Adolesc Psychiatry.* 2009;48(10):1005–1013.

Thompson EA, Eggert LL, Randell BP, et al. Evaluation of indicated suicide risk prevention approaches for potential high school dropouts. *Am J Public Health.* 2001;91:742–752.

Treatment for Adolescents with Depression Study (TADS) Team. Fluoextine, cognitive-behavioral therapy, and their combination for adolescents with depression: treatment for adolescents with depression study (TADS) randomized controlled trial. *JAMA.* 2004;292:807–820.

Treatment for Adolescents with Depression Study (TADS) Team. The treatment for adolescents with depression study (TADS): long-term effectiveness and safety outcomes. *Arch Gen Psychiatry.* 2007;64:1132–1144.

Verona E, Sachs-Ericsson N, Joiner TE, Jr. Suicide attempts associated with externalizing psychopathology in an epidemiological sample. *Am J Psychiatry.* 2004;161:444–451.

SUGGESTED WEBSITES FOR SUICIDE

National Center for Mental Health Check-Ups at Columbia University. This website offers extensive information on youth mental health, psychiatric illness, and suicidality for parents, teachers, clinicians, and policy makers. A newsletter is available. Address: http://www.teenscreen.org/

Centers for Disease Control and Prevention, Suicide. A US Department of Health and Human Services website offering information, prevention, toolkits, and curriculum guides for families and providers, with the aim of enhancing public health. Address: http://www.cdc.gov/ViolencePrevention/suicide/index.html

Suicide Prevention Resource Center. A clearinghouse of over 490 web pages and 250 library resources on suicide prevention information. This site is also a portal to other valuable resources about suicide prevention. The site includes individual state suicide prevention pages, news and events, an online library, training, and links to other websites. Address: http://www.sprc.org/

American Foundation for Suicide Prevention. The leading national not-for-profit organization exclusively dedicated to understanding and preventing suicide through research, education, and advocacy, and to reaching out to people with mental disorders and those impacted by suicide. Address: http://www.afsp.org/

National Institute of Mental Health. An organization providing national research leadership in an effort to prevent suicide. Address: http://www.nimh.nih.gov/health/index.shtml

SUGGESTED READINGS FOR CLINICIANS

Jobes, DA. *Managing Suicidal Risk: A Collaborative Approach.* New York: The Guilford Press; 2006.

Miller AL, Rathus JH, Linehan MM. *Dialectical Behavior Therapy with Suicidal Adolescents.* New York: The Guilford Press; 2007.

REVIEW QUESTIONS

The following questions are related to Vignette 1.

1. What factors increase Jeremy's suicide risk?
   a. Male gender
   b. Depression
   c. Potentially viable methods for suicide in the home
   d. All of the above
   e. None of the above

2. What would be a reasonable disposition plan for Jeremy?
   a. Send to the nearest emergency department
   b. Evaluate for possible antidepressant and refer for psychotherapy
   c. Start SSRI and follow up within 1 week
   d. b and c
   e. Any of the above

3. Which of the following issues add to Jeremy's suicide risk?
   a. Parental divorce
   b. Break-up with girlfriend

  c. Poor grades
  d. All of the above
  e. None of the above

Answers: 1-d, 2-e, 3-d

The following questions are related to Vignette 2.
1. Which of the following should be included in your assessment of Sarah's suicide risk?
    a. Determining whether Sarah has access to potentially lethal medications, knives or other sharp items, firearms, and anything else that she might use to harm herself
    b. Asking Sarah to generate several things that she could do to keep herself safe in the event that she feels suicidal
    c. Finding out whether Sarah is ever at home alone or unsupervised by an adult
    d. All of the above

2. Which of the following factors most significantly increases Sarah's risk for suicide?
    a. Her race; African Americans are more likely to commit suicide than other racial groups
    b. Her gender
    c. The presence of one or more psychiatric conditions
    d. None of the above

3. What information you've gotten from Sarah thus far would warrant breaking confidentiality and talking to her mother about her suicide risk?
    a. Sarah thinks about death on a near-daily basis
    b. Sarah has considered methods by which she could kill herself
    c. Sarah has found medications in her home that she believes could be lethal if taken in overdose
    d. All of the above
    e. None of the above

4. Sarah should be asked to sign a "no harm" agreement as it will significantly decrease the odds of her committing suicide.
    a. Yes, evidence suggests that "no harm" agreements are an effective tool in reducing suicide risk
    b. No, there is no evidence to support that "no harm" agreements are an effective tool in reducing suicide risk
    c. Sarah should be asked to sign a "no harm" agreement only in the context of other interventions that have been shown to be more effective in reducing risk. Providers should know that "no harm" agreements do not provide any assurance of safety and do not protect them from liability
    d. b and c

Answers: 1-d, 2-c, 3-d, 4-b and c

Aggression by Children and Adolescents

Introduction

The evaluation of aggression in children and adolescents is complex because aggression and violence by themselves are not necessarily pathologic behaviors. Aggression may be *adaptive* and serve important social and biologic goals, such as when a child (hereafter "child" means a child or an adolescent up to age 18 years) is rough-housing with a sibling or aggressively defends himself or herself from an attacker. Adaptive aggression is normal, has a place in society, and does not require treatment. *Maladaptive* aggression, on the other hand, is a dysfunctional behavior, which is ultimately harmful to the individual. As Connor notes, compared to adaptive aggression, maladaptive aggression is often inappropriate to the social context; is more intense, frequent, or long-lasting than its apparent cause warrants; and often, but not always, appears to be impulsive and unregulated.

Families of children with these types of behaviors can easily become overwhelmed and often need assistance from primary care providers, mental health professionals, or other community supports. Because types and causes of aggression vary, the evaluation and treatment of these behaviors is complex and often requires multidimensional strategies ranging from the simple to the extreme. This chapter will clarify these complexities and present a suggested approach to the clinical management of maladaptive aggression. The use of the term *aggression* in this chapter will hereafter denote maladaptive aggression unless otherwise noted.

Background

Historically, socially unacceptable aggression in children has been addressed both by the justice and by the mental health systems. The American *justice system's* formal involvement with child aggression began with the establishment of the first juvenile court in Chicago in 1899. The court originally began as an outgrowth of a broad urban reform movement, which viewed maladaptive behaviors in children as the product of poverty and other negative social forces typically found in large, industrialized urban cities. Such a view contributed to juvenile courts historically operating under the doctrine of *parens patriae,* or parent of the people. When a child's welfare appeared at risk, the court tried to facilitate rehabilitation through referral to social service agencies. In focusing on the child's welfare, the juvenile court system has generally promoted the distinction between juvenile and adult offenders. In the last 50 years, there have been legal challenges to this policy, which have led to modifications of how juvenile offenders are treated. The first of these challenges occurred in the 1960s through suits that claimed the juvenile system, by operating separately from the adult justice system, denied due process to child offenders by limiting their access to legal protections available to adult offenders.. More recently, in the 1980s and 1990s, increased juvenile crime and attendant media coverage have led to modifications of juvenile law codes allowing juveniles, under certain circumstances, to be tried as adults in criminal courts.

Like the justice system model, the *mental health model* also developed out of progressive reforms of the early twentieth century. Psychiatrists, psychologists, and social workers, operating as members of clinical teams in newly formed *child guidance clinics,* intervened with maladjusted children in local communities. Initially the child guidance movement concentrated on efforts of *prevention* as a means of social reform; over time, however, the clinics shifted toward individual *treatment* of identified children. As this shift occurred, there was a change in the recognized typical social characteristics of the maladjusted child away from poor, immigrant children of lower social classes toward increasing numbers of children from higher income, better educated families.

In contemporary American society, the juvenile justice and mental health systems continue to have intersecting roles in interventions with aggressive children; for example, as Teplin and colleagues found in 2002, up to 75% of juvenile offenders have at least one diagnosable psychiatric disorder. In order to address such needs, there have been efforts to place mental health professionals in correctional facilities, but these services remain underdeveloped and inadequately funded and staffed.

Clinical Features

Aggression is not a diagnosis but rather a behavior pattern that has a variety of presentations and determinants. Adaptive aggression can be a normal aspect of early social development (i.e., a toddler hitting someone to get back a toy) or be needed to preserve one's safety. Aggression is maladaptive when it occurs with inappropriate intensity, duration, or frequency. Although a wide variety of subtypes of pathologic aggression have been postulated, two dichotomous subtypes appear to the authors to be the most clinically relevant categorizations: (1) hot versus cold aggression and (2) direct versus indirect aggression.

"Hot" and "Cold" Aggression

"Hot" aggression refers to impulsive, aggressive, and defensive behaviors that arise in response to an actual or perceived attack or provocation. This type of aggression is best conceptualized as a defensive fear-driven response to threat and frustration. It is associated with high central nervous system (CNS) autonomic arousal and irritability due to activation of the fight, flight, and freeze response; behaviorally there is an uncoordinated, poorly modulated response to the threat with high risk of self-harm and low probability of successful outcome or reward. Children with "hot" aggression often display biases that, in the setting of socially provocative or ambiguous situations, lead them to make exaggerated, inappropriate, and aggressive responses to peers and adults, whom they may inappropriately believe to have hostile intentions toward them. "Hot" aggression is associated with a history of developmental disturbances, physical abuse, social instability, or neuropsychiatric problems, such as inattention and impulsivity.

Children with "cold" aggression are commonly described as having callous-unemotional traits and appear to have little CNS autonomic arousal or visible signs of fear, irritability, and anger when engaged in aggressive acts. This type of aggression is pursued in order to obtain a desired goal or favorable outcome such as food, property, social status, or pleasure in inflicting harm. Unlike in "hot" aggression, the execution of "cold" aggressive acts occurs in an organized, patterned, goal-directed, and controlled manner, which increases the likelihood of successful outcome. "Cold" aggression theories in humans postulate that this behavior can be reinforced in the context of social environments that provide social role modeling and external reinforcements for such behavior, such as gangs or violence-prone communities. "Cold" aggression has a later age of onset than does "hot" aggression, and is felt to be quite unresponsive to medication treatments.

Direct and Indirect Aggression

Both the cold and hot forms of aggression may manifest in either physical or nonphysical ways. Physical aggression and violence are easily recognized behaviors—they constitute a "direct" form of aggression in which the individual is directly physically manipulating or harming another individual. Nonphysical expressions of aggression, often termed "indirect" aggression, are only recently becoming recognized clinically as aggressive acts.

Indirect aggression, as described by Vaillancourt, is a form of maladaptive behavior that involves manipulating social relationships in aggressive ways to intentionally hurt target victims. In contrast to direct aggression, which peaks at around 30 months of age in the general population, indirect aggression increases in its occurrence throughout childhood and may peak, for females at least, somewhere in late adolescence or young adulthood. Examples of indirect aggression include motivating others to dislike a person, betraying others' trust by divulging their secrets, using subtle speech or body language to convey derogatory interpersonal messages, and spreading rumors about others, as for example, with regard to promiscuous sexual behavior, frigidity, or sexual orientation. Indirect aggression is more commonly seen in females compared to males, and when accounted for in community samples, it narrows the gender gap in terms of the overall prevalence of aggression in children.

Children who utilize indirect aggression often gain status and popularity within certain peer circles, but at the same time they are likely to be disliked by their victims, other lower-status individuals, and their larger peer networks. Thus, in terms of social adaptation, indirect aggression has features of both competence and impairment. Clinical referral of children who utilize indirect aggression is not very common. What is more common is to receive referrals on children who themselves are victims of indirect aggression and therefore experience anxiety and depression, or may plan out "cold" aggressive actions as a response to feeling victimized. As interest, knowledge, and research on the effects of indirect aggression grow, especially as regards the occasional serious negative outcomes that occur from it, schools and other community organizations have begun taking this type of aggression very seriously by enacting rules and punishments to attempt to limit its use.

Epidemiology

Aggression in infants and toddlers is common, contributes to healthy social adaptation, and usually does not continue to be a significant concern for children as they mature. Conflicts naturally arise in normal interactions, and assertiveness is one way infants and toddlers learn to establish relationships and boundaries in their evolving social lives. In a random community sample of 572 toddlers aged 17 months, 72% could be classified as having either modest or high aggression. When followed up to 42 months of age, these initially aggressive toddlers showed greater persistence of aggression when compared to the 28% of the sample rated as having "little or no physical aggression." As children age further, however, most learn nonphysical forms of conflict resolution so that by the time they enter first grade, the rates of aggression in community samples are much lower.

School-aged children who participate in aggressive acts tend to repeat their aggression and are consistently rated by their teachers through their school years as being more aggressive than their peers. Outcomes for this subset are concerning: data from an original birth cohort of 1265 subjects studied over a period of 25 years found that the children who displayed the highest levels of aggression between age 7 and 9 years had, as adults, significantly worse criminal, mental health, substance-abuse, and relational outcomes compared to their less aggressive counterparts, with rates between 1.5 and 19 times higher than the least disturbed 50% of children studied. This association of conduct problems with poor adult outcomes was similar for females and males.

Combined rates of indirect and direct aggression are similar for males and females until around age 7. After this, the data indicate that males are about 3.5 times as likely as females to commit direct physical violence, while females are more likely to utilize indirect forms of aggression. The median age for onset of significant antisocial behaviors has been estimated at about 7 years in males and 13 years in females. African American children are about 1.5 times as likely as Caucasian American children to commit violent acts—other ethnicities have not been compared nationally. According to "Youth Violence: A Report of the Surgeon General", child violence is fairly common in that 30% to 40% of males and 16% to 32% of females have committed at least one seriously violent act (aggravated assault, robbery, gang fights, or rape) by age 17. The peak age of onset of seriously violent offences is 16.

US criminal levels of aggression in juveniles, such as murder and aggravated assault, peaked in the mid-1990s after a period of rapid increase from the mid-1980s. Since then, violent crime in juveniles has decreased by half. Despite this overall improvement, there have been a number of highly publicized crimes, such as the school shootings at Columbine in 1999, which have reminded the public of the seriousness of child aggression and violence. Individuals who continue their violence through adulthood are more likely to have had an early onset of violent acts (before puberty), and are more likely to be engaged in a risky lifestyle involving drug use, precocious sex, and gun involvement.

Etiology

Historically, there has been considerable debate between nativist perspectives, on the one hand, and social learning perspectives, on the other, as to the causes of aggression. From a nativist view, aggression is an innate drive and natural behavioral consequence of a biologically driven competition for limited resources. From a social learning view, however, aggression is not innate but is learned through the modeling of other people's aggressive behaviors, whether in the home, at school, or as portrayed in the media.

The approach of much contemporary work on aggression synthesizes these two perspectives through elaborating current understandings of the role *gene–environment interactions* play in the development and expression of aggression. According to this view, while an individual begins the developmental process with certain species-wide innate propensities like the potential for aggression, the direction and development of these propensities depend in large part on the interactions between these innate factors and the individual's environment. Some children, due to both genetic and environmental factors, have a more difficult time compared to others in learning functional alternative strategies to aggression when faced with certain environmental conditions. Childhood maltreatment and exposure to aggressive adults, for instance, are potent environmental factors shown in the work of Dorothy Lewis to favor the development persistent aggressive behavior. Lewis's work also stresses, however, how innate vulnerabilities can modulate the expression of aggressive behaviors in individuals exposed to maltreatment. For example, in children with pre-existing CNS dysfunction, exposure to maltreatment is particularly potent in promoting aggression.

In the following discussion of risk factors for the development of aggression, it will be helpful to keep in mind this dynamic and complex interplay between individual and environmental factors. It is also important to note that while the risk factors presented later in the text are predictive of an increased probability of aggression, in most cases they represent associations rather than known causal factors.

Risk/Resilience Factors

A number of *individual factors* have been identified as predisposing children to aggressive behavior, as summarized in Table 22-1. Prenatal alcohol exposure is associated with antisocial behavior and impulsive aggression, while prenatal nicotine exposure is associated with

TABLE 22-1	Essential Risk Factors for Aggression and Related Behaviors
• **Individual risk factors** Genetic susceptibility Prenatal toxin exposure "Difficult" temperament Cognitive deficits Affect dysregulation • **Family risk factors** Maltreatment and neglect Inadequate (i.e., coercive) parenting Family dysfunction and marital conflict	• **Community factors** Peer rejection Antisocial peer group affiliation Neighborhood violence and poverty Media violence exposure

attention-deficit/hyperactivity disorder (ADHD), conduct disorder (CD), and other adverse behavioral outcomes. Certain inborn temperaments have also been linked to aggressive behaviors in young people. According to Connor, children with temperaments described as "difficult," "novelty seeking," or "sensation seeking" in preschool are at increased risk for later psychopathology including CD and aggression. This association is more often seen in males versus females, and when associated with concomitant environmental stressors such as family dysfunction.

Deficits in cognitive function and performance have also been identified as important markers of increased risk of antisocial behavior. Deficits in prefrontal cortex–mediated executive functioning leading to impairments in impulse control and behavioral regulation have been associated with chronic aggression. Additional cognitive factors associated with conduct problems and aggression include low verbal and performance IQ and academic underachievement. Children with impairments in mood regulation often display chronic irritability, easy frustration, anger, dysphoria, and aggression. Children with high mood reactivity and sustained negative mood may have social information processing deficits that bias them to "hot" aggression defensive responses to perceived threats from others.

Maltreatment is an important source of increased risk of aggression in children. In an influential paper in 1989, Widom reported that children exposed to maltreatment and neglect are at a significant increased risk of the development of aggressive behaviors. Other factors that influence the relationship between maltreatment and aggression include the type of maltreatment exposure, the age of occurrence, and IQ level. Genetics also plays a role in how one responds to maltreatment. For example, Caspi and colleagues have been able to demonstrate that whether or not a child exposed to maltreatment develops problems with significant aggression as an adult depends in part on which of two different forms of the gene monoamine oxidase A (MAOA) the individual has.

Inadequate parenting practices are another important family risk factor. Patterson's *Coercive Family Process* links the development of conduct problems to a pattern of inconsistent disciplining and follow-through, which leads to conflict and inadvertent reinforcing of childhood aggressive behavior through parents being either overly punitive or acquiescing to their child's demands as a way to end the conflict. Additional parenting factors associated with the development of behavioral problems include insufficient supervision, poor delineation of boundaries, and low levels of parent positive praise and involvement. Bidirectional influences are also important. Children with difficult temperaments and disruptive behaviors are likely to elicit negative responses from their parents and other adults with whom they have contact. Additional family risk factors include family stressors such as marital conflict, domestic violence, separation, and divorce; parent psychopathology and criminality; single parenting without sufficient supports; and family poverty.

Negative *community factors,* such as unfavorable school, neighborhood, and social environments, also increase the risk of aggression. Neighborhoods with high resident turnover and limited community resources lack *collective efficacy,* placing children from families with low socioeconomic status (SES) at risk for delinquent behaviors. Chronic exposure to neighborhood violence is strongly correlated with increased aggression, especially during adolescence. Connor notes that early childhood social rejection by peers and a later congregation of aggressive children into groups promote further learning of antisocial behaviors and impede the development of prosocial skills, especially during adolescence. Ameliorating factors for these negative peer influences include supportive family relationships and academic competence. One last important community factor is children's exposure to media violence (MV). Singer and colleagues have reported that the amount of time elementary school children watched television was closely correlated with their self-reported levels of violent behavior. Children who have emotional and behavioral disorders, live in homes where violence is permitted, or witness violence in their neighborhood appear to be at greater risk to be influenced by MV. Suggested causal mechanisms of MV promoting aggressive behaviors in children include the following: (1) MV increases "hot" aggression through sensitization of the threat response system, (2) MV increases "cold" aggression through loss of empathy and habituation to the suffering of others, and (3) MV encourages the use of violence as an acceptable method of working through conflicts and problems.

Diagnostic Considerations

The clinical assessment and treatment of aggression often occur in mental health settings where treatments rely on assigning *Diagnostic and Statistical Manual of Mental Disorders, Fourth Edition* (*DSM-IV*) psychiatric diagnoses and initiating interventions based on those diagnoses. This is frequently not ideal for several reasons. First, most maladaptive juvenile aggressive behaviors occur in individuals who are not psychiatrically ill, and therefore nonpsychiatric theories of etiology and intervention are usually required. Second, an aggressive act may be an adaptive behavioral response to a threatening encounter (such as a child pushing away a peer who is teasing them); therefore, even in a child with a previous *DSM-IV* diagnosis, aggression may be developmentally or situationally appropriate. Lastly, the presence of aggressive behavior is not very diagnostically helpful because the presentations of a number of *DSM-IV* illnesses can include aggression as a clinical feature. However, with these caveats in mind, if aggression occurs in the setting of a treatable *DSM-IV* psychiatric illness, as summarized in Table 22-2, then treating that underlying illness has a good chance of impacting the degree of occurrence of aggression. The following section summarizes the associations between aggression and a number of *DSM-IV* disorders as noted by Connor.

Three childhood disorders are commonly grouped together as disruptive behavior disorders, and often present with aggression: CD, oppositional defiant disorder (ODD), and ADHD. ODD is a common disruptive behavior disorder characterized by negativistic and hostile behavior that usually involves verbal conflicts rather than physical aggression. ODD behaviors, however, can be associated with later progression to CD in some children, and therefore may predict later aggressive behaviors. Childhood-onset (prior to age 10) conduct-disordered children are more likely to be males, act alone, show evidence of neuropsychiatric disease, commit violence, and have a lifetime course of psychopathology. Adolescent-onset conduct-disordered children show greater female numbers, are less likely to be physically violent, and are more likely to desist from aggression once they achieve adult autonomy, responsibilities, and opportunities. ADHD is a risk factor for adolescent and adult aggression, and is

TABLE 22-2 *DSM-IV* Disorders with Clinical Features of Aggression

- **Disruptive behavior disorders**
  CD—greater psychopathology if childhood onset
  ODD—more likely to be associated with verbal versus physical aggression
  ADHD—aggression more likely to be seen in hyperactive/impulsive subtype

- **Mood disorders**
  Depression—in children, irritability may lead to acting out behaviors including aggression
  Bipolar disorder—irritable mood, psychomotor agitation, and psychosis can lead to aggression

- **Anxiety disorders**
  Anxiety disorders—generally seen as a protective factor for aggression; exception is PTSD

- **Additional *DSM-IV* disorders**
  Substance abuse—substances associated with aggression include alcohol and cocaine
  Mental retardation—aggression may be related to medical illness or environmental precipitant
  ASD—aggression may be related to verbal impairment, behavioral rigidity, or change in routine
  Psychotic disorders—aggression risk increases with age, low SES, male gender, and SUD
  Traumatic brain injury—increased risk if history of aggression or concurrent family dysfunction
  Seizure disorders—aggression most likely seen during "postictal" state of confusion

CD, conduct disorder; ODD, oppositional defiant disorder; ADHD, attention-deficit hyperactivity disorder; PTSD, posttraumatic stress disorder; ASD, autistic spectrum disorder; SUD, substance use disorder.

commonly found among conduct-disordered children. The hyperactivity/impulsivity subtype has a stronger relationship to aggression than does the inattentive subtype.

Childhood mood disorders may also present with aggressive features. Anger, irritability, and hostility can all be features of depression. Compared to depressed adults, children may lack the developmental (particularly cognitive) capacity to suppress negative feelings, which can lead to externalizing behaviors such as aggression when depressed. Aggression may also occur with bipolar disorder in children. Symptoms that appear to increase the risk of aggression in bipolar-disordered children include irritable mood, psychomotor agitation, distractibility, disinhibition, and psychosis. The degree and persistence of behavioral disturbance in bipolar disorder can be quite intense especially when symptoms of CD and/or ADHD are present.

Anxiety disorders are not commonly associated with aggression. If fact, anxiety broadly defined can be considered a protective factor for the expression of antisocial behaviors such as aggression. However, sometimes a heightened perception of threat leads to defensive posturing and acting out, and in that way anxiety could lead to aggressive reactions to threatening situations. This is particularly pertinent to posttraumatic stress disorder (PTSD). PTSD can dysregulate cortical and subcortical brain structures that process and organize adaptive behavioral responses in the face of perceived or actual threats. Such dysregulation can lead to maladaptive behavioral responses such as rage, hostility, and aggression when an individual encounters reminders of past trauma. This "cued" maladaptive fear response may occur outside the individual's conscious awareness and, therefore, may clinically be difficult to identify as the antecedent of the behavioral episode.

Other *DSM-IV* disorders may present with aggression as a prominent clinical feature. These include substance-abuse disorders (SUD), mental retardation, autistic spectrum disorders (ASD), psychotic disorders, and neuropsychiatric disorders, such as traumatic brain injury or seizure disorder. Substances that are frequently associated with an increased risk of aggression include alcohol, cocaine, and phencyclidine (PCP). The behavioral effects of a drug may vary according to whether its blood level amount is increasing (intoxication) versus decreasing (withdrawal). For example, alcohol intoxication (versus withdrawal) has a greater associated with aggression; conversely, opiate withdrawal (versus intoxication) is more likely to be associated with aggression.

Cognitively impaired children are more likely to present with impulsive "hot" aggression than "cold" aggression. Potential precipitants for aggression in cognitively impaired children include seizures, task-related anxiety or avoidance behaviors, environmental irritants, poorly planned goal-directed actions, communication difficulties, underlying psychiatric disorders such as depression, and medication side effects. In verbally impaired ASD children, aggressive or self-injurious behaviors may be related to untreated medical conditions causing pain or discomfort. ASD females may have aggression temporally related to their menstrual cycles. Behavioral rigidity is common in ASD children; changes in routine or environment may precipitate disruptive behaviors as a result.

Psychotic disorders, including schizophrenia, are rare in children but become more common in middle and late adolescence. Factors associated with adolescent psychosis, which appear to increase the risk for violence and aggression, include proximity to family and friends, low SES, male gender, and substance abuse. Traumatic brain injury may lead to disinhibited social behaviors including provocative speech and actions, but as Connor notes, aggressive behaviors are usually not seen unless they were present to some degree before the injury. Seizure-related "ictal" aggression is a rare phenomenon, but "postictal" aggression is more common and may be associated with individuals feeling vulnerable, confused, and threatened by their environment directly following a seizure.

Assessment and Treatment

Assessment and Treatment of the Acutely Aggressive Child

Clinicians are sometimes asked to intervene in acute childhood aggression, a circumstance in which a child has recently committed a violent act, is currently violent, or is about to be violent. In the presence of an immediate or imminent threat of aggression or violence, a brief evaluation focused on ensuring immediate safety becomes the first priority. Safety during the evaluation can be ensured by removing access to weapons and by having multiple care providers present during the assessment. According to Hilt and Woodward's approach summarized in Table 22-3, a calm, soft spoken, respectful demeanor that gives careful attention to

---

TABLE 22-3   Essential Assessment for Acute Aggression

- Use a soft voice and calm respectful manner to help defuse anger.
- Ensure no weapons are present.
- Destimulate the environment if possible (less noise and light).
- Remove any valuable breakable objects/equipment from the room.
- Strongly consider offering the child food or drink.
- Offer child control through "forced choices" (i.e., sit here or there?).
- Get sequence of what happened before aggressive act(s).
- Listen and empathize.
- Reassure family it is your job to "make sure everyone is safe."
- Halt any flare of parent–child arguments by interviewing separately if needed.
- Tell child how you plan to honor any reasonable requests.
- Do health screening/mental status assessment, that is, substance intoxication, delirium, mania, and psychosis.
- Consider offering child distracting toys/sensory modalities while waiting.
- Consider medications if situation not improving.

TABLE 22-4	Essential Pharmacotherapy for Acute Aggression

- Risperidone—0.25 mg (school age) to 2 mg (late adolescent) PO
- Olanzapine—2.5 mg (school age) to 10 mg (late adolescent) PO
- Lorazepam—0.05 mg/kg/dose PO/IM/IV (maximum 2 mg/dose)
- Diazepam—0.04–0.2 mg/kg/dose PO/IM/IV (maximum 10 mg/dose)
- Diphenhydramine—1 mg/kg/dose to maximum 50 mg PO/IM/IV
- Ziprasidone—10–20 mg IM if >16 years, 10 mg IM if 12–16 years
- Haloperidol—0.025–0.075 mg/kg/dose IM (maximum 5 mg)

PO, oral intake; IM, intramuscular; IV, intravenous administration.
Note: Above-suggested dosages in authors' decreasing order of preference; must have consent/assent
for treatment; otherwise medicine use is considered a restraint.
From: Hilt and Woodward, 2008.

ensure that the child's current concern is "heard" will also help keep an acute situation from boiling over.

Once the child feels heard and attended (by such things as carefully listening to the child's concerns and offering the child some food or drink), the next assessment priority is getting a brief history from the caregiver about the situation. If the caregiver makes argument-inciting accusations in the child's presence, the interview should stop and later be resumed away from the child. Brief inquiries into potential biologic contributions to the current agitated state may uncover abuse of substances, an underlying psychosis or mania, or an acute mental status change suggestive of a delirium. Armed with this basic information, a clinician can move toward providing further calming measures and, if appropriate, rapid treatment for any specific disorders present (such as medical treatment of an encephalitic delirium).

Medications may be used as acute aggression or agitation treatments after establishing an assessment-based plan of care (such as a need to treat anxiety), after nonmedication strategies have been tried and found to not help, and after obtaining both parental consent and patient assent for use of a medication. Medications should never be given for discipline or convenience. Oral medications are strongly preferred over injections due to greater acceptability to the child and a similar time for onset of action for the suggested medications in Table 22-4. Injection of a medication implies that such administration is not a treatment, but rather the administration of a chemical restraint.

Although there are differing opinions about selecting agitation treatment medications, generally the authors recommend the use of an antipsychotic over a benzodiazepine for acute situations due to a lower risk of paradoxical agitation reactions in children. Children already taking a benzodiazepine or an antipsychotic may benefit from an additional dose of that medication rather than trying any new medication. Restraint, either physical or chemical, should be considered only when the child is actively trying to harm themselves or others, and if employed, their use should follow all applicable state and federal guidelines. A pharmacologic approach to the pharmacotherapy of acute aggression is shown in Table 22-4.

Assessment of the Recurrently or Chronically Aggressive Child

Historical elements sought from both the child and the parent should focus on aggression subtypes (i.e., hot versus cold and direct versus indirect), risk factors, and related psychiatric diagnoses, as outlined earlier in this chapter and in Table 22-5. If a parent seems able to offer only limited historical details as to the circumstances of their child's aggressive actions, it may help to explicitly focus on obtaining a chain analysis of events leading up to at least one particular incident. By looking closely at the sequence of events, an aggressive act may be revealed to

---

TABLE 22-5   Essentials of Assessment for Recurrent Aggression

- Assume a politely neutral stance to both parent and child.
- Obtain the full sequence of events from child and parent before at least two aggressive acts.
- Look for impulsive versus planned aggression pattern.
- Look for the communicative meaning to the aggression.
- Investigate biologic contributions.
- Determine substance abuse, developmental impairment, delirium, and head injury.
- Assess modeling of aggression in the family and/or a history of bullying.
- Get collateral information from the school or other caregivers.
- Assess a history and mental status screen for *DSM-IV* disorders.

---

come at the end of a series of frustrations about which the parent was previously unaware. It helps to maintain a politely neutral stance while getting the child's view of events, since children are unlikely to speak freely about themselves if they perceive their interviewer as a parental ally who is looking to label them as "bad."

A parent who is very frustrated with their aggressive child may not be the most accurate historian. Especially in the presence of parental exasperation, another observer such as a school-teacher or relative may add significantly to understanding the problem at hand. Questionnaires sent to school teachers or to other caregivers may be a means of gathering such collateral information in a time-efficient manner for the provider.

Determining if the child's aggression pattern is predominantly "hot" versus predominantly "cold" is useful because the recommended treatments are often quite different for these two aggressive subtypes (as outlined in the next section). For instance, children who use aggression deliberately to get what they want and who come from a family in which needs are not met unless one is manipulative to obtain them would likely need treatments that are targeted toward "cold" aggression.

The child's mental status may also provide diagnostic clues that there is a psychiatric disorder contributing to aggression. Mental status assessment in children mostly involves close observation of the child, coupled with some targeted questions about mood and thought processes. For instance, a child observed to have downcast eyes, low energy level, withdrawn body posture, and irritable mood should be screened for a depressive disorder that may be contributing to aggression. A child who behaves in an extremely impulsive and hyperactive fashion in the office should be screened for ADHD as contributing to the occurrence of aggression.

Diagnostic Tools

Medical testing has a very minor role in evaluating childhood aggression. Unless there are specific concerns with brain functioning, diagnostic aids like an electroencephalogram (EEG), head imaging, cerebrospinal fluid (CSF) studies, or blood tests are not useful. Medical evaluations are warranted, however, in the presence of fever or headache, neurologic abnormalities, physical dysmorphology, or delirium.

Questionnaires or psychological testing may aide the evaluation of aggressive children. A general behavioral health screening questionnaire, such as the Child Behavior Checklist (CBCL) or the brief Pediatric Symptom Checklist (PSC-17), may provide clues to the presence and type of an underlying psychiatric disorder. If there is already a concern for a specific psychiatric disorder, specific assessment scales for that condition, such as the Vanderbilt Scale for ADHD, could be useful for identifying treatable conditions. If there is a concern that the child's frustrations stem from an intellectual impairment or a learning disability, obtaining formal psychological testing by a licensed psychologist (using intelligence tests such as the "Wechsler's Intelligence Scale for Children" [WISC] or the "Bayley Scale of Infant and Toddler Development") would enable the child to receive academic assistance from the school. Objective monitoring of the symptoms of aggression over time could be done with a rating scale such as the Children's Aggression Scale (CAS) or through the use of other standardized questions.

Treatment of the Recurrently or Chronically Aggressive Child

Treatment of chronic, recurrent aggression proceeds most successfully by first identifying if a child has any underlying DSM-IV diagnoses. Specific diagnoses, when present, enable the provider to select evidence based treatments which can either directly or indirectly reduce aggression. For instance, treating major depression or PTSD, if present, can proceed along the best available evidence base for those disorders, and the treatment as conducted will often reduce the observed, associated aggressive behaviors. Another well-recognized example of the utility of correctly identifying all DSM-IV disorders that are present is when aggressive symptoms of ODD are comorbid with ADHD. Multiple studies have shown that prescribing a stimulant medication for ODD comorbid with ADHD may reduce aggressive behaviors.

The second stage in treatment would be to determine whether a child's aggression is serving an important communicative function and to address any underlying message that can be discovered. A common example of this is the child who has a developmental or severe communication disorder and who is aggressive when they can find no other means of expressing themselves—aggression in this population could mean something as simple as that the child is hungry or has pain. Other forms of aggression such as communication can be found in the developmentally normal child, who may have difficulty expressing a particular frustration in any other way. For instance, a child who is suffering from being bullied at school, is afraid to talk about it, and is subsequently acting out aggressively toward younger peers needs to have their underlying stressor identified and addressed.

The third stage in treatment, if other efforts have not helped, would be a target symptom–based approach based on a characterization of the child's aggression pattern. Subtyping aggression, as outlined earlier in this chapter, becomes especially important for this approach. Aggression that is predominantly "cold" in nature is generally not going to be treatable with medications—psychosocial treatments focused on intervening with the child's environment are preferred. As authors like Weisz have noted, there have been hundreds of studies of different psychosocial treatments designed to address child aggression, though relatively few of these are widely disseminated and available in communities. Some of the evidence-based specific therapies to look for by name in treating "cold aggression" include multisystemic therapy (MST), functional family therapy (FFT), and multidimensional treatment foster care. Also, there are a large number of well-researched parent-management training programs, such as the Parent–Child Interaction Training (PCIT), the Incredible Years, and the Positive Parenting Program (Triple P) that may be more available in a community from individual therapists. The parent-management training approach in general asserts that parents should (1) learn basic behavioral principles with child rearing, (2) learn how to define and track the prosocial and antisocial behaviors to target, and (3) practice and then carry out behavior modification programs at home. Performing individual one on one counseling for a child without treating the child's environment through one of the above-mentioned approaches is unlikely to be helpful, particularly with prepubertal children. If working with a skilled child therapist is not an option, there are a number of self-guided parent-management training options (i.e., books and videos) available that may be worth pursuing (see the "Suggested Readings" section).

Recurrent "hot" aggression problems often involve reactions to abnormal threat perceptions in the environment, such as the cortical processing changes that were described earlier with PTSD. For these children the essential treatment goal would be to relearn how to emotionally process environmental stimuli so as to not react in only aggressive ways. Although it can take years to achieve success, it is possible to do so through such things as participation in social skills groups, emotion coaching, individual supportive counseling, trauma-focused cognitive behavior therapy (CBT), and caregiver training to provide highly skillful responses to a child's emotional outbursts.

Medications are not the primary means to treat "hot" aggression, but if there are recurrent aggressive outburst symptoms that are consistently maladaptive and impede progress in therapy, then medications may be worth trying. Low doses of medications that downregulate the autonomic nervous system, such as alpha-agonists or beta-blockers, may for some children help to mitigate their fight or flight reactivity. If the child's abnormal threat perceptions are enhanced by the presence of an anxiety disorder, then it may be appropriate to try giving the child an SSRI.

There are a number of medications that are sometimes used to nonspecifically treat recurrent, "hot," maladaptive aggression. As per the 2003 "Treatment recommendations for the use of antipsychotics for aggressive youth" (TRAAY) guidelines, in the case of extreme reactive aggression (particularly with a dissociative or psychotic component) antipsychotics like risperidone may be helpful in reducing the extremes of aggression explosiveness. Since antipsychotics have significant side effects with long-term use, periodic monitoring is essential as well as repeated trials of discontinuing the medication after stabilization has occurred. Pappadopulos and colleagues have summarized that the alpha-agonists, lithium, and valproic acid are other medications with some demonstrated effectiveness in treating nonspecific, maladaptive "hot" aggression. Benzodiazepines, though sometimes given to treat an acute aggressive episode, are not preferred for long-term aggression care due to the tolerance and dependence that develop. Since each of these medications has significant risks to review and monitor carefully with long-term use, initiation of one of these medications should be done with great caution, and in the authors' opinion should be done only in the setting of a significant functional impairment.

Particularly when medications are prescribed in a symptom-focused, rather than diagnosis-focused, manner, children should be carefully monitored so as to stop any medication that fails to achieve the desired outcome. For symptom-focused indications, like reducing the frequency of impulsive aggression, one should establish the exact treatment targets ahead of time and monitor these targets carefully over time. If a medication fails to improve the targeted problem, which might be the average number of aggressive incidents per day, then the medication must be stopped. All too often, medications are continued indefinitely due to a compassionate desire to "do something" in the setting of recurrent aggression, despite the fact that these medicines either do not help or only yield a temporary benefit. With appropriate long-term monitoring, it is possible to use medications given as symptom-focused treatments safely and effectively.

Conclusions

Aggression is a common behavior in children that may be either adaptive or maladaptive in nature. Increasing understanding has led to categorization of aggression as "hot" versus "cold" and "direct" versus "indirect," distinctions that influence treatment planning. A wide variety of biologic, psychological, and social factors influence the expression of maladaptive aggression, and need to be considered in any treatment planning. Psychosocial treatments for aggression are strongly preferred over medication treatments, unless there is an underlying psychiatric diagnosis like ADHD or major depression for which a medication is indicated. In these cases, combined treatment with both medication and psychotherapy or behavioral training is considered the optimal approach. Vigorous treatment is indicated, as aggression in childhood is a risk for aggression throughout the lifespan.

CASE VIGNETTES

VIGNETTE 1: AN 8 YEAR OLD BOY WITH HOT AGGRESSION

Daniel is an 8-year-old boy who was recently suspended from school after an incident in math class when he suddenly started verbally abusing his teacher and several classmates. This escalated into him knocking over chairs and running out of the class into the hallway. At his pediatrician's, Daniel initially denied remembering what had triggered this behavior. Careful questioning, however, revealed that before this explosion, he had been doing a math problem on the board, which was too difficult for him to solve. After he got back to his desk, he felt like the classmates behind him were "snickering." That is when he felt like he "couldn't take it anymore" and started yelling.

Daniel had a normal birth and delivery, and early developmental milestones were on time. He has had no significant illnesses. He has always been a very active, intense, and "touchy" child who is forgetful and distractible, and does not adapt well to new situations. He has difficulty keeping friends due to getting angry when things do not go his way. Over the years, as his social isolation has grown, he has become a target of his peers, who often pick on him and tease him. His school performance has always been below what his parents believe he is capable of.

Daniel's aggression problems started in kindergarten; in the last year, however, aggression has escalated, and his parents are becoming increasingly concerned. Like the recent episode in math class, many of these aggressive episodes seem to be related to becoming frustrated with a situation. While he typically refuses to accept blame at the time of these incidents, often after he has calmed down, he will appear sad, apologize, and promise to be better.

Daniel's aggression is consistent with the "hot" aggression subtype. Daniel shows that he is having difficulty managing frustrations in his relationships and with school work (for which he may need extra assistance) without becoming aggressive. He may have a learning disability, a mood disorder, or an attention disorder that is contributing to his frustrations.

The provider recommended several things: (1) to investigate for ADHD through the use of symptom rating scales at home and school, (2) to request that the school evaluate him for a learning disability, (3) for mom to complete a CBCL general mental health questionnaire to look for likelihood of other disorders, and (4) to refer Daniel to a local child therapist for parenting assistance and help evaluate for treatable disorders.

Daniel was eventually diagnosed with ADHD and a nonverbal learning disability; he was enrolled in special education and had a trial of stimulant medication. Daniel's parents reported the stimulant medication reduced his explosiveness by about 50%. He was also diagnosed with ODD by his therapist. The therapist engaged the parents in parent-management training, which emphasized creating a consistent, structured, and predictable home environment with clear guidelines for expected behaviors and consequences. She also emphasized to the parents the importance of improving the quality of their relationship with Daniel and worked with the family in improving their emotional regulation and relationship skills by utilizing the work of John Gottman. The school implemented several special education modifications including having a tutor help Daniel with math. At a subsequent pediatrician visit 3 months later, the parents reported that though Daniel was still occasionally having bad days at school, overall things were better and he seemed much happier.

VIGNETTE 2: A 13 YEAR OLD BOY WITH COLD AGGRESSION

Gregory is a 13-year-old boy who, his mother says, has long-standing aggressive and anti-social behaviors. The most recent event occurred while at swimming lessons at the community swimming pool. According to one of the lifeguards, Gregory had loaned his swim goggles to another boy in exchange for getting to listen to a boy's iPod. Later, when the boy asked for his iPod back, Gregory refused to give it to him. The lifeguard intervened because of the argument, and the iPod was returned, but as the boy walked away, Gregory tripped him, causing him to hit his head on the concrete. When confronted, Gregory showed no concern for the boy's injury and denied tripping him. At home, Gregory continued to calmly stick to his version of what happened, and said that the boy deserved what happened anyway for "changing his mind about the trade." Gregory told the doctor that he did not have any problem with aggression and that the only problem was people are always treating him unfairly.

Gregory had a normal birth and delivery, and early developmental milestones were on time. His parents never lived together. During his early life, Gregory often was taken care of by his father's family as the mother was addicted to cocaine and the father was frequently in and out of jail. When Gregory was 5 years old, the mother succeeded in becoming sober and since then has been a responsible parent for him. From age 5 on, Gregory's mother noted he was aggressive with other children. She initially thought this was because Gregory had never had any consequences for his behaviors. Over the years, however, Gregory's mother has become more and more worried as Gregory has continued to show a disregard for rules and other people's feelings. He has frequently been in trouble for intentionally hurting and bullying peers, stealing, lying, leaving home and class without permission, and trying to con peers and adults. At school, teachers are frustrated that Gregory does not show remorse when others are hurt and with his nonchalant attitude toward negative consequences for misbehavior. Academically, they say he can "do the work when he chooses to," but add that he resents being told what to do and often complains of being bored with routine assignments.

Gregory's aggression is consistent with the "cold" aggression subtype. He shows callous-unemotional traits and little autonomic arousal, visible signs of fear, irritability, or anger when engaged in aggressive acts. He uses his aggression intentionally in order to obtain desired goals. It is possible that in his early years while he was not living in a consistent home environment, the primary way he got his needs met was through aggression, a lesson he has not been able to unlearn since. He also may have a biologic predisposition to having low physiologic arousal to emotional stimuli.

Gregory's pediatrician had Gregory's mother and teachers complete CBCL rating scales, which indicated his only clinically significant problems were with rule-breaking and aggressive behaviors. She referred Gregory to a child therapist, who identified these same areas of concern and diagnosed Gregory with a CD. The therapist initiated behavior therapy with Gregory, while Gregory's mother began parent-management training, which emphasized creating a consistent and structured home environment with clear guidelines for expected behaviors. The school chose to temporarily transfer Gregory to a self-contained classroom where his behavior could be monitored more closely. He also began attending a local youth center after school where he was able to begin taking boxing lessons. Despite these interventions, Gregory continued to have significant conduct problems, which led his therapist to seek additional social supports through a university-based MST program. With this additional family and community support, Gregory's behaviors began to be more socially appropriate, which eventually allowed him to be transferred back to the regular classroom setting and avoid being referred to the juvenile court system.

BIBLIOGRAPHY

Caspi A, McClay J, Moffitt TE, et al. Role of genotype in the cycle of violence in maltreated children. *Science.* 2002;297:851–854.

Connor DF. *Aggression and Antisocial Behavior in Children and Adolescents.* New York: The Guilford Press; 2002.

Fergusson DM, Horwood LJ, Ridder EM. Show me the child at seven: the consequence of conduct problems in childhood for psychosocial functioning in adulthood. *J Child Psychol Psychiatry.* 2005;46:837–849.

Hilt RJ, Woodward TA. Agitation treatment for pediatric emergency patients. *J Am Acad Child Adolesc Psychiatry.* 2008;47(2):132–137.

Lewis DO. From abuse to violence: psychophysiological consequences of maltreatment. *J Am Acad Child Adolesc Psychiatry.* 1992;31(3):383–391.

Lochman JE, Dodge KA. Social-cognitive processes of severely violent, moderately aggressive, and non-aggressive boys. *J Consult Clin Psychol.* 1994;62:366–374.

Pappadopulos E, MacIntyre JC, Crismon ML, et al. Treatment recommendations for the use of antipsychotics for aggressive youth (TRAAY), Part II. *J Am Acad Child Adolesc Psychiatry.* 2003;42:145–161.

Pappadopulos E, Woolston S, Chait A, et al. Pharmacotherapy of aggression in children and adolescents: efficacy and effect size. *J Am Acad Child Adolesc Psychiatry.* 2006;15(1): 27–39.

Patterson GR. *Coercive Family Process.* Eugene, OR: Castalia; 1982.

Satcher D. *Youth Violence: A Report of the Surgeon General,* 2001. Available at: http://www.surgeongeneral.gov/library/youthviolence/default.htm. Accessed June 1, 2009.

Seguin JR, Zelazo PD. Executive function in early physical aggression. In: Tremblay RE, Hartup WW, Archer J, eds. *Developmental Origins of Aggression.* New York: The Guilford Press; 2005.

Singer MI, Slovak K, Frierson T, et al. Viewing preferences, symptoms of psychological trauma, and violent behaviors among children who watch television. *J Am Acad Child Adolesc Psychiatry.* 1998;37:1041–1048.

Teplin LA, Abram KM, McClelland GM, et al. Psychiatric disorders in youth in juvenile detention. *Arch Gen Psychiatry.* 2002;59:1133–1143.

Tremblay RE, Nagin DS, Seguin JR, et al. Physical aggression during early childhood: trajectories and predictors. *Pediatrics.* 2004;114:e43–e50.

Vaillancourt T. Indirect aggression among humans: social construct or evolutionary adaptation? In: Tremblay RE, Hartup WW, Archer J, eds. *Developmental Origins of Aggression.* New York: The Guilford Press; 2005: 158–177.

Weisz JR, Hawley KM, Doss AJ. Empirically tested psychotherapies for youth internalizing and externalizing problems and disorders. *Child Adolesc Psychiatr Clin N Am.* 2004;13:729–815.

Widom CS. The cycle of violence. *Science.* 1989;244:160–166.

SUGGESTED READINGS FOR PARENTS

The Explosive Child
Author: Ross Greene, PhD
Publisher: Harper Paperbacks; 2005

1-2-3 Magic: Effective Discipline for Children 2–12
Author: Thomas Phelan, PhD
Publisher: Parent Magic, Inc.; 3rd edition, 2004

Parenting Your Out-of-Control Teenager: 7 steps to Reestablish Authority and Reclaim Love
Author: Scott P. Sells, PhD
Publisher: St. Martin's Griffin; 2002

Raising an Emotionally Intelligent Child
Author: John Gottman, PhD, and Joan Declaire
Publisher: Simon and Schuster; 1998

SUGGESTED READINGS FOR CLINICIANS

Aggression and Antisocial Behavior in Children and Adolescents
Author: Daniel F. Connor.
Publisher: The Guilford Press; 2002

SUGGESTED WEBSITE

American Academy of Child and Adolescent Psychiatry oppositional defiant disorder resources:
http://www.aacap.org/cs/ODD.ResourceCenter

REVIEW QUESTIONS

1. *Maladaptive* aggression is characterized by which of the following?
   a. Aggression of an inappropriate duration
   b. Aggression of an inappropriate intensity
   c. Aggression that leads to achieving a goal
   d. Both a and b

2. Which of the following statements about child aggression are true?
   a. More than 90% of childhood aggression relates to a psychiatric diagnosis.
   b. It is uncommon for children under 5 years old to be aggressive.
   c. Both juvenile justice and mental health systems address child aggression.
   d. Males are twice as likely as females to show either direct or indirect aggression.
   e. None of the above.

3. Which of the following are characteristics of "hot" aggression?
   a. Is usually a response to an actual or perceived attack or provocation
   b. Is more likely to respond to medications than is "cold" aggression
   c. Is associated with high central nervous system autonomic arousal and irritability
   d. All of the above

4. Which of the following are examples of *indirect* aggression?
   a. Physical assault
   b. Yelling at a peer
   c. Starting a false rumor about a peer
   d. Pouring water on someone's clothes

5. Which of the following psychiatric diagnoses are recognized to be associated with child aggression?
   a. Oppositional defiant disorder
   b. Conduct disorder
   c. Autistic spectrum disorder
   d. ADHD
   e. All of the above

Answers: 1-d, 2-c, 3-d, 4-c, 5-e

23

Ann Childers, MD

Nutritional Aspects of Psychiatric Disorders

Let food be thy medicine, and medicine thy food.—Hippocrates

Introduction

Nutrition, the keystone of life, is a frequently overlooked aspect of child and adolescent psychiatry, and medicine in general. Traditional foods that ensured health, fertility, and survival over millions of years, and that determined our modern genotype, are scarcely found on a modern American table. The burden of modern diet–related illness has created vast markets for the vitamin and mineral fortification of processed foods, nutrient supplements, and "neutraceuticals." These approaches do not entirely solve the problem, and may present new ones. Vitamins, minerals, and fatty acids work synergistically and in balance with one another. Too much of one nutrient may cause a deficiency of another. For example, too much zinc may result in a copper deficiency, and too much omega 6 essential fatty acid can result in a relative deficiency of omega 3 essential fatty acid. Furthermore, nutrients are best utilized by the body in the contexts from which they arise, from plants and animals with which humans evolved. While synthetic vitamins, chelated minerals, and nutrients extracted from foods in commercial settings have shown usefulness, they are less likely to be as safe and effective as nutrients acquired from a diet of whole foods.

The study of nutrition as it relates to mental health is at its embryonic stage, particularly as it relates to children and adolescents. The evidence base is limited, and most studies suffer from methodologic limitations. Nonetheless, field researchers persist in investigating the role of nutrition in health, the scientific literature is increasingly addressing how nutrition affects mental health, and emerging evidence leaves tantalizing clues as to how medical providers may benefit patients using promising approaches with a few to no side effects.

Given the scope and complexity of this important subject, not all aspects of nutrition and mental health can be addressed here. What follows is an overview of nutrition as it applies to the mental health of children and adolescents, with suggestions as to how the medical provider can use nutrition to augment psychiatric treatment.

Conduct Disorder and Antisocial Personality Disorder

General Background

Aggressive behaviors in children and adolescents are marked by irritability, restlessness, impulsivity, and a tendency toward violence. While such traits are observed in children and adolescents with conduct disorder, these traits overlap with other diagnoses of childhood and adolescence known as the disruptive behavior disorders, including attention deficit hyperactivity disorder (ADHD) and oppositional defiant disorder (ODD). The influence of nutrition on these conditions is just beginning to come into focus.

In 2002, a landmark study was published in the *British Journal of Psychiatry* by Bernard Gesch. "The Young Prisoners Study" reported that offenders were often inclined to choose foods lacking in essential nutrients which could influence their behaviors. Therefore, he conducted a double-blind, placebo-controlled study of the effect of dietary supplementation with physiologically adequate amounts of vitamins, minerals, and fatty acids. He divided a population of 231 prisoners ages of 18 and 21 years into two groups, one receiving placebo and one receiving a selection of vitamins, minerals, and fatty acids (here referred to as "nutrients") for 4 months. Investigators then tracked offenses among the inmates. At the conclusion of the study, prisoners receiving placebo showed no change in baseline behaviors, while prisoners receiving nutrients improved markedly. Among those receiving nutrients, there were 26% fewer violations overall, with serious breaches of conduct, including violence, reduced by 37%.

Iron Deficiency

Studies of specific nutritional deficiencies in conduct disorder are small, but the evidence that exists is intriguing. Iron is a mineral essential to brain health. It is a cofactor in the metabolism of tyrosine to dopamine and functions in the enzyme system involved in the production of serotonin, dopamine, norepinephrine, and epinephrine. Studies by Webb and Oski suggest that iron deficiency may play an important role in the aggressive behaviors and conduct disorder by male adolescents and Rosen has found iron deficiency among incarcerated adolescents to be nearly twice that found among nonincarcerated peers.

Hypoglycemia

Hypoglycemia has been linked to criminal and violent behavior. Studies from Finland report that criminals with a history of violence are more inclined to experience hypoglycemia, particularly when under the influence of alcohol, which enhances the action of insulin, further reducing blood sugar levels. By promoting high insulin levels, foods containing highly refined and processed starches and sugars have the potential to cause hypoglycemic symptoms 2 to 4 hours after they are ingested. This is most likely to occur when insulin remains in the bloodstream long after glucose has been metabolized, leading to a hypoglycemic "overshoot." The child or adolescent whose brain is starved for glucose may complain of hunger, blurred vision. He or she may exhibit slurred speech, irritability, and may act out aggressively.

Glycemic load is defined as an indicator of glucose response or insulin demand that is induced by total carbohydrate intake. There is a correlation between the glycemic load of a child's meals and snacks and the child's propensity for hypoglycemia. Fiber and fats, which modify glycemic loads, are frequently absent from cereals and snacks marketed to children. For example, when served with fat-free milk, highly refined boxed cereals are free to promote elevated blood sugar and hypoglycemic overshoots via the action of insulin produced in the pancreas. Teachers observe the resultant midmorning slump when children cannot attend to lessons and are inclined to misbehave.

The best approach is to serve meals and snacks that are balanced in terms of fat, complex carbohydrates, and protein. For example, a piece of whole-milk cheese, in which carbohydrate is combined with fat and protein, is a preferred snack choice to a primarily carbohydrate food, such as a cracker or an apple. The former choice holds greater potential to promote satiety and blood sugar stabilization over time. Fiber is also recognized for its ability to slow the release of sugar to the bloodstream, thereby stabilizing blood glucose as well; however, bran from most commercially processed whole grains is also high in phytates, which prevents the absorption of minerals from the diet. Fermenting (e.g., sourdough) and soaking ("sprouted") grains, nuts, beans, and lentils prior to cooking reduce the phytate content.

Grain, bean, and lentil products prepared in this fashion should be included as part of a healthy meal plan.

Hypocholesterolemia

The correlation of low total serum cholesterol levels and death from suicides and accidents in adults is well documented. Adult subjects with total cholesterol concentrations lower than 160 mg/dL are found to score higher on aggressive hostility, anxiety, phobia, and psychoticism in several studies. Similar trends appear in a recent study of youth. In a 2005 study of non-African American children, Zhang showed children and adolescents with low total serum cholesterol, defined as less than 145 mg/dL, displayed more violence and were nearly threefold more likely to be suspended from school than peers with higher cholesterol levels. From these findings, Zhang postulates that low total serum cholesterol is either a risk factor for aggression, or perhaps a risk marker for other biologic variables that predispose to aggression. Other investigators examining this issue speculate cholesterol modulates serotonin, and the absence of adequate cholesterol reduces serotonin availability.

Lithium

Lithium is the mineral salt best known to psychiatrists. First recognized in 1949 as a medical approach for bipolar disorder, lithium has since found a number of other psychiatric uses, including the management of anger in intermittent explosive disorder and as an adjunct to antidepressant treatment for major depressive disorder. Children with bipolar disorder, conduct disorder, and extremely aggressive behavior have been shown to improve with lithium treatment.

Lithium is found in a number of food sources, such as vegetables and grains. It is also found in the water supplies in many areas in the United States (US). The role, if any, that dietary lithium plays in humans is not entirely understood. During gestation, lithium concentrates in organs and, as gestation progresses, becomes less concentrated. Autopsy studies show lithium to be most concentrated in the cerebellum, followed by the cerebrum and the kidneys. Unexplained gender differences exist, with women concentrating 10% to 20% more lithium in the cerebrum and cerebellum than men.

The concentration of lithium in tissue and blood may impact human behavior. Dawson and colleagues examined the relationship between lithium in tap water and urine and found an inverse association with rates of psychiatric admissions and homicides. The lower the lithium levels in the water (and subsequently in the urine), the higher the rates of psychiatric problems and serious crimes. Other investigators have found similar results. Using crime rate data from 1978 to 1987, Schrauzer and Shrestha found highly significant inverse associations between water lithium levels and the rates of homicide, suicide, and forcible rape. Significant inverse associations were also found between water lithium levels and possession of narcotics, burglary, theft, and in juveniles, running away. Subsequently, they also found that the lithium content in the scalp hair of incarcerated violent criminals was lower than that of nonincarcerated controls. While these data do not demonstrate cause and effect, they suggest a role for lithium.

Omega 3 Essential Fatty Acids EPA and DHA

Fatty acid deficiencies are common in children with behavior and learning problems. Signs of fatty acid deficiency include thirst, frequent urination, rough, dry or scaly skin, dry, dull or "lifeless" hair, dandruff, and soft or brittle nails. Follicular karatosis, or hard, dry skin around hair follicles, are characteristic. Temper tantrums and sleep problems have been found on standardized rating scales to be more common in children with lower fatty acid concentrations.

Fatty acids are called "essential" if they cannot be manufactured by the body and need to be obtained exogenously. Ideally, the intake of omega 3 essential fatty acids is in balance with omega 6 essential fatty acids in ratios ranging from 1:1 to 1:4. But, the modern Western diet promotes an abundance of omega 6 fatty acids, from commercial vegetable oils and grain-fed livestock, with scant intake of omega 3 fatty acids from rich sources such as oils from wild (not farmed) fish, fats from wild game, and fats from pasture-finished livestock, including chickens and dairy animals. Modern trends in food production result in omega 3 to omega 6 essential fatty acids intake ratios that range from 1:13 to 1:20 in favor of omega 6.

Nutritionally adequate supplies of the omega 3 essential fatty acids eicosapentaenoic acid (EPA) and docosahexaenoic acid (DHA) can only be obtained from animal sources. While alpha linoleic acid (ALA), an essential fatty acid found in plants sources such as flaxseed, can be converted to EPA and DHA in humans, conversion is too limited to prevent deficiency. For this reason, vegan children and vegetarian children for whom fish or other rich animal sources are not included in meals are at particular risk for deficiencies in EPA and DHA.

Omega 3 essential fatty acids comprise as much as 30% of human neuronal membranes. The functions of omega 3 fatty acids are wide ranging and include neurotransmission enhancement, neuroprotection, and anti-inflammatory roles. Thus, in 2006, the American Psychiatric Association (APA) issued a consensus statement regarding the role of the omega 3 essential fatty acids EPA and DHA in mental health. The APA now recommends "Patients with mood, impulse control, or psychotic disorders should consume 1 g EPA + DHA per day." Fish oil supplements provide rich sources of omega 3 fatty acids. For children who do not swallow capsules well, flavored liquids, small flavored capsules, and chewable forms are available.

Side effects of fish oil are rare, and generally mild. The most common complaints are gastroesophageal reflux and belching. These side effects can usually be avoided by ensuring oils are fresh, cooling oil preparations in the refrigerator, and dosing at bedtime. The literature generally indicates that omega 3 essential fatty acids are safe for use in diabetics, but some data suggest they may alter glucose metabolism. There is one report of hypomania in a depressed adult who took 330 mg DHA and 220 mg EPA three times per day. Symptoms of hypomania resolved 2 days after discontinuation of DHA and EPA. While concerns have been raised as to the potential for bleeding and bruising, fish oil supplementation does not appear to be responsible in most cases. There is a report of an adult taking warfarin who experienced a significant change in coagulation status when fish oil was doubled from 1000 mg to 2000 mg per day; so caution should be exercised in patients taking anticoagulants.

Attention Deficit Hyperactivity Disorder

Attention deficit hyperactivity disorder (ADHD) has been related to a multitude of factors, including diet, sensitivities to food additives, heavy metal and other toxicities, low protein/high carbohydrate diets, mineral imbalances, essential fatty acid deficiencies, phospholipids deficits, amino acid deficits, thyroid disorders, vitamin B complex–related disorders, and phytochemicals. As attributions are numerous, many with scant scientific support, only a few key nutrients of interest will be discussed here.

Omega 3 Essential Fatty Acids EPA and DHA

More research exists on ADHD and essential fatty acids than any other nutrient. Interest in the role of these fatty acids in ADHD spans three decades and suggests that fatty acid deficiency may be common in people with ADHD and particularly affect their performance in the classroom. However, deficiencies have also been linked with behavior, learning, and health problems in boys both with and without a diagnosis of ADHD. Treating individuals with low omega-3 fatty acids with 1 g of EPA + DHA each day, as recommended by the APA, is unlikely to do harm, and may result in symptom improvement over subsequent months.

Additives and Preservatives

The notion that a link exists between consumption of food dyes and preservatives and hyper-activity has been resurrected in recent years. Most often derived from petroleum products and coal tar, brightly colored dyes are added to foods to give the impression of freshness, sweetness, and/or ripeness. Dyes in colors attractive to children are abundant in candy, gum, cereals, sport drinks, popsicles, gelatin, cookies, frostings, and many other food items. Swanson and Kinsbourne, citing the Food and Drug Administration (FDA), note that Americans now consume five times as much food dye as they did 30 years ago.

In 1973, Dr. Benjamin Feingold, a pediatric allergist, suggested that artificial food colorings caused hyperactivity in children. His theories ignited a firestorm of controversy in the US. It took another 30 years for researchers to confirm Dr. Feingold's suspicions. In 2004, Schab and Trinh performed a meta-analysis of previous studies and demonstrated that food colorings worsen hyperactivity in children with hyperactivity syndromes. Then, on September 6, 2007, the *Lancet* reported definitive findings from a double-blind, placebo-controlled study performed at the University of Southampton. In this study, 153 three-year-old and 144 eight- to nine-year-old normal children from a range of socioeconomic backgrounds had all artificial colors, flavors, and preservatives removed from their diets. Children in the active group were next presented with a challenge drink containing artificial food colorings and sodium benzoate, a preservative common to soft drinks and processed foods in the US. Included among these colorings were four common coal tar–derived azo dyes: Sunset yellow (F D & C Yellow # 6), Tartrazine (F D & C Yellow # 5), Quinoline yellow (F D & C Yellow # 10), and Allura red AC (F D & C Red # 40). The addition of food colorings to sodium benzoate was significantly associated with hyperactivity in this normal population of children. In light of this study, Dubik noted in the *AAP Grand Rounds*, "Thus, the overall findings of the study are clear and require that even we skeptics, who have long doubted parental claims of the effects of various foods on the behavior of their children, admit we might have been wrong." They recommended "a trial of a preservative-free, food-coloring-free diet is a reasonable intervention" for hyperactive children.

Iron Deficiency

Symptoms of iron deficiency can mimic ADHD, or complicate its treatment. Iron deficiency in the US is common and appears to be on the increase, despite iron fortification of cereals and other foods. As reported by Looker in 2002, data from the National Health and Nutrition Examination Survey (NHANES) 1999–2000 reveal that iron deficiency affects from 1 in 20 to 1 in 14 children between the ages of 1 and 11 years. Adolescent girls tend to be more affected than boys, with 9% of 12- to 15-year-olds and 16% of 16- to 19-year-olds affected. Children who are iron deficient, with or without anemia, experience cognitive and behavioral difficulties that may interfere with normal development. Iron deficiency renders affected individuals more susceptible to absorption of lead and cadmium; the presence of pica heightens this risk. Additionally, symptoms of lead toxicity overlap with symptoms of ADHD. Iron deficiency is more common among adolescent girls after menarche, particularly when menorrhagia is present. Athletes and the obese are also at particular risk. Children and adolescents deficient in iron may complain of fatigue, poor concentration, and impulsivity along with a decline in school performance. Iron deficiency may be accompanied by involuntary limb movements during sleep (nocturnal myoclonus) and restless legs syndrome (RLS), which erodes the quality of sleep. Children affected by these conditions are frequently hyperactive and impulsive in the classroom as they struggle to remain alert. Iron-deficient adolescents may decline in scholastic and athletic performance, as well as exhibit conduct problems.

Some studies suggest iron deficiency is prevalent among children and adolescents with ADHD. Konofal and colleagues measured ferritin levels of 53 children and young adolescents diagnosed with ADHD who had been medication-free for 2 months. They found ferritin levels to be abnormally low (average of 22 ng/mL) in 84% of the ADHD population and only 18% of controls (average of 44 ng/mL). One third of the iron-deficient ADHD population had extremely low levels of serum ferritin. Furthermore, lower ferritin levels corresponded with more severe ADHD symptoms per a standardized ADHD rating scale.

Preliminary studies also show restoring iron decreases ADHD symptoms in children who are iron deficient. In a 2005 case study, Konofal and colleagues described an iron-deficient (serum ferritin 13 ng/mL), but not anemic (Hgb 12.9 mg/dL), 3-year-old male with symptoms of ADHD and disturbed sleep. After 8 months of iron supplementation, ferritin increased to 102 ng/mL and the child's ADHD symptoms improved per parent's and teacher's scores on standardized ADHD rating scales. Sleep also improved. In 2008, these investigators conducted a similar intervention for 23 nonanemic but iron-deficient (ferritin levels <30 ng/mL) children of ages 5 to 8 years who met the criteria for ADHD. In this placebo-controlled study, 18 children received 80 mg oral iron sulfate per day over 12 weeks, while 5 children received a placebo. After 12 weeks, the children receiving iron supplementation showed significant decreases in ADHD symptoms compared to their controls as measured by standardized rating scales; decreases reportedly comparable to treatment with stimulants. These preliminary studies are worth taking seriously. When the lower limit of ferritin is defined as 30 ng/mL or higher, children evaluated for ADHD appear to be at increased risk for iron deficiency. Additionally, restless leg syndrome (RLS) is frequently comorbid with ADHD. According to the American Academy of Family Physicians, iron deficiency plays a role in RLS as well, and persons with ferritin levels less than 50 ng/mL are at heightened risk. Given this, it seems reasonable to investigate iron stores in children and adolescents evaluated for ADHD. Where suspicion of iron deficiency is low, children and adolescents with presumed ADHD may undergo an initial screening with a serum ferritin and a C-reactive protein (CRP). If ferritin is above 50 ng/mL but CRP is high, the ferritin value may be falsely elevated due to inflammation. In this case, further laboratory investigation into iron status is appropriate. Where suspicion of iron deficiency is high, obtaining an iron panel along with ferritin and CRP is recommended. Recommended dietary allowances for iron are presented in Table 23.1.

Zinc

According to the US Department of Agriculture (USDA), zinc deficiency is common; up to 62% of young children in the US do not get enough zinc in their diets. Zinc is important for various aspects of cellular metabolism. Without adequate zinc, neurotransmitter synthesis is

TABLE 23-1	Recommended Dietary Allowances for Iron for Infants, Children, Adolescents, and Adults			
Age	Males (mg/day)	Females (mg/day)	Pregnancy (mg/day)	Lactation (mg/day)
7 to 12 months	11	11	N/A	N/A
1 to 3 years	7	7	N/A	N/A
4 to 8 years	10	10	N/A	N/A
9 to 13 years	8	8	N/A	N/A
14 to 18 years	11	15	27	10
19 to 50 years	8	18	27	9
51+ years	8	8	N/A	N/A

Source: Dietary Supplement Fact Sheet: Iron Office of Dietary Supplements—National Institutes of Health—http://ods.od.nih.gov/factsheets/iron.asp.

TABLE 23-2	Recommended Dietary Allowances for Zinc for Infants, Children, Adolescents, and Adults			
Age	Male	Female	Pregnancy	Lactation
Birth to 6 months	2 mg^a	2 mg^a		
7 month to 3 years	3 mg	3 mg		
4 to 8 years	5 mg	5 mg		
9 to 13 years	8 mg	8 mg		
14 to 18 years	11 mg	9 mg	13 mg	14 mg
19+ years	11 mg	8 mg	11 mg	12 mg

^{a}Adequate intake (AI).

Source: Institute of Medicine, Food and Nutrition Board. Dietary Reference Intakes for Vitamin A, Vitamin K, Arsenic, Boron, Chromium, Copper, Iodine, Iron, Manganese, Molybdenum, Nickel, Silicon, Vanadium, and Zinc. Washington, DC: National Academy Press, 2001.

compromised. Several controlled studies show that a deficiency of zinc is associated with ADHD, which improves when zinc sulfate supplements are provided. Animal proteins, including beef, lamb, pork, crabmeat, turkey, chicken, lobster, clams and salmon, are the richest and most bioavailable dietary sources of zinc. Infants and children are at particular risk for zinc deficiency when diets are poor in meat. While plant sources are common, absorption and utilization of zinc from these sources is poor. Also, diets high in phytates, such as high plant fiber diets, are also shown to enhance the elimination of diet-acquired zinc, increasing the likelihood of deficiency. There appears to be at least one food-coloring connection to zinc deficiency as well. In 1990, Neil Ward showed that children with ADHD lose zinc when exposed to the food dye tartrazine (FD & C Yellow #5).

Zinc supplements should be used with caution as copper and zinc are maintained in the body in equilibrium and an oversupply of zinc may result in low copper status. Too much zinc also results in altered iron function, reduced immune function, and reduced levels of high-density lipoproteins (HDLs). Zinc can be found in most multiple vitamin and mineral supplements. A standard children's multiple vitamin can be used as a zinc supplement so long as manufacturers balance the mineral content. Recommended dietary allowances for zinc are provided in Table 23.2.

Magnesium

The fourth most abundant mineral in the human body, magnesium plays a major role in neurotransmitter synthesis. It is involved in hundreds of enzymatic processes that support healthy development involving both structure (e.g., bones) and function (e.g., muscle and nerve performance) of bodily function. Magnesium assists in proteins synthesis and is involved in carbohydrate metabolism, blood pressure control, and immune function. Magnesium is a vital component of virtually every aspect of the body.

Magnesium deficiency has been linked to multiple conditions. In 1997, Kozielec found signs of magnesium deficiency in children with ADHD compared with healthy controls. In 2002, Grimaldi reviewed the relevant literature and concluded that magnesium deficiency may be the central and common pathway resulting in Tourette syndrome and comorbid conditions, including, but not limited to, asthma, ADHD, obsessive–compulsive disorder, anxiety, depression, migraine, self-injurious behavior, rages, seizure, heart arrhythmia, sensitivity to sensory stimuli, and an exaggerated startle response.

Magnesium deficiency is characterized by tension, agitation, nervous excitability, stress, tremors, tics, and fatigue. Latent tetany is a feature of magnesium deficiency, and children and adolescents with this condition may experience muscle tension with soreness, and bruxism. Magnesium is important for muscle relaxation. Muscle dysfunction arising from a deficiency in this mineral may extend to the gastrointestinal system, leading to a poor appetite. Impaired peristalsis associated with constipation is not uncommon and magnesium deficiency should be considered in the differential diagnosis of children with a history of frequent vomiting, gastritis and/or encopresis with constipation. Hypo- or hyperglycemia, tremors, weakness, fatigue, muscle cramps in lower extremities, involuntary muscle contractions, numbness, and tingling may signal magnesium deficiency. In rare events in which magnesium deficiency progresses to a severe degree, personality changes may occur, with seizures and arrhythmias in later stages.

Nutrient-dilute diets high in refined starches and sugars and low in whole food magnesium sources incline children and adolescents toward magnesium deficiency, as do psychotropic medications that enhance the release of catecholamines. The association of heavy alcohol use with magnesium deficiency is well known. The desirable ratio of intake of calcium to magnesium is about 2:1; an imbalance of intake favoring an excess of calcium also hastens magnesium deficiency via an increased catecholamine release. Anxious children and children enduring excessive environmental stress require more magnesium than calmer children; inadequate stores impose additional stress with enhanced release of catecholamines, resulting in a vicious cycle that promotes further stress and deficiency.

Routine serum magnesium laboratory test is an unreliable estimate of magnesium stores. Hypokalemia raises suspicions for hypomagnesemia, as up to 60% of patients with hypomagnesemia are also hypokalemic. A red blood cell (RBC) magnesium test is a fair estimate of body magnesium stores, but normal RBC magnesium levels do not rule out hypomagnesemia. Perhaps the most accurate way to gauge magnesium is via the magnesium-loading test. This test requires a baseline 24-hour urine sample, followed by an injection of magnesium, and repeat of the 24-hour urine. While more accurate, this latter method is not a popular choice for reasons of inconvenience, and in the case of children, involvement of a needle poke.

For the child or adolescent with a history suggestive of magnesium deficiency and whose kidney function is within normal limits, it is not unreasonable to begin a trial of a magnesium supplement in the absence of laboratory testing. There are many adequate over-the-counter formulations on the market. Magnesium-citrate, -malate, -taurinate, and -glycinate are among the best-studied formulations. Magnesium hydroxide is less desirable as it is not well absorbed and may result in diarrhea. Slow-release preparations containing calcium in a 2:1 ratio with magnesium work well for many children, particularly those with poor calcium intakes. Warm baths in Epsom salts a few times a week encourage skin absorption of magnesium, and can be relaxing before bedtime. Daily bathing in Epsom salts should be avoided, however, to prevent drying of skin. Recommended dietary allowances for magnesium are provided in Table 23.3.

TABLE 23-3	Recommended Dietary Allowances for Magnesium for Toddlers, Children, Adolescents, and Adults			
Age (years)	Male (mg/day)	Female (mg/day)	Pregnancy (mg/day)	Lactation (mg/day)
1–3	80	80	N/A	N/A
4–8	130	130	N/A	N/A
9–13	240	240	N/A	N/A
14–18	410	360	400	360
19–30	400	310	350	310

Source: Institute of Medicine. Food and Nutrition Board. Dietary Reference Intakes: Calcium, Phosphorus, Magnesium, Vitamin D and Fluoride. National Academy Press. Washington, DC, 1999.

In physically healthy children and adolescents, loose stools are the most common limiting factor when dosing a magnesium supplement. Less commonly, nausea and vomiting may occur, particularly if the dose is given on an empty stomach. Using the guidance in Table 23.3, the practitioner may wish to give the full daily requirement of magnesium at night, to encourage relaxation and sleep, or if this is not tolerated, divide the daily requirement into twice daily dosing. Magnesium can be taken with food which may prevent nausea. Magnesium should be given cautiously to patients with poor kidney function as it can accumulate to toxic levels. Adding vitamin B_6 in a daily multiple vitamin assists with absorption and utilization of magnesium. While complete results take weeks to months to realize, improvement in many symptoms of magnesium deficiency occur within days of starting repletion therapy.

General Recommendations for Disruptive Behavior Disorders

When children and adolescents present for evaluation of disruptive behavior disorders, it is helpful to obtain a general idea of diet, including all meals and snacks. Nutritionally oriented laboratory tests may include serum ferritin level with CRP, and an RBC magnesium level. If the ferritin level is low, a serum lead level could be considered. If cholesterol is low, investigation of thyroid function may be warranted as hyperthyroidism can lower cholesterol and induce psychiatric symptoms such as hyperactivity and mania. Celiac disease can also lower cholesterol via malabsorption; children and adolescents with this condition may also present with psychiatric symptoms, including disruptive behaviors.

In general, children and adolescents with disruptive behavior disorders such as ADHD should eat balanced meals and avoid sugar-sweetened beverages. In 2009, Johnson summarized a statement from the American Heart Association (AHA) noting that these beverages are the primary source of added sugars in Americans' diets, "Excessive consumption of sugars has been linked with several metabolic abnormalities and adverse health conditions, as well as shortfalls of essential nutrients." Per the NHANES III, the AHA reports that the average American consumes 22 teaspoons sugar daily, with 14- to 18-year-olds consuming a whopping average of 34.3 teaspoons per day. The AHA recommends that children ages 4 to 8 years consume no more than three teaspoons of added sugar from all sources (e.g., catsup, hamburger buns) for every 1600 calories consumed. By comparison, one 12-oz. can of soda pop contains the equivalent of 10 teaspoons or more.

Breakfast should be a daily event, as it protects against the decline of attention in the morning. David Benton and colleagues monitored children's ability to concentrate on work in the classroom. Children who ate breakfast or received a midmorning snack were better able to attend to their work than those who did not eat in the morning.

Strive to eliminate "empty calorie" foods and beverages high in refined sugars, starches, colorings, additives, and preservatives. A good rule of thumb is, if it causes tooth decay it should be eaten sparingly and with caution. There should be a complete protein source at every meal. Eggs are a good example, as they are inexpensive and hold the highest biological value for protein. Meats, fish, and poultry are recommended as well. While milk, soy, and eggs are convenient sources of protein, they interfere with iron absorption and should not be served in the same meal with red meats. Because most modern soy products (e.g., tofu) interfere with absorption of a broad range of minerals and can interfere with thyroid function in susceptible individuals, it is recommended that soy products be served sparingly. The iron bioavailability of green vegetables is heightened when they are cooked in cast iron, combined with ascorbic acid (vitamin C), and/or combined with red meat. Salads and whole-grain breads relinquish fat-soluble vitamins A, K, and E more easily when accompanied by fats such as dairy butter and extra virgin olive oil. Among breads, sourdough and sprouted grain breads are recommended as the involved fermenting and/or sprouting may promote favorable blood sugar levels.

Probiotic organisms are essential to digestion and the absorption of nutrients by the gut. Probiotics do not remain in the gut indefinitely and must be replenished each day. Children and adolescents can obtain healthy bacteria from foods containing live cultures, such as yogurt, kefir, and other lacto-fermented foods. Probiotics may be taken in pill form as well.

It is recommended that children and adolescents not be restricted in terms of natural (not highly processed) dietary fats and cholesterol from whole foods. Nonoxidized natural fats and cholesterol are essential to healthy development. Consumption of nutritional fats begins in infancy with mother's milk which is rich in nonoxidized cholesterol, and delivers about 50% of its energy as fats. For growing children and adolescents, a diet consisting of 40% fat can be encouraged. It has been demonstrated that children on low-fat diets may consume significantly less energy, up to 25% less, resulting in short stature and inadequate nutrient intake. Fats are required for absorption of fat-soluble vitamins and minerals necessary for growth and development; and, as previously discussed, fats moderate the glycemic loads of carbohydrates. Highly processed, oxidized, and hydrogenated fats, partially hydrogenated vegetable oils (trans fats), and oxidized cholesterol found in processed foods, along with oils processed at high temperatures, are shown to increase oxidative stress, denature neuronal membranes, and promote chronic illness. Such denatured fats and cholesterols should be avoided.

A daily multivitamin with extra vitamin D is included as part of the Healthy Eating Food Pyramid proposed by Harvard School of Public Health. Although food is the preferred source of nutrients, a daily tablet of a standard multiple vitamin with minerals can provide added insurance against deficiencies. If a child is not iron deficient, a preparation without iron is preferred. Essential fatty acids are important as well. One to two grams of fish oil per day can be recommended safely in most cases.

Mood and Anxiety Disorders

While disorders of mood and anxiety are distinct, they share overlapping clinical presentations and biological underpinnings. Nutritional considerations are similar for both, and for this reason they will be combined together under this section.

Caffeine and Theobromine

Caffeine consumption may contribute to negative affective states in young people, including arousal, irritability, interference with sleep. In her 2008 study of depressed youth, Whalen found that caffeine exacerbated youth's anxiety. Caffeine withdrawal has also been associated with negative affect. Caffeine is hidden in unexpected places, such as noncola soda pop, coffee-flavored ice cream, energy jerky, energy gum, and some types of candy. Chocolate is another stimulant common to foods. While most chocolate contains little caffeine, it contains theobromine. The darker the chocolate, the higher the theobromine concentration.

Vitamin B$_{12}$ and Folate

Perhaps the best-studied nutrients in relationship to depression are the B vitamins. A deficiency of folate and vitamin B$_{12}$ (also known as cobalamin) are correlated with depression in the general population. Folate and vitamin B$_{12}$ are major determinants of one-carbon metabolism, in which S-adenosylmethionine (SAM) is formed. SAM donates methyl groups that are crucial for neurological function. For example, B$_{12}$ and folate are active in the formation of neurotransmitters, phospholipids that are a component of neuronal myelin sheaths, and cell receptors. B$_{12}$ also functions in folate metabolism, and a deficiency in B$_{12}$ can result in a secondary folate deficiency. B$_{12}$ deficiency may be accompanied by a number of psychiatric manifestations, including irritability, personality changes, depression, and psychosis. Children and adolescents who are obese, who have eating disorders and/or are vegetarian are at particular risk for B_{12} deficiencies. The richest sources of B_{12} are meats from fish and animals, particularly mollusks and organ meats. While less-robust, fortified cereals are important sources of B_{12} for vegetarians. Adequate absorption of B_{12} relies on a healthy, functioning digestive system. In the stomach, in the presence of hydrochloric acid and protease (protein-splitting) enzymes, B_{12} is split from proteins in foods. Once released, B_{12} attaches to intrinsic factor to form a complex that can be absorbed by the digestive tract.

If deficiency is suspected, a B_{12} level can be drawn. If the level is abnormally low, the child or adolescent can be treated with B_{12}; but, if it is in the low-normal range, and if the patient has healthy renal function, drawing a serum methylmalonic acid (MMA) level can clarify whether the patient is deficient. A high MMA indicates B_{12} deficiency, but the magnitude does not correlate with the severity of deficiency. In patients with impaired renal function, MMA accumulates in the blood, resulting in a chronically high level irrespective of B_{12} status.

There are several ways to replete vitamin B_{12}. While effective, the injectable form will raise objections from young patients. Oral B_{12} is available. Nasal mists such as CaloMist and Nascobal are usually well tolerated and are available by prescription. A transdermal patch is also available. Therapeutic noninjectable doses tend to be higher than doses delivered by injection, as far less B_{12} from noninjectable forms actually reach the bloodstream.

Folate deficiency has long been linked to depression in the general population. Folate is actively involved in the synthesis of monoamine neurotransmitters. Liver is a robust natural source of folate. Other natural sources include, but are not limited to, beans, legumes, and green vegetables. Synthetic folate can be found in fortified foods and multiple vitamins. Recommended dietary allowances of B_{12} are presented in Table 23.4.

Iron

Children with depressive symptoms should be screened for iron deficiency, as symptoms of iron deficiency in children and adolescents overlap with symptoms of depression. Children and adolescents with iron deficiency alone without anemia may experience impaired cognitive functioning and memory, decreased athletic performance, a decline in school performance and lowered endurance. As iron deficiency approaches anemia, symptoms may also include, but are not limited to, fatigue, lethargy, disturbed sleep, depressed mood, and headaches.

Magnesium

As previously mentioned, low intakes of magnesium are widespread in the US, affecting as much as 70% of the population. When compounded by excess calcium and stress, a dietary magnesium deficiency may cause insomnia, agitation, anxiety, confusion, irritability, weakness,

TABLE 23-4	Recommended Dietary Allowances for Vitamin B_{12} for Children, Adolescents, and Adults		
Age (years)	Males and Females (µg/day)	Pregnancy (µg/day)	Lactation (µg/day)
1–3	0.9	N/A	N/A
4–8	1.2	N/A	N/A
9–13	1.8	N/A	N/A
14–18	2.4	2.6	2.8
19 and older	2.4	2.6	2.8

Source: Institute of Medicine. Food and Nutrition Board. Dietary Reference Intakes: Thiamin, riboflavin, niacin, vitamin B_6, folate, vitamin B_{12}, pantothenic acid, biotin, and choline. National Academy Press. Washington, DC, 1998.

and in severe cases, hallucinations. By addressing intraneuronal magnesium deficits, restoring magnesium may assist in resolving symptoms of depression and anxiety.

Omega 3 Essential Fatty Acids EPA and DHA

Preliminary studies of the omega 3 essential fatty acids EPA and DHA show promise as an adjunct for treatment of affective disorders in adults, including bipolar disorder and major depressive disorder. Few such studies in children and adolescents exist, but preliminary reports are intriguing. Nemets and colleagues in 2006 studied a population of 20 children between the ages of 6 and 12 years with major depressive disorder. Ten received omega 3 fatty acids and 10 received placebo. After 1 month of treatment, 7 out of 10 children receiving omega 3 fatty acids had a greater than 50% reduction in depression symptoms on standardized rating scales. While there was modest improvement in the placebo group, none had a 50% reduction in symptoms. At study exit, four children receiving omega 3 fatty acids reached full remission of depression, while no child in the placebo group remitted.

Vitamin D

As mentioned, deficiencies in Vitamin D may be related to psychological problems like seasonal affective disorder (SAD), depression, and other disorders. The psychiatric effects of vitamin D deficiency may be moderated through the parathyroid. When vitamin D is low, parathyroid hormone (PTH) becomes elevated. Studies in adults show PTH is at its ideal physiologic concentration when serum vitamin D levels are at 32 ng/mL or greater. As vitamin D levels decline below this point, PTH levels rise. Depending on the severity, an increase in PTH places patients at various risks for psychiatric problems such as dementia, depression, psychosis, and anxiety that are related to PTH, and resolve when PTH is corrected. Those with excessive secretion of PTH (hyperparathyroidism) have abnormally high blood levels of calcium and may complain of fatigue, lethargy, and memory problems.

Children and adolescents taking anticonvulsant drugs appear to be at increased risk for vitamin D deficiency. For example, the anticonvulsant phenytoin is known to increase the clearance of a number of vitamin D metabolites and to induce vitamin D deficiency. Patients who are taking phenytoin and/or phenobarbital are at risk for bone fractures due to low levels of vitamin D. In a controlled study by Riancho, blood levels of vitamin D in children taking anticonvulsants were dramatically lower in winter months. Bone strength has been shown to be increased in children taking anticonvulsant drugs who were supplemented with an activated form of vitamin D and calcium over 9 months.

Children and adolescents with vitamin D deficiency may be depressed and/or anxious and fatigued. They may complain of bone pain and joint aches. Some complain of sternal tenderness with point pressure due to osteomalacia. They may have periodontal bleeding with brushing. In fact, the NHANES II found an inverse correlation between serum vitamin D concentrations and periodontal disease in adults. Vitamin D also affects the skin. The faces of people with vitamin D deficiency often appear pale, which improves once vitamin D is restored. Screening for vitamin D deficiency can be done during a well-child examination, or as part of a psychiatric assessment. Screening consists of obtaining a serum 25 hydroxyvitamin D (25(OH)D) level and serum calcium. If calcium is elevated, the child should not receive vitamin D treatment until the underlying cause is ascertained and treated. The optimal serum range for vitamin D is 50 to 80 ng/mL. Serum vitamin D values below 40 ng/mL or above 100 ng/mL deserve attention. If vitamin D is at or slightly above 100 ng/mL, serum calcium is normal and the individual does not take vitamin D supplements or eat vitamin D–rich foods (e.g., liver), but spends considerable time in the sun, there is probably no concern. However, if the level is elevated and the individual takes supplements, the practitioner should examine the supplement types and sources, and advise cutting back vitamin D intake until levels reach the optimal range.

TABLE 23-5	Essentials of Nutritional Assessment

- Take a nutritional history. Interview parents and children about children's eating habits at home, school, and in other environments. Determine how much chocolate and caffeine the child obtains from all sources, and at what times of the day.
- Ask parents and children about food allergies, and whether they notice emotional and/or behavioral changes, for better or worse, when children eat certain foods. The family's observation that some foods impact emotions and behavior will assist with engagement and compliance when you make dietary recommendations later.
- Inquire as to the child's medical history. Is the child a picky eater? Does the child have a history of weight loss, chronic illness, diarrhea, or malabsorption? Has the child been iron deficient or anemic in the past? Is menorrhagia present? Has there been a recent surgery? Does the child have an eating disorder? Is the child vegetarian or vegan?
- Obtain height, weight, and Body Mass Index (BMI), and document these on growth charts. Observe and document the child's body habitus in the mental status examination.
- Include serum ferritin plus CRP, and 25(OH)Vitamin D plus calcium in the initial laboratory workup. You may wish to consider an RBC magnesium test as well.
- If the child is vegetarian or vegan, obtain a blood sample for a B_{12} and/or methylmalonic acid test.
- For younger children with histories of anemia and/or low ferritin levels, consider testing for lead.

Conclusions

The evolving field of nutrition is just beginning to find its place in mental health. Emerging evidence shows that modern processed and denatured foods with artificial additives take their toll on both physical and mental health. Children and adolescents require nutrient-dense intakes to accomplish healthy development, yet foods marketed to this population are among the most processed, chemical-laden, and least nourishing. Medical practitioners are in a unique position to educate families to reverse this trend, endowing lifelong mental and physical benefits to our young patients and their families. The essentials of nutritional assessment are summarized in Table 23.5, and the essentials of nutritional treatment are summarized in Table 23.6.

TABLE 23-6	Essentials of Nutritional Treatment

- Educate parents about the importance of nutrition to their child's mental health. Teach parents and children the elements of a balanced diet plan.
- Encourage parents to avoid artificial food additives, including preservatives, flavor enhancers, and colorings. Recommend they shop the perimeter of the grocery store to avoid processed foods. Whole foods, with plentiful vegetables, some fruits and whole (not fat-free or low-fat) natural protein sources are best.
- Provide standard written materials regarding the nature of a nutritious diet.
- Encourage parents to avoid processed foods and return to a diet of whole foods. Suggest slow food conveniences such as a crockpot to ease preparation.
- Parents should involve their children in family meals, and demonstrate healthy eating. Encourage parents to shop with their children, allowing children to choose fruits and vegetables to eat at mealtimes. Parents can have their children assist with meal preparation. Growing a family garden and/or visiting local farms will enhance the child's food education.
- As a general approach for children not allergic to fish: recommend daily fish oil to provide 1 g EPA + DHA per day. This may be given at bedtime.
- One standard iron-free multiple vitamin and mineral supplement per day can be recommended. Look for vitamin tablets without artificial colors.

CASE VIGNETTES

VIGNETTE 1: TRACIE, A PRESCHOOLER WITH HYPERACTIVITY RESPONSIVE TO IMPROVED NUTRITION

Tracie is a 3 year and 2 month old white female who presents for a complaint of hyperactivity. She is accompanied by her 25-year-old mother. In addition to her hyperactivity and impulsivity necessitating an Individual Education Plan through her school district, Tracie's developmental history is significant for her mother's iron deficiency anemia during her second and third trimester. Her mother complains that Tracie sleeps only a few hours a night. On more than one occasion she escaped from the house and was found on a busy street. Her mother now uses a harness and tether to keep her daughter with her. She describes a diet rich in carbohydrates, sugar, and food coloring, with little protein and low in natural dietary fats and cholesterol. On examination the child appears well developed, well nourished, of normal weight and with pallor. She is hypermotoric and curious, opening drawers, grabbing the computer keyboard and mouse, reaching for computer keys, touching whatever interests her in the moment. When commanded by her mother, Tracie sits a moment but then moves on to something else. Eye contact is fleeting, but better maintained with her mother than with the examiner. Language is articulate and logical but sparse. Laboratory assessment was ordered to determine ferritin and lead levels. A whole foods diet was recommended beginning with eggs each morning. For sleep, melatonin 3 mg by mouth at bedtime was prescribed. At a follow-up visit 2 weeks later, the mother notes that her daughter sleeps through the night, and can sit on her lap and maintain attention throughout their reading of a book. While Tracy remains more active than other children her age, she is more easily redirected. Her use of language is increased; she is more interpersonally interactive, and asks more questions. The laboratory assessment showed that Tracie was iron deficient (ferritin 20 ng/mL), but not lead toxic. Therefore, her pediatrician started iron repletion therapy.

VIGNETTE 2: COREY, A SCHOOL-AGED CHILD WITH VITAMIN AND MINERAL DEFICIENCY

Corey is a 9-year-old African American male admitted to psychiatric residential treatment with diagnoses of ADHD and conduct disorder and restless legs syndrome. The stimulant dose needed to adequately control his symptoms of ADHD is higher than what would be predicted by his weight. He presents with holes in the upper part of his shirt, which he chews over the course of a day. The hospital staff observes that he chews other nonfood items as well, such as paper, pencils, and pens. His mood is depressed and he appears anxious. Prior to admission he describes a diet of chips, sweetened caffeinated sodas, starchy entrees and snack foods, with little in the way of produce or proteins. He spends most of his time indoors. He complains of insomnia. He appears well developed and of normal weight, but with translucent-appearing skin. There is tenderness with sternal pressure suggestive of osteomalacia. Conjunctiva are pale. Laboratory assessment includes 25(OH)Vitamin D, calcium complete blood count (CBC), and ferritin. The 25(OH)Vitamin D is significantly deficient at 12 ng/mL, and ferritin suggests iron deficiency (15 ng/mL). CBC is within normal limits. Vitamin D repletion regimen is put in place and his pediatrician determines that his iron deficiency is dietary and begins iron repletion. While receiving meals in residential treatment, his overall nutrition improves. Within 3 months, Corey no longer chews nonfood items. His skin is a rich dark color and his bone tenderness is resolved. He appears calmer, more relaxed. Sleep is improved. His stimulant dose is lowered to the dose expected for weight. Within 8 months, teachers note that his concentration is improved. His parents notice a positive change in his demeanor.

BIBLIOGRAPHY

Arnold LE, DiSilvestro RA. Zinc in attention-deficit/hyperactivity disorder. *J Child Adolesc Psychopharmacol.* 2005;15:619–627.

Bayard M, Avonda T, Wadzinski J. Restless Legs Syndrome. *Am Fam Physician.* 2008;78:235–243.

Benton D, Maconie A, Williams C. The influence of the glycaemic load of breakfast on the behaviour of children in school. *Physiol Behav.* 2007;92:717–724.

Burgess JR, Stevens L, Zhang W, et al. Long-chain polyunsaturated fatty acids in children with attention deficit hyperactivity disorder. *Am J Clin Nutr.* 2000;71:327–330.

Dawson EB, Moore TD, McGanity WJ. Relationship of lithium metabolism to mental hospital admission and homicide. *Dis Nerv Syst.* 1972;33:546–556.

Dietrich T, Joshipura KJ, Dawson-Hughes B, et al. Association between serum concentrations of 25-hydroxyvitamin D_3 and periodontal disease in the US population. *Am J Clin Nutr.* 2004;80:108–113.

Dubik M. Food colorings, preservatives, and hyperactivity. *AAP Grand Rounds.* 2004;12:54–55.

Etcheverry P, Hawthorne KM, Liang LK, et al. Effect of beef and soy proteins on the absorption of non-heme iron and inorganic zinc in children. *J Am Coll Nutr.* 2006; 25:34–40.

Gesch CB, Hammond SM, Hampson SE, et al. Influence of supplementary vitamins, minerals and essential fatty acids on the antisocial behaviour of young adult prisoners: randomized, placebo-controlled trial. *Br J Psychiatry.* 2002;181:22–28.

Golomb BA, Stattin H, Mednick S. Low cholesterol and violent crime. *J Psychiatr Res.* 2000;34:301–309.

Grantham-McGregor S, Ani C. A review of studies on the effect of iron deficiency on cognitive development in children. *J Nutr.* 2001;131:649S–668S.

Grimaldi BL. The central role of magnesium deficiency in Tourette's syndrome: causal relationships between magnesium deficiency, altered biochemical pathways and symptoms relating to Tourette's syndrome and several reported comorbid conditions. *Med Hypothesis.* 2002;58:47–60.

Harvard School of Public Health. The Nutrition Source: Vitamin D and Health. http://www.hsph.harvard.edu/nutritionsource/what-should-you-eat/vitamin-d/ Accessed January 20, 2010.

Hunt JR. Bioavailability of iron, zinc, and other trace minerals from vegetarian diets *Am J Clin Nutr.* 2003;78(suppl):633S–639S.

Johnson RK, Appel LJ, Brands M, et al. Dietary sugars intake and cardiovascular health: a scientific statement from the American Heart Association. *Circulation.* 2009;120:1011–1020.

Konofal E, Cortese S, Lecendreux C, et al. Effectiveness of iron supplementation in a young child with attention-deficit/hyperactivity disorder. *Pediatrics.* 2005;116:e732–e734.

Konofal E, Lecendreux M, Arnulf I, et al. Iron deficiency in children with attention deficit/hyperactivity disorder. *Arch Pediatr Adolesc Med.* 2004;158:1113–1115.

Konofal E, Lecendreux M, Deron J, et al. Effects of iron supplementation on attention deficit hyperactivity disorder in children. *Pediatr Neurol.* 2008;38:20–26.

Kozielec T, Starobrat-Hermelin B. Assessment of magnesium levels in children with attention deficit hyperactivity disorder (ADHD). *Magnes Res.* 1997;10:143–148.

Kumar J, Muntner P, Kaskel F, et al. Prevalence and associations of 25 hydroxyvitamin D deficiency in US children: NHANES 2001–2004. *Pediatrics.* 2009;124:e362–e370.

Looker AC. Iron Deficiency—United States, 1999–2000. *MMWR Weekly.* 2002;51:897–899.

Milner JA, Allison RG. The role of dietary fat in child nutrition and development: summary of an ASNS Workshop. *J Nutr.* 1999;129:2094–2105.

Nemets H, Nemets B, Apter A, et al. Omega-3 treatment of childhood depression: a controlled, double-blind pilot study. *Am J Psychiatry.* 2006;163:1098–1100.

Ong KH, Tan HL, Lai HC, et al. Accuracy of various iron parameters in the prediction of iron deficiency in an acute care hospital. *Ann Acad Med Singapore.* 2005;34:437–440.

Pinhas-Hamiel O, Doron-Panush N, Reichman B, et al. Obese children and adolescents: a risk group for low vitamin B_{12} concentration. *Arch Pediatr Adolesc Med.* 2006;160:933–936.

Riancho JA, del Arco C, Arteaga R, et al. Influence of solar irradiation on vitamin D levels in children on a nticonvulsant drugs. *Acta Neurologica Scand.* 1989;65:171–173.

Richardson AJ, Montgomery P. The Oxford-Durham study: a randomized, controlled trial of dietary supplementation with fatty acids in children with developmental coordination disorder. *Pediatrics.* 2005;115:1360–1366.

Richardson AJ, Puri BK. The potential role of fatty acids in attention deficit hyperactivity disorder. *Prostaglandins Leukot Essent Fatty Acids (Edinburgh).* 2000;63:79–87.

Rosen GM, Deinard AS, Schwartz S, et al. Iron deficiency among incarcerated juvenile delinquents. *J Adolesc Health Care*. 1985;6:419–423.

Schab DW, Trinh NH. Do artificial colors promote hyperactivity in children with hyperactive syndromes? A meta-analysis of double-blind placebo-controlled trials. *J Dev Behav Pediatr*. 2004;25:423–434.

Schrauzer GN, Shrestha KP. Lithium in drinking water and the incidences of crimes, suicides, and arrests related to drug addictions. *Biol Trace Elem Res*. 1990;25:105–113.

Seelig MS. Consequences of magnesium deficiency on the enhancement of stress reactions; preventive and therapeutic implications (a review). *J Am Coll Nutr*. 1994;13:429–446.

Swanson JM, Kinsbourne M. Food dyes impair performance of hyperactive children on a laboratory learning test. *Science*. 1980;207:1485–1487.

Trimble MR, Corbett JA, Donaldson D. Folic acid and mental symptoms in children with epilepsy. *J Neurol Neurosurg Psychiatry*. 1980;43:1030–1034.

U.S. Department of Health and Human Services, U.S. Department of Agriculture. Dietary Guidelines for Americans 2005. http://www.health.gov/dietaryguidelines/dga2005/document/pdf/DGA2005.pdf Accessed January 20, 2010.

Virkkunen M. Reactive hypoglycaemic tendency among habitually violent offenders. *Neuropsychobiology*. 1982;8:35–40.

Ward NI, Soulsbury KA, Zettel VH, et al. The influence of the chemical additive tartrazine on the zinc status of hyperactive children: a double-blind, placebo-controlled study. *J Nutr Med*. 1990;1:51–58.

Webb TE, Oski FA. Behavioral status of young adolescents with iron deficiency anemia. *J Special Ed*. 1974;8:153–156.

Whalen DJ, Silk JS, Semel M et al. Caffeine consumption, sleep, and affect in the natural environments of depressed youth and healthy controls. *J Pediatr Psychol*. 2008;33:358–367.

Zhang J, Muldoon MF, McKeown RE, et al. Association of serum cholesterol and history of school suspension among school-age children and adolescents in the United States. *Am J Epidemiol*. 2005;161:691–699.

SUGGESTED READING

Richardson, A. *They Are What You Feed Them: How Food Can Improve Your Child's Behaviour, Learning and Mood*. 2006; Harper Thorsons, publisher.

SUGGESTED WEBSITES FOR CLINICIANS AND PARENTS

National Institutes of Health Office of Dietary Supplements
  http://dietary-supplements.info.nih.gov/
Food and Behaviour Research
  www.fabresearch.org
Cereal Facts—Yale University
  www.cerealfacts.org
Crime Times
  www.crimetimes.org

REVIEW QUESTIONS

1. In its 2006 consensus statement the American Psychiatric Association recommends omega 3 essential fatty (EPA + DHA) acid supplementation for patients with:
   a. Mood disorders only
   b. Developmental disabilities only
   c. Mood disorders, impulse control disorders, and developmental disabilities
   d. Mood, impulse control, and psychotic disorders
   e. None of the above

2. Which breakfast is most likely to sustain stable blood sugars throughout the morning?
   a. French bread topped with grape jelly, served with a glass of cranberry juice
   b. Scrambled eggs, buttered sourdough toast and orange wedges, served with a glass of full fat milk

    c. Fruit flavored nonfat cream cheese on a bagel, served with a glass of 100% pure apple juice

    d. Unsweetened cornflakes with skim milk, served with a glass of 100% pure organic grape juice

    e. Fat-free breakfast pastries, served with a glass of tomato juice

3. Deficiency in which of the following is reported to promote psychosis?

    a. Vitamin B_{12}

    b. Bromine

    c. Vitamin D

    d. a and c

    e. none of the above

4. Vegan children are at particular risk for deficiencies in which nutrients?

    a. B_{12}, iron, and the omega 3 essential fatty acids DHA and EPA

    b. Folate, copper, and ascorbic acid

    c. B_6, potassium, and ALA

    d. Vitamin E, vitamin A, and omega 6 essential fatty acids

    e. All of the above

5. Which of the following associations have been reported in the scientific literature?

    a. Iron deficiency with diagnoses of ADHD and restless legs syndrome

    b. EPA and DHA supplementation with improvement in depressive symptoms

    c. Vitamin, mineral, and fatty acid supplementation with reduction of violent behavior in young prisoners

    d. Artificial food colorings and preservatives with ADHD symptoms in normal children

    e. All of the above

Answers: 1-d, 2-b, 3-d, 4-a, 5-e.

Caring for Children and Adolescents with Mental Health Problems in the General Health Setting

Introduction

The responsibility for the identification and management of mental health disorders has historically resided within the specialty mental health disciplines of social work, psychology, and psychiatry. In the past few decades, a number of factors have shifted the care of and responsibility for children with mental health disorders to other child service sectors such as child welfare, education, juvenile justice, and most importantly, general health care settings such as primary care clinician offices.

This shift in care can present several challenges to providers in these nontraditional service sectors. Clinicians from various disciplines may be faced with the question of how to best provide care for patients with disorders about which they may have received little formal training. In many settings, mental health treatment is not seen as the primary task of the sector; rather, mental health disorders are seen as disruptive to the mission of the organization. The stigmatizing nature of mental health disorders has often suppressed organized efforts to address these prevalent and impairing conditions. To further complicate the delivery of care, the world of mental health is very different from traditional medical care, and clinicians may find the assessment, treatment, and referral processes difficult to navigate.

The purpose of this chapter is to highlight the role of nonmental health specialists generally and primary care clinicians specifically in the management of these disorders. Because the literature is more extensive on primary care settings as compared to juvenile justice or child welfare, the majority of this chapter will focus on primary care clinicians and their practices. However, many of the lessons are relevant for other child service sectors. Throughout the chapter we will emphasize resources that can help facilitate efficient and high-quality evaluation and treatment for targeted mental health problems within primary care settings. A separate section will be devoted to office preparedness in order to assist clinicians by anticipating potential pitfalls and offering practical suggestions to address them.

The most appropriate management of many mental health disorders continues to reside within the specialty of mental health services. Primary care clinicians are encouraged to define the types of problems that they can safely manage alone or in close collaboration with a specialist, and when they should refer.

The Care of Mental Health Disorders in General Health and Other Settings

As the initial point of contact into the health care system, primary care clinicians are often asked by families to evaluate behavioral and developmental problems. In fact, as many as 20% of children and adolescents in primary care have a significant psychosocial problem that requires attention. Mental health disorders are associated with increased use of general health care services and can be among the greatest frustrations for primary care clinicians.

The Value of Primary Care–Centered Approaches

A number of important factors unique to primary care make it an ideal location for the management of patients with psychosocial concerns. Mental health disorders may be conceptualized like other chronic health conditions that benefit from the care and coordination provided by the child's medical home. As defined by the American Academy of Pediatrics (AAP), the ideal medical home is accessible, family centered, continuous, comprehensive, coordinated, compassionate, and culturally effective. The medical home model suggests that children receive the highest quality care when service delivery is coordinated and located in a central, accessible location rather than within fragmented systems of care. Benefits of this type of care model include the provision of a single, often familiar, clinician to oversee the patient's care, coordination of multiple types of information from diverse settings, longitudinal monitoring and communication, and the ability to keep comprehensive records in a single location.

The stigma associated with mental health disorders is commonplace, and feelings of shame or embarrassment often translate into barriers for accessing care. The pre-existing relationship of the primary care clinician with families can mitigate some of these feelings for patients and families alike. Through the delivery of services within the primary care setting, patients and families can feel more comfortable discussing their concerns in an environment with which they are already familiar. Primary care relationships in the home community through schools and social service agencies may also provide a stable foundation upon which to manage complex psychosocial problems and often lead to interaction with diverse agencies and professionals.

The Challenges of Care Delivery Within the Primary Care Sector

Many clinicians are committed to the provision of care for children with mental health disorders within their practices. Yet despite these potential strengths, primary care clinicians may not adequately address concerns raised by families due to several barriers within the primary care service sector. Primary care clinicians are called upon to address a wide variety of psychosocial problems that may be difficult to anticipate within a busy primary care practice. Patients and parents may suppress concerns because of the stigma accompanying mental health disorders. Parents of children with mental health disorders are often affected by similar conditions themselves, compounding the processes of assessment and management. Clinicians are also responsible for the management of psychosocial problems with a wide range of severity. While some problems may represent a normal developmental process, they may still be of concern for families and require attention on the part of the clinician. In other cases, symptoms may be significant enough to warrant the diagnosis of a mental health disorder.

Many clinicians express concern that they did not receive comprehensive training in mental health issues. Recent updated guidelines in many different primary care fields have emphasized the importance of training and ongoing continuing education for mental health disorders. Some providers may feel as though there is "little they can do" in the office setting and may choose not to elicit concerns or to avoid them when they arise. Many clinicians are understandably cautious to initiate management because limited specialty resources are accessible in many communities for ongoing support and backup. Thankfully, a number of practical and easy-to-use resources have been developed and are readily available for use in the primary care setting. These resources will be discussed in more detail later in the chapter.

Lastly, primary care clinicians who bill for assessment and treatment services often find that care is inadequately reimbursed by insurance companies. The longer visit time required to adequately address complex problems may be difficult to fit into a busy primary care practice. In some instances, third-party payers may challenge payment under the assumption that services fall under the realm of mental health carveouts. Recent statewide and national initiatives to reform the insurance system and treat mental health disorders with the same respect as medical diagnoses may begin to offer a solution to these issues. Continued advocacy from both primary care and mental health specialists is vital for enhancing insurance coverage for mental health disorders.

In summary, primary care clinicians are often called upon to address mental health concerns within their practices, but the presence of certain barriers can present challenges to the delivery of care. By anticipating the difficulties that families and clinicians alike may face, the evaluation and treatment process can proceed more smoothly when psychosocial concerns arise or are elicited. The following sections will highlight the management of mental health disorders with the primary care setting, from the classification of symptoms to the processes of assessment, treatment, referral, emergency care, and prevention.

Consider the scenario of Brittany Clark and her pediatrician Dr. King. Their story will continue throughout the chapter, highlighting key points in the assessment and management of mental health concerns within the primary care setting.

Dr. King, a pediatrician in a busy primary care office, quickly reviews the chart for her next patient, Brittany. Dr. King has just seen a 2-year-old with constipation, and the patient scheduled after Brittany is in the office because of an asthma flare. Brittany is a 9-year-old girl whom Dr. King has seen regularly for the last few years. Brittany is here today because of trouble in school. According to Dr. King's schedule, she has 15 minutes to spend with Brittany and her mother. Dr. King realizes that she may need to spend more time with Brittany than her schedule today allows. She plans to obtain a brief history, ask the parents and Brittany's teacher to complete some questionnaires, and schedule a visit 3 days later. Dr. King schedules the visit at the end of the day so that Brittany won't miss school and Dr. King can devote more time to the visit if necessary.

KEY POINTS: Primary care clinicians are called upon to evaluate children and adolescents with diverse complaints. Flexible scheduling and triage is often necessary to find time to obtain more information and thoroughly address complex concerns.

Classification of Mental Health Problems

The clustering of signs and symptoms into a diagnostic classification system can be useful for many reasons. It can serve as a way for parents and professionals to conceptualize their concerns and to better communicate with each other. Accurate diagnosis can allow for conversations about treatment and, in some cases, a discussion about the child's future. The unique demands of primary care call for different approaches to diagnostic assessment than those traditionally employed in mental health settings.

The *DSM* Approach

For clinicians in the fields of mental health, the classification system detailed in the *Diagnostic and Statistical Manual of Mental Disorders* (*DSM*) is most widely used. With a fifth revision in preparation, *DSM-IV* provides information on symptom clusters, epidemiology, and clinical course, plus detailed information regarding diagnostic criteria for mental health disorders. For many disorders listed in the *DSM-IV*, diagnosis requires not only the presence of symptoms but also the occurrence of distress or impairment associated with those symptoms. A section in the *DSM-IV* entitled "Disorders Usually First Diagnosed in Childhood" describes conditions commonly diagnosed within the childhood and adolescent years. These include attention-deficit hyperactivity disorder (ADHD), autism spectrum disorders, oppositional defiant disorder, and disorders of sleep, feeding, and elimination. For other conditions such as anxiety and mood disorders, the clinician relies on adult criteria as detailed in *DSM-IV*.

The diagnostic criteria set forth by *DSM-IV* have been endorsed by a number of professional organizations as guidelines to follow in the primary care setting. For example, the AAP recommends that all clinicians, primary care clinicians and specialists alike, utilize the *DSM-IV* criteria for the diagnosis of ADHD. Similar recommendations have been made for the diagnosis of autism spectrum disorders and depression.

Aspects of Classification Unique to Primary Care

While the *DSM* framework offers salient diagnostic guidelines for primary care, certain aspects of management in the office setting cannot be fully addressed using the *DSM* system. Mental health clinicians, for whom the *DSM* system was designed, focus their practice on individuals with manifest mental health disorders. In contrast, primary care clinicians spend more time with families whose concerns exist along a continuum that may range from typical development to an overt mental health disorder. Challenges regarding coding and reimbursement for symptoms that do not meet the threshold for a mental health diagnosis can further complicate the process of addressing these concerns in the office setting.

An additional diagnostic challenge for the primary care clinician involves the substantial amount of comorbidity that exists among children with behavioral disorders. Nearly one third of children with ADHD may also meet the diagnostic criteria for oppositional defiant disorder, and learning disorders, anxiety, and mood disorders are more common than in the general population. Among children with autism spectrum disorders, there is a relatively high prevalence of ADHD and/or anxiety symptoms. Diagnostic uncertainty may exist for young children in whom symptoms can be difficult to categorize. For example, early-onset bipolar disorder can be difficult to distinguish from ADHD and disruptive behaviors disorder in younger children. Added to the behavioral comorbidity is the extensive medical comorbidity present among many children seen in health care settings. Children with chronic medical conditions are at risk for mental health disorders, but psychosocial concerns may be difficult to identify in the midst of significant medical illness.

Primary Care–Oriented Diagnostic Approaches

Primary care–based diagnostic frameworks have been developed to assist nonmental health clinicians in the office setting. These resources help clinicians classify symptoms to begin to provide or access care in the setting of subthreshold symptoms, environmental challenges, and the reality of greater diagnostic uncertainty.

DSM-PC

The *Diagnostic and Statistical Manual for Primary Care (DSM-PC) Child and Adolescent Version* was designed by experts in the fields of child psychiatry, psychology, and pediatrics. The purpose of the *DSM-PC* is to assist primary care clinicians in describing and identifying behavioral conditions in the office setting. Codes for billing were also proposed to begin to allow for improved reimbursement for the management of behavioral concerns from primary care offices. The *DSM-PC* was designed to be compatible with the classification of mental disorders described in *DSM-IV* but also to better capture the diagnostic challenges faced by primary care clinicians.

The *DSM-PC* manual is divided into two main sections. The *situations section* describes environmental concerns that can affect child development. Subsections include challenges to the primary support group (domestic violence and divorce), changes in care giving (foster care and physical or mental illness in a parent), housing and education challenges (illiteracy and discord with peers or teachers), and community or social challenges (discrimination and religious concerns). This section also highlights risk and protective factors to help clinicians consider how the effect of certain stressors may be amplified or attenuated by environmental factors. The *child manifestations section* groups presenting symptoms into behavioral clusters that help the clinician determine a differential diagnosis. Examples of child manifestation clusters include impulsive/hyperactive or inattentive behaviors, emotions and moods, and negative/antisocial behaviors. Common presentations that take into account the child's age and development are provided, and common comorbid conditions are also listed.

Based on the premise that symptoms vary along a continuum, symptoms are presented in the *DSM-PC* framework under three different categories:

1. *Developmental variations:* symptoms that fall within the range of typical development but that can result in stress or concern for parents. A teenager whose parents are concerned about occasional moodiness is an example of a developmental variation. While the behavior is within the range of typical development, it may still cause substantial stress for the family.

2. *Problems:* symptoms that cause disruption of the child's functioning but are not sufficiently severe or impairing to the degree that a mental disorder should be diagnosed. A preschooler whose parents present with concerns about high energy level without other symptoms of ADHD is an example in this category. While the child may have behavior problems in preschool, his or her symptoms do not meet criteria for the diagnosis of a disorder.

3. *Disorders:* symptoms that are significantly severe and impairing to warrant the diagnosis of a disorder, as detailed in *DSM-IV*. A school-aged child who presents with classic obsessive and compulsive symptoms and a resulting inability to do schoolwork is an example in this category. Obsessive–compulsive disorder is diagnosed when the *DSM-IV* criteria are met and the symptoms cause marked difficulty for the child.

Bright Futures in Practice: Mental Health

Another primary care–oriented approach was created as part of the Bright Futures program. *Bright Futures in Practice: Mental Health* seeks to define mental health in the context of the developing child and to promote healthy outcomes for children and adolescents. It serves as an extension of *Bright Futures: Guidelines for Health Supervision of Infants, Children, and Adolescents*, which outlines preventive care strategies for pediatric health supervision visits. In *Bright Futures in Practice: Mental Health*, a major emphasis is placed on the early identification of psychosocial problems and mental health disorders. Collaborative care between families, professionals, and communities is emphasized.

The *Bright Futures in Practice: Mental Health* is divided into two volumes. Volume I, a practice guide, includes developmental chapters that highlight problems that can arise during the developmental stages of infancy, early childhood, middle childhood, and adolescence. The bridges section seeks to assist clinicians with the continuum of care from the identification of conditions to the management of common behavioral and mental disorders in primary care. Criteria for diagnosis are based on the *DSM-IV* and *DSM-PC* frameworks. Volume II is a mental health toolkit that contains hands-on resources for screening, education, and management. As a key resource for clinicians, the mental health tool kit will be discussed in more detail later in the chapter.

Common Factor Approach

Traditional management strategies have focused on the importance of accurate diagnosis to ensure specific, evidence-based treatments. As discussed earlier in the text, several factors unique to primary care can render this approach difficult. The common factor approach is based on the theory that communication interventions, termed "practice elements," can be utilized early in the course of symptoms to help groups of individuals with similar types of undifferentiated concerns rather than a specific diagnosis. In short, communication strategies for undifferentiated concerns can help improve both early symptoms and subsequent diagnostic strategies. Common factors that are important for determining the treatment process include characteristics of the patients and clinicians, their interactions, and the expertise of the clinician to foster behavior change.

A common factor approach that enhances communication between clinician and family can be successfully integrated into the traditional model of assessment and treatment for mental health in primary care. Using this model, early interventions can begin at the onset of the assessment process and be fine-tuned during the diagnostic process. Initial treatments such as parent education, reassurance, behavior plans, or communication strategies can be pursued for children who do not meet diagnostic criteria for a specific disorder but whose concerns warrant intervention and are causing distress. When problems are more differentiated or focused, interventions specific to certain types of disorders may be offered, even if the diagnosis is uncertain or symptoms are subthreshold. Examples of these types of interventions, or "practice elements," include limit setting, rewards, and time out for disruptive and noncompliant behaviors. For disorders in which diagnosis implies specific treatments, such as stimulant medication for ADHD, the diagnostic framework of the *DSM-PC* and *DSM-IV* is suggested, although the communication strategies, involvement of families, and ongoing counseling of the common factor approach can still be engaged. Throughout the process, it is important to remember that more severe symptoms necessitate a faster progression toward formal diagnosis, specific evidence-based treatments or practice elements, and possibly specialty care. A potential difficulty with the use of the common factor approach by primary care clinicians is the current emphasis by third-party payers on formal diagnosis and mental health credentialing in order for behavioral services to be reimbursed.

> Dr. King learns that Brittany began struggling in school this year. She has always gotten good grades, but this year her grades have slipped. She seems distracted and can't focus on her work. She has been missing assignments. Brittany's teacher has wondered about the possibility of ADHD. Mrs. Clark has noticed similar problems at home. Mrs. Clark mentions that their family is going through a difficult time. Brittany's grandmother has become ill and is now living with Brittany and her family. Brittany has been taking care of her younger brother while her mother cares for her grandmother. Brittany is also concerned about her grandmother's health and worries that she may soon pass away.
>
> **KEY POINTS:** Despite a busy office practice, primary care clinicians can successfully evaluate complex behavioral symptoms and related risk factors. Consideration of the presenting symptoms in the context of the child's environment and across multiple settings is crucial.

The Assessment Process

The fast pace of the primary care setting can make it a challenging place to address psychosocial concerns. In response, screening and assessment tools have been designed to allow families and clinicians to begin a dialogue about symptoms, elicit symptoms that are not apparent, and better define diagnoses. In many cases, consensus on the use of a specific type of tool does not yet exist, although there is growing support for the use of formal instruments to assess psychosocial health during routine well-child visits.

TABLE 24-1	The Essentials of Assessment in Primary Care Settings

In addition to a careful history, assessment tools provide essential information as follows:
- Screening tools
  - Identify symptoms that warrant further evaluation
  - Are administered to a general population
  - Example: Pediatric Symptom Checklist-17 (PSC-17)
- Symptom tools
  - Quantify and group symptoms into a recognizable pattern
  - Are administered when clinical concerns arise
  - Example: Center for Epidemiologic Studies—Depression Scale for Children (CES-DC), Vanderbilt Rating Scales for attention-deficit hyperactivity disorder, parent and teacher versions (VADPRS and VADTRS), Screen for Children's Anxiety and Related Emotional Disorders (SCARED)
- Monitoring tools
  - Allow clinicians to track symptoms in response to treatment
  - Are administered after diagnosis is confirmed
  - Example: VADPRS and VADTRS Follow-Up Scales

Screening and Assessment Tools

Defining terms and the specific uses of formal instruments is important when considering how to best elicit psychosocial concerns in the primary care setting. Universal screening tools are given to broad groups of children to identify the need for more targeted evaluation and elicit undisclosed symptoms (Table 24-1). This may include all children or all children presenting for well visits in general health care settings. In contrast, specific assessment tools are used to validate diagnoses and define the degree of impairment once concerns have been elicited either by history or through a screening tool. Some can also be used as a monitoring tool to evaluate the patient's response to treatment over time, although most assessment tools have not been tested for this purpose. It is important to remember that each type of questionnaire was developed for a specific purpose, and the characteristics of the instrument will be valid only when the questionnaire is used for the purpose for which it was designed. Questionnaires can also be helpful to obtain information from other sources such as teachers or care providers. While questionnaires provide a useful supplement to clinical information, the results of questionnaires must be combined with historical information and the clinician's impressions before a diagnosis is determined. The results of questionnaires alone are not sufficient to establish a diagnosis.

Universal Screening Questionnaires

Universal screening questionnaires may be useful for clinicians to use routinely at health supervision visits or when they have general concerns about the presence of a disorder. Clinicians are cautioned to first develop a plan to effectively manage clinically significant universal screening results before general screens are administered to groups of children. Practical issues to consider before using general screening tools include determining methods to address clinically significant findings and the specific linkages with specialists that must be made before initiating any program to identify children. More information on these issues is provided in the section entitled "Office Preparedness" at the end of this chapter.

An example of a universal screening questionnaire is the Pediatric Symptom Checklist (PSC). It is a 35-item questionnaire completed by parents that focuses on cognitive, emotional, and behavioral concerns in children. The accompanying PSC-Youth Report (Y-PSC) can be completed by children 11 years or older. Respondents rate the presence of symptoms from "never," to "sometimes," to often." Higher scores suggest that further assessment is warranted, and cutoff ranges have been determined based on the child's age. The checklists and scoring system can be found in *Bright Futures in Practice: Mental Health*. An abbreviated 17-item version of the PSC has also been developed (PSC-17).

Specific Assessment Tools

A specific assessment tool can be used when concerns steer the provider toward the consideration of a particular diagnosis. Specific assessment tools can be used to validate conditions commonly seen in primary care including ADHD and depression. The Vanderbilt ADHD Diagnostic Rating Scales, designed for both parents and teachers to complete, can be used by primary care clinicians in the evaluation of children for ADHD. Respondents rate the presence of symptoms from "never," to "occasionally," to "often," to "very often." Behaviors are divided into the following categories: inattention, hyperactivity/impulsivity, oppositional defiant disorder and conduct disorder, and anxiety or depression symptoms. A brief "performance" section is included to assess the degree of impairment associated with symptoms. Rating scales are available for initial diagnosis and for follow-up, such as for symptom monitoring once medication has been initiated. The rating scales and scoring information are available in the public domain through the National Association for Children's Healthcare Quality or through the AAP's ADHD toolkit.

Several rating scales are available to help providers better define the presence of depressive symptoms. A useful resource for primary care clinicians is the Guidelines for Adolescent Depression in Primary Care (GLAD-PC). These recommendations include information on assessment tools and are summarized in the GLAD-PC toolkit, which is available electronically. The Columbia Depression Scale includes 22 yes/no questions derived from the depression section of the Diagnostic Interview Schedule for Children (DISC), a structured clinical interview designed to aid in the diagnosis of mental health disorders in youth. It is available in teen and parent versions. The 6-item Kutcher Adolescent Depression Scale is a brief version of the complete KADS. It contains six items completed by the adolescent, who rates depressive symptoms from "hardly ever" to "all of the time" on a four-point scale. Information on both of these scales can be accessed through the GLAD-PC toolkit and can be reproduced with permission. The Center for Epidemiological Studies—Depression Scale for Children (CES-DC) is a 20-item self-report scale in the public domain designed to assess for the presence of depressive symptoms. The scale and scoring system can be accessed in *Bright Futures in Practice: Mental Health*.

Dr. King feels that Brittany appears more withdrawn and distracted than at previous visits. Brittany agrees that she's having a hard time paying attention in school, but that she isn't sure why. She agrees that things at home have been stressful. Dr. King scores the Vanderbilt ADHD Diagnostic Rating Scale completed by Mrs. Clark and her teacher. Brittany's scores are in the clinically significant range for ADHD-predominantly inattentive type, but also for anxiety/depression. She shares these results with Brittany and her mother and decides to speak privately with Brittany to better understand her feelings about the stressors at home.

KEY POINTS: When symptoms arise, rating scales can be helpful in confirming diagnostic impressions and obtaining information from other sources. Results from rating scales can serve as a starting point to discuss symptoms not readily apparent.

The Interview Approach

In many respects the approach to understanding mental health signs and symptoms is similar to other medical concerns. Information about when the problem started is important. Some problems may arise after a major stress, such as divorce or a family move. Other problems, such as ADHD symptoms, will have been a constant theme throughout the child's development. Information on the severity of and impairment due to symptoms is important to help determine the presence of a disorder and the degree of intervention required. The frequency of symptoms is also important. It can be helpful to understand whether the child's symptoms have a particular meaning to the family. For example, a mother who has been diagnosed with bipolar disorder may be worried that her adolescent daughter's moodiness is an early warning sign of the same diagnosis. Understanding her underlying concerns can help the clinician address worries that may not be elicited unless specifically addressed.

As environment is a crucial aspect to development, clinicians must gain an understanding of the children's functioning at home and in educational and social settings. Important information includes who lives in the home, who provides care for the child, and if any stressors for the family are present. If necessary, information on functioning at school can be obtained through questionnaires completed by teacher or through phone consultation after a signed release from the parent has been obtained. Older children and adolescents should be interviewed separately, especially to discuss sexual relationships, use of drugs or alcohol, and thoughts of harm to self or others. In some cases it may be necessary to ask about concerns related to physical or sexual abuse. A question such as "Has anyone ever touched your body in a way that made you feel uncomfortable?" can also be adapted to young children.

Throughout the interview, the clinician must remain sensitive to the family's concerns. For some families, discussing mental health concerns is very stressful and may elicit feelings of shame or failure. Clinicians can use these opportunities to educate families about mental health, a process termed *psychoeducation*. Families can be reassured that psychosocial problems among children and adolescents are common and that effective treatments exist. Throughout the interview, a collaborative approach is often the most useful. Families often have ideas about what might be helpful for them. By asking for this information directly, clinicians can avoid making recommendations that families are unlikely to follow or have already tried unsuccessfully.

Certain interview techniques may be useful when psychosocial concerns are elicited. In contrast to many clinical problems encountered in primary care when a concise history is sufficient, mental health symptoms may be best elicited with open-ended questions. Asking about a child's talents or strong points should be included in these open-ended questions. Parents often appreciate a strength-based approach, which allows them to talk about the child's successes in addition to the areas in which there are problems.

For children and families struggling with problems that involve behavior change, the technique of motivational interviewing (MI) can be particularly helpful. MI is a collaborative, goal-directed style of interviewing in which the client's desire to change is elicited and supported. Initially developed for the treatment of adults with substance abuse problems, MI is an empirically supported intervention that can be used with both adolescents and parents for a number of clinically relevant issues. Proponents of MI suggest that individuals are most likely to change if it is their idea. While the responsibility for change is placed with the adolescent or parent, the clinician's role is to help facilitate the process. Specific MI techniques include expressing empathy, enhancing confidence, and asking for permission to offer advice. An example might include "I've worked with other families who have had concerns similar to yours. Would you like to hear about some strategies that have been helpful for other children I've worked with?" MI works best for families who are ambivalent toward change; when a family is ready to make a change, the clinician is advised to partner with the family to take the next step. Formal training in MI is essential for effective implementation. Further information on training in MI can be found through the Motivational Interviewing Network of Trainers.

Management of Mental Health Disorders in Primary Care

Once concerns are identified or a disorder is diagnosed, the clinician and family will begin to develop plans for intervention. The process of describing their concerns in a supportive environment can be an important first step for families. The management process should involve patient and family education about mental health issues to reduce stereotypes that can negatively affect treatment. The most effective interventions are designed when the clinician and family together target goals for treatment in a collaborative fashion. The types of treatment to be considered include office-based interventions, psychotherapeutic interventions, and medications (Table 24-2). Often a combination of these interventions is most helpful. Some interventions can be effectively delivered by the primary care clinician; in other cases the clinician will choose to manage the patient in consultation with a mental health specialist or may refer the patient for specialized care. In each of these scenarios, the involvement of the primary care office as a medical home throughout the treatment process is valuable.

Office-Based Interventions

For many psychosocial problems, effective interventions can begin in the office setting. This is especially true for problems that do not meet the full criteria for a mental health disorder. Clinicians are encouraged to partner with families to develop specific goals for treatment. Parent-oriented handouts that address common developmental or behaviors concerns can be accessed through the *Bright Futures* and *Bright Futures in Practice: Mental Health* programs.

TABLE 24-2 The Essentials of Treatment in Primary Care

Primary care clinicians provide treatment to children whose symptoms cover a wide range of severity. A graded approach to treatment is essential in the primary care setting.
- First steps: parent and child education
  - Useful to address parent concerns
  - Examples: Bright Futures handouts, books, websites
- Intermediate interventions: targeted programs and courses
  - Useful to address more significant symptoms
  - Examples: Triple P—Positive Parenting Program, Community-Based Parenting Programs, Hospital-Based Educational Seminars
- Specialized treatment: Mental Health Specialty referral
  - Useful to address significant symptoms and mental health disorders
  - Examples: psychologist, psychiatrist, social worker, or therapist
- When to refer to a mental health professional
  - Diagnostic clarification
  - Custody determination
  - Self-harm behaviors
  - Substance abuse
  - Parental request
  - Lack of improvement or worsening symptoms
  - Complex psychiatric conditions (such as bipolar disorder, schizophrenia, and conduct disorder)
  - Clinician request

Examples include how to handle anger, principles of limit setting, and tips for homework completion. The AAP toolkits mentioned earlier in the text contain helpful information for patient and family education and management strategies for ADHD and depression.

Behavioral interventions are frequently used by mental health specialists to help shape the development of prosocial behaviors, and similar principles can be modified for use in the primary care setting. Behavioral interventions are aimed at increasing the frequency of positive behaviors and decreasing negative ones. Techniques used in behavioral modification include reinforcing desired behaviors with small rewards. Undesirable behaviors may be addressed by applying neutral or negative consequences, such as planned ignoring or taking away privileges. Token systems and sticker charts can be used to immediately reinforce behaviors and can serve as a means to earn small rewards after the child does well for a period of time. Behavioral problems that respond well to these types of interventions include disruptive behaviors and disorders of sleep and elimination.

Parent training programs can also be coordinated or initiated from the primary care office. The Triple P—Positive Parenting Program utilizes a targeted approach for managing behavioral problems in the primary care setting. The program encompasses five-tiered levels of intervention designed to increase parental competence and prevent the development of severe emotional problems. Level 1 Triple P is specifically aimed at prevention strategies targeting all parents interested in child development. Levels 2 and 3 Triple P are designed to be delivered within the primary care setting to address common behavioral problems such as noncompliance, sleep problems, and aggressive behaviors. The interventions are designed to be delivered in a few brief office visits to help parents manage a problem behavior.

Psychotherapeutic Interventions

Whereas behavioral interventions seek to shape behavior by modifying the environment, psychotherapeutic interventions address internal thoughts, emotions, and behaviors to affect change. Psychotherapy may involve the individual child or adolescent, his or her family, or groups of individuals with similar problems. In general, psychotherapy is provided by mental health specialists such as psychologists, psychiatrists, and social workers. The primary care clinician may refer individuals with mental health concerns to these specialists for evaluation, or treatment, or both. The reader is referred to Chapter 26, "Evidence-Based Psychotherapies," for more information.

Psychopharmacologic Interventions

Primary care clinicians are increasingly being asked to prescribe medications for mental health conditions in the office setting. Medications can be helpful for the management of certain mental health disorders. In some cases, such as ADHD, medication may be the most effective form of treatment. In other cases, such as anxiety disorders and depression, medications can be effective treatment on their own but may be more effective when combined with psychotherapeutic interventions. The use of medications should be considered only when symptoms are severe and impairing and when the diagnosis is well established. However, in many situations, medications alone do not provide adequate treatment.

In general, medications should be prescribed at the lowest effective dose possible to improve symptoms and minimize side effects, and doses can be increased slowly if necessary. A single medication to manage symptoms is preferable, when possible. Increasing the dose of a single medication to find effective levels is almost always preferable to adding medications. When medications are begun, it is useful to partner with families to determine which symptoms will be targeted with medication, as families benefit from a clear understanding of which problems should be expected to respond well to medications and which will not. Target symptoms and potential side effects should be monitored closely during treatment. The use of medications should be coordinated among all providers involved in the patient's care.

Recent "black box warnings" regarding antidepressants and the American Heart Association's concern about adverse effects of stimulants on cardiac functioning have caused unease among some primary care clinicians. Early concerns have largely been refuted, and many psychotropic medications can be safely used in the primary care setting with appropriate monitoring. Clinicians will need to determine their level of comfort when prescribing psychotropic medications. Children with certain medical conditions may be predisposed to particular adverse events, and in some cases, certain medications should be avoided or used only after consultation with a specialist.

The Referral Process

Although clinicians are able to effectively address a variety of concerns in the office setting, certain problems will necessitate a referral to a mental health specialist. Throughout the referral process, families benefit from the continued involvement of the primary care clinician, who frequently provides a key role in the facilitation of mental health services. Innovative models of care are increasingly providing coordinated specialty care in collaboration with the child's medical home and preferentially in the same facility.

Indications for Referral

Clinicians or parents may request the services of mental health specialists in various situations. Psychologists, social workers, and psychiatrists can be helpful in the assessment process when a diagnosis is not straightforward. Psychiatrists can provide assistance with medication management, which can be useful when patients are taking multiple medications or when medications with side effects are being considered. Both of these services can be provided in a consultative manner, or care can be transferred to the specialist for primary management. Certain types of treatment, such as intensive behavioral management and psychotherapeutic interventions, are generally conducted only by trained mental health specialists.

In many cases, primary care clinicians refer to mental health specialists when symptoms are particularly severe. Examples include moderate-to-severe anxiety and mood disorders. Symptoms such as mania, psychosis, and suicidal thoughts or actions are best managed emergently by trained mental health providers. Families may request a referral to a mental health specialist directly, and the primary care clinician can help by facilitating the referral. The primary care clinician may feel that the family's concerns are outside the scope of his or her practice, and a referral may be useful. Situations that involve custody determinations are likely best managed by a mental health professional trained in forensic assessments. Although a parent may feel that the primary care clinician is an ideal provider to offer these recommendations, the assessment process can be a difficult one, and information should be obtained from both parents. If families inquire about a determination of custody, clinicians may request that the assessment is made by an independent, court-appointed evaluator.

Innovative Management Patterns

Innovative care models are being developed and adapted to enhance the management of mental health issues in primary care. These include the chronic care model, collaborative care, and colocation.

Chronic Care Model

The delivery of primary care has evolved to emphasize common problems addressed in the office setting, namely, the management of acute conditions and the delivery of preventative health for children. Visit times are usually short and focused. However, the ongoing and often complicated concerns of the family struggling with mental health issues can strain a system designed to manage the common acute problems encountered in the primary care office. By conceptualizing mental disorders like other chronic conditions, the needs of families can be better anticipated. Initially proposed for chronic medical conditions, the chronic care model has been adapted to address the challenges of providing management of mental disorders within the primary care setting.

One of the key themes of the chronic care model is the engagement of the clinician and patient in a collaborative relationship in which the needs of the patient are specifically addressed longitudinally. Self-management is promoted by encouraging the patient to identify problems important to him or her, to set goals, and to plan for treatment in a collaborative manner with the clinician. Clinicians provide support to facilitate behavior change, which is often needed for a family to successfully manage ongoing problems. The chronic care model emphasizes five principles important to the delivery of high-quality care for chronic illness

1. The use of specific protocols for clinical conditions or situations
2. Restructuring of the office to allow for patients who need more time, resources, and close follow-up
3. Attention to patients' need for information and to support behavior change
4. The ability to access specialty care
5. Information systems that facilitate care and track patients over time

Research in adult patients with depression has shown that this type of model can be cost-effective and provide high-quality chronic care for adults with mental disorders.

Collaborative Care and Decision Support

As with the chronic care model, similar themes of collaboration between clinicians and patients are found in the collaborative care model. In this approach, clinicians and patients collaboratively determine the clinical concerns and treatment approaches. Other key aspects include patient education and support and enhanced access to specialty care when complex needs arise. In order to address the issue of enhanced access to specialty care, decision-support programs have been designed to link primary care clinicians with mental health specialists for ongoing consultation and clinical support.

A number of decision-support programs are being developed nationally. One of the more well studied programs is the Massachusetts Child Psychiatry Access Project (MCPAP), which began as an initiative to support primary care providers managing children with mental health disorders. In this model, primary care clinicians contact the program by paging the child psychiatrist and discussing their case. If the clinician and specialist determine that a referral is necessary, the program facilitates the referral in a timely manner. Communication with the referring physician occurs through telephone contact and the specialist's transcribed report. Once evaluated by the program, children deemed to be stable are returned to the referring clinician. Other services provided by the program include phone consultation between the primary care clinician and psychiatrist and continuing education programs. Initially funded locally by a one-time grant, the program now serves primary care practices statewide with funding obtained through the state budget.

A second program developed by Campo et al. addresses the need for "stepped" care provided by specialists to address mental health issues in primary care. The program links providers from a metropolitan child psychiatry facility in Pennsylvania with a rural pediatric practice and a primary care–based counseling center. The model involves a psychiatric advanced practice nurse, social worker, and child psychiatrist with funding from the pediatric practice and the on-site counseling center. The advanced practice nurse serves as the liaison between the clinicians and the specialist and is involved in care coordination and direct patient care, including assessment, triage, and family education. The social worker provides focused psychotherapeutic services, and the psychiatrist is available for case review and consultation 1 day/week. Care for routine concerns is provided individually by the primary care clinician. Depending on the complexity, cases are managed jointly with the collaborative care team or individually by a specialty mental health provider.

Colocation Models

The colocation of mental health providers in primary care offices has the potential to address many of the barriers to care described previously. However, colocated mental health services can be a difficult practice model for primary care clinicians to envision, both logistically and financially. Williams et al. review three approaches used by practices in North Carolina that have proven to be successful in terms of logistics, billing, and patient and provider satisfaction. Successful models include the use of the following:

1. Mental health specialist (master's-level psychological associate) employed by the primary care practice
2. Mental health specialist (doctoral-level psychologist) with an independent practice located within the primary care office
3. Community mental health center employee (clinical social worker) located within a private pediatric practice

The important point is that there are many different ways to implement colocated mental health services. By finding the model that is a best fit for their needs, practices are most likely to be successful.

Finally, a brief comment is warranted regarding the growing use of telemental health (TMH) programs to improve mental health care within primary care. Multiple types of TMH programs have been developed to suit the needs of traditional mental health clinics, novel settings such as day care and mobile health care clinics, and primary care practice. TMH is well suited to the three aforementioned innovative models. It allows patients with chronic illnesses more access to specialty consultation so that they may become more active partners in their own care. In the collaborative care and decision-support model, the psychiatrist can participate by videoconferencing rather than telephone, making the collaboration with the primary care physician, an advanced practitioner, or a care manager more personalized and akin to an in-person consultation. And the videoconferencing equipment needed to conduct a session is compact, allowing virtual colocation of the psychiatrist in the primary care clinic.

Dr. King learns that Brittany is experiencing significant anxiety in response to the stressors at home. She is also worried about how this has affected her grades. Dr. King discusses her impressions with Brittany and her mother. Together they decide that a referral to a therapist in the community is the best course of action. Despite several weeks of therapy, Brittany becomes increasingly anxious. Brittany's therapist contacts Dr. King, who prescribes an SSRI. With combined treatment, Brittany's symptoms improve. She is followed regularly by Dr. King and her therapist, who keep in regular contact.

KEY POINTS: The primary care setting can allow for the delivery of comprehensive, collaborative care for mental health conditions.

Emergencies

Mental health emergencies are stressful and frightening for everyone involved, from patients and families to providers. A child may present with emergent symptoms before being diagnosed with a mental health condition, although in retrospect, symptoms may have been present for some time. In children who have been diagnosed previously with a disorder, symptoms may worsen or evolve. For example, depressive symptoms may evolve to include suicidal thinking. A subset of children diagnosed with ADHD may develop manic symptoms that resemble bipolar disorder. Certain medications may cause behavioral activation or increase the likelihood of suicidal thinking. It should be noted that once a diagnosis is made, it is not necessarily static, and clinicians should be aware that the severity and type of symptoms experienced may change over time.

Situations that demand emergency care largely include those in which there is substantial concern regarding potential harm to the child. These include

- Behaviors with a high potential for self-harm
  - Self-injurious acts
  - Suicidal thinking
  - Suicide attempt
- Psychosis
- Potential abuse or neglect

These concerns necessitate immediate action by the clinician. In many cases the clinician will refer for care through an emergency room, through either a general medical hospital or, if available, a psychiatric facility. The level of care needed will then be determined. For most children with risk of harm, inpatient psychiatric admission will be recommended. For children already linked with the mental health system, contacting their mental health provider is essential. Concerns that involve abuse or neglect may be managed by the primary care clinician after contacting children's services or by a regional child advocacy center, if available. Cases that involve serious mental health issues are best managed with the help of mental health professionals. Children and families should be counseled from the start of treatment that these types of concerns must be discussed with appropriate authorities and should note that confidentiality of parent or child reports cannot be maintained when harm to a child is involved.

Other symptoms, depending on their severity, may require emergent evaluation by a mental health specialist, but do not necessarily always warrant hospitalization. Children with manic symptoms, severe depression, or any type of symptom that is debilitating for the patient or family deserve a prompt assessment. In some cases this can be accomplished by a telephone call between the primary care clinician and the mental health specialist, who can help triage the patient to the type of care needed. If the symptoms are significant enough to raise concerns about safety, inpatient admission should be considered.

During the assessment and treatment process, families should be educated regarding types of symptoms to be concerned about and what to do if they are present. The clinician should be contacted if symptoms worsen or new symptoms develop. The family should be given an action plan detailing what to do and who to call if they have concerns. These include an after-hours contact number for the clinician, community resources such as a suicide hotline, and information about emergency care.

Office Preparedness

The task of managing mental health conditions within primary care may seem daunting. Evidence suggests that clinicians continue to be interested in providing these services to families, and many are already doing so successfully. Moreover, families value the coordinated care that primary care clinicians can provide. However, evidence also indicates that clinicians may feel overwhelmed by the scope of problems that they encounter. This section will focus on ways to anticipate and address potential issues before they arise so that the clinician and his or her entire office staff can be best prepared.

Practice Organization

In most cases, primary care practices are logically structured to address the common problems they encounter: acute concerns and preventative care. In order to address the complexity of mental health concerns, practices may consider ways to restructure visits when mental health concerns are suspected. Possible approaches include allowing a small percentage of visits to be of longer duration than typical acute care visits. When time does not allow for concerns to be adequately discussed at the present visit, the clinician may acknowledge the importance of the family's concerns and suggest that an appointment be scheduled in the near future. These visits may be scheduled at the end of the day so that other appointments are not affected if the visit runs longer than expected. If specific concerns are elicited when the appointment is made, questionnaires might be sent to the family prior to the visit. Examples include a general screen for emotional symptoms such as the PSC, or a specific screen for disorders such as ADHD or depression, depending on the parents' concerns. Practices may choose to send a letter to the parents explaining the purpose of the questionnaires and that extra time has been set aside for their visit to address their concerns.

Once the visit is scheduled, certain steps can allow the visit to proceed more smoothly. A staff member may entertain younger siblings or the individual child should it be necessary to talk privately with parents. As the visit comes to an end, clinicians may ask the parents to sign a release form to exchange information with teachers, care providers, or other professionals. Pertinent questionnaires, handouts, and other resources (discussed later in the text) should be readily available. Having a file drawer or website with downloadable copy that contains these materials can be useful; an individual clinician with a specific interest in these conditions may be responsible for maintaining and updating these materials for the practice.

To best ensure continued care, follow-up should be determined at the visit close. Clinicians may request that the subsequent visit be longer than the standard visit time. In some cases, follow-up or monitoring can be done successfully using telephone calls, by either the clinician or the nurse. Efforts are under way to promote reimbursement for time spent managing complex problems by phone, and clinicians may choose to bill for these services. Some third-party payers will cover the cost of these services, and clinicians may need to consider if they will choose to bill the family if this service is not covered. Practices may address this issue with insurance companies when contracts are negotiated. Front desk staff should be aware of referral procedures for patients with different types of insurance including medical assistance, private insurance, and Health Maintenance Organizations (HMO). Given the complexities of this process, the practice may appoint a receptionist to "specialize" in these types of referrals or consider referral software such as Rachel3000 (http://novuscom.net/~amir608/rachel/).

Staff Training

The effective management of mental health problems involves the entire office staff. Oftentimes, calls from families come first to receptionists and nurses. Unlike concerns about ear pain or sore throats, parents may describe vague symptoms, or may even schedule a visit for a different reason. Careful listening may be required to determine when parents have concerns that they may not voice directly. Staff should be aware that visits with complex concerns often cannot be adequately addressed with the time slot of an acute visit; they may be instructed to check with the clinician to ensure an extended visit time. Staff should be aware of the potential acuity of mental health problems, and patients with symptoms that raise significant concerns about safety should be given an appointment promptly. Staff should be trained to recognize mental health emergencies and should be instructed to contact the clinician promptly if concerns arise. Information on emergency care and suicide hotlines should be readily available, when needed. Lastly, the education of staff members includes emphasizing their role in reducing the stigma associated with mental health disorders. Families' concerns should be addressed with empathy, compassion, and professionalism. Training can include using appropriate language and ways to ask questions in a sensitive and nonstigmatizing manner. The importance of confidentiality and its boundaries should also be discussed.

Key Steps to Facilitate Care

The completion rate for referrals to mental health providers is often low, due in large part to the barriers discussed earlier in the text. Several key steps can make it more likely that a specialty appointment will be completed. These steps include the following:

1. Discuss reasons why a referral is recommended and what types of services can be expected.
2. For families who decline a referral, explore their concerns. In some cases, education, support, and reassurance will help reluctant families to seek care.
3. For families who agree to the referral, choose a provider based on factors that will best facilitate care. These factors include insurance coverage, location, and treatment goals.
4. Use referral forms that enhance communication between referring clinicians and specialists. Effective referral forms may include specific reasons for the referral, contact information for the referring clinician, and a summary of pertinent background information including medical history, medications, and laboratory testing, if applicable. Signed consent forms to exchange information can be included with the referral to encourage communication. The GLAD-PC toolkit includes a brief report form that can be completed by the specialist with blanks that prompt information about their summary findings and prescribed medications.
5. Determine the specific roles of the specialist and primary care provider throughout the treatment process. A brief checkbox in this regard is included on both the referral and the report form included in the GLAD-PC toolkit.
6. Assist the patient in making the referral appointment and providing reminders and follow-up calls.

Resources

Having resources readily available can be helpful to the busy clinician. Several resources have been discussed throughout the chapter, and a few will be highlighted here.

As an extension of *Bright Futures Guidelines for Health Supervision of Infants, Children and Adolescents, Bright Futures in Practice: Mental Health* includes suggestions for office-based interventions for common problems encountered in primary care. Resources for clinicians are provided in a way that they can be accessed at health supervision or problems-focused visits, and a number of patient handouts are included. A list of selected organizational resources is also provided. For providers with Internet access, the link to *Bright Futures in Practice: Mental Health* can be added to their "Favorites" section for easy access. Volume II is a mental health toolkit specifically designed for this purpose. Handouts that are used frequently can be copied for easy use. Other assessment tools and parent handouts should be easily accessible. These may include resources found in the AAP's ADHD and Autism toolkits and the GLAD-PC toolkit, which are available electronically or in print through the AAP. Also available from the AAP is Pediatric Care Online, an electronic resource that contains parent handouts, algorithms, and the AAP's comprehensive *Textbook of Pediatric Care*, along with its companion volume *Toolkit for Primary Care*.

As mental health care is often provided within the community setting, a list of mental health clinicians, community organizations, and regional programs can be helpful. Early intervention programs, Big Brother/Big Sister programs, and parenting classes can be helpful resources for families. Some communities offer school-based services for counseling and psychiatric care. Locations for emergency care and hotlines for suicide, domestic violence, and substance abuse are also important. Many resources can be found in the yellow pages under the headings "human services" and "social services" or on the Internet. Social work agencies can also be very helpful with service coordination. Clinicians may wish to establish ties with community providers whom they can contact with questions or when emergent situations arise. The American Academy of Pediatrics' Task Force on Mental Health has developed *Strategies for System Change in Children's Mental Health: A Chapter Action Kit* to assist clinicians in providing efficient, coordinated care to children and families with mental health concerns. Included in the kit are forms to collect summary information from community mental health providers and a referral form to solicit collaboration from mental health specialty providers.

Clinicians may also find it useful to have easy access to appropriate billing codes for behavioral or mental health conditions and to use appropriate terminology to best ensure reimbursement. A quick guide to pertinent billing codes can be found in *Bright Futures in Practice: Mental Health, Volume II* (Selected General Medicine and Behavioral Current Procedural Terminology [CPT] Codes). Other resources regarding diagnosis and correct terminology include the *DSM-PC* and *DSM-IV*. Clinicians may find that certain ICD-10 codes are better reimbursed by some insurance companies. Asking the practice manager to track reimbursement for common mental health problems can be useful. Clinicians are encouraged to appeal denials promptly. Clear documentation that substantiates the level of billing is important. A sample form entitled "Documentation for Reimbursement" can be used to enhance documentation and is included in the *Bright Futures in Practice: Mental Health, Volume II*.

Consider the use of the resources presented earlier in the text in the following scenario. Practitioners in a family practice office decide to address the problem of poorly coordinated mental health services:

A family practice office is becoming frustrated with the low rate of completed mental health referrals for children in their community. While they have a well-established relationship with the adult providers in their area, a select few offices in their community accept referrals for children. The process for referrals is cumbersome. When the clinician refers a child, the receptionists search for mental health centers that accept the patient's insurance. This results in several phone calls and a substantial time delay for scheduling the appointment. Occasionally, families are no longer interested in the referral when the appointment is finally made with the appropriate mental health provider.

In order to improve their referral rate, the family practice office decides to make some changes in their process. They first sample 20 random charts to see how many referrals are completed. They realize that in many cases they often do not receive feedback from the mental health provider once the referral is made. They surmise that this is because they have not forwarded a release of records request.

They decide to change their processes. They denote a single receptionist as the "mental health specialist." This receptionist becomes responsible for all mental health referrals, and she develops an expertise in understanding insurance guidelines. The practice discusses changes in the referral process with three key mental health centers in the community. Together they decide that the new process will involve faxing the referral sheet from the American Academy of Pediatrics' Chapter Action Kit with a signed consent to exchange information. This allows for a collaborative relationship to develop between the family practitioners and mental health providers.

Three months later the family practitioners re-evaluate their process changes. They sample 20 charts of patients referred for mental health treatment. Fifteen of the 20 charts contain documentation from the mental health provider, and 14 of 20 patients completed their referral.

KEY POINTS: Practice-based resources can be used to partner with mental health specialists. Benefits of this approach include improved communication and coordinated referrals

Prevention

The prevention of mental health conditions is complex. On the one hand, evidence is accumulating that certain conditions have a strong genetic component. On the other hand, evidence also suggests that environment plays a crucial role in child development. Prevention can be aimed at various environmental factors such as promoting positive parenting, enhancing community ties, and preventing violence. Working to reduce the stigma associated with mental illness can also be helpful in encouraging families to seek care early, when concerns first arise.

Discussed earlier in the text because of its role in office-based interventions, the Triple P—Positive Parenting Program is designed to promote positive parenting strategies. Level 1 Triple P involves the distribution of information to interested parents about parenting practices. The program includes information in the form of anticipatory guidance about how to solve common behavior problems. By empowering parents, the goal is for them to intervene before common problems progress to a more serious condition.

A similar strategy is employed by the Connected Kids program, accessible through the AAP website. Connected Kids is a program aimed at violence prevention through directed anticipatory guidance by offering a strength-based approach to promote healthy emotional development. The program aims to help parents understand typical development and to encourage prosocial behaviors while discouraging undesirable ones. It builds on the Bright Futures format of health supervision visits, prompting clinicians to introduce and reinforce developmentally appropriate topics. Topics are divided into four age ranges: infancy, early and middle childhood, and adolescence. Informational brochures are available on pertinent, developmentally appropriate topics such as the importance of play, independence, bullying, drug abuse, and healthy relationships. The program can be used as a launching pad to introduce these topics in a neutral way to families.

Early childhood programs have been found to foster child development. Two such programs include the Head Start Program and Early Intervention. Head Start is a federally funded child development program designed to serve low-income families. Children who participate in Head Start have been shown to experience educational benefits and improved social–emotional development. The Early Intervention Program, ensured by the Individuals with Disabilities Education Act, is a federally mandated program that provides for early recognition and treatment of children with developmental delays. These programs can provide valuable community support and service coordination to families in need. Research suggests that the most effective programs combine specific, child-centered goals with a focus on parent–child interaction and the development of healthy relationships. The book *From Neurons to Neighborhoods: The Science of Early Childhood Development* provides an exhaustive review of influences on early child development with an emphasis on the promotion of healthy development and implications for public policy.

Conclusions

The comprehensive care provided by primary care clinicians is highly valued by patients and families. As such, the primary care setting offers many benefits to families seeking care for mental health concerns. Although presence of barriers makes the provision of care for mental health disorders more challenging, primary care clinicians have several tools available to allow them to successfully navigate the processes of assessment, treatment, and referral. Throughout the process of care, themes of collaboration, information sharing, and communication are crucial. By anticipating the needs of patients and families, primary care clinicians can respond effectively and empathetically to mental health concerns, while continuing to efficiently provide care for the wide range of problems that infants, children, and adolescents may encounter.

BIBLIOGRAPHY

American Academy of Pediatrics. Policy statement: medical home initiative for children with special needs project advisory committee. *Pediatrics.* 2002;110:184–186.

American Academy of Pediatrics, Committee on Quality Improvement, Subcommittee on Attention-Deficit/ Hyperactivity Disorder. Clinical practice guideline: diagnosis and evaluation of the child with ADHD. *Pediatrics.* 2000;105:1158–1170.

American Academy of Pediatrics. Connected kids: safe, strong, secure. Available at: http://www.aap.org/connectedkids/. Accessed December 14, 2009.

American Psychiatric Association. *Diagnostic and Statistical Manual of Mental Disorders, Text Revision. Fourth Edition.* Washington, DC: American Psychiatric Association; 2000.

Bridge JA, Iyengar S, Salary CB, et al. Clinical response and risk for reported suicidal ideation and suicide attempt in pediatric antidepressant treatment: a meta-analysis of randomized controlled trials. *J Am Med Assoc.* 2007;297:1683–1696.

Campo JV, Shafer S, Strohn J, et al. Pediatric behavioral health in primary care: a collaborative approach. *J Am Psychiatr Nurs Assoc.* 2005;11:276–282.

Connor DF, McLaughlin TJ, Jeffers-Terry M, et al. Targeted child psychiatric services: a new model of pediatric primary clinician-child psychiatry collaborative care. *Clin Pediatr.* 2006;45:423–434.

Hagan JF, Shaw JS, Duncan P, eds. *Bright Futures Guidelines for Health Supervision of Infants, Children, and Adolescents—Third Edition.* Available at: http://www.brightfutures.aap.org. Accessed December 14, 2009.

Hettema J, Steele J, Miler W. Motivational interviewing. *Annu Rev Clin Psychol.* 2005;1:91–111.

Jellinek M, Patel BP, Froehle MC, eds. *Bright Futures in Practice: Mental Health.* Available at: http://www. brightfutures.org/mentalhealth/. Accessed December 14, 2009.

Kelleher KJ, McInerny TK, Gardner WP, et al. Increasing identification of psychosocial problems: 1979–1996. *Pediatrics.* 2000;105:1313–1321.

Leslie LK, Newman TB, Chesney J, et al. The Food and Drug Administration's deliberation on anti-depressant use in pediatric patients. *Pediatrics.* 2005;116:195–204.

Perrin JM, Friedman RA, Knilans TK, the Black Box Working Group, the Section of Cardiology and Cardiac Surgery. Cardiovascular monitoring and stimulant drugs for attention deficit/hyperactivity disorder. *Pediatrics.* 2008;122:451–453.

Sanders MR. Triple P—positive parenting program: towards an empirically supported validated multilevel parenting and family support strategy for the prevention of behavior and emotional problems in children. *Clin Child Fam Psychol Rev.* 1999;2:71–90.

Shonkoff JP, Phillips DA, eds. *From Neurons to Neighborhoods: The Science of Early Child Development.* Washington, DC: National Academy Press; 2000.

Vetter VL, Elia J, Erickson C, et al. Cardiovascular monitoring of children and adolescents with heart disease receiving stimulant drugs. A scientific statement from the American Heart Association's Council on Cardiovascular Disease in the Young Congenital Cardiac Defects Committee and the Council of Cardiovascular Nursing. *Circulation.* 2008;117:2407–2423.

Wagner EH, Austin BT, Von Korff M. Organizing care for patients with chronic illness. *Milbank Q.* 1996;74:511–544.

Williams J, Shore SE, Meschan Foy J. Co-location of mental health professionals in primary care settings: three North Carolina models. *Clin Pediatr.* 2006;45:537–543.

Wissow L, Anthony B, Brown J, et al. A common factors approach to improving mental health capacity of pediatric primary care. *Adm Policy Ment Health.* 2008;35:305–318.

Wolraich M, Felice ME, Drotar D. *The Classification of Child and Adolescent Mental Disorders in Primary Care: Diagnostic and Statistical Manual for Primary Care (DSM-PC)*. Elk Grove, IL: American Academy of Pediatrics; 1996.

Wong M, Atkins D, Taylor J, et al. Diagnosis of Attention-Deficit/Hyperactivity Disorder. Summary, Technical Review: Number 3; 1999. Available at: http://www.ahrq.gov/clinic/epcsums/adhdsutr.htm. Accessed December 14, 2009.

Zuckerbrot RA, Cheung AH, Jensen PS, et al., the GLAD-PC Steering Group. Guidelines for adolescent depression in primary care (GLAD-PC): I. Identification, assessment, and initial management. *Pediatrics*. 2007;120:e1299–e1312.

SUGGESTED READINGS

Committee on Psychosocial Aspects of Child and Family Health and Task Force on Mental Health. The future of pediatrics: mental health competences in pediatric primary care. *Pediatrics*. 2009;124:410–421.

Parker SJ, Zuckerman BS, Augustyn MC, eds. *Developmental and Behavioral Pediatrics: A Handbook for Primary Care*. 2nd ed. Philadelphia, PA: Lippincott Williams & Wilkins; 2005.

Wolraich M, Felice ME, Drotar D. *The Classification of Child and Adolescent Mental Disorders in Primary Care: Diagnostic and Statistical Manual for Primary Care (DSM-PC)*. Elk Grove, IL: American Academy of Pediatrics; 1996.

SUGGESTED WEBSITES

- **Bright Futures Mental Health.** An electronic resource that consists of two volumes. Volume I contains information on the evaluation and management of mental health concerns commonly seen in the primary care setting. Volume II is a toolkit that contains evaluation and management resources for clinicians, with an emphasis on collaborative care. Address: http://www.brightfutures.org/mentalhealth/
- **Caring for Children with ADHD: A Resource Toolkit for Clinicians.** A resource available in both print and electronic versions. Developed by the American Academy of Pediatrics, the toolkit contains information on the evaluation and management of children with ADHD in the primary care setting. Resources to enhance parent education and collaboration with schools are emphasized. Address: http://www.aap.org/healthtopics/adhd.cfm
- **Guidelines for Adolescent Depression in Primary Care (GLAD-PC) Toolkit.** An electronic resource that focuses on the evaluation and management of depression in the primary care setting. Address: http://www.glad-pc.org
- **Pediatric Care Online.** An electronic resource available to members of the American Academy of Pediatrics. Pediatric Care Online offers a collection of handouts, algorithms, and useful links, including an electronic version of the American Academy of Pediatrics' *Textbook of Pediatric Care*. Address: http://www.pediatriccareonline.org/pco/ub/home
- **Magination Press.** An electronic resource from the American Psychological Association. Magination Press offers collections of books for children about anxiety, divorce, emotions, ADHD, and other mental health–oriented topics. Address: http://www.maginationpress.com
- **Motivational Interviewing.** This electronic site contains information for clinicians about the technique of motivational interviewing. Information on the Motivational Interviewing Network of Trainers is also provided. Address: http://www.motivationalinterview.org/

REVIEW QUESTIONS

1. Behavioral symptoms in young children
   a. Are predictive of a mental health disorder later in life
   b. Can easily be sorted into diagnostic categories
   c. Are mediated by positive and negative influences within the child's environment
   d. Require a precise diagnosis before treatment can begin

2. Benefits of the management of mental health concerns in the primary care setting include
   a. The ease of billing for mental health services within the primary care service sector
   b. The delivery of services in a familiar environment
   c. Increased ability to coordinate care within the medical home
   d. Both b and c

3. A referral to a mental health provider is indicated
    a. When diagnostic uncertainty arises
    b. If symptoms worsen or do not improve
    c. Any time symptoms are elicited
    d. Both a and b

4. Interventions that can be delivered effectively by primary care clinicians include all of the following except
    a. Cognitive–behavioral therapy
    b. Psychotropic medications
    c. Behavioral strategies
    d. Providing educational resources for parents

5. The "black box" warning placed on certain psychotropic medications
    a. Indicates that only mental health clinicians should prescribe them
    b. Suggests that the risk outweighs the benefit for most patients
    c. Means that prescribing clinicians should engage patients in a dialogue regarding potential risks
    d. States that these medications are not appropriate for patients younger than 18 years of age

Answers: 1-c, 2-d, 3-d, 4-a, 5-c

CHAPTER

25

Ajit N. Jetmalani, MD

Psychopharmacology

Introduction

Research over the past 30 years has elucidated many neurobiological processes associated with psychiatric disorders. These findings have coincided with a growing understanding of early-onset psychopathology leading to new conceptualizations of mental illness, its etiology, and treatment. Many psychiatric disorders are now known to represent developmental anomalies that begin in childhood and persist over the lifespan. Psychotropic medications have increasingly been used to treat children and adolescents with these neuropsychiatric disorders, however, Roberts and colleagues note that, "50% to 75% of drugs used in pediatric medicine have not been studied adequately to provide appropriate labeling information." In 1997, the United States (U.S.) Congress passed the "Food and Drug Administration Modernization Act" which encouraged pharmaceutical companies, with the promise of 6-month exclusivity, to develop pediatric studies to evaluate medication efficacy. Over the past decade, the National Institute of Mental Health (NIMH), National Institute of Child Health and Human Development (NICHD), and the pharmaceutical industry have launched a range of pediatric studies focused on the short-term efficacy of various medications, including psychotropics. Pharmacotherapy is now an integral part of biopsychosocial treatment planning for youth with neuropsychiatric disorders. This chapter presents concepts and practical information to guide optimal prescribing for youth in the context of the rapidly expanding, and at times confusing, research.

General Principles of Psychopharmacology

The following sections focus on the essential elements underlying the successful utilization of psychotropic medications with youth. They are based in part on the Practice Parameter on the Use of Psychotropic Medication in Children and Adolescents recently published by the American Academy of Child and Adolescent Psychiatry (AACAP). Their 12 principles are summarized in Table 25-1.

TABLE 25-1	Use of Psychotropic Medications in Children and Adolescents

Principles of Prescribing:

Assessment
- Before initiating pharmacotherapy, a psychiatric evaluation is completed.
- Before initiating pharmacotherapy, a medical history is obtained, and a medical evaluation is considered when appropriate.
- The prescriber is advised to communicate with other professionals involved with the child to obtain collateral history and set the stage for monitoring outcome and side effects during the medication trial.

Treatment and Monitoring Plan
- The prescriber develops a psychosocial and psychopharmacological treatment plan based on the best-available evidence.
- The prescriber develops a plan to monitor the patient, short and long term.
- Prescribers should be cautious when implementing a treatment plan that cannot be appropriately monitored.

Assent and Consent for Treatment
- The prescriber provides feedback about the diagnosis and educates the patient and family regarding the child's disorder and the treatment and monitoring plan.
- Complete and document the assent of the child and consent of the parents before initiating medication treatment and at important points during treatment.
- The assent and consent discussion focuses on the risks and benefits of the proposed and alternative treatments.

Implementation of Treatment
- Implement medication trials using an adequate dose and for an adequate duration of treatment.
- The prescriber reassesses the patient if the child does not respond to the initial medication trial as expected.
- The prescriber needs a clear rationale for using medication combinations.
- Discontinuing medication requires a specific plan.

Comprehensive Biopsychosocial Evaluation

A thorough psychiatric assessment should precede the initiation of pharmacotherapy. The biopsychosocial model provides an optimal framework for integrating aspects of the evaluation into a formulation from which is derived a treatment plan. Biological factors begin with the child's genetic potential and progress through intrauterine life to environmental insults and developmental setbacks. Psychological components include a core capacity for interpersonal relationships and the ability to understand others and express oneself verbally and nonverbally. Psychological factors also relate to executive functioning skills that overlap with biological endowment such as the ability to regulate sensory inputs and organize responses to internal and external stressors. Social components include contextual aspects of youths' lives at home, school, and the community, including any traumatic experience. A formulation is not a simple reiteration of these factors but integrates the most salient factors into a statement of how the youth came to his/her current status in life. It is intended to help the clinician to individualize decision making. For example, if diagnosis drives treatment planning for an autistic child living in a chaotic home, treatment might consist only of a medication trial. By contrast, if a biopsychosocial formulation drives treatment planning, recommendations might include support services, in-home parent training, coordination with the school, as well as a medication trial. This approach protects children against more restrictive, and traumatizing, interventions.

Establishing a Strong Treatment Alliance

Implementing a medication plan with a strong treatment alliance is the major goal for clinicians. A treatment alliance can be defined as the working relationship among a child, his parents or guardians, and the clinician. It has several pivotal aspects. The engagement of the child and family as a partnership is key to achieving compliance, satisfaction, and outcomes. Presenting a confident and empathic demeanor while addressing the chief complaint, will improve adherence to any medical prescription. A child and his/her parents will view the areas of concern from their individual perspectives, which may vary from the clinician's perspective. Keeping everyone engaged in the treatment process requires the clinician to balance these perspectives and share responsibility for the child's treatment with the family. When developing a treatment plan, time must be set aside for questions both to minimize misunderstandings and to create a shared treatment vision.

Completing the informed-consent procedure is another alliance building opportunity. A family that hears a well-reasoned plan from a clinician will have greater confidence in the plan and will better participate in the decision-making process. This process should focus on creating a set of outcome expectations and their means of measurement so as to engage the family in data gathering during a medication trial. Setting shared expectations up-front will yield better communication throughout treatment and satisfaction with outcome.

Understanding Pharmacokinetics and Pharmacodynamics

Pharmacokinetics are the effects of the body on medications. *Pharmacodynamics* are the effects of medication on the body. Several variables may affect both pharmacokinetics and pharmacodynamics of medications in youth compared to adults.

Pharmacokinetics include the effects on drug metabolism of the rates and the extent of absorption, the range of distribution in bodily compartments (tissues and fluids), the efficiency and extent of degradation into smaller bioactive or inactive compounds, and the eventual rate and extent of excretion. In pediatric psychopharmacology, distribution, metabolism, and excretion diverge from adult kinetics. The main factors involve differences in fluid to tissue ratios, relatively higher ratios of hepatic and renal capacity to size, available circulating proteins that bind drugs, and development of cytochrome P450 enzymes. Overall, compared to adults, children may metabolize medications more rapidly based on weight. Unfortunately, weight-based prescribing guidelines are of limited predictive utility for most psychotropic medications. Understanding the cytochrome system is particularly important in understanding the potential interactive effects of drugs that are inducers (increase enzyme activity), substrates (subject to breakdown), and inhibitors (reduce effectiveness of enzymes) in order to avoid interactions that may lead to uncomfortable, or even lethal, complications. Finally, due to genetic polymorphism in the P450 system, a small portion of the population is defined as "slow metabolizers." They risk accumulating high levels of medications at usual therapeutic doses. An Indiana University School of Medicine website maintains a list of cytochrome enzyme categories of commonly used drugs that can assist physicians in identifying drug–drug interactions.

Pharmacodynamics refers to the physiological effects of drugs on the body. Drug effects include actions on enzymes, agonist and antagonist actions on receptors, storage, release and reuptake of neurotransmitters, secondary effects on receptor numbers and sensitivity, and membrane permeability. Drugs may also induce immune system reactions by direct cell toxicity, effects on replication, or cellular metabolism. These actions are further influenced by the protein binding of drugs which affect their bioavailability.

Medications have a dose–response curve which describes the range of their effects at various blood concentrations. Some medications also have a therapeutic window, that is, a narrow range of serum levels within which a drug exerts therapeutic effects without toxicity. For example, lithium has a narrow therapeutic window of 0.7 to 1.2 meq/L. Serum levels below this range are generally ineffective and levels above this range cause serious complications.

Evidence-Based Treatment (EBT)

Randomized clinical trials (RCT) now support the efficacy of psychotropic medications for a variety of pediatric psychiatric disorders. Classification systems have been developed to rate the quality of research cited as EBTs. In 1995, the International Psychopharmacology Algorithm Project Report categorized levels of evidence as follows:

Class A includes medications with good empirical support, based on consistently positive results in RCTs.

Class B consists of drugs with fair empirical support showing positive, but inconsistent, results in RCTs or positive results from small sample trials.

Class C includes drugs with minimal empirical support, based primarily on accumulated clinical experience from case reports and open-label studies.

Many medications are rated in the B and C categories, or even unrated, particularly for children under the age of 11 years. Furthermore, medications that are shown to be *efficacious* in short-term controlled studies may not prove *effective* in a longer-term or "real life" settings.

Consensus Guidelines for Care

Ideally, all pharmacotherapy would be evidence-based derived from large RCTs. Until such Level A studies are available, physicians should rely on best practices developed by the AACAP, and/or various state or academic centers. One such set of guidelines based on a combination of empirical data and consensus guidelines is available from the Texas Children's Medication Algorithm Project (CMAP) for several disorders such as major depressive disorder, attention-deficit hyperactivity disorder (ADHD), and ADHD comorbid with anxiety, depression, tics, or aggression. There is some evidence that such an approach produces more uniform and effective outcomes. For example, the Multimodal Treatment of Children with ADHD study found that algorithm-driven pharmacologic care produced better outcomes than did community care. However, such approaches often do not consider comorbid disorders, despite their frequency in child and adolescent psychiatric disorders.

Current Controversies

Prescribing medications for neuropsychiatric disorders of children and adolescents has raised many controversies related to their safety, the use of such medications with vulnerable youth, and the lack of evidence regarding their long-term risks and benefits.

Developmental Effects of Psychotropic Medication

In 2007, Leckman and King discussed the rapid increase in prescriptions of selective serotonin re-uptake inhibitors (SSRIs) for children and the lack of studies examining their impact on central nervous system (CNS) development and functioning. The limited studies with laboratory animals exposed to SSRIs suggested negative impact on anatomic development and functioning. Such findings mandate physicians to weigh such potential undiscovered risks against current need in deciding whether to prescribe these medications during developmentally sensitive periods.

In contrast to these potential risks, there is some evidence that treatment of early-onset disorders may be protective. For example, schizophrenia is a neurodegenerative disorder with gray and white matter abnormalities. Research with neural cell cultures and the brains of humans who have suffered a first episode of psychosis suggests that the second-generation antipsychotics (SGAs) may have a *neuroprotective role* in schizophrenia compared to no treatment, and even compared to treatment with first-generation antipsychotics (FGAs). The

SGAs appear to enhance neurotrophic factors and antioxidation effects due to decreased apoptosis of neurons. These encouraging findings are tempered by conflicting studies with nonhuman primates. Overall, a neuroprotective role for the SGAs is intriguing, but unproven. A discussion of such potential benefits and risks for CNS development should be integrated into the informed-consent process.

Early Childhood Prescribing

The past decade has seen a dramatic increase in the prescription of psychotropic medications for preschool children. The Preschool ADHD Treatment Study (PATS) found that low doses of methylphenidate could help very young children diagnosed with ADHD without major side effects. In a separate study, risperidone was found to help young autistic children to regulate disruptive behaviors. Multiple psychotropic medications are used off-label for various problems experienced by preschoolers. In response, the Preschool Psychopharmacology Working Group of the AACAP developed guidelines for pharmacotherapy with young children, including the formulation of algorithms for several diagnoses and overall recommendations. In brief, these recommendations emphasize the preferential use of psychotherapy, reserving medication for major functional impairment, conducting an appropriate consent procedure with the parents regarding the lack of an evidence base for such prescribing, and tracking outcomes.

Prescribing for Children in Foster Care

Children and adolescents placed in foster homes are particularly vulnerable. Zito and colleagues reviewing data in Texas noted that 37.9% of youth in foster care were prescribed psychotropic medications, and of these 41.3% were prescribed three or more medications. These rates were considerably higher than the general Medicaid population of youth living with their families. The meaning of these findings is subject to interpretation; but concerns about polypharmacy has led several states to legislate independent monitoring of psychotropic prescribing practices for youth in foster care. The impact of such monitoring is not yet known. Meanwhile, physicians must ensure that evidence-based and consensus-guideline care remains the criterion for psychopharmacotherapy with all youth, regardless of residence.

Polypharmacy

Polypharmacy has become commonplace. There are conditions in which more than one psychotropic medication is indicated, for example, bipolar disorder. But, in many, perhaps most, cases of polypharmacy, the risks are not counterbalanced by evidence of efficacy. Many commercial insurers and states' departments of health now monitor such practices. In 2007, the Texas Department of State Health Services developed the following screens which may suggest problem prescribing practices for youth: absence of a diagnostic assessment; concurrent use of more than three psychotropic medications; prescribing of two or more medications in the same class (use of a long-acting and immediate-release stimulant of the same chemical entity does not apply); polypharmacy is utilized prior to monotherapy; the psychotropic doses exceed recommended guidelines. The Practice Parameter on the Use of Psychotropic Medications in Children and Adolescents developed by the AACAP further notes the need to develop a treatment and monitoring plan with the family that includes an approach for patients who do not respond typically, alternatives to polypharmacy, and discontinuation of ineffective medications.

Cardiovascular Risks of Stimulants

Since the late 1980s, the potential cardiotoxicity of the stimulants has been noted. In February 2005, Health Canada suspended the marketing and distribution of Adderall-XR after reports of sudden unexplained death in children with and without cardiac defects who were prescribed Adderall-XR. This ban was rescinded in August 2005 and a warning was issued regarding the risk of sudden unexplained death in patients with known cardiac anomalies who were taking Adderall-XR. In 2008, Vetter and colleagues published a scientific statement from the American Heart Association (AHA) summarizing the evaluation that should be conducted when prescribing stimulants. The recommendation that all children should receive a screening electrocardiogram (ECG) caused a controversy because of the expense and the lack of data demonstrating risk reduction. Furthermore, the American Academy of Pediatrics (AAP) and the AACAP have noted that there is no established relationship between stimulants and cardiac death. The AAP recommends that clinicians carefully assess all children for cardiac abnormalities, including those for whom ADHD treatment is being considered, and does not recommend routine screening ECGs.

This controversy will likely continue. In 2009, Gould and colleagues found that of 564 cases of sudden cardiac death among youths 7 to 17 years old, 10 were prescribed methylphenidate compared to only 2 of the matched 564 youth who died accidentally. These results may be interpreted as supporting the AHA's concerns. Thus at this point of scientific knowledge, physicians must make their own decision regarding the use of screening ECGs based on thorough consideration of elements of history and physical exam.

Antidepressants and Suicide Risk

In April 2004, the Food and Drug Administration (FDA) published a review of SSRI studies with children and adolescents that in the aggregate indicated that the SSRIs were associated with twice the rate of suicidal thinking and behavior compared to placebo, 4% versus 2% respectively. There were no completed suicides. In response, the FDA issued a "black-box" warning for all antidepressants. This risk has now been confirmed in several other studies. Subsequent to the black-box warning, Gibbons and colleagues found that the rate of SSRI prescriptions fell 22% in the Netherlands and the United States. At the same time, completed suicides rose 49% in the Netherlands and 14% in the United States. This temporal relationship suggests a cause and effect relationship between untreated depression and suicide. During this period, a large multicenter study, The Treatment for Adolescents with Depression Study (TADS), found efficacy for fluoxetine combined with Cognitive Behavioral Therapy (CBT) in speeding the recovery from moderate to severe depression. An additional finding was that the fluoxetine group had higher rates of suicidal ideation, but not completed suicide, which was completely ameliorated for the patients who also received CBT. Thus, ongoing caution is warranted in using SSRIs with youth, and most of these youth should concurrently be engaged in psychotherapy.

Patterns of Publishing

Finally, physicians depend on the findings of empirical studies to guide their care. Unfortunately, withholding negative outcomes was common until recently. Eric Turner and colleagues have reviewed the impact of selective publication of positive studies on effect size for selected treatments. They note that of 74 registered studies, 31% were never published. Further analysis confirmed a clear pattern of withholding negative findings which greatly distorted the effect size of various drug trials upward by 32%. In 2005, the FDA mandated that all studies that are submitted to the FDA in support of medication efficacy should be prospectively registered to preclude the obfuscation of negative outcomes. Hopefully, increased scrutiny by the FDA and individual investigators will remedy this scientific duplicity.

Psychotropic Medications

This section presents essential information for prescribing psychotropic medications with youth, including both major classes of medications and those with idiosyncratic uses. Most of these medications are not FDA-approved for pediatric populations. Many are supported by systematic studies, but others are used "off-label" without an evidence base. Finally, while *neurobiological mechanisms* are based on current research and theory, the actual *therapeutic mechanisms* of psychiatric medications, in youth and adults, remain unknown.

Stimulants

Stimulants are the most studied psychotropic medication class among the youth. The two major types of stimulants are methylphenidate and amphetamines. In controlled studies, all stimulants are equally efficacious. However, an individual youth may respond differentially to a particular type of stimulant, for example, amphetamines rather than methylphenidates, or even to a specific medication within a type, for example, Metadate rather than Ritalin. Table 25-2 summarizes relevant prescribing information for the available stimulant preparations.

Indications

Stimulants are FDA-approved for the treatment of ADHD. Amphetamines are approved for children over 3 years old and methylphenidate for children over 6 years old.

Mechanism of Action

Stimulants are sympathomimetic drugs structurally similar to catecholamines. They boost norepinephrine and dopamine signals in a number of different ways. According to Stahl, methylphenidate blocks the norepinephrine and dopamine reuptake pumps making more of these neurotransmitters available in the synaptic cleft. In contrast to methylphenidate, amphetamines are also a competitive inhibitor and pseudosubstrate for the presynaptic norepinephrine and dopamine transporters. Therefore, amphetamines not only block neurotransmitter reuptake but are also transported into the neuron itself. Ultimately, both mechanisms optimize dopamine and alpha$_2$A activity in the prefrontal cortex with resulting increase in attention and decrease in impulsivity.

The parts of the CNS that are hypothesized to be affected in ADHD are also the areas where stimulant medications exert their effects. The most important areas appear to be the frontal and prefrontal cortex, the seat of attention, focus, memory, and other executive functions such as information processing, planning, organizing, and self-regulation. As Stahl notes, dopamine and norepinephrine modify the signal to noise ratio of data processed by the frontal and prefrontal cortex thereby improving inhibitory capacities of these cortical structures. Additionally, the prefrontal cortex sends long nerve tracts to other parts of the CNS, including the basal ganglia and the cerebellum, to further coordinate planning and motor activity. Stimulants are likely active in improving transmission in these tracts.

Major Complications and Their Management

The well-known potential side effects of stimulants are summarized in Table 25-2. Most of theses can be managed by adjusting the dose and/or timing of administration. The more concerning potential major complications are discussed below.

Cardiotoxicity and the aforementioned risk of sudden death are the major concern. The AHA, AAP, and AACAP all recommend gathering a more detailed medical history for the child and family along with a cardiac examination, as summarized in Table 25-3. Blood pressure, pulse rate and rhythm, and cardiac tolerance should be assessed at each follow-up visit. The use of a pretreatment ECG remains controversial. Potential cardiac risks, including the risk of sudden death, should be discussed with guardians as part of the informed-consent process.

Appetite suppression and growth inhibition are due to the anorectic effects of stimulants. In 2007, Caron reported that after 3 years of methylphenidate treatment, children 7 to 9 years of age showed decreases in growth rates without evidence of growth rebound. These children

TABLE 25-2 Stimulant Medications

Drug	Dosing	Common Side Effects	Duration of Action
Methylphenidate			
Methylphenidate (Ritalin, Methylin, Methylin Chewables, Methylin Liquid, Metadate ER, generic methylphenidate)	Initiate 5 mg BID to TID Increase by 5–10 mg increments up to 60 mg max. Estimated dose range 0.3–0.6 mg/kg/dose.	Insomnia, headache, stomachache, decreased appetite, weight loss, repetitive behaviors, growth retardation, tics, irritability, dysphoria, and rebound agitation. Also, psychotic symptoms with visual hallucinations possible.	About 3–4 hours.
Dexmethylphenidate (Focalin) (Isolated dextroisomer of methylphenidate)	Half the dose noted for methylphenidate.	Same as above. May be less prone to causing sleep or appetite disturbance.	About 3–4 hours.
Dexmethylphenidate (Focalin XR 50% short acting and 50% long acting)	Double the dose of regular release Focalin. Once daily.	Same as above.	About 8 hours.
Methylphenidate (Ritalin SR)	Start with 20 mg daily. May combine with short acting for quicker onset (only available as 20 mg dose).	Same as above.	Onset delayed for 60–90 minutes. Duration supposed to be 6–8 hours, but can be quite individual and unreliable.
Methylphenidate (Ritalin LA) *50% immediate release beads and 50% delayed release beads* (Metadate CD) *30% immediate release and 70% delayed release beads*	Initiate at 10–20 mg daily. Adjust weekly in 10 mg increments to maximum of 60 mg taken once daily.	Same as above.	Onset in 30–60 minutes. Duration about 8 hours.
Methylphenidate (Concerta) *22% immediate release and 78% gradual release*	Starting dose is 18 mg once daily up to a max of 72 mg daily.	Same as above but less rebound risk.	Onset in 60–90 minutes. Duration about 10–14 hours.

Dextroamphetamine

Drug	Dosage	Side Effects	Onset/Duration
Dextroamphetamine (Dextrostat, Dexedrine)	For ages 3–5 years: Initiate at 2.5 mg. Increase by 2.5 mg at weekly intervals. 6 years and older: initiate at 5 mg once or twice daily. 40 mg/day max.	Insomnia, headache, stomachache, decreased appetite, weight loss, growth retardation, tics, repetitive behaviors, irritability, dysphoria, rebound agitation. May also elicit psychotic symptoms and mania at higher rate than methylphenidate.	Onset in 30–60 minutes. Duration about 4–5 hours.
Dextroamphetamine (Dexedrine Spansules)	Single daily dosing up to a maximum of 40 mg/day.	Same as above.	Onset in 30–60 minutes. Duration about 5–10 hours.

Amphetamine Salts

Drug	Dosage	Side Effects	Onset/Duration
Amphetamines salts (Adderall)	Age 6 years and older, initiate at 5 or 10 mg, up to 30 mg per dose.	Same as above.	Onset in 30–60 minutes. Duration about 4–5 hours.
Amphetamine salts (Adderall-XR) *50% immediate release beads and 50% delayed release beads*	Age 6 and older: Starting dose is 5 or 10 mg. May be adjusted in 5–10 mg increments up to 40 mg per day.	Same as above.	Onset in 60–90 minutes (possibly sooner). Duration 10–12 hours.

TABLE 25-3	American Heart Association History Guidelines for Stimulant Use

Child's History
- History of fainting or dizziness (particularly with exercise)
- Seizures
- Rheumatic fever
- Chest pain or shortness of breath with exercise
- Unexplained, noticeable change in exercise tolerance
- Palpitations, increased heart rate, or extra or skipped heart beats
- History of high blood pressure
- History of heart murmur other than innocent or functional murmur or history of other heart problems
- Intercurrent viral illness with chest pains or palpitations
- Current medications (prescribed and over the counter)
- Health supplements (nonprescribed)

Family History
- Sudden or unexplained death in someone young
- SCD or "heart attack" in members <35 years of age
- Sudden death during exercise
- Cardiac arrhythmias
- HCM or other cardiomyopathy, including dilated cardiomyopathy and right ventricular cardiomyopathy (right ventricular dysplasia)
- LQTS, short-QT syndrome, or Brugada syndrome
- WPW or similar abnormal rhythm conditions
- Event requiring resuscitation in young members (<35 years of age), including syncope requiring resuscitation
- Marfan's Syndrome

SCD, sudden cardiac death; HCM, hypertrophic cardiomyopathy; LQTS, long QT syndrome; QT, QT interval; WPW, Wolff-Parkinson-White Syndrome

may be over an inch shorter than their untreated peers at maturity. Remedies include the use of nutritious snacks in the evening, dietary supplements at lunch and after school, medication "holidays" on weekends and summers if possible. Additionally, the clinician may consider a medication that does not last into the dinner hour; the downside is that children may then struggle with completing their homework.

Tics may be caused by or exacerbated by stimulants. The child and family will need to make a risk–benefit decision with the clinician to decide whether to stop the stimulant, ignore the tics as long as they are not stigmatizing, or to treat the tics with a second medication. This decision will largely be based on how successful the child is with stimulants.

Finally, the stimulants are cleared by the kidneys. This makes them readily compatible with many other psychiatric and somatic medications that are hepatically metabolized.

Prescribing Essentials

All stimulants demonstrate comparable efficacy in controlled studies, although individual children may respond preferentially to a specific medication. Recent advances in drug-delivery technology for the stimulants have made available a wide range of dosing forms and properties allowing the physician to individualize treatment. Medication selection is based on factors such as dosing frequency, compliance, feasibility of medication administration during the school day, duration of action, side-effect profiles, and cost. For most children, the longer-acting preparations are preferable for convenience and compliance, particularly to avoid having to take medication at school.

Longer-acting preparations also lead to less rebound and withdrawal effects and are less likely to cause anxiety and mood fluctuations. On the other hand, if a child is sleeping poorly or eating poorly, a shorter-acting preparation may be preferable. Some children respond better to a rapid-onset stimulant at the beginning of the day. In these cases, augmenting a long-acting stimulation preparation with a rapid-onset preparation in the morning will provide optimal benefits. Children who experience irritability when their medication wears off may benefit from a small dose of a short-acting stimulant in the late afternoon. As per the CMAP, if one type of stimulant is not tolerated or effective, it is reasonable to try one more medication of the same type before switching to a different type of stimulant. The concomitant use of methylphenidate and an amphetamine is not consistent with guideline care.

Antidepressants

Antidepressant medications are used to treat numerous psychiatric disorders in children and adolescents, including: depression, obsessive–compulsive disorder (OCD), other anxiety disorders, trauma-related symptoms, bulimia, enuresis, ADHD, and smoking cessation. There are many types of antidepressants which are classified based on their mechanisms of action rather than their chemical structure. The various antidepressants, their chemical effects, and clinical guidelines are summarized in Table 25-4.

Indications

Tricyclic antidepressants (TCAs) include imipramine, desipramine, amitriptyline, nortriptyline, protriptyline, and doxepin. They are highly effective in treating adult depression.

The TCAs with FDA-approval for youth include: doxepin (over 12 years), clomipramine (over 10 years), and imipramine (over 6 years). The TCAs were the first antidepressants to be used to treat depression, obsessive–compulsive and other anxiety disorders in children and adolescents. Other uses with youth have included enuresis, ADHD, sleep disorders, and pain syndromes. Systematic studies with youth have focused on their use for depression, and to a lesser extent anxiety. Double-blinded placebo-controlled trials have found the TCAs to be no more effective than placebo in treating juvenile-onset major depression. Use in anxiety disorders has shown limited effectiveness as well, except for clomipramine which has demonstrated efficacy for the treatment of OCD. Interestingly, they have demonstrated efficacy for ADHD. Eighteen controlled studies involving 953 children demonstrated at least moderate benefit compared to placebo. TCAs are now considered a third-line treatment of ADHD, limited by their adverse effects and narrow therapeutic window, and thus potential toxicity. The TCAs are not used much for depressive or anxiety disorders any more. The exception is clomipramine, although side effects limit its use to refractory OCD.

SSRIs include citalopram, escitalopram, fluoxetine, fluvoxamine, paroxetine, and sertraline. The SSRIs are not more effective than the TCAs in treating depressed adults, but they have many fewer serious and annoying side effects leading to their popularity. The SSRIs that are approved by the FDA for use in pediatric populations include fluoxetine (8 years and older), sertraline (6 years and older), escitalopram (12 years and older), and fluvoxamine (8 years and older). The SSRIs have an established evidence base for use with youth including fluoxetine and escitalopram for major depression, sertraline for anxiety disorders, and fluvoxamine for OCD. While not FDA-approved for use in pediatric populations, citalopram has shown efficacy in randomized controlled trials for the treatment of depression and anxiety in youth.

Atypical antidepressants include bupropion, venlafaxine, and mirtazapine. All have FDA-approval and indications for the treatment of depression in adults. Bupropion is also indicated for the treatment of smoking cessation. However, there are few randomized controlled studies demonstrating efficacy for these atypical antidepressants for any psychiatric disorder in youth. A single study has shown bupropion to be more efficacious than placebo but less efficacious

TABLE 25-4 Antidepressant Medications

Drug	Chemical Effect	Average Daily Dose	Side Effects	Indications
Tricyclic Antidepressants (TCAs)				
Amitriptyline (tertiary amine) (Elavil)	5HT, ±NE	Children: 1–3 mg/kg/day Adolescents: 25–100 mg/day	Cardiac arrhythmia, potentially lethal in overdose, anticholinergic side effects, orthostasis, sedation, GI intolerance, weight gain, sexual dysfunction. May increase risk of suicidal behavior.	Not FDA-approved for use in children. Historic uses: Insomnia, night terrors, enuresis, ADHD, chronic pain.
Imipramine (tertiary amine) (Tofranil)	Primary effects on NE	For enuresis, initial dose usually 25 mg/day ages 6 years and older. May increase by 25 mg/day/week not to exceed 75 mg/day.	As above.	FDA-approved for treatment of enuresis for youth 6 yrs and older.
Clomipramine (tertiary amine) (Anafranil)	5HT (more potent than other TCAs) +NE	Recommended starting dose is 25 mg/day. May increase 25 mg/day/wk up to 100–200 mg/day or 1.4 mg/pound whichever is smaller. Recommended max dose 200 mg/day.	As above.	FDA-approved for pediatric OCD in youth 10 years and older.
Doxepin (tertiary amine) (Sinequan)	5HT, NE, H1, H2, M	For sleep 10–25 mg 1 hour before bedtime. For depression start 10–25 mg/day. Increase slowly up to 50–100 mg/day. Usually more than 100 mg/day not needed in teens.	As above. Considered to have the least cardiotoxic potential of the TCAs.	FDA-approved for depression in children over age 12. May also be helpful for pruritis, insomnia, and anxiety.
Nortriptyline (secondary amine) (Pamelor)	NE, ±5HT	Suggested doses for Children: 1–3 mg/kg/day in 3–4 divided doses. Adolescents: 30–150 mg/day in 3–4 divided doses.	Same as for amitriptyline, but anticholinergic effects less pronounced.	Not FDA-approved for use in children.
Desipramine (secondary amine) (Norpramin)	Primary effects on NE	For children 6–12 years old, the suggested dose ranges from 10 to 30 mg per day in divided doses. For adolescents, daily dosages range from 25 to 50 mg but may be increased up to 100 mg, if needed.	Same as for imipramine, but anticholinergic effects less pronounced. Occasional insomnia. While sudden death from arrhythmias is rare, concerns persist.	As above.

Selective Serotonin Reuptake Inhibitors (SSRIs)

Citalopram (Celexa)	5HT reuptake inhibitors	5–40	May increase risk of suicidal behavior. Activation and agitation.	Not FDA-approved in children, although widely used in pediatric populations.
			Serotonin syndrome.	
			Weight gain.	
			Sexual side effects.	
Escitalopram (Lexapro)		2.5–20		FDA-approved for depression in children 12 years and older.
Fluoxetine (Prozac)		5–60 mg/day.		FDA-approved for depression and OCD in youth 8 years and older.
Sertraline (Zoloft)		25–200 mg/day Divided dosing.		FDA-approved for OCD in youth 6 years and older. Off-label used for depression and PTSD.
Fluvoxamine (Luvox)		25–200 mg/day divided dosing.		FDA-approved for OCD in youth 8 years and older.
Paroxetine (Paxil)		No pediatric dosing recommendations.		Not FDA-approved for children and not recommended for off-label use with pediatric populations.

Atypical Antidepressants

Bupropion (Wellbutrin)	DA and NE reuptake inhibitor	Starting dose is 37.5 mg increasing gradually (wait at least 3 days) to a maximum of 2–3 doses, no more than 150 mg/dose.	Irritability, decreased appetite, and insomnia. Lowers seizure threshold especially for individuals with eating disorders and seizure disorders, and particularly with short acting dose preparation over 200 mg (adult data) May increase risk of suicidal behavior.	Not FDA-approved in children, though used in pediatric populations for ADHD and depression.

(continued)

467

TABLE 25-4   **Antidepressant Medications** (*continued*)

Drug	Chemical Effect	Average Daily Dose	Side Effects	Indications
Atypical Antidepressants				
Bupropion (Wellbutrin SR)	DA and NE reuptake inhibitor	Usually dosed twice daily. Starting dose is 100 mg/day increasing gradually to a maximum of 100 mg bid in youth. Maximum recommended dose in adults 200 mg bid.	As above.	As above.
Buproprion (Wellbutrin XL)	DA and NE reuptake inhibitor	Usually dosed once daily. Starting dose is 150 mg/day Usual maximum dose 300 mg/day in youth. Maximum dose in adults 450 mg/day.	As above.	As above.
Venlafaxine (Effexor, Effexor XR)	5HT and NE reuptake inhibitor	No dosing information available for children. Start at lowest dose 25 mg once daily. Common maintenance dose in youth 25–100 mg/day. Usual maximum dose 225 mg/day for adults.	GI intolerance, sexual dysfunction, activation, mania, sleep disturbance, hypertension. May increase risk of suicidal behavior.	Not FDA-approved in children, though used in pediatric populations as third-line antidepressant for refractory depression. Consider use for ADHD.
Mirtazapine (Remeron)	5HT, NE reuptake inhibitor	No dosing information available for children. Start at lowest dose possible 15 mg once daily. Maximum recommended dose in adults 45 mg/day.	Somnolence, weight gain, rare agranulocytosis. May increase risk of suicidal behavior. Sedation is more common in low doses.	Not FDA-approved in children, though used in pediatric populations as third-line antidepressant for refractory depression and to take advantage of its therapeutic and side effects of sedation.
Trazodone (Desyrel)	5HT 2A reuptake inhibitor	Suggested initial dosing for insomnia 25 mg qhs. May increase in 25 mg increments to 100–150 mg qhs.	Somnolence. Priapism is rare, more common in younger boys then in teens.	Not FDA-approved in children, though commonly used in pediatric populations for insomnia.

5HT, serotonin; NE, norepinephrine; DA, dopamine; H, histamine; M,muscarinic; SI, suicidal ideation; FDA, Food and Drug Administration; GI, gastrointestinal; OCD, obsessive compulsive disorder; ADHD, attention-deficit hyperactivity disorder.

than stimulants in treating youth with ADHD. Clinical lore posits that bupropion may be less likely to induce mania, and many clinicians prefer it for the treatment of bipolar depression. Mirtazapine and venlafaxine are usually reserved for youth who have failed two SSRI trials. Venlafaxine is reputed to have a quicker onset of therapeutic action and be more effective in treatment-resistant depression, but there are no systematic studies regarding its use in early-onset major depression. Thus, it is currently indicated as a third or fourth-line intervention in medication algorithms for depressed youth. Venlafaxine does have demonstrated efficacy in the treatment of youth with anxiety and open-label studies suggest efficacy in the treatment of ADHD. Mirtazapine has also found a role for depressed youth suffering insomnia or weight loss. To date there are no systematic studies supporting the use of mirtazapine in pediatric populations. There are some open-label studies supporting its use in anxiety. Finally, trazodone is FDA-approved for the treatment of depression in adults. It is also commonly used to treat anxiety in adults and insomnia in both adults and youth. The sedative effects have immediate onset. In children, the safety and efficacy of trazodone have not been established. Nonetheless, it is widely used.

Mechanism of Action

Two related theories are posited regarding the etiology of depression. The *monoamine deficiency hypothesis* posits that the normal amount of monoamine neurotransmitter activity becomes reduced, depleted, or dysfunctional for unclear reasons leading to depression. Interestingly, neurotransmitters can regulate the number of their own receptors via chemical instructions to the cell's DNA to synthesize a greater or lesser number of its own receptors. The *neurotransmitter receptor hypothesis* then posits that deficient activity of monoamine neurotransmitters causes "upregulation" of postsynaptic monoamine neurotransmitter receptors, that is, an increase in neurotransmitter receptor synthesis. The converse, "downregulation," refers to a process by which intracellular enzymes instruct the cell's DNA to slow down the synthesis of the neurotransmitter's receptor. These processes appear to occur at both the presynaptic somatodendritic areas near the cell body and in the synapse itself near the axon terminal and are hypothesized to reverse the depressed state.

Whether or not these processes are really etiologically related to the onset and remission of depression, they are associated with the actions of antidepressant medications and temporally related to remission of depression. Antidepressants inhibit neurotransmitter reuptake by blocking the transporter at the presynaptic somatodendritic area and at the terminal end of the neuron. This process produces immediate effects on the availability of synaptic neurotransmitters, yet clinical effects are delayed by days to weeks consistent with the onset of action of antidepressants. Reuptake inhibition in the somatodendritic end of the neuron is thought to be the primary mechanism accounting for the therapeutic effects of the SSRIs and reuptake inhibition of axonal receptors is thought to be the therapeutic mechanism for the TCAs.

TCAs block the presynaptic reuptake of both norepinephrine and serotonin, the degree of which varies by chemical structure of the TCA. Tertiary amines (e.g., amitriptyline, imipramine, doxepin) primarily block serotonin reuptake, and secondary amines (e.g., desipramine, nortriptyline, protriptyline) principally block norepinephrine reuptake. The TCAs have a wide range of receptor affinities including muscarinic, histaminic, and alpha-adrenergic receptors which confers considerable potential for adverse effects. The TCAs are hepatically metabolized substrates for several cytochrome P450 isoenzymes (e.g., 1A2, 2C9, 2C19, 2D6, 3A3/4) and subject to many drug interactions. Drugs that either inhibit or induce the same hepatic enzymes will influence the serum concentration of the TCAs which impacts efficacy and side effects. The rate of metabolism can be patient-variable. Patients who are considered "slow hydroxylators" should receive lower doses.

The SSRIs are structurally dissimilar, yet they share many pharmacological properties due to their relatively selective serotonin (5-hydroxytryptamine, 5-HT) reuptake inhibition in the synaptic gap. Some SSRIs also have weak effect on dopamine, particularly at higher doses which may affect their side-effect profile. All of the SSRIs are metabolized by the liver, but their cytochrome P450 isoenzyme profiles differ which has major implications for side effects. These factors are summarized in Table 25-4.

Atypical antidepressants differ in their mechanisms of action. *Bupropion* has a unique and poorly understood mechanism. In addition to its inhibition of norepinephrine reuptake, bupropion appears to be an indirect dopamine agonist. Structurally, it is similar to the psychostimulants. These properties may relate to its efficacy in ADHD. *Venlafaxine* is pharmacologically similar to the SSRIs, but also includes norepinephrine properties giving it TCA qualities, putatively without the same potential for toxicity. *Mirtazapine* also enhances both serotonergic and noradrenergic activity by blocking alpha$_2$ adrenergic presynaptic receptors which results in increased norepinephrine and serotonin neurotransmission. In addition to being a moderate alpha$_2$ adrenergic antagonist, it is a potent histamine antagonist and a moderate muscarinic antagonist. These effects result in sedation as well as hyperphagia, giving it a niche in the treatment of depressed youth with severe insomnia or weight loss. Finally, trazodone is a serotonin 2A and 2C receptor blocker, as well as a serotonin reuptake blocker. However, moderate to high doses are required to produce these effects limiting its use as an antidepressant. Lower doses exploit trazodone's potent antagonism of 5HT2A, histamine 1, and alpha 1 adrenergic receptors, thereby producing considerable sedation and making trazodone useful as a sleep agent.

Serious Complications and Their Management

Suicidal thinking and behaviors led the FDA to issue a "black-box" warning regarding the antidepressant treatment of youth. Subsequent studies have supported this concern. All physicians should discuss these risks during the consent process with a balanced presentation of the pros and cons of pharmacological treatment versus no pharmacological treatment, and alternative approaches to treatment, that is, psychotherapy for milder depression or anxiety. Such discussion should emphasize the preferential approach of combined pharmacological and psychotherapy treatment for moderate to severe illness. Frequent follow-up sessions can also minimize the risk for suicidality during treatment.

Agitation may result from SSRIs due to their effects on dopamine systems, perhaps via flooding and weakly engaging dopamine receptors, producing akathisia and other extrapyramidal effects that are difficult to differentiate from worsening of the original condition or emerging mania. Reduction in dose or changing to another agent is advised, rather than the addition of a medication to offset these effects.

Serotonin syndrome is a rare, idiosyncratic reaction to serotonergic medications. This potentially fatal condition affects multiple organ systems, including *somatic* (myoclonus), *cognitive* (confusion/hallucination), and *autonomic* (hyperthermia, hypertension, diaphoresis, nausea, diarrhea). Treatment consists of emergent support and cessation of any medication that increases serotonin in the CNS such as the SSRIs and TCAs.

Discontinuation syndromes resemble flu-like symptoms, confusion, or even "electric shock-like sensations." Shorter-acting SSRIs such as paroxetine, sertraline, and fluvoxamine have greater potential for such withdrawal symptoms than fluoxetine. A slow taper of these SSRIs usually prevents this syndrome. If withdrawal side effects persist, despite a slow taper, consideration should be given to adding low-dose fluoxetine during the taper. The downside of this strategy is a drug–drug interactions, or serotonin syndrome.

Drug Interactions are common for the SSRIs, TCAs, and bupropion as they are potent inhibitors of various P450 enzymes. SSRIs may also induce enzyme activity and are then metabolized by these enzymes (substrates). The informed-consent process should include educating the family about the risks of combining drugs at therapeutic doses and discussing with their pharmacist or primary clinician the addition of any prescribed or over-the-counter agent.

TCAs have a narrow therapeutic window. Thus, higher doses, drug interactions, and slow metabolism can lead to cardiotoxicity and lethality. In the 1980s, a series of sudden deaths were reported in children prescribed desipramine. Although a causal association was never proven, the risk of cardiotoxicity along with the development of safer classes of antidepressants led most physicians to discontinue the routine use of TCAs with youth. Treatment with TCAs should be preceded by an ECG and a follow-up ECG with any major change in dosage or the addition or elimination of medication that affect the metabolism of the TCAs, for example, anticonvulsants. Serum levels may be useful to avoid toxicity. Bupropion is contraindicated in patients with epilepsy or eating disorders due to its potential to decrease the seizure threshold in patients with these disorders. *Venlafaxine* is similar to the short-acting SSRIs in that a discontinuation syndrome may develop after only 1 week of therapy. *Mirtazapine's interaction* with selected histamine and 5-HT receptors leads to hyperphagia and weight gain. Finally, trazodone's most notable serious side effect is priapism. Although not a frequently reported side effect in boys, they may be more likely than adult males to develop this side effect.

Prescribing Essentials

As discussed above, the SSRIs are the first-choice antidepressant for pediatric indications.

The choice of a specific SSRI is determined by other medications being taken, half-life, drug interactions, family history of response, and costs. Citalopram and escitalopram are preferred for youth prescribed medication for somatic illness due to its low rate of protein binding and low cytochrome P450 inhibitor properties. If family history raises concerns about activation, a drug with a shorter half-life is preferable as it will clear the system more quickly. Alternatively, a longer half-life will be beneficial for teens who erratically take their medication or for a child with a history of SSRI withdrawal.

As noted in Table 25-4, SSRIs are dosed once to twice daily depending on their half-lives and ages of the patient; younger age may necessitate twice daily dosing. Transition from one antidepressant to the next should involve cross tapering with the exception of fluoxetine discontinuation, as this drug's half-life is many days. Caution is warranted when cross tapering fluvoxamine with other SSRIs or TCAs due to the prominent cytochrome P450 inhibition.

Anxiolytics

Anxiolytics are comprised primarily of drugs of the benzodiazepine family. Other anxiolytics include the azapirones (buspirone) and antihistamines (hydroxyzine). They are the least studied and utilized psychotropics with youth. Their properties are presented in Table 25-5.

Indications

Benzodiazepines were developed as anticonvulsants but have had a long history with adults in the treatment of anxiety disorders, insomnia, musculoskeletal disorders, alcohol withdrawal, and the acute treatment of neuroleptic-induced akathisia. They include, in increasing order of duration of action alprazolam, oxazepam, lorazepem, diazepam, and clonazepam. Some benzodiazepines are FDA-approved for the treatment of seizures in pediatric populations including clonazepam for infants, children, and adolescents, diazepam for youth ages 6 months and older, and lorazepam for children 12 years and older. None has been FDA-approved for the treatment of pediatric anxiety, but they are widely used based on physicians' experience. They have an important role in treating severe anxiety and acute insomnia related to anxiety disorders, trauma, and mood disorders. Clinical lore suggests that children may require higher doses than adults due to their more rapid hepatic metabolism. This has not proven true and

TABLE 25-5   Anxiolytics

Drug	Chemical Effect	Average Daily Dosing	Side Effects	Indications
Benzodiazepines				
Clonazepam (Klonopin)	GABA	0.1–0.2 mg/kg/day in three divided doses	Sedation, ataxia, disinhibition, risk of tolerance addiction, and withdrawal.	FDA-approved for seizures in youth. FDA-approved for anxiety in adults.
Diazepam (Valium)	GABA	0.12–0.8 mg/kg/day in 3–4 divided doses		
Lorazepam (Ativan)	GABA	0.02–0.1 mg/kg every 4 to 8 hours		
Alprazolam (Xanax)	GABA	No pediatric dosing guidelines	As above. Risk of abuse may be greater due to short half-life.	Not FDA-approved in children. FDA-approved for anxiety in adults.
Oxazepam (Serax)	GABA	10–15 mg t.i.d. in adolescents	As above except less sedation than other benzodiazepines.	Not FDA-approved in children. FDA-approved for anxiety in adults.
Nonbenzodiazepines				
Buspirone (BuSpar)	5HT	0.3–0.6 mg/kg/day in two divided doses	Dizziness, headache, lightheadedness, nausea.	As above.
Hydroxyzine (Vistaril, Atarax)	H1 antagonist	0.5–1.0 mg/kg q 6–8 hours	Sedation, dizziness, lethargy.	FDA-approved for anxiety in both children and adults. Also used for nausea, preanesthetic.

GABA, γ-aminobutyric acid; 5HT, serotonin; FDA, Food and Drug Administration.

lower doses are indicated to minimize side effects. Due to the potential for tolerance and addiction, these medications are appropriate for acute treatment (2 to 3 weeks) while SSRIs are introduced and used over the long term. An exception might be adolescents with intractable panic or OCD who may benefit from chronic use of a benzodiazepine.

Other anxiolytics used to treat youth with anxiety disorders include *buspirone* and *hydroxyzine*. Despite established efficacy in the treatment of adults, buspirone is not FDA-approved for children, nor has it been systematically studied with youth, and does not appear to have a role in treating pediatric anxiety. *Hydroxyzine* has been used to treat anxiety symptoms since the 1950s. Its original FDA-approval was for "anxiety and tension associated with psychoneurosis," and "acute hysteria." Other FDA indications include: preoperative anxiety, alcohol withdrawal, as well as pruritus, nausea, and vomiting. It is used "off-label" for insomnia. Hydroxyzine is FDA-approved for treating anxiety in children over 6 years old. It is less potent than the benzodiazepines and does not carry the same risks of dependence and addiction. Its effectiveness as an antianxiety agent for long-term use (over 16 weeks) has not been assessed.

Mechanism of Action

Several neurotransmitters are involved in the production of anxiety symptoms at the level of the amygdala and numerous anxiolytic drugs have actions on these specific neurotransmitter systems to relieve anxiety symptoms. γ-aminobutyric acid (GABA) is intimately involved in these actions. GABA is the principal inhibitory neurotransmitter in the brain and serves a regulatory role in reducing the activity of many neurons, including those in the amygdala. One theory of the etiology of anxiety disorders is that the "set point" for GABA sites is "switched" so that individuals respond with anxiety to neutral antagonist and agonist stimuli.

Benzodiazepines exert their anxiolytic effects by potentiating the inhibitory effects of GABA in the amygdala and prefrontal cortex. GABA receptor sites have a central chloride channel and binding sites for both GABA and benzodiazepines—the latter referred to as the GABA-A allosteric modulatory site. When GABA binds to the GABA receptor sites, it opens the inhibitory chloride ion channels to a limited extent allowing the flow of chloride ions. When a benzodiazepine binds to this site in the absence of GABA, it has no effect. But, when it binds to the same site in the presence of GABA, it increases the frequency of opening of these inhibitory chloride channels producing an anxiolytic effect. Some benzodiazepines undergo hepatic metabolism via oxidation (e.g., diazepam, flurazepam) while others are metabolized by glucuronide conjugation (e.g., lorazepam, oxazepam).

Buspirone is an azapirone anxiolytic without anticonvulsant, sedative, or muscle-relaxant properties and with a poorly understood mechanism. It is a serotonin 1A partial agonist that is thought to exert its anxiolytic effects through binding to both presynaptic and postsynaptic 5HT1A receptors, thereby enhancing the input of serotonin to key amygdala nuclei so as to blunt fear-associated outputs. Its delayed onset of action suggests that their effects are not due to occupancy of receptor sites, but due to adaptations in neurotransmitter receptors, similar to the antidepressants. Similar mechanisms may account for the anxiolytic effects of the SSRIs. Buspirone is metabolized hepatically and is a substrate for the cytochrome P450 3A4 isoenzyme. Its half-life is short (2 to 3 hours in adults) but is increased in patients with hepatic dysfunction. Buspirone is not recommended for patients with severe renal or hepatic impairment. Unlike benzodiazepines, the anxiolytic effect of buspirone is delayed up to 2 to 4 weeks.

Hydroxyzine is an antihistamine that blocks histamine 1 receptors. Antihistamines treat anxiety symptoms by decreasing hyperarousal, vigilance, and hyperalertness, but seem to have little effect on anxiety per se. Hydroxyzine usually provides some immediate relief with the first dose, typically within 15 to 20 minutes.

Major Complications and Their Management

Benzodiazepines are highly lipophilic and, therefore, have a rapid onset of action, which can induce a euphoric effect. Those benzodiazepines with rapid onset of action, such as alprazolam, are the most likely to induce euphoria and have the greatest risk of abuse. These drugs also have short and intermediate half-lives which are associated with a greater risk of rebound or withdrawal effects. Compounds with a prolonged onset of action, like clonazepam, do not induce a euphoric response and are less likely to have withdrawal side effects. These drugs usually have longer half-lives which avoids the peak and valley effects of shorter-acting benzodiazepines, but are also associated with a risk of accumulation, especially in slow metabolizers, for example, a delayed sedative effect. Additionally, clonazepam may interact with the SSRIs. For example, fluoxetine inhibits cytochrome P450 3A4 and this inhibition may affect the clearance of clonazepam. For some patients, lorazepam's intermediate half-life leads to inter-dosing withdrawal symptoms. Oxazepam may be less sedating than the other benzodiazepines which may make it more useful for treating daytime anxiety.

Some patients may experience paradoxical or disinhibitory reactions. Such disinhibition includes acute excitement, giddiness, loquaciousness, hyperactivity, hostility, rage, and sexually inappropriate behaviors. Failure to recognize this reaction may lead to even higher doses of benzodiazepines in an attempt to control apparent core behavioral or mood symptoms.

All benzodiazepines have the potential to induce sedation and ataxia which can be controlled by dosage reduction. Withdrawal reactions may be life threatening in patients with a history of long-term use. These situations warrant an extended taper or a switching to longer-acting agent, such as clonazepam, to safely taper the shorter-acting benzodiazepam.

Hydroxyzine is well tolerated with sedation that is usually transient. Toxicity is unusual and fatal overdoses uncommon. Overdose can result in an anticholinergic syndrome with prominent confusion and hallucinations. When combined with analgesics or hypnotics, the synergistic depressant effects on the CNS can be fatal.

Prescribing Essentials

The choice of an anxiolytic is based on clinical considerations, other medications taken, and family preferences. For example, if a teen has a history of substance use, hydroxyzine may be preferred. Parents may advocate for buspirone if their own anxiety had been treated with this medication. Other factors considered are time to onset of action and duration of action. Both the benzodiazepines and hydroxyzine should be used for short-term treatment to provide initial symptom relief while awaiting the therapeutic benefits of an SSRI. Optimal anxiety control may necessitate multiple daily dosing particularly if the youth shows evidence of interdose withdrawal symptoms during the use of an agent with a short half-life. Agents with longer half-lives may not show prominent side effects immediately, but they may be evident after several weeks of treatment as the agent accumulates in tissue. Thus, the time to onset of action and half-life determine the frequency of dosing. Hydroxyzine's half-life averages 14 hours in adults, but it can be as short as 5 hours in children, necessitating dosing two to four times per day.

Presently, there are no data demonstrating that buspirone is an effective anxiolytic for children and many psychiatrists question its efficacy for youth. At best, buspirone may be considered a third or fourth-line treatment for pediatric anxiety.

Antipsychotic Medications

Antipsychotic, or neuroleptic, medications were developed for schizophrenia and other psychotic illnesses, but have found a role in many major mental illnesses. Their widespread popularity in the treatment of child and adolescent disorders is multidetermined including the recognition of early-onset disorders previously thought to begin in adulthood such as bipolar disorder, the need for adjunctive treatment for childhood-onset disorders with severe behavioral disturbances such as that occurs in autism, and the lack of or partial effectiveness of psychotherapies for severe disorders. These medications are classified as first-generation antipsychotics (FGAs) and second-generation antipsychotics (SGAs). The FGAs, also known as "typical," "traditional," or "conventional" antipsychotics, are defined by their blockade of dopamine-2 (D2) receptors. SGAs, or "atypical" antipsychotics, are defined by their blockade, or antagonism, of both D2 and serotonin-2A receptor sites. Features of the antipsychotics are summarized in Table 25-6.

Indications

The primary indications for all antipsychotics with adults are for the treatment of schizophrenia and bipolar mania. Only a few antipsychotic medications are FDA-approved for use in children. Among the FGAs, those approved for youth include: *haloperidol* (≥3 years old) for the treatment of aggression and tic disorders; *pimozide* (≥12 years old) for tic disorders; and *thioridazine* (≥2 years old) for psychosis, impulsivity, and aggression. However, neither pimozide nor thioridazine is used routinely anymore due to the risk of sudden death from lengthening of the QTc interval and Torsades de Pointes syndrome.

All of the SGAs are FDA-approved for the treatment of adults with schizophrenia and mania, except for clozapine which is not approved for bipolar disorders. Those that are FDA-approved for the treatment of acute mania and schizophrenia in youth include risperidone (≥5 years old), aripiprazole (≥13 years old), and olanzapine (≥13 years old). Additionally, risperidone is FDA-approved for, and aripiprazole is awaiting approval for, the treatment of aggression and hyperactivity in autistic patients. Other SGAs do not have FDA-approval for use with children and adolescents. Despite these limited FDA indications, all of the SGAs are widely used off-label with youth suffering disturbances of thinking and affective regulation, and impulse control that impair their functioning and ability to meet developmental expectations, often placing themselves and/or others in danger. These disturbances are thought to be associated with abnormalities in the limbic system which require medical–psychiatric interventions when environmental adjustments and psychotherapy are ineffective alone. The choice of SGA for an individual child is largely determined by physicians' balancing their experience in treating specific disorders with the known side-effect profiles.

The FGAs may be seeing a rebirth. The Treatment of Early-Onset Schizophrenia Spectrum (TEOSS) disorders found that molindone was as effective as risperidone and olanzapine in treating psychotic symptoms with a lower risk of metabolic side effects. Although molindone is no longer available in the United States and Canada, these findings open the door for physicians to consider other FGAs with youth. The NIMH-funded Clinical Antipsychotic Trials of Intervention Effectiveness (CATIE) study with adults found that perphenazine was as effective as olanzapine, quetiapine, and risperidone in treating the positive and negative symptoms of schizophrenia and average health care costs were 20% to 30% lower for perphenazine. Thus, there now appears to be a larger number of options for physicians to consider in individualizing treatment for severe disturbances in childhood and adolescence.

Mechanism of Action

The antipsychotics have been widely studied in terms of their effect on the CNS's neurochemisty and the pathways mediating these neurotransmitters. As Stahl so elegantly elaborates, all antipsychotics affect D2 dopamine receptors. FGAs primarily block D2 receptors and SGAs variably block D2 receptors and act in a range of ways on serotonergic, histaminic, and muscarinic receptors, as summarized in Table 25-6. These actions appear to account for the heterogeneous therapeutic and side-effect profiles of these medications. D2 receptors are found in four primary dopamine pathways: *nigrostriatal, mesolimbic, mesocortical, and*

TABLE 25-6 Antipsychotic Medications

Receptor Affinity	First-Generation Antipsychotics (FGA)		Second-Generation Antipsychotics (SGA)					
	Haloperidol	Molindone	Aripiprazole	Clozapine	Olanzapine	Quetiapine	Risperidone	Ziprasidone
Half-life (hours)	20	3	72	16	30	7	3	7
Dosing (varies by age and condition)	0.25–5 mg daily	5–15 mg t.i.d. or q.i.d.	5–15 mg daily	25–300 mg daily	2.5–20 mg daily	25–300 mg divided	0.25–4 mg divided	20–60 mg twice daily
Side Effects	Haloperidol	Molindone	Aripiprazole	Clozapine	Olanzapine	Quetiapine	Risperidone	Ziprasidone
Anticholinergic	0	0	0	+++	++	0+	0	0
EPS: Akathisia	+++	++	++	+	+	+	+	+
EPS: Tardive dyskinesia	++	+/++	0+	0	0+	0+	0+	0+
Cardiovascular: Orthostasis	0	+	0+	+++	++	++	+	0
Cardiovascular: ↑ QTc	0+	+	0+	+	0+	+	+	++
Metabolic: ↑ Lipids	0+	0+	0+	++	++	+	+	0+
Metabolic: Diabetes	0+	0+	0+	+++	++	++	+	0+
Metabolic: Weight gain	+	0+	+	+++	+++	++	++	+
↓ Seizure threshold	0+	0+	0+	++	0+	0+	0+	0+
↑ Prolactin	++	++	→	0	++	0	+++	+

Monitoring

	Haloperidol	Molindone	Aripiprazole	Clozapine	Olanzapine	Quetiapine	Risperidone	Ziprasidone
	Baseline and follow-up AIMS, BMI, monitor blood pressure, lipids.	Baseline and follow-up AIMS, BMI, monitor blood pressure, lipids.	Baseline and follow-up AIMS, BMI, monitor blood pressure, lipids, fasting blood sugars.	Baseline and follow-up AIMS, BMI, monitor blood pressure, lipids, fasting blood sugars CBC.	Baseline and follow-up AIMS, BMI, monitor blood pressure, lipids, fasting blood sugars.	Baseline and follow-up AIMS, BMI, monitor blood pressure, lipids, fasting blood sugars.	Baseline and follow-up AIMS, BMI, monitor blood pressure, lipids, fasting blood sugars prolactin level, consider prolactin.	Baseline and follow-up AIMS, BMI, monitor blood pressure and pulse, ECGs.

A1, alpha agonist; DA, dopamine; 5HT, serotonin; M, Muscurinic; EPS, extrapyramidal symptoms; NMS, neuroleptic malignant syndrome; CBC, complete blood count; BP, blood pressure; ECG, electrocardiogram; BMI, Body Mass Index; AIMS, Abnormal involuntary movements.

tuberoinfundibular. The *mesolimbic* pathway regulates the limbic system. Dysfunction in this system is thought to account for the "positive" symptoms of schizophrenia (delusions and hallucinations) as well as affective symptoms such as mania, anger, and hostility. D2 blockade is associated with resolution or decrease of such "positive" symptoms. The *mesocortical* pathway is involved in the regulation of cognition, particularly involving frontocortical activities which moderate executive functions such as attention, affect, and motivation. Dysfunction in this pathway appears to be associated with the negative symptoms of schizophrenia, such as inattention, amotivation, and flattening of affect. Interestingly, D2 blockade here may make negative symptoms worse while improvement appears indirectly associated with the SGAs' serotonergic effects. The *nigrostriatal* pathway mediates motor functions. D2 blockade leads to extrapyramidal motor side effects including akathisia, dystonia, pseudoparkinsonian symptoms, and tardive dyskinesia. The *tuberoinfundibular* pathway inhibits release of prolactin. D2 blockade leads to an increased release of prolactin.

In terms of specific SGAs, aripiprazole and ziprasidone have unique actions. At low and high doses aripiprazole acts predominantly as a D2 *agonist*, not antagonist, to decrease dopamine activity. It may increase serotonin effects at high doses. Clinically, aripiprazole at low and high doses may agitate patients. Ziprasidone is predominantly a serotonin agonist at low doses and may also cause agitation if initiated at low doses. On the positive side, both aripiprazole and ziprasidone may augment antidepressant effects of the SSRIs at low doses, likely due to their serotonergic activity. For youth with psychotic disorders who are agitated or unable to sleep, olanzapine or quetiapine may be preferred due to their sedating antihistaminic activity.

These neuroleptic medications can have profound positive effects on disturbing and impairing symptoms, indeed they may be life-altering, even life-saving, for many youth. However, such optimism must be tempered by the legitimate concerns expressed in the medical and scientific communities regarding their unknown potential long-term effects on the developing brain. Studies of such effects would be difficult to conduct, but are clearly needed.

Major Complications and Their Management

The FGAs are associated with movement disorders, which in part led to the popularity of the SGAs. Prophylactic use of vitamin E, 400 to 2000 IU/day, is recommended for adults with all neuroleptics to help protect against the development of tardive dyskinesia. Anticholinergic agents are used to contain the extrapyramidal symptoms that develop with both groups of antipsychotics. They are not usually used prophylactically but only when symptoms develop. Although the SGAs have a preferable motor side-effect profile, their potential to cause metabolic syndrome has led to the reconsideration of use of the FGAs.

Metabolic syndrome can occur with any of the neuroleptics. Among the FGAs, it is more likely with the less-potent antipsychotics. The SGAs appear more likely than the FGAs to cause metabolic syndrome in youth. Clozapine, olanzapine, risperidone, and quetiapine carry higher risk than aripiprazole and ziprasidone. The symptoms of metabolic syndrome include abdominal obesity, dyslipidemia, glucose intolerance, and hypertension. A common root for these symptoms appears to be insulin resistance which increases with obesity. However, some patients develop elevated lipids and diabetes without weight gain. Children taking SGAs should have regular evaluation of Body Mass Index (BMI = weight (kg) × height (meters)^2). By definition, a child who measures greater than the 95th percentile for BMI and waist size, has a blood pressure over the 95th percentile for age, and has a fasting blood sugar over 110 mg/dL, and triglycerides over 150 mg/dL suffers metabolic syndrome. Prevention of this syndrome is difficult for families as it warrants careful dietary control of caloric intake and exercise. Correll and colleagues provide an extensive review of managing metabolic syndrome.

Hyperprolactinemia is common with the SGAs, especially risperidone. Symptoms may include decreased menstruation, nipple discharge, breast enlargement, sexual dysfunction, and pubertal development. Mildly elevated prolactin levels may spontaneously normalize over 6 to 12 months. Levels under 200 ng/dL may be addressed by lowering the SGA dose, or by switching to aripiprazole which lowers prolactin levels. Persistently elevated levels warrant further evaluation for other abnormalities, such as a pituitary tumor.

Neuroleptic Malignant Syndrome (NMS) is a rare but potentially fatal disorder resulting from D2 blockade in the hypothalamus. Classic presentations include hyperthermia, muscular rigidity, autonomic instability, confusion, elevated white blood cell count, and elevated creatinine phosphokinase (CPK) due to rhabdomyolysis. Treatment involves discontinuation of the offending medication and supportive measures such as hydration. Some clinicians use dopamine agonists such as bromocriptine, and muscle relaxants such as dantrolene to offset the rigidity. However, the efficacy of these treatments has not been systematically examined.

Cardiac complications include QT prolongation and Torsades de Pointes which can be fatal. The Center for Education and Research on Therapeutics (CERT) at the University of Arizona maintains a website that lists medications that are associated with cardiovascular complications. This website lists the following antipsychotics as having an established risk for prolonged QT and Torsades de Pointes: chlorpromazine, haloperidol, pimozide, and thioridazine. It lists several SGAs as having a possible risk for these complications, including clozapine, ziprasidone, risperidone, and quetiapine. These medications warrant evaluation of youth's cardiovascular status and then monitoring for complications, including follow-up ECGs.

Prescribing Essentials

The AACAP's Practice Parameter for the Assessment and Treatment of Children and Adolescents with Schizophrenia notes that neuroleptic medication is the core primary treatment for schizophrenia and psychotic disorders in youth, similar to the recommendations for adults with such disorders. The TEOSS study with youth, the CATIE study with adults, and the Cost Utility of the Latest Antipsychotic Drugs in Schizophrenia Study (CUtLASS) raise questions about the comparable efficacy, effectiveness, side effects, and costs of the FGAs and SGAs in the treatment of positive and negative symptoms of schizophrenia. Such considerations may apply to the use of the neuroleptics for other severe psychiatric illness of youth. However, the length of these studies precludes conclusions regarding their comparable risks for tardive dyskinesia, which was a major consideration in the preferential use of the SGAs over the past two decades. While investigators in the laboratory and clinicians in the field develop best practices regarding the preferential uses of the FGAs and SGAs, the prescribing clinician appears to have gained the option of using a broader range of neuroleptics to individualize treatment.

A major consideration in the use of all neuroleptics is that primary psychotic symptoms may decrease within 1 to 2 weeks of initiation of treatment, but full benefits on cognitive, affective, and behavioral symptoms may take weeks to realize. It is usually recommended to wait at least 4 to 6 weeks to determine efficacy of an antipsychotic, and many patients may require up to 16 to 20 weeks of treatment to show a response. Physicians may be eager to see benefits sooner and often augment or "jump start" treatment with another agent, for example, the addition of an FGA to an SGA, or the addition of a benzodiazepine or lithium. A switch to clozapine is cautiously used for cases that are clearly refractory to usual, as well as rather unconventional, approaches due to the side-effect profile of this medication and the need for frequent serum monitoring for agranulocytosis.

Mood Stabilizers

The class of medications termed mood stabilizers refers to agents that can stop the cycling between depression and euphoria in bipolar disorder. These medications include lithium and selected antiepileptic drugs (AEDs) that have been well studied in adults and have an emerging evidence base with children and adolescents. The mood stabilizers are often used in combination with other psychotropics due to the difficulties in treating the extreme poles of bipolar disorder. Properties of mood stabilizers are presented in Table 25-7.

Indications

The treatment of bipolar disorder is complicated as the medications that treat the manic phase of illness may not treat the depressed phase, and medications that treat the depressed phase may induce cycling. Lithium is the classic mood stabilizer. It is the only non-AED drug that is FDA-approved for the treatment of bipolar disorder and has been approved for youth over 12 years old. Most of the AED mood stabilizers have obtained FDA-approval for pediatric seizure disorders, including: carbamazepine at any age, oxcarbazepine for youth over 4 years old, and valproate for youth over 2 years old. None of these AEDs has been FDA-approved for the treatment of early-onset bipolar disorder. However, an evidence base is developing. Valproate has shown efficacy in several but not all smaller studies. The efficacy of carbamazepines is equivocal but also not well studied with youth. A meta-analysis indicated a large effect size, but more recent study has questioned its efficacy with youth. Oxcarbazepine has not been well studied with adults and a recent study with youth did not show benefits over placebo. However, this AED continues to be widely used in clinical practice for the treatment of youth with bipolar disorder. Case studies, open label, and small studies with adults and youth suggest that lamotrigine may be effective in the treatment of the depressive phases of bipolar disorder without the risk of inducing cycling as can occur with antidepressants, but controlled studies are lacking. Despite initial suggestions of efficacy for gabapentin and topiramate in the treatment of bipolar disorder in adults, subsequent studies have not supported their role as mood stabilizers.

Mechanism of Action

The exact mechanisms of action for the mood stabilizers are unknown, but recent evidence is intriguing as to the potential pathologic processes underlying bipolar disorder and the focus for stabilizing its cycling. Lithium appears to affect multiple systems. Traditional theories note how lithium alters sodium transport across cell membranes and alters the metabolism of the catecholamines and serotonin. More recent evidence indicates that lithium alters intracellular signaling through actions on second messenger systems such as phosphatidyl inositol and G proteins. Lithium is also thought to affect gene expression involved in regulating growth factors and neuronal plasticity.

The mechanism of action of valproate is thought to include the blockade of voltage-sensitive sodium channels and the increase of GABA in the CNS. The other AED mood stabilizers are also thought to exert their effects through the blockade of voltage-sensitive sodium channels and possibly through the inhibition of glutamate.

Major Complications and Their Management

Bone marrow suppression can occur with valproate and carbamazepine resulting in agranulocytosis and even aplastic anemia. However, it should be noted that a transient reduction in the white blood cell count is common early in the course of treatment and should not necessitate drug discontinuation. Some clinicians recommend lowering of the dose and using a slower titration to achieve successful treatment. Thus, the use of these AED mood stabilizers requires that a complete blood count is obtained at baseline and then at 2 weeks, at 1 and 3 months, and then every 6 months.

Hepatotoxicity can occur with valproate and carbamazepine due to a chemical hepatitis evidenced by elevations in liver enzymes. Therefore, liver function tests should be obtained prior to treatment, then again at 2 weeks, at 1 and 3 months after the initiation of treatment,

TABLE 25-7 Mood Stabilizers

Drug	Mechanism of Action	Average Daily Dose	Side Effects	Monitoring
Lithium carbonate (Lithobid, Eskalith)	Unknown. May act to modulate glutamate activity as well as modification of gene expression.	Children: 15–60 mg/kg/day in 3–4 divided doses. Adolescents: 600–1800 mg/day in 3–4 divided doses or 2 divided doses for sustained release products.	Hypothyroidism, nephrotoxicity, sedation, thirst, polyuria, polydipsia, weight gain, GI intolerance, tremor, seizures, acne, decreased cognitive ability.	Serum levels. Acute mania: 0.8–1.5 mEq/L. Maintenance: 0.5–1 mEq/L. TSH, Renal panel, Urinalysis prior to treatment and at 1, 3, and every 6 months thereafter.
Valproate, valproic acid (Depakote, Depakene)	Reduces high-frequency neuronal firing and sodium-dependent action potentials; enhances GABA.	30–60 mg/kg/day in 2–3 divided doses.	Sedation, thrombocytopenia, alopecia, nausea, weight gain, tremor, GI upset, hepatotoxicity, neutropenia, agranulocytosis, decreased cognitive ability.	Serum level. 50–125 µg/mL. CBC, Liver enzymes pre treatment, and at 2 weeks, 1 month, 3 months, and every 6 months thereafter.
Carbamazepine (Tegretol, Carbatrol)	Inhibits voltage-dependent sodium channels and decreases glutamate activity.	Children: 10–20 mg/kg/day in 3–4 divided doses. Adolescents: 400–800 mg/day in 2–3 divided doses.	Dizziness, rash, Stevens–Johnson syndrome (life-threatening toxic epidermal necrolysis), impaired coordination, slurred speech, ataxia, drowsiness, nausea, vomiting, agranulocytosis, hepatotoxicity, decreased cognitive ability.	Serum level: 8–12 µg/mL. CBC, Liver enzymes pretreatment, and at 2 weeks, 1 month, 3 months, and every 6 months thereafter.
Oxycarbazepine (Trileptal)	Inhibits voltage-dependent sodium channels and decreases glutamate activity.	Age 4–16 year: 8–10 mg/kg generally not to exceed 600 mg/day, given in a BID regimen. See PDR for weight-related final dose targets.	Same as carbamazepine but less risk of neutropenia and add risk of hyponatremia, decreased cognitive ability.	Baseline sodium and monitor of signs and symptoms of hyponatremia.
Lamotrigine (Lamictal)	Inhibits voltage-dependent sodium channels and decreases glutamate activity.	12.5 mg daily for weeks 1 and 2. 25 mg daily for weeks 3 and 4. 50 mg daily for week 5. 100 mg daily for week 6. Target dose: 100 mg to 200 mg daily.	Stevens–Johnson syndrome (life-threatening toxic epidermal necrolysis), decreased cognitive ability.	No serum monitoring when used for psychiatric purposes as no established relationship of serum level to efficacy or toxicity.

GABA, γ-aminobutyric acid; GI, gastrointestinal; PDR, Physicians' Desk Reference; TSH, thyroid stimulating hormone; CBC, complete blood count.

and then at every 6 months throughout the course of treatment. It should be noted that low-level elevations in liver function tests do not mandate cessation of treatment. Monitoring, and perhaps consultation with a hepatologist, is recommended.

Nephrotoxicity can occur during lithium treatment and may be irreversible. Therefore, monitoring of serum creatinine and blood urea nitrogen and urinalysis should occur at baseline and at 2 weeks, 1 month, 3 months, and every 6 months thereafter.

Thyroid suppression is relatively common with lithium treatment resulting in elevations of thyroid stimulating hormone (TSH) which does not necessarily require treatment. However, over time, functional hypothyroidism may occur and necessitate treatment. Thus, TSH levels should be obtained prior to treatment and at 1 month, 3 months, and then at 6-month intervals throughout the duration of treatment. In cases of clinical hypothyroidism when lithium is the only effective mood-stabilizing agent, treatment with thyroid hormone is generally effective.

Neurotoxicity is a potential complication of all mood stabilizers and may be dose-dependent. This may include cognitive dulling which can be particularly difficult for children's academic performance. Additionally, lithium overdose may cause permanent CNS injury, particularly to the cerebellum with resultant chronic ataxia.

Skin lesions are also common and may be serious. Lithium may cause or exacerbate cystic acne. Lamotrigine and carbamazepine are associated with Stevens–Johnson syndrome. This condition is more likely in patients concomitantly prescribed other medications especially valproate. The risk increases with rapid titration of lamotrigine. Slow titration appears to minimize risk. Recommendations are for increases of only 25 mg weekly, possibly more slowly when other drugs are concomitantly prescribed.

Prescribing Essentials

The Practice Parameter for the Assessment and Treatment of Children and Adolescents with Bipolar Disorder published by the AACAP generally follows the consensus guidelines developed by the Texas Medication Algorithm Project (TMAP) for adults with bipolar disorder. The TMAP provides algorithms for the manic phase of bipolar I disorder and the depressed phase of bipolar I and bipolar II disorders. It did not develop an algorithm for the hypomania of bipolar II disorder as it deemed that insufficient data existed to propose an algorithm. In brief, these guidelines recommend lithium, valproate, or an SGA for euphoric mania/hypomania; valproate or an SGA for dysphoric mania/hypomania and mixed states; and then either carbamazepine or olanzapine for individuals who do not respond to or have intolerable side effects with the primary recommendations. For patients in a depressed phase, lamotrigine is recommended alone or as an addition to a successful mood stabilizer, followed by quetiapine monotherapy, and then a combination of olanzapine and fluoxetine. For nonresponders to these primary and secondary choices, less commonly used two-drug combinations, or polypharmacy, is recommended. Clearly, the use of mood stabilizers to treat bipolar disorder and other causes of mood dysregulation requires considerable expertise in psychopharmacology. One important, and common, example is the use of lamotrigine with other AED mood stabilizers. Valproate decreases lamotrigine's metabolism and thereby increases its serum level up to 50%. Therefore, the dose of lamotrigine must be *decreased* by half when prescribed concurrently with valproate. Conversely, lamotrigine's serum level is decreased up to 50% when used concurrently with carbamazepine necessitating an *increased* dose of lamotrigine to maintain therapeutic levels. Estrogen-containing birth control pills also lower lamotrigine levels by up to 40%.

Discontinuation of mood stabilizers should also be conducted carefully. A slow titration of the dose of lithium and AED mood stabilizers to therapeutic levels may reduce the frequency and severity of metabolic and other side effects. Because these drugs have frequent cognitive side effects, differentiating illness from side effects is challenging. Deterioration in language, academics, organization, and other cognitive functions should be considered as possible medication side effects and may require decrease of dosage or change in medication. If discontinuation of lithium or the AED mood stabilizers is required, they should be tapered slowly to avoid precipitating a manic episode and a seizure in the case of the AEDs.

Other Psychotropic Medications

A variety of other medications are routinely used in the treatment of child and adolescent psychiatric disorders. A few of these agents will be briefly discussed. Their properties are summarized in Table 25-8.

Atomoxetine is classified as a norepinephrine reuptake inhibitor. It was developed as an antidepressant, although never marketed, nor FDA-approved, as such. Atomoxetine is the first nonstimulant medication that has been FDA-approved for the treatment of ADHD. Although its exact mechanism of therapeutic action is unknown, atomoxetine causes selective inhibition of presynaptic norepinephrine transporters, resulting in increases of both norepinephrine and dopamine in the prefrontal cortex. It may induce mild increases in blood pressure and pulse, but no ECG changes have been described. A target dose is 1.2 mg/kg administered as a single daily dose in the morning or in two divided doses in the morning and late afternoon/early evening. Atomoxetine may find a special niche for youth diagnosed with ADHD and comorbid tics or anxiety. It is also useful when a 24-hour effect is required. Interestingly, when prescribed at bedtime, atomoxetine may improve enuresis and insomnia.

Clonidine and guanfacine are central α2-adrenoreceptor agonists thought to reduce sympathetic outflow from the brain stem. They are widely used in child and adolescent psychiatry to treat hyperarousal associated with hyperactivity, impulsivity, anxiety, and trauma-related states, possibly by regulation of excitatory glutamate activity in the frontal cortex. Guanfacine's more selective effect on the alpha-2a receptor in the frontal lobes may account for its additional benefits in regulating attention and decreasing sedation. The availability of a long-acting form, Intuniv, allows for single daily dosing which precludes children having to take medication during school hours. By contrast, clonidine's sedating effects, mediated by antihistaminic action make it helpful in settling aroused youth so that they can fall asleep. However, both clonidine and guanfacine may cause mid-phase insomnia and exacerbate enuresis. These medications also have a role in treating tics. Their mechanism for decreasing tics is unclear. It is theorized that the agonist action on alpha-2a receptors improves the inhibitory capacity of the frontal cortex which may in turn improve the voluntary control of tics. Other uses have included the control of aggression toward self and others in youths with developmental disorders or head injuries.

There is some concern about combining these medications with stimulants due to the risks of cardiac arrhythmias, but no advisories have been issued regarding additional ECG monitoring. Both medications should be used cautiously with other drugs that can cause orthostasis. Neither drug should be withdrawn abruptly due to the risk of rebound hypertension.

Diphenhydramine is an antihistamine used to treat a variety of symptoms. Its hypnotic effects are due to antagonism of histamine 1 receptors. Diphenhydramine and two related drugs, benztropine and trihexyphenidyl, reduce the extrapyramidal side effects (EPS) caused by neuroleptics. The mechanism is indirect as dopamine and acetylcholine have a reciprocal relationship in the nigrostriatal pathway that mediates the development of EPS through excessive acetylcholine, or cholinergic, activity. Dopamine inhibits acetylcholine. When dopamine receptors are blocked by neuroleptic medication, this removes the inhibition. The resulting

TABLE 25-8 Other Medications With Psychotropic Properties

Norepinephrine Reuptake Inhibitor	Dosing	Common Side Effects	Duration of Effects
Atomoxetine (Strattera)	Initiate at 0.5 mg/kg. The targeted clinical dose is 1.2 mg/kg but titrate slowly at weekly intervals. Medication must be used each day.	Decreased appetite, gastrointestinal upset (can be reduced if medication taken with food), sedation (can be reduced by dosing in evening), lightheadedness.	Starts working within a few days to 1 week, but full effect may not be evident for a month or more. Duration of effect 24 hours.
		Risk of suicidal ideation and mania.	
Alpha-2 Agonists			
Clonidine (Catapres)	Starting dose is 0.025–0.05 mg/day in evening. Increase by similar dose every 5–7 days, adding to morning, mid-day, possibly afternoon, and again evening doses in sequence. Total dose of 0.1–0.3 mg/day divided into 3–4 doses.	Sleepiness, hypotension, headache, dizziness, stomachache, nausea, dry mouth, depression, nightmares. Severe rebound hypertension if abruptly discontinued.	Onset in 30–60 minutes. Duration about 3–6 hours.
Clonidine (Catapres) Patch	Corresponds to daily doses of 0.1 mg, 0.2 mg, and 0.3 mg respectively. Can not cut patch.	Same as Catapres tablet but 50% of children will have contact dermatitis.	Duration 4–5 days, so avoids the vacillations in drug effect with tablets.
Guanfacine (Tenex)	Starting dose is 0.5 mg/day in evening and increases by similar dose every 7 days as indicated in divided doses 2–3 times per day. Daily dose range 0.5–4 mg/day. DO NOT skip days.	Compared to clonidine, lower chances/severity of side effects, especially fatigue and depression. Also less headache, nausea, stomachache, dry mouth. Rebound hypertension if doses are missed.	Duration about 6–12 hours.
Guanfacine (Intuniv)	Starting dose a 1 mg/day. Do not increase more than 1 mg/day/week.	Compared to clonidine, lower chances/severity of side effects, especially fatigue and depression. Also less headache, nausea, stomachache, dry mouth. Rebound hypertension if doses are missed.	Elimination half-life thought to be approximately 17 hours.
	Maximum recommended dose 4 mg/day. Higher doses not studied.		

increased cholinergic activity produces EPS. An anticholinergic agent then suppresses this activity, ameliorating EPS that is coincident with the use of neuroleptics. An overdose of these medications can produce an anticholinergic syndrome with frightening visual hallucinations, confusion, flushing, dryness of the mucosa, and blurred vision.

Amantadine is another agent used to treat EPS, but by a direct mechanism. It acts by direct stimulation of D2 receptors to offset the blockade induced by the neuroleptics. The risk is exacerbation of psychosis. Other uses include the treatment of ADHD in children with developmental disabilities as shown by King and colleagues and possibly mood stabilization in bipolar disorder as reviewed by Stahl.

Conclusion

The past decade of research has significantly increased evidence-based pharmacological options for the treatment of youth with psychiatric illnesses. Furthermore, research increasingly indicates that the combination of medication with evidence based psychotherapy is superior to either treatment alone for youth suffering from many psychiatric illnesses. However, the long-term benefits, potential prophylaxis, and risks of these medications are not known. Longitudinal study is clearly needed. A biopsychosocial formulation and treatment planning, with objective measures of outcomes, improve effectiveness and reduce complications of pediatric psychopharmacology.

CASE VIGNETTES

VIGNETTE 1: A PREPUBERTAL BOY WITH COMORBID ADHD AND PTSD

Jack is a 7-year-old boy living with his biological mother and 5-year-old sister, and attending a special education 1st grade classroom. His mother brings him to clinic due to recent violence towards his younger sister requiring stitches in the emergency room (ER). Jack's mother describes her son as having an intense violence-filled fantasy life and behaves as if he is "possessed" with anger. His father who had terrorized the family with domestic violence is now incarcerated for assault. His mom reports that Jack and his sister have witnessed the father's aggression towards their mother on multiple occasions. The family is now in a stable living situation and mother is seeking employment, but feels exhausted trying to deal with Jack.

Further history reveals that Jack has had several trials of antipsychotic medications and stimulants from a prior provider. Risperidone and olanzapine caused intense hunger which resulted in multiple awakenings and eating during the night. Any efforts to secure the kitchen were met with screaming tantrums keeping everyone awake. Quetiapine caused daytime somnolence. Aripiprazole caused EPS. Stimulant medication trials showed mixed effectiveness. In lower doses, Jack was less hyperactive and focused well. However, when the dose was raised high enough to stop the aggressive behavior, Jack became more irritable and suffered insomnia. As Jack's family lives in a rural community, his family physician referred them for a telepsychiatry consultation with a child and adolescent psychiatrist.

On mental-status examination, the psychiatrist noted that Jack had no dysmorphia, was hyperactive, running all around the room, and intrusive as he opened all the cabinet drawers. He was easily distracted. Moreover, he easily startled to extraneous noises outside the office. Jack appears hypervigilant and aroused, but with no indications of hallucinations. He did not seem to understand many of the questions that his mother and the psychiatrist asked. Mother appeared tired and depressed, although she did try to redirect her son.

Using a biopsychosocial formulation, the psychiatrist realized that Jack's diagnostic profile was complicated by the family's chaotic lives as the mother tried to settle her family and return to the work force. He worked with social services to provide some help at school and in the home to strengthen the mother's efforts. Then the psychiatrist was able to complete Jack's evaluation. He diagnosed Jack with ADHD, a receptive language disorder, and posttraumatic stress disorder (PTSD). His mother was diagnosed with depression. The psychiatrist recommended a trial of either a SSRIs or alpha-2a agonist to contain Jack's anxiety and hyperarousal. His mother refused an SSRI because she felt that "I don't want my child to become suicidal." The addition of clonidine and then guanfacine to his stimulant caused unacceptable daytime sedation. His mother then allowed a trial of sertraline. Jack continued to take his stimulant and sertraline. Jack's aggression and tantrums decreased in frequency and duration over the ensuing 6 weeks. His mother was encouraged and agreed to engage in a course of parent behavioral training for disruptive children. Jack started Trauma-focused CBT, modified for his age and delays, by a local therapist under supervision of the telepsychiatrist.

This case illustrates three important points. First, a biopsychosocial formulation is needed to understand the context of a child's presentation, particularly when the family has been traumatized. Second, about a third of children diagnosed with ADHD also suffer anxiety disorders which can confuse the clinical picture, but also require treatment. Third the tendency to rely on the use of antipsychotics to treat agitation in youth, and particularly those with developmental delays, can lead clinicians away from salient diagnostic considerations that should focus on treatment. In this case, Jack had anxiety symptoms due to PTSD. Treatment with an SSRI, which is FDA-approved for the treatment of anxiety in children and PTSD in adults, proved to be an effective intervention.

VIGNETTE 2: A DEPRESSED TEEN IN FOSTER CARE

Jill is a 14-year-old girl living with her foster mother and father while attending a public high school in the 9th grade. Jill has had a year-long history of poor grades, changes in her peer group, and minimal attention to her appearance since being removed from her family after her 16-year-old sister accused their stepfather of sexually abusing her. She believes her sister accused her stepfather because she was angry at him for having her arrested for selling drugs. Her family history is positive for depression in multiple maternal family members. Her biological mother's depression was effectively treated with venlafaxine.

Because of Jill's depression, low energy, fatigue, and insomnia she is referred to her pediatrician. Her history, physical examination, and laboratory assessment (thyroid, complete blood count, iron level, vitamin D) do not suggest a physiologic cause for her symptoms. A drug screen was negative. Her pediatrician prescribes fluoxetine, because her caseworker did not want Jill taking a medication that is not FDA-approved for use in children. After 8 weeks of treatment, Jill improved minimally. She is then referred to a therapist for psychotherapy with CBT. By the sixth session, Jill showed no further improvement. Her therapist was concerned and asked her pediatrician to review the medication options. He switched her from fluoxetine to sertraline, which did not help over 8 more weeks and she had started to refuse to get up in the morning for school. The pediatrician considered aripiprazole or lamotrigine as the next step, but was uncertain, and Jill's caseworker refused to approve either. Jill was then referred to a child psychiatrist.

The child psychiatrist considered venlafaxine due to Jill's nonresponse to two SSRIs. However, he knew that the TORDIA (Treatment of Resistant Depression in Adolescents) study found that adolescents who are resistant to SSRI treatment and had a history of self-injurious behavior had an increased rate of suicidality with venlafaxine. However, Jill had no such prior history and her mother had a positive response to venlafaxine. Furthermore, the Texas CMAP for depressive disorders recommends a trial of an atypical antidepressant after two failed SSRI trials. Jill's caseworker was convinced to allow a venlafaxine trial when the psychiatrist emphasized that he was trying to avoid polypharmacy and following consensus guideline care from the CMAP the TORDIA study.

Subsequently, the psychiatrist reviewed his original biopsychosocial formulation. He noted the context in which Jill's depression arose. He then offered to have joint sessions with Jill and her sister to help them to reconcile and to cope better with the disruption to their family. With this new treatment plan Jill slowly improved without complications.

This vignette underscores the dilemma in treating refractory depression in youth. It can be very challenging given the evidence that antidepressants can indeed induce suicidality in youth but the equally concerning finding that failure to treat may have similar outcomes. Caseworkers are understandably cautious regarding the welfare of their wards. Pediatricians are increasingly pressured to treat psychiatric disorders, but without psychiatric consultation. While there is some movement to resort to polypharmacy to treat apparently refractory depression, atypical antidepressants should be considered before resorting to augmentation strategies, particularly as consensus guidelines include the use of such atypical antidepressants. Polypharmacy risks not just drug–drug interactions, but further complications such as weight gain and metabolic effects. By utilizing evidence-based or consensus guideline interventions, working closely with caseworkers, and providing psychoeducation to the child's team regarding state-of-the-art treatment for depression, a shared vision for treatment can be created.

BIBLIOGRAPHY

American Academy of Child and Adolescent Psychiatry. Practice parameter for the assessment and treatment of children and adolescents with bipolar disorder. *J Am Acad Child Adolesc Psychiatry.* 2007;46(1):107–125.

American Academy of Child and Adolescent Psychiatry. Practice parameter for the assessment and treatment of children and adolescents with schizophrenia. *J Am Acad Child Adolesc Psychiatry.* 2001;40 (7 suppl):4S–23S.

American Academy of Child and Adolescent Psychiatry. Practice parameter on the use of psychotropic medication in children and adolescents *J Am Acad Child Adolesc Psychiatry.* 2009;48:961–973.

The University of Arizona Center for Education and Research on Therapeutics (CERT) QT Drug Lists by Risk Groups. Available at http://www.azcert.org/medical-pros/drug-lists/drug-lists.cfm. Accessed January 28, 2010.

Brent DA, Emslie G, Clarke G. Switching to another SSRI or to venlafaxine with or without cognitive-behavioral therapy for adolescents with SSRI-resistant depression: the TORDIA randomized controlled trial. *J Am Med Assoc.* 2008;299:901–913.

Campo JV, Perel J, Lucas A, et al. Citalopram treatment of pediatric recurrent abdominal pain and comorbid internalizing disorders: an exploratory study. *J Am Acad Child Adolesc Psychiatry.* 2004;43:1234–1242.

Caron M, Volkow ND, Swanson JM, et al. Effects of stimulant medication on growth rates across 3 years in the MTA follow-up. *J Am Acad Child Adolesc Psychiatry.* 2007;46:1015–1027.

Correll CU, Carlson HE. Endocrine and metabolic adverse effects of psychotropic medications in children and adolescents. *J Am Acad Child Adolesc Psychiatry.* 2006;45:771–791.

Correll CU. Antipsychotic use in children and adolescents: minimizing adverse effects to maximize outcomes. *J Am Acad Child Adolesc Psychiatry.* 2008;47:9–20.

Emslie GJ, Hughes CW, Crismon ML, et al. A feasibility study of the childhood depression medication algorithm: the Texas Children's Medication Algorithm Project (CMAP). *J Am Acad Child Adolesc Psychiatry.* 2004;43:519–527.

Flockhart DA. Drug interactions: Cytochrome P450 drug interaction table. Indiana University School of Medicine; 2007. Available at http://medicine.iupui.edu/clinpharm/ddis/table.asp. Accessed August 2, 2009.

Food and Drug Administration. Clinical Trials Protocol Registration System, U.S. Public Law 110–85. Available at http://prsinfo.clinicaltrials.gov/fdaaa.html. Accessed February 14, 2010.

Gibbons RD, Brown CH, Hur K, et al. Early evidence on the effects of regulators' suicidality warnings on SSRI prescriptions and suicide in children and adolescents. *Am J Psychiatry.* 2007;164:1356–1363.

Gibbons RD, Brown CH, Mann JJ. SSRI prescribing rates and adolescent suicide: is the black box hurting or helping. *Psychiatric Times.* 2007;24:1–6.

Gleason MM, Egger HL, Emslie GJ, et al. Psychopharmacological treatment for very young children: contexts and guidelines. *J Am Acad Child Adolesc Psychiatry*. 2007;46:1532–1572.

Gogtay N. Cortical brain development in schizophrenia: insights from neuroimaging studies in childhood-onset schizophrenia. *Schizophr Bull*. 2008;34:30–36.

Gould MS, Walsh BT, Munfakh JL, et al. Sudden death and use of stimulant medication in youths. *Am J Psychiatry*. 2009;166:992–1001.

Greenhill L, Kollins S, Abikoff H, et al. Efficacy and safety of immediate-release methylphenidate treatment for preschoolers with ADHD. *J Am Acad Child Adolesc Psychiatry*. 2006;45:1284–1293.

Health Canada Website. Health Canada suspends the market authorization of ADDERALL, a drug prescribed to Attention Deficit Hyperactivity Disorder (ADHD) in children. Available at http://www.hc-sc.gc.ca/ahc-asc/media/advisories-avis/_2005/2005_01-eng.php. Accessed February 14, 2010.

Jobson KO, Potter WZ. International psychopharmacology algorithm project report. *Psychopharmacol Bull*. 1995;31:457–459.

Jones PB, Barnes TRE, Davies L, et al. Randomized controlled trial of the effect on quality of life of second- vs first-generation antipsychotic drugs in schizophrenia: cost utility of the latest antipsychotic drugs in schizophrenia study (CUtLASS 1). *Arch Gen Psychiatry*. 2006;63:1079–1087.

King BH, Wright MD, Handen BL. Double-blind, placebo-controlled study of amantadine hydrochloride in the treatment of children with autistic disorder. *J Am Acad Child Adolesc Psychiatry*. 2001;40:658–665.

Leckman J, King R. A developmental perspective on the controversy surrounding the use of SSRIs to treat pediatric depression. *Am J Psychiatry*. 2007;164:1304–1306.

Lieberman JA. Comparative effectiveness of antipsychotic drugs: a commentary on Cost Utility of the Latest Antipsychotic Drugs in Schizophrenia Study (CUtLASS 1) and Clinical Antipsychotic Trials of Intervention Effectiveness (CATIE). *Arch Gen Psychiatry*. 2006;63:1069–1072.

Lieberman JA, Bymaster FP, Meltzer HY, et al. Antipsychotic drugs: comparison in animal models of efficacy, neurotransmitter regulation, and neuroprotection. *Pharmacol Rev*. 2008;60:358–403.

Lieberman JA, Stroup TS, McEvoy JP, et al. Effectiveness of antipsychotic drugs in patients with chronic schizophrenia. *N Engl J Med*. 2005;353:1209–1223.

March JS, Silva SG, Compton S, et al. The Child and Adolescent Psychiatry Trials Network (CAPTN). *J Am Acad Child Adolesc Psychiatry*. 2004;4:515–518.

McCracken JT, McGough J, Shah B, et al. Risperidone in children with autism and serious behavioral problems. *N Engl J Med*. 2002;347:314–321.

Michelson D, Faries D, Wernicke J, et al. Atomoxetine in the treatment of children and adolescents with attention-deficit/hyperactivity disorder: a randomized, placebo-controlled, dose-response study. *Pediatrics*. 2002;108:e83.

Olfson M, Crystal S, Huang C, et al. Trends in antipsychotic drug use by very young, privately insured children. *J Am Acad Child Adolesc Psychiatry*. 2010;49:13–23.

One Hundred Fifth Congress of the United States. U.S. Department of Health & Human Services Website. Food and Drug Administration Modernization Act of 1997. Title I—Improving Regulation of Drugs, Section 111. Pediatric Studies of Drugs. http://www.fda.gov/RegulatoryInformation/Legislation/FederalFoodDrugandCosmeticActFDCAct/SignificantAmendmentstotheFDCAct/FDAMA/FullTextofFDAMAlaw/default.htm#SEC.%20111. Accessed February 13, 2010.

Roberts R, Rodriguez W, Murphy D, et al. Pediatric drug labeling—improving the safety and efficacy of pediatric therapies. *J Am Med Assoc*. 2003;290:905–911.

Sikich L, Frazier JA, McClellan, et al. Double-blind comparison of first and second generation antipsychotics in early-onset schizophrenia and schizoaffective disorder: finding from the treatment of early-onset schizophrenia spectrum disorders (TEOSS) study. *Am J Psychiatry*. 2008;165:1420–1431.

Stahl SM, Munter N. *Stahl's Essential Psychopharmacology: Neuroscientific Basis and Practical Applications*. 3rd ed. New York, NY: Cambridge University Press; 2008:102–103.

Texas Department of Health Services. CMAP: Attention-Deficit/Hyperactivity disorder algorithm. Available at http://www.dshs.state.tx.us/mhprograms/adhdpage.shtml. Accessed February 14, 2010.

Texas Department of Health Services. Bipolar disorder algorithm. Available at http://www.dshs.state.tx.us/mhprograms/pdf/TIMABDalgos2005.pdf. Accessed February 14, 2010.

Texas Department of Health Services. Major depressive disorder algorithm. Available at http://www.dshs.state.tx.us/mhprograms/mddpage.shtml. Accessed February 12, 2010.

Texas Department of Health Services. Psychotropic medication utilization parameters for foster children. Available at http://www.dshs.state.tx.us/mhprograms/pdf/PsychotropicMedicationUtilizationParametersFoster Children.pdf. Accessed February 14, 2010.

The MTA Cooperative Group. A 14-month randomized clinical trial of treatment strategies for attention-deficit/hyperactivity disorder. Multimodal Treatment Study of Children with ADHD. *Arch Gen Psychiatry*. 1999;56:1073–1086.

The TADS Team. The Treatment for Adolescents With Depression Study (TADS) long-term effectiveness and safety outcomes. *Arch Gen Psychiatry*. 2007;64:1132–1143.

Turner EH, Matthews AM, Linardatos E, et al. Selective publication of antidepressant trials and its influence on apparent efficacy. *N Engl J Med*. 2008;358:252–260.

Vetter VL, Elia J, Erickson C, et al. Cardiovascular monitoring of children and adolescents with heart disease receiving medications for attention deficit/hyperactivity disorder. A scientific statement from the American Heart Association Council on Cardiovascular Disease in the Young Congenital Cardiac Defects Committee and the Council on Cardiovascular Nursing. *Circulation*. 2008;117:2407–2423.

Vitry AI. Comparative assessment of four drug interaction compendia. *Br J Clin Pharmacol*. 2007;6:709–714.

Wagner KD, Ambrosini P, Rynn M, et al. Efficacy of sertraline in the treatment of children and adolescents with major depressive disorder: two randomized controlled trials. *J Am Med Assoc*. 2003;29:1033–1041.

Wagner KD, Robb AS, Findling RL, et al. A randomized, placebo-controlled trial of citalopram for the treatment of major depression in children and adolescents. *Am J Psychiatry*. 2004;161:1079–1083.

Walkup JT, Albano AM, Piacentini J, et al. Cognitive behavioral therapy, sertraline, or a combination in childhood anxiety. *N Engl J Med*. 2008;359:2753–2766.

Weisz JR, Jensen PS. Efficacy and effectiveness of child and adolescent psychotherapy and pharmacotherapy. *Ment Health Serv Res*. 1999;1:125–157.

Zhou F, Liang Y, Salas R, et al. Corelease of dopamine and serotonin from striatal dopamine terminals. *Neuron*. 2005;46(1):65–74.

Zito JM, Safer DJ, Sai D, et al. Psychotropic medication patterns among youth in foster care. *Pediatrics*. 2008;121:e157–e163.

SUGGESTED READINGS

Helping parents, youth and teachers understand medications for behavioral and emotional problems: A resource book of medication information handouts. 3rd Edition.
Editor: Mina Dulcan
Publisher: American Psychiatric Publishing 2006, paperback 759 pages, CD included.

Straight talk about psychiatric medications for kids
Author: Tim Wilens
Publisher: Guilford 2008, paperback 325 pages.

Pediatric Psychopharmacology: A practical Guide
Editors: Jefferson Prince, Jeffrey Bostic, Kristen Smith Russell
Publisher: Humana Press 2010, 325 pages.

Stahl's Essential Psychopharmacology: The Prescriber's Guide
Author: Steven Stahl
Publisher: Cambridge University Press 2009, 654 pages.

Issues and viewpoints in Pediatric Psychopharmacology
Authors: Mark Riddle, John Walkup, Benedetto Vitiello
Published: International Review of Psychiatry, April 2008.

Child and Adolescent Psychiatry Alerts.
M.J. Powers and Co., Publishers
65 Madison Ave.
Morristown, NJ 07960

Biological Therapies in Psychiatry
Alan Gelenberg, MD, Editor
Healthcare Technology Systems
PO Box 42650
Tucson, AZ 85733-2650

SUGGESTED WEBSITES

Flockhart's P450 Table: http://medicine.iupui.edu/clinpharm/ddis/
NIMH Mental Health Medications: http://infocenter.nimh.nih.gov/subject.cfm?category=35
Texas Algorithm: http://www.dshs.state.tx.us/mhprograms/adhdpage.shtm
Arizona Cert. QT Drug Lists by Risk Groups. http://www.azcert.org/medical-pros/drug-lists/drug-lists.cfm
The Brown University Child & Adolescent Psychopharmacology Update. http://www3.interscience.wiley.com/journal/122688820/issue

REVIEW QUESTIONS

1. Pharmacokinetic factors include all of the following except:
   a. The effects of the rates and extent of absorption
   b. Range of distribution in various bodily compartments (tissues and fluids)
   c. Modification of membrane permeability
   d. The rate and extent of excretion

2. Second-generation antipsychotics (SGAs) increase the risk of metabolic syndrome which includes all the following findings except:
   a. Abdominal obesity
   b. Insulin resistance
   c. Cardiac conduction delay
   d. Elevated blood pressure

3. Which statement is accurate about SSRIs?
   a. SSRIs cause a 4% risk of attempted suicide.
   b. Fluoxetine and escitalopram are FDA approved for the treatment of depression in children over the age of 6.
   c. Fluoxetine may be stopped abruptly without risk of withdrawal.

4. Which of the following has been associated with Stevens–Johnson syndrome:
   a. Valproate and lithium
   b. Carbamazepine and lamotrigine
   c. Lithium and gabapentin
   d. Oxcarbazepine and topiramate

5. How often should prolactin levels be monitored for youth treated with antipsychotic medications?
   a. Weekly
   b. Monthly
   c. Quarterly
   d. Annually

6. Alpha agonists
   a. Are FDA-approved for treating ADHD and PTSD
   b. Tend not to lower blood pressure in children and adolescents
   c. Are used to treat tics and psychosis
   d. Are used to treat enuresis
   e. Are associated with mid-phase insomnia

7. Stimulant medications
   a. Do not cause a loss of stature in long-term use
   b. Increase risk of substance abuse in long-term use
   c. Are FDA-approved for use in children as young as 2 years old
   d. All are equally efficacious in controlled studies
   e. Not as effective as atomoxetine

8. Venlafaxine and bupropion
   a. Work through alpha-2a agonism
   b. Are associated with hypertension
   c. Are available in long-acting forms
   d. Are both FDA-approved for treating ADHD
   e. May be used for treating tics

9. Atomoxetine
   a. Is a norepinephrine reuptake inhibitor
   b. Is a serotonin reuptake inhibitor
   c. Is a dopamine reuptake inhibitor
   d. Is a norepinephrine and serotonin reuptake inhibitor
   e. None of the above

10. Benzodiazepines
    a. Are not FDA-approved for use in children
    b. Have been shown in controlled studies to be efficacious in treating pediatric anxiety
    c. Work through histamine blockade
    d. Are highly lipophilic
    e. Are less effective in treating anxiety than buspirone

11. Which of the following may decrease the risk of developing tardive dyskinesia in patients treated with neuroleptics?
    a. Vitamin A
    b. Vitamin B1
    c. Vitamin C
    d. Vitamin D
    e. Vitamin E

12. Which of the following is FDA-approved for treating schizophrenia and mania in youth?
    a. Aripiprazole
    b. Olanzapine
    c. Risperidone
    d. All of the above
    e. None of the above

Answers: 1-c, 2-c, 3-c, 4-b, 5-d, 6-e, 7-d, 8-c, 9-a, 10-d, 11-e, 12-d

Evidence-Based Psychotherapies

Introduction

"Evidence-based practice" is a term used to describe the integration of scientific research and best clinical practice. Various health experts, institutions, or professional guilds like the American Academy of Pediatrics (AAP), the American Medical Association (AMA), the National Registry of Evidence-Based Programs and Practices (NREPP), the Cochrane Collaboration, the American Psychological Association (APA), the Institute of Medicine (IOM), and the American Academy of Child and Adolescent Psychiatry (AACAP) have independently developed definitions and/ or position statements regarding evidence-based practice. According to these expert guidelines, evidence-based treatments should be based on data from several independent, randomized, double-blinded, placebo-controlled studies demonstrating statistically significant superiority over an alternative intervention. The traditional example of evidence-based practice in medicine is the pharmacologic treatment of illness based on rigorous medication trials. Similarly, evidence-based psychotherapy refers to psychosocial treatments for which systematic controlled studies have established efficacy. During the past two decades, rigorous research methods have been used to investigate the efficacy of psychotherapy and related interventions for mental disorders of childhood and adolescence. There are now hundreds of studies establishing the efficacy of psychotherapies for multiple juvenile disorders. However, these efficacious therapies have not yet been fully implemented in community settings. The purpose of this chapter is to provide clinicians an overview of the evidence-based psychotherapies that have been developed for children and adolescents and the status of their dissemination in the community.

Background

Research on the efficacy of psychotherapy for children began in the 1950s and 1960s. In a review of contemporary treatments, Leavitt concluded that they did not seem more effective than "tincture of time." These early approaches that were based on anecdotal reports and case studies have given way to evidence-based practice as in other areas of health care. Multiple professional organizations have developed guidelines to define "evidence-based psychotherapies." However, there is no consensus yet among these guidelines in establishing the levels of evidence.

The Cochrane Collaboration and the APA have developed definitions of evidence-based practice, requirements for which include (1) randomized controlled research, (2) research designs with adequate sample size and defined study populations, and (3) independent replication. In 1995, the APA Task Force expanded these requirements in defining evidence-based effectiveness to consider feasibility, generalizability, cost, and benefit. Hoagwood and colleagues note that *efficacious* treatments are based on carefully controlled research protocols generally conducted in an academic setting with homogenous study populations and multiple exclusionary criteria, while *effective* treatments are based on research in naturalistic settings with heterogeneous populations and fewer exclusionary criteria using real-world practitioners rather than research therapists. Therefore, what is *efficacious* in controlled studies may not be *effective* in clinical practice, and ideally evidence-based treatments examined in research settings would later be examined in community settings.

In 2001, the IOM released a report titled "Crossing the Quality Chasm." In this report the IOM noted that "between the health care we have and the care we could have lies not just a gap, but a chasm." The report called for a major revision of the health care system. Notably, one of the key elements cited for change included the need for health professionals to use evidence-based practices that integrate the best research with clinical expertise and patient values.

In October 2006, the AACAP published a policy stating that the "ultimate goal" of evidence-based practice is to base clinical decision-making in the areas of causation, diagnosis, prognosis, treatment, and practice parameters on empirical evidence. Child and adolescent psychiatry as one of the youngest medical specialties acknowledges through this policy that many treatments in the mental health care of pediatric populations need more rigorous assessment of efficacy. As many children and adolescents present with multiple diagnoses, complex psychosocial factors, and unique developmental paths that are rarely addressed in efficacy research, further investigation of effectiveness is also needed. This policy statement encourages clinicians to use all available empirical data in developing individual treatment plans.

Currently, the institutional implementation of evidence-based practice is occurring on a national basis. California, Colorado, Hawaii, Michigan, New York, and Ohio belong to the Child and Family Evidence-Based Practices Consortium. As a group, they are involved in a wide range of evidence-based program and policy development. The consortium provides a forum for sharing experiences and ideas on the implementation of evidence-based practice. Other states, such as Connecticut, Oregon, and Washington, require the implementation of evidence-based treatments for youth whose care is supported by state funding. Ironically, private insurance companies often do not support evidence-based psychotherapies.

Classifications of Evidence-Based Treatments

Currently, there is no consensus regarding the criteria for classifying evidence-based psychotherapies. Rating systems have been developed by various guilds and organizations to evaluate evidence-based practice, including the AAP, the APA, the US Preventive Services Task Force, and the Cochrane Collaboration. These systems vary in defining the research methodologies that constitute levels of evidence. The NREPP provides an online searchable database of interventions available for the prevention and treatment of mental health and substance-use disorders. This resource aids consumers, agencies, and organizations in implementing data-supported programs. Two examples of these rating systems are described as follows in the organizations' own words.

The APA defines four levels of criteria:

Criteria 1 level or "well-established" treatments are based on positive data from at least two good group-design experiments conducted at two independent research settings. Resulting data should show results that are statistically superior to control groups such as placebo, medication treatments, other psychological treatments, or well-established treatments.

Criteria 2 level or "probably-efficacious" treatments are based on data from at least two good experiments showing the treatment is superior to a wait-list control group. If one or two experiments by the same research team meet the well-established treatment criteria, this also qualifies as probably efficacious.

Criteria 3 level or "possibly-efficacious" treatments need to be supported by only one good study showing a treatment to be efficacious in the absence of conflicting studies.

Criteria 4 level or "experimental" treatments are defined by lack of any studies using a well-established methodology.

The US Preventive Services Task Force uses the following system for ranking evidence regarding treatment efficacy:

Level I treatments require evidence obtained from at least one randomized controlled study.

Level II-1 treatments require evidence obtained from well-designed, controlled trials without randomization.

Level II-2 treatments are based on evidence obtained from well-designed, cohort, or case–control analytic studies, preferably from more than one center or research group.

Level II-3 treatments are based on evidence obtained from multiple time series with or without intervention. Also, dramatic results from uncontrolled studies might be regarded as Level II-3 evidence.

Level III treatments are based on opinions of respected authorities, drawn from clinical experience and descriptive studies, or reports of expert committees.

Categories of Psychotherapies

The development of evidence-based psychotherapy has built on the existing knowledge of psychotherapeutic process. Traditionally, psychotherapies have been classified according to (1) participants or (2) theoretic construct.

Participant-Based Approaches

Therapies based on participants include individual, group, and family therapies. Modeled after adult psychotherapies, individual therapy with children denotes a child meeting with a therapist on an individual basis without the presence of a parent, although additional psychotherapeutic sessions with the parent may be needed. This form of therapy assumes that a child or an adolescent will be able to work with a therapist without the assistance of a parent. Lewis emphasizes that there is no indication for individual psychotherapy with younger children without concomitant parental interventions, such as parental guidance and counseling, parent skills training, or family therapy. Sometimes parental interventions may be limited to simple support to ensure that parents continue to involve their child in treatment. In adolescence, the role for parental intervention and involvement is more variable. The available research has supported the involvement of parents in some specific therapies such as *Interpersonal Therapy for Adolescents,* but not for others such as *Group Cognitive–Behavioral Therapy.*

During the past 10 years, several hundred publications have presented an evidence base for various forms of group psychotherapy. Participants in group psychotherapy may be similar or diverse diagnostically, but usually are of the same developmental stage. Group psychotherapy has become an integral part of inpatient and outpatient treatment planning. A meta-analysis by Hoag and Burlingame in 1997 examined 56 outcome studies on the effects of group treatment for children and adolescents. The results showed that group psychotherapy was more efficacious than placebo controls or wait-list control groups. Group psychotherapies for children and adolescents are frequently constructed around specific problems. For example, group therapy is a mainstay of treatment for substance-use disorders and is often incorporated into treatment for depression, anxiety, bereavement, poor social skills, and impulse-dyscontrol problems. In most problem-oriented groups, group membership consists of youth in the same developmental phase so that they share similar challenges and so that core techniques are applicable to the entire group. In some group treatments, however, groups of families are formed, and in this case, ages of youth may vary. Group therapy is increasingly difficult to find for privately insured individuals due to poor financial reimbursement. Ironically, in some public agencies, group treatments are used to reduce individual treatments that are considered more costly.

Family psychotherapy refers to interventions aimed at changing maladaptive or harmful interactions among family members so as to improve the functioning of individuals as well as the family as a whole. Parental skills training and psychoeducation should not be considered a form of family therapy because they do not focus on family relationships. Family therapy for children and adolescents is especially indicated for families whose parents have already received skills training but are unsuccessful because of their individual resistance or family dysfunction. Family interventions have an evidence base for treating pediatric depression, anxiety, substance abuse, attention-deficit hyperactivity disorder (ADHD), bipolar disorder, and psychosis. Current approaches to child treatment stress the integration of family therapy into the comprehensive treatment plan. For example, family therapy is an integral intervention in multimodal treatment plans for ADHD and anxiety disorders. Family psychotherapies may include many different constellations of family members. In its most traditional format, family therapy includes members of the nuclear family. The constellation of family members included in treatment sessions may change as therapy progresses. Family therapy may start with parental sessions with one or both parents and progress to include all family members.

Theory-Based Approaches

Psychotherapies are frequently categorized according to a theoretic perspective. The US Department of Health and Human Services' Surgeon General's report of 1999 states that the major specific psychotherapeutic interventions for children are *Psychodynamic Psychotherapy*, *Supportive Psychotherapy*, *Cognitive–Behavioral Psychotherapy*, *Interpersonal Psychotherapy*, and *Family Systemic Interventions*. With the exception of the last approach, these therapies originally were developed for adults and then adapted for children based on developmental considerations.

Psychodynamic psychotherapies, also termed insight-oriented psychotherapies, rely on theories of intrapsychic development and functioning. There are several such theories with different foci. The most traditional and older therapies posit that children show maladaptive behaviors because of overwhelming or unresolved intrapsychic conflicts. These conflicts can be caused by multiple sources ranging from mother–child relationship problems to environmental trauma and, according to the psychoanalytic theories, the child's psychosexual development. For example, a 6-year-old child who witnessed his mother being robbed at gunpoint on a bus may develop transient hysterical blindness anytime he sees a bus. A young child may become anxious about his anger at his mother for not gratifying his wishes because his anger conflicts with his need for her love. *Psychodynamic Therapy* for older children or adolescents requires a level of psychological development that allows conscious awareness of conflict and the ability to tolerate anxiety-provoking interpretations that connect feelings and behaviors during therapy. This higher level of psychological development and verbal skills is also needed in order for the youth to maintain a working relationship with his or her therapist during difficult times throughout the treatment process and to not act out in a self-destructive or socially harmful manner. For example, a teenager whose parents have had a contentious divorce may enter treatment because she feels uncomfortable in dating and has started cutting herself. After connecting her psychological discomfort with her guilty distortions that she caused her parents' divorce, such a youth may be able to better tolerate a romantic relationship. In psychodynamic approaches with younger children, often referred to as *Play Therapy*, conscious insight into troubled feelings may not be gained. However, unconscious conflicts may be resolved in the metaphor of the play themes acted out in treatment sessions. Mastery over a psychic insult (a perception of danger to the ego) may be gained through the expression of internal experiences during play coupled with appropriate interpretations. This mastery over a threatened ego and confusing emotions may then generalize to a youth's outer world, evidenced by movement from a regressed position of self-protection to an adaptive position of meeting developmental challenges.

Psychoanalytic and psychodynamic therapies do not have a strong evidence base supporting their use in children, as there are no randomized controlled studies of their efficacy. Lewis notes that play therapy with preschool or school-aged children in the absence of any other interventions is not an effective treatment for preschool and school-aged children.

Supportive Psychotherapy originated in psychoanalytic theory. However, in contrast to psychoanalytic therapies, *Supportive Psychotherapy* focuses on supporting the individual's psychological strengths and defenses, not uncovering unconscious conflicts or exploring the meaning of maladaptive behaviors that is anxiety provoking for the patient. The focus is on containing the individual's anxiety. Supportive interventions are typically used when a patient is in crisis or not psychologically minded and so is not able to make use of insight-oriented interventions. When the crisis has been stabilized, psychodynamic techniques may be useful for many patients who seek change in their lives or to understand themselves. In *Supportive Therapy*, a therapist may help a child to better understand his or her parents' divorce and maintain positive relationships using statements such as "Your parents say you did not cause their divorce; it is nobody's fault," and then helping the child to develop strategies to maintain relationships with each parent. A depressed teen might be gently confronted about her overreaction to breaking up with her boyfriend with supportive statements such as "It is difficult now, but you have shown the ability to cope with a previous breakup; this does not have to affect your other relationships and schoolwork. How did you get through the past breakup?" A therapist will encourage a child to use verbal skills in dealing with a school bully and help him to develop copies strategies based on the child's abilities in other areas, for example, "You are good at using words, so let's think about some statements you can use in these situations." The therapist may also provide limited advice, such as when to involve adults when being bullied. In addition, *Supportive Psychotherapy* utilizes direct environmental interventions. The therapist may suggest to children and parents specific ways of changing their physical environment to meet the challenges of perceived problems. In the bullying example, a therapist might suggest that the child avoid walking home alone after school, speaking to the principal, talking to the parents of the bully, or even enrolling the child in martial art training.

While supportive psychotherapeutic techniques are commonly used in the treatment of both adults and children, there is little evidence of their efficacy in pediatric populations. For example, a 2007 study of treatments for bulimia led by le Grange showed that teenagers with bulimia are more likely to recover if they are in family-based therapy than if they are in individual supportive therapy.

Cognitive therapies are based on social learning theory and also integrate several psychotherapeutic techniques based on operant and classical conditioning. According to Aaron Beck, *Cognitive Therapy* (CBT) describes five major interrelated elements that contribute to psychological difficulties: interpersonal-environmental context, an individual's unique physiology, emotional functioning, behavior, and cognition. These elements form the complex system that is addressed by *Cognitive Therapy*. Depressed children and adolescents, similar to depressed adults, display Beck's "depression triad," that is, negative attitudes (or distortions) regarding themselves, their environment, and the future. "Catastrophizing" and perceiving situations only in "black and white" are other maladaptive attributional styles used by depressed youth. Cognitive therapists consider a youth's particular circumstances and intervene at both cognitive and behavioral levels to influence thinking, acting, feeling, and somatic reaction patterns. According to McClure and Friedberg, the framework for *Cognitive Therapy* sessions includes the following six components: (1) mood or symptom check-in, (2) homework review, (3) agenda setting, (4) addressing session content, (5) homework assignments, and (6) eliciting feedback. Successfully integrating each of these elements in a *Cognitive Therapy* session facilitates effective and efficient interventions. Through cognitive treatments, a child learns the relationships between his or her cognitions (thoughts or thinking style), feelings (emotions), and behaviors (actions). Ultimately, changing underlying cognitions can reduce depressed or anxious emotions and maladaptive or inappropriate behaviors. Thus, the cognitive therapies do not rely on exploration of underlying conflicts, intrapsychic origins of the depressed or anxious feelings, or the youth's self-expression through verbal or play interaction.

Multiple systematic studies support the use of CBT in the treatment of various juvenile psychiatric disorders, including depression, anxiety, and obsessive–compulsive disorder (OCD). Using the APA criteria, CBT for these disorders are considered "well-established" and effective.

Behavioral therapies are a mainstay of evidence-based treatments for a variety of childhood disorders. These therapies are now widely accepted in mainstream practice, as they have an evidence base in treating various psychiatric disorders from self-harming behaviors that occur in autism to avoidant behaviors characteristic of anxiety. Behavioral therapies, most notably implemented as *Behavior Modification,* are based on the behavioral concepts of classical and operant conditioning. *Classical Conditioning* is the type of learning made famous by Pavlov's experiments with dogs. An example of behavior modification using classical conditioning is the use of the bell and pad for an enuretic child. The major theorists in the development of *Operant Conditioning* are Edward Thorndike, John Watson, and Burrhus F. Skinner. Positive reinforcement or the use of "rewards" is an example of *Operant Conditioning* used to shape behaviors. A *Token Economy* is a system in which a child is positively reinforced, or "receives tokens," for demonstrating specific adaptive behaviors. Teaching parents about such behavioral interventions is major part of *Parent Skills Training.* Because behavioral therapies, in general, have a strong evidence base for treating children, they should be part of a clinician's approach to caring for children with disturbed behavior.

Review of Evidence-Based Psychotherapies

As research has progressed in the treatment of child psychiatric disorders, the number of evidence-based psychotherapies has increased, particularly for the most common disorders such as ADHD, depression, and anxiety. Therapies for these disorders have been examined in both single site and large multisite studies. Other disorders, such as eating disorders, still lack an evidence base to guide clinicians, as studies have not met the criteria of any rating system to support efficacy. The following review uses the APA's system for classifying evidence-based psychosocial treatments for children and adolescents.

Attention-Deficit Hyperactivity Disorder
ADHD is the most extensively studied psychiatric illness of childhood. Since the 1937 classic study, "The Behavior of Children Receiving Benzedrine," thousands of treatment studies have been published. Pharmacotherapy is the most commonly used efficacious and effective treatment. Stimulant medications, and more recently atomoxetine, have met the APA standard of a "well-established" evidence-based psychotherapy. There is a growing body of work, however, supporting behavioral interventions, such as *Behavioral Management Training* (BMT) and *Behavior Contingency Management* (BCM) in the classroom, as "well-established" treatments. Nonetheless, in recent research, the combination of pharmacotherapy and psychosocial interventions has not been shown to be more effective than medication alone in cases of ADHD without comorbidity. The idea of using a combination of treatments for ADHD has existed for the past three decades. Satterfield first reported on the use of *Multimodal Therapy* for ADHD, which showed evidence that multiple treatment interventions are more effective than any treatment used in isolation. These findings, however, were not replicated in the 1999 Multimodal Treatment Study of Children with ADHD (MTA Study), which has served as the "gold standard" for clinical practice in the treatment of ADHD. However, for ADHD comorbid with oppositional defiant disorder (ODD), the addition of psychosocial interventions to algorithm-based pharmacologic treatment did improve outcomes. While the AMA, AAP, and AACAP support pharmacotherapy as the sole treatment of uncomplicated ADHD, with

behavioral interventions a secondary or augmenting treatment, the APA Task Force contends that behavioral treatments should be employed as the initial or primary treatment for ADHD and that medications should be added as adjunctive treatment when behavioral interventions are not efficacious.

The AAP guidelines have included BCM in the classroom setting as a "well-established" treatment based on the review by Pelham and Fabiano of 23 studies supporting BCM. This review also found that *Behavioral Parent Training* (BPT) met the criteria for a "probably-efficacious" treatment, and with liberal interpretation of the APA Task Force criteria, barely met the standard for "well-established" treatments. This review also concluded that there was no evidence supporting cognitive interventions for ADHD or peer-group interventions such as social skills training or summer treatment programs. Also important is that Pelham and Fabiano note that most ADHD treatment studies have investigated boys under 13 years of age. Therefore, by strict criteria, there is no "well-established" or "probably-efficacious" ADHD psychosocial treatment for teens or girls.

Disruptive Behavior Disorders

Disruptive behavior disorders (DBDs) apply to a broad range of psychiatric behaviors. The *DSM-IV-R* category of DBDs includes three major diagnoses: ADHD, ODD, and conduct disorder (CD). Research studies tend to separate treatments for ADHD from that for CD and ODD, and so in this section, we focus on CD and ODD. In 1998, Brestan and Eyberg identified 12 treatments that met the criteria for being either "probably efficacious" or "well established." In a 2008 review in the *Journal of Child and Adolescent Psychology* on evidence-based psychotherapies for disruptive behaviors, 15 psychotherapies were identified as "efficacious" and only one treatment met the standard for a "well-established" treatment, the *Parent-Management Training Oregon Model* (PMTO). The majority of these treatments are psychoeducational interventions for parents. Of the six parent-management training interventions cited by Eyberg, Nelson, and Boggs, only one is targeted for elementary or high school youth. Four of the interventions are designed for a skills training group therapy format. Treatments created for preschool and early-school-aged children include *Helping the Noncompliant Child, The Incredible Years, Parent–Child Interaction Therapy, Triple P,* and PMTO. For adolescents, *Multisystemic Therapy* (MST) and *Multidimensional Treatment Foster Care* (MTFC) have been extensively studied.

MST is designated a "probably-efficacious" treatment by APA standards. It is a community-based intervention that cannot be self-taught but requires specialized training by program staff. MST is a resource-intensive, multimodal intervention that requires multiple treatment team members to maintain fidelity to the model. MST targets adolescents with serious antisocial and conduct-disordered behaviors. It supports families through family therapy, cognitive–behavioral interventions, behavior therapies, parent training, pragmatic family therapies, and pharmacologic interventions. MTFC is a "probably-efficacious" community-based program targeting youth with severe and chronic delinquent behavior. Prospective foster parents are provided over 20 hours of specialized training from experienced foster parents in the use of token economies and other behavior-shaping modalities. Foster parents also receive daily telephone supervision from program supervisors. Youth in MTFC programs receive weekly sessions from individual therapists who help them to develop problem-solving skills and promote prosocial behaviors. Biologic parents or guardians who will accept the youth from MTFC homes after treatment is completed are also provided intensive parent-management training to ensure continuity of care.

The only treatment that qualified as a "well-established" treatment for disruptive behavior is the PMTO for children 3 to 12 years old. Two independent research teams, one led by Patterson and the other by Bernal, provided data showing that the PMTO was superior to an alternative treatment. This intervention focuses on teaching parents basic behavior-intervention theory. Therapists meet with parents on a regular basis for an average of 10 to 17 hours over the treatment intervention with additional twice-weekly phone check-ins.

It is notable that in contrast to ADHD, psychosocial treatment studies for ODD and CD outnumber medication studies. The AACAP Practice Parameters for the Assessment and Treatment of Children and Adolescents with Conduct Disorders states that medication alone as an intervention for CD is an insufficient treatment plan. Furthermore, Conner and colleagues suggest that youth with CD and ODD should not be treated with psychotropic medication unless psychosocial interventions have failed. Generally, medication for disruptive behaviors is indicated only when other comorbid disorders are present. Training manuals and texts regarding most of the efficacious treatments for DBDs are readily available either online or in hard copy.

Depressive Disorders

The evidence base for the treatment of depressed youth has steadily increased during the past two decades. CBT and *Interpersonal Therapy* (IPT) are the two most studied therapies for childhood and adolescent depression. CBT delivered in individual, group, and parental/family venues is recognized as a "well-established" treatment. Enough systematic research has been completed on IPT that it is rated as "probably efficacious" for adolescents. Additionally, behavioral approaches currently considered "experimental" will likely meet "probably-efficacious" levels in the near future.

The Treatment of Adolescent Depression Study (TADS) study reinforced the existing support for CBT in the treatment of depression. This multisite, randomized controlled study compared the use of fluoxetine, CBT, and combination of both for 327 adolescents ages 12 to 17 years. In adolescents with moderate to severe depression, treatment with fluoxetine alone or in combination with CBT accelerates recovery. One of the main advantages of adding CBT to a medication regimen was that it appears to reduce suicide risk by providing a tool for a depressed youth to use if suicidal impulses ensue. Taking benefits and harms into account, combined treatment appears to be superior to either treatment alone. CBT has been well incorporated into real-world practice. Therefore, child psychiatrists in practice can readily offer comprehensive and effective combined treatment to depressed youth without assistance from other clinicians. Such "one stop treatment" is efficient for youth and families and contains costs to some degree.

Obsessive–Compulsive Disorder

Exposure and Response Prevention (ERP) is considered the most efficacious psychotherapy for the treatment of OCD. ERP is considered a specific type of CBT that is used to decrease the fears and cognitive distortions of OCD. In the initial phase of treatment, youth with OCD are guided by their therapist to identify and rank fears and anxieties that interfere with daily functioning. Next, a patient is exposed to a feared stimulus and then prevented from engaging in compulsive compensatory behaviors, such as hand washing after flushing a toilet. Initially, this activity will elicit intense anxiety; however, with repeated exposure to an anxiety-provoking stimulus and prevention of the usual maladaptive response, these fears usually diminish or resolve. ERP can be administered as an individual or a group psychotherapy. It can also be part of a family therapy intervention in which parents and the child can be coached in using ERP techniques in the home. Therapy sessions can range from 30 minutes to 2 hours. The usual number of sessions can range from 12 to 20. Occasional "booster" sessions may be indicated if OCD symptoms return after remission or persist at a more intense level after initial treatment.

The most rigorous research on the efficacy of CBT in the treatment of OCD is the Pediatric OCD Treatment Study (POTS). This investigation, conducted at three academic centers, compared CBT alone versus medical management with sertraline alone versus CBT and sertraline combined. A total of 112 patients ranging in age from 7 to 17 years diagnosed with OCD were included. The investigators concluded that "children and adolescents with

OCD should begin treatment with the combination of CBT plus a serotonin reuptake inhibitor (SSRI) or CBT alone." Like many psychiatric disorders, OCD is best treated with a combination of both psychotherapy and psychotropic medications; but unlike most psychiatric disorders, treatment of OCD with an evidence-based psychotherapy alone is more efficacious than treatment with medication alone.

Anxiety Disorders

Anxiety disorders comprise the most common mental illness in children and adolescents. A review of evidence-based psychotherapies by Silverman, Pina, and Viswesvaran in 1998 found that for the past 10 years, no psychotherapy has met the criteria for a "well-established" treatment. In general, CBT has the most evidence to support its use in treating anxiety symptoms. Since 1994, 14 studies using various forms of CBT for anxiety including individual, group, and parent groups have met the "probably-efficacious" level of evidence. Most recently, the Child/Adolescent Anxiety Multimodal Study (CAMS) by Walkup and colleagues compared CBT to sertraline in a multisite, randomized controlled trial of 488 children aged 7 to 17 years. In children with separation anxiety, social phobia, or generalized anxiety disorder, approximately 60% responded to CBT alone, 55% responded to sertraline alone, and 24% responded to placebo. A combination of both CBT and medication produced an 80% response, clearly superior to either CBT or medication treatment alone. All therapies were superior to placebo. If another study replicates these findings, then CBT will meet the APA criteria for a "well-established" psychotherapy. The next generation of studies will likely increase the support for psychotherapy for anxiety disorders.

As in the treatment of depression, child psychiatrists should be able to independently treat youth with anxiety disorders providing both evidence-based CBT and pharmacotherapy. Training manuals and textbooks on the psychotherapies for anxiety disorders in children are readily available.

Trauma-Related Disorders

Approximately 25% of youth in the United States experience a traumatic event by the age of 16. Exposure to trauma leads to many types of negative reactions. Less than 50% of youth who are traumatized graduate from high school, and more than 50% of these traumatized students have a psychiatric illness. These findings highlight the need for early identification and intervention to minimize morbidity and mortality. No medication is FDA approved for treating trauma symptoms in youth. Based on the efficacy and FDA approval of sertraline for the treatment of adult posttraumatic stress disorder, pharmacotherapy for pediatric trauma symptoms has been categorized as "possibly efficacious" or "experimental." Therefore, psychotherapy should be considered a primary treatment for traumatized children.

A review by Silverman noted that between 1993 and 2004, there were eight studies that showed efficacy of *Trauma-Focused Cognitive–Behavioral Therapy* (TF-CBT). TF-CBT was the only treatment found to meet the criteria for a "well-established" treatment as it has been shown to be superior to psychosocial placebo, wait-list placement, and another treatment in at least two independent research settings and by two independent investigatory teams. TF-CBT, like other cognitive–behavioral interventions, utilizes individual sessions focusing on cognitive techniques to restructure thinking and behavioral procedures to alter maladaptive responses to specific stimuli, in this case to alter responses to previous traumatizing stimuli. Additionally, TF-CBT also virtually exposes individuals to their traumatizing experiences through narrative therapy, drawings, and other exercises. These safe in vitro experiences are then followed by skills training that includes techniques such as developing substitute behaviors for maladaptive responses, using strategies to distract oneself from emotional trauma responses, and relaxation techniques.

For other therapies addressing trauma, school-based group CBT met the criteria for a "probably-efficacious" treatment. "Possibly-efficacious" therapies included *Client-Centered*

Psychotherapy, Family Therapy, Child–Parent Psychotherapy, Eye Movement Desensitization and Reprocessing (EMDR), and *Resilient Peer Treatment*. Treatment manuals and textbooks on TF-CBT are readily available.

Eating Disorders

Compared to other childhood psychiatric disorders, the evidence base for the treatment of eating disorders is slim. Keel and Haedt reviewed the literature and found that most studies were limited by major design flaws needed to determine efficacy. Thus, there are no individual, group, or community-based interventions that meet efficacy criteria for youth. Only family therapy for anorexia nervosa is considered a "well-established" intervention, albeit based on research of just two studies by Russell in 1987 and Robin and colleagues in 1999. Also, a randomized controlled study in 2007 by le Grange and colleagues showed that a family-based intervention for bulimic adolescents was more efficacious than supportive psychotherapy. There are no other systematic studies on the treatment of bulimic youth. Studies with adults suggest that CBT or IPT may be useful, but relevance to youth remains unclear. Only one treatment manual is available.

Substance-Use Disorders

Initial treatments developed for youth with substance-use disorders were based on adult models of treatment. Drug-abusing youth were frequently placed in residential programs and then transitioned to 12-step outpatient programs. Early efficacy research on these programs was plagued by methodological limitations, including small sample size, lack of control groups, no randomization, inadequate measurement of drug use, and reliance on self-report of drug use. Subsequently, Dishion questioned the effectiveness of 12-step groups for youth and further suggested that they may be harmful as they may serve as "peer deviancy training." However, Kaminer notes that there are insufficient controlled studies to support this view. Nevertheless, research over the past two decades has focused less on residential and 12-step interventions and has moved to family interventions. Evidence-based family interventions typically focus on improving communication by emphasizing family members' interrelatedness and "joining" the family to enhance engagement. Then, families identify maladaptive interaction patterns, and "restructure" to develop new, more adaptive patterns.

A review by Waldron and Turner in 2008 examined 46 different interventions with 2300 adolescents. Three treatments met the criteria for "well-established" level of care including *Multidimensional Family Therapy, Functional Family Therapy,* and a group intervention. "Probably-efficacious" treatments included many family interventions, including MST, *Brief Strategic Family Therapy,* and *Behavioral Family Therapy.* Individual CBT and the *Adolescent Community Reinforcement Approach* (ACRA) were noted to be promising, but more research is needed to evaluate their efficacy. *Motivational Interviewing* (MI) is considered a "well-established" treatment for adults, but there is no evidence yet supporting its efficacy with teens.

Interventions for youth substance-use disorders require specialized training. For example, in order to be certified in *Functional Family Therapy,* therapists must take specialized classes and be proctored for several cases. MST also requires multiple trainings and regular monitoring to ensure fidelity to the model. Additionally, it requires a team of clinicians including a case manager, psychiatrist, and consultation group. Private clinicians, therefore, will likely not be able to provide comprehensive evidence-based treatment for substance-use disorders on their own. Texts are readily available describing the aforementioned treatment interventions.

Autism

Treatments for autism have been controversial since Bruno Bettelheim's pronouncement in the 1960s that autism was caused by "refrigerator mothers." Despite evidence that early intervention is associated with better outcomes, many health policies will not ensure treatment for autism. In 2008, Rogers and Vismara reviewed evidence-based treatments for autism. They note a relative paucity of randomized controlled trials for autism compared to other psychiatric disorders, but also demonstrated efficacy in the available long-term and short-term studies.

Rogers and Vismara reviewed studies between 1998 and 2006. They found four studies that utilized randomized controlled designs, but with small samples. Only the *Lovaas Method,* known as *Applied Behavioral Analysis* (ABA), met the criteria for a "well-established" treatment. No treatment met the criteria for "probably efficacious," and three treatments met the criteria for being "possibly efficacious." ABA uses positive interactions through the use of favored activities and reinforcement of any attempts to communicate with child-specific reinforcers. Further behavior shaping is promoted through positive reinforcement of successive approximations and prompting and fading procedures. ABA is a resource-intensive intervention that requires 35 to 40 hours per family per week, making it beyond the reach of most families.

Autism requires a multidisciplinary, multimodal approach to treatment. A child psychiatrist is usually not the core treatment provider, but is part of a treatment team. Team members include a mental health professional who specializes in the assessment and treatment of autism, a primary care clinician, social workers, special education teachers, and community case coordinators. The schools comprise the major venue for interventions. *The Treatment and Education of Autistic and Related Communication-Handicapped Children* (TEACCH) program is a prime example of school-based interventions. These school programs provide consistent environmental structure, teachers who are knowledgeable about an autistic child's need for predictable routines, and more visual approaches to learning as opposed to verbal communication. There are many manuals and books available on autism treatment. Some of the treatments and trainings require the involvement of a clinician who has specialized training in the interventions.

Discussion

Considerable gains have been made in understanding child and adolescent psychopathology and the therapeutic approaches to treating these disorders and improving youth's lives (Table 26-1). Efficacious treatments are now available for many of the most common pediatric psychiatric disorders. However, effectiveness has generally not been addressed, and these evidence-based psychotherapies have generally not been disseminated outside of major academic settings. Psychotherapies that are efficacious when provided in research settings by rigorously trained and supervised therapists to narrowly defined samples face many challenges to fidelity when implemented in community settings with variably trained therapists and a broad range of patients with comorbidities and aversive psychosocial circumstances. Furthermore, the cost of maintaining fidelity to a model may be prohibitive so that communities decide to drop an efficacious therapy from their programs. Mental health training programs need to update their curricula to emphasize newer evidence-based treatments over traditional nondirective treatments, such as play therapy or supportive interventions. Most evidence-based psychotherapies are matched with specific diagnoses, but there may be benefits to basing treatments on symptom clusters so as to disseminate their use in mental health settings where psychiatric diagnosis is not emphasized.

Chorpita observes multiple barriers to the dissemination of evidence-based psychotherapies. Clinicians dislike using complex manuals with multiple sections that do not appear relevant to their patients' needs. Lack of compatibility with existing payment structures will decrease a clinician's likelihood of using these interventions if they cannot be reimbursed. Private insurance companies often will not pay for evidence-based psychotherapies, such as in-home skills training

TABLE 26-1	Essentials of Evidence-Based Psychotherapies

- Clinicians should implement treatment with a well-established evidence-based psychotherapy, when available.
- If a well-established psychotherapy is not available for a specific disorder or age range, the next best empirically supported psychotherapy should be used.
- Efficacy does not ensure effectiveness.
- Until the effectiveness of selected psychotherapies is established, efficacious psychotherapies should be faithfully implemented in community setting.
- If an available efficacious treatment is precluded from implementation in a setting or community, for example, due to funding or other factors, the core therapeutic aspects of the treatment should be utilized, as possible—in the interest of dissemination.
- For all evidence-based psychotherapies with youth, parents or guardians should be involved in psychoeducation relevant to the child's needs, the specific disorder, and its treatment. Parents may need their own psychotherapy.
- The evidence supporting a specific evidence-based psychotherapy may change over time. Clinicians should regularly update their knowledge and skills regarding the relevance and application of evidence-based psychotherapies.

or ABA. The complexity of new evidence-based psychotherapies can impede their dissemination as the requirements for implementation and documentation are not compatible with the realities of community practice. Evidence-based therapies are not available for all juvenile disorders and represent a policy problem for large systems seeking to adopt them. Finally, many of the treatment protocols are difficult to obtain or require extensive trainings that clinicians find difficult to incorporate into their busy practices.

Even with these many challenges to implementing evidence-based psychotherapies, new studies and existing data continue to be examined for efficacy in research settings and effectiveness in the community. Academic centers, states, governmental agencies, and stakeholders continue to demand evidence-based treatments for their young patients and families. Clinicians and families need to know what treatments youth will receive when referred to a mental health specialist, and the scientific basis for these interventions.

Conclusions

Psychotherapeutic interventions are an integral part of any comprehensive treatment plan for youth with psychiatric disorders. Evidence-based therapies are now available to treat many disorders of childhood and adolescence. But gaps exist, for example, the lack of evidence-based treatments for adolescents with ADHD or treatments for autistic children. When available, efficacious therapies should be used in both academic and nonacademic settings with attention to maintaining fidelity to the interventions and overcoming the obstacles to full implementation. Much work remains to be done to integrate available evidence-based therapies into mainstream practice and to continue to investigate optimal evidence-based interventions for all disorders. As many efficacious treatments require both pharmacotherapy and psychotherapy, child and adolescent psychiatrists are in an optimal position to offer youth and families a full package of services. However, for multidisciplinary, multimodal therapies, treatment will be shared among two or more clinicians. Close collaboration is needed among clinicians and with parents to ensure successful outcomes, and to further build an evidence base.

CASE VIGNETTES

VIGNETTE 1: ADOLESCENT-DIRECTED TREATMENT FOR DISRUPTIVE MIDDLE-SCHOOL STUDENT

John is a 13-year-old adolescent in a single-parent home living with his mother and two younger brothers. He has been referred to a local community mental health center for increasing aggression and depression. His mother is worried that since his father went to prison for drug dealing, John has been hanging out with the wrong crowd and becoming well known by the police. When confronted about his delinquent behavior, he threatens suicide. His sleep cycle is reversed. He would stay up all night and sleep during the day. His mother has tried to set behavior limits at home without success. John's mother participated in an evidence-based parent-management training program for disruptive youth and earnestly tried to apply what she learned in the home. However, John's level of depression and aggression remained unchanged, and the school was threatening to expel him because of continued disruptive behaviors. There is an extensive history of depression and suicide in the family. He has never been treated with medication. He has been refusing to come to the local mental clinic saying, "I don't want to talk to any stupid shrinks."

The consulting psychiatrist at the local mental health clinic reviewed John's case. He suggested John receive medication management from his primary care provider, since he was refusing to come to the mental health clinic. John's mother was able to get him to see his primary care doctor who prescribed John an antidepressant that "would help treat his insomnia." John agreed to take this prescription because he wanted to sleep better. John's behaviors started to change, and he was able to complete the school year without further incident. He was able to establish a normal sleep pattern and was less irritable. Despite his treatment with an antidepressant, however, he continued to have thoughts of death and began to isolate himself in his bedroom at home, which was unusual for him during summer vacation. His mother again approached him about going to the mental health clinic. He relented stating, "I'll go one time, but I still don't want to talk to any stupid shrink." At his intake appointment he found he wouldn't have to attend individual therapy if he wanted to attend the teen group. He was readily agreeable to this. After completing the assigned group sessions, he was less isolative and no longer complained about feeling suicidal to his mother.

For some youth, attending a group is preferable to seeing a therapist for individual therapy. The use of group therapy for depression is a "well-established" treatment for adolescent depression. These groups provide skills coaching for youth with depressive and suicidal thoughts. While medication is helpful for some youth with depression, the combination of antidepressants and psychotherapy is considered superior to medication alone as demonstrated by this case vignette.

VIGNETTE 2: COMBINATION TREATMENT FOR SHY THIRD GRADER

Ally is a 9-year-old girl from an upper-middle-class family. She is the only child of a lawyer and stay-at-home mother. As an infant she was hospitalized for an extended period for viral meningitis and, since this time, was viewed by her parents to be quite fragile. Her mother is well known to her elementary school for attending class with her daughter while in kindergarten and first grade. Now in third grade, this is the first year of school that her mother has not been in the classroom during school hours. Ally is very shy and has difficulty making friends. She is constantly afraid that she may get injured on the playground and is always complaining of daily stomachaches. Bedtimes are difficult. She often has tantrums when it is time to sleep. Often her parents would find her awake well past midnight. She cries when asked to answer questions in class and is avoidant of social contact with others not in her class. Ally's pediatrician completed a medical workup for her chronic stomach problems. He could not find an "organic" cause for her gastrointestinal (GI) complaints and made a tentative diagnosis of anxiety disorder. He recommended a trial of sertraline, but her parents were fearful of the black box warning associated with the use of antidepressants in children.

Her pediatrician made a referral to a child psychologist for assessment and treatment of her intense anxiety. The child psychologist confirmed the diagnosis of generalized anxiety disorder, and a course of CBT was started. After 4 months of weekly individual psychotherapy using a standard CBT curriculum for school-age youth, Ally showed a decrease in her anxiety symptoms. She was able to answer questions in class without crying and play with a select group of friends during recess. However, she continued to be plagued by frequent attacks of GI distress and insomnia. With her symptom relief came more parental trust in her pediatrician, and with the support of Ally's psychologist, they asked for a trial of sertraline. Several months after being treated with this antidepressant, Ally was able to fall asleep at bedtime without trouble, though she still complained of stomachaches a couple of times a month. As with depression, treatment of anxiety in children is more effective when using the combination of both psychotropic medication and CBT.

BIBLIOGRAPHY

American Academy of Child and Adolescent Psychiatry. *Policy Statement: Evidence-Based Practice.* AACAP Website. Available at: http://www.aacap.org/cs/root/policy_statements/evidence_based_practice. Accessed May 20, 2010.

American Academy of Pediatrics. Policy statement: classifying recommendations for clinical practice. *Pediatrics.* 2004;114:874–877

American Medical Association. Physician Consortium for Performance Improvement (PCPI) position statement. *The Evidence Base Required for Measures Development;* 2009. Available at: http://www.ama-assn.org/ama1/pub/upload/mm/370/pcpi-evidence-based-statement.pdf. Accessed January 16, 2010.

American Psychological Association Task Force on Psychological Intervention Guidelines. *Template for Developing Guidelines: Interventions for Mental Disorders and Psychosocial Aspects of Physical Disorders.* Washington, DC: American Psychological Association; 1995.

American Psychological Association Task Force on Promotion and Dissemination of Psychological Procedures. Training in and dissemination of empirically validated psychological treatments. *Clin Psychol.* 1995;48:3–23.

Arnold LE, Chuang S, Davies M, et al. Nine months of multicomponent behavioral treatment for ADHD and effectiveness of MTA fading procedures. *J Abnorm Child Psychol.* 2004;32:39–51.

Beck AT, Alford BA. *Depression: Causes and Treatment.* 2nd ed. Philadelphia, PA: University of Pennsylvania Press; 2009:12–43.

Bernal ME, Klinnert MD, Schultz LA. Outcome evaluation of behavioral parent training and client-centered parent counseling for children with conduct problems. *J Appl Behav Anal.* 1980;13:677–691.

Brestan EV, Eyberg SM. Effective psychosocial treatments of conduct-disordered children and adolescents: 29 years, 82 studies, and 5,272 kids. *J Clin Child Psychol.* 1998;27:180–189.

Chorpita BF, Becher KD, Daleiden EL. Understanding the common elements of evidence-based practice: misconceptions and clinical examples. *J Am Acad Child Adolesc Psychiatry.* 2007;46:647–652.

Conner DF, Calson GA, Chang KD, et al. Juvenile maladaptive aggression: a review of prevention, treatment, and service configuration and a proposed research agenda. *J Clin Psychiatry.* 2006;67:808–820.

Dishion TJ, Poulin F, Barraston B. Peer group dynamics associated with iatrogenic effects in group interventions with high-risk youth. *New Dir Child Adolesc Dev.* 2005;91:79–92.

Eyberg SM, Nelson MM, Boggs SR. Evidence-based psychosocial treatments for children and adolescents with disruptive behavior. *J Clin Child Adolesc Psychol.* 2008;37:215–237.

Hamilton J. Clinicians' guide to evidence-based practice. *J Am Acad Child Adolesc Psychiatry.* 2005;44:494–498.

Hoagwood K, Hibbs E, Brent D, et al. Introduction to the special section: efficacy and effectiveness in studies of child and adolescent psychotherapy. *J Consult Clin Psychol.* 1995;63:683–687.

Hood KK, Eyberg SM. Outcomes of parent–child interaction therapy: mother's reports of maintenance three to six years after treatment. *J Clin Child Adolesc Psychol.* 2003;32:419–429.

Institute of Medicine. *Crossing the Quality Chasm: A New Health System for the 21st Century.* Washington, DC: National Academy Press; 2001.

Kaminer Y. Challenges and opportunities of group therapy for adolescent substance abuse: a critical review. *Addict Behav.* 2005;30:1765–1774.

Katz LY, Cox BJ, Gunasekara S, et al. Feasibility of dialectical behavior therapy for suicidal adolescent inpatients. *J Am Acad Child Adolesc Psychiatry.* 2004;43:276–282.

Keel PK, Haedt A. Evidence-based treatments for eating problems and eating disorders. *J Clin Child Adolesc Psychol.* 2008;37:39–61.

Leavitt EE. Psychotherapy with children: a further evaluation. *Behav Res Ther.* 1963;60:326–329.

le Grange D, Crosby RD, Rathouz PJ, et al. A randomized controlled comparison of family-based treatment and supportive psychotherapy for adolescent bulimia nervosa. *Arch Gen Psychiatry.* 2007;64:1049–1056.

Lewis M. Intensive individual psychodynamic psychotherapy: the therapeutic relationship and the technique of interpretation. In: Lewis M, ed. *Child and Adolescent Psychiatry. A Comprehensive Textbook.* Baltimore, MD: Williams & Wilkins; 1991:796–805.

March JS, Franklin M, Nelson A, et al. Cognitive–behavioral psychotherapy for pediatric obsessive–compulsive disorder. *J Clin Child Psychol.* 2001;30:8–18.

McClellan JM, Werry JS. Evidence-based treatments in child and adolescent psychiatry: an inventory. *J Am Acad Child Adolesc Psychiatry.* 2003;42:12.

Friedberg RD, McClure JM, Garcia JH. *Clinical Practice of Cognitive Therapy for Children and Adolescents: Nuts and Bolts.* New York, NY: Guilford Press; 2002:45–68.

MTA Cooperative Group. A 14-month randomized clinical trial of treatment strategies for attention-deficit/ hyperactivity disorder. *Arch Gen Psychiatry.* 1999;56:1073–1086.

National Registry of Evidence-Based Programs and Practices (NREPP). *Evidence-Based Practice in the Context of NREPP.* Available at: http://www.nrepp.samhsa.gov/about-evidence.asp. Accessed January 19, 2010.

Nixon RD, Sweeney L, Erickson DB, et al. Parent–child interaction therapy: a comparison of standard and abbreviated treatments for oppositional preschoolers. *J Consult Clin Psychol.* 2003;71:251–260.

Patterson GR, Chamberlain P, Red JB. A comparative evaluation of a parent-training program. *Behav Health.* 1982;13:638–650.

Pelham WE, Fabiano. Evidence-based psychosocial treatments for attention-deficit hyperactivity disorder. *J Clin Child Adolesc Psychol.* 2008;37:184–214.

Robin AL, Siegel PT, Moye AW, et al. A controlled comparison of family versus individual therapy for adolescent with anorexia nervosa. *J Am Acad Child Adolesc Psychiatry.* 1999;38:1482–1489.

Rogers SJ, Vismara LA. Evidence-based comprehensive treatments for early autism. *J Clin Child Adolesc Psychol.* 2008;37:8–38.

Russell GFM, Szmukler GI, Dare C, et al. An evaluation of family therapy in anorexia nervosa and bulimia nervosa. *Am J Psychiatry.* 1987;44:1047–1056.

Satterfield JH, Satterfield BT, Schell AM. Therapeutic interventions to prevent delinquency in hyperactive boys. *J Am Acad Child Adolesc Psychiatry.* 1987;26:56–64.

Silverman WK, Ortiz CD, Viswesvaran C, et al. Evidence-based psychosocial treatments for children and adolescents exposed to traumatic events. *J Clin Child Adolesc Psychol.* 2008;37:156–183.

Silverman WK, Pina AA, Viswesvaran C. Evidence-based psychosocial treatment for phobic and anxiety disorders in children and adolescence. *J Clin Child Adolesc Psychol.* 2008;37:105–130.

Steiner H. Practice parameters for the assessment and treatment of children and adolescents with conduct disorder. *J Am Acad Child Adolesc Psychiatry.* 1997;36:122S–139S.

The Cochrane Collaboration. *Evidence-Based Medicine and Health Care.* Available at: http://www.cochrane.org/docs/ ebm.htm. Accessed December 15, 2009.

The Pediatric OCD Treatment Study (POTS) Team. Cognitive–behavioral therapy, sertraline, and their combination for children and adolescents with obsessive-compulsive disorder. *JAMA.* 2004;292:1969–1976.

The TADS Team. The treatment for adolescents with depression study (TADS): long-term effectiveness and safety outcomes. *Arch Gen Psychiatry.* 2007;64:1132–1144.

US Department of Health and Human Services. *Mental Health: A Report of the Surgeon General.* Washington, DC: US Government Printing Office; 1999.

US Department of Health and Human Services. *U.S. Preventive Services Task Force Grade Definitions.* Available at: http://www.ahrq.gov/clinic/uspstf/grades.htm#post. Accessed January 16, 2010.

Walkup JT, Albano AM, Piacentini J, et al. Cognitive behavioral therapy, sertraline, or a combination in childhood anxiety. *N Engl J Med.* 2008;359:2753–2766.

Waldron HB, Turner CW. Evidence-based psychosocial treatments for adolescent substance abuse. *J Clin Child Adolesc Psychol.* 2008;37:238–261.

Webster-Stratton C, Hammond M. Treating children with early-onset conduct problems: a comparison of parent and child training interventions. *J Consult Clin Psychol.* 1997;65:93–109.

SUGGESTED READINGS/RESOURCES/MANUALS

Overview of Evidence-Based Psychotherapies

The second special issue on evidence-based psychosocial treatments for children and adolescents: a ten-year update. *J Clin Child Adolesc Psychol.* 2008, Jan–Mar issue.

Handbook of Evidence-Based Therapies for Children and Adolescents Bridging Science and Practice
Editors: Ric Steele, David Elkin, and Michael Roberts
Publisher: Springer, 2008
Hardback 590 pages

Evidence-Based Psychotherapies for Children and Adolescents
Editors: Alan Kazdin and John Weisz
Publisher: Guilford Press, 2003
(A good review for clinicians of several evidence-based psychotherapies used in children and adolescents)
Hardback 476 pages

Psychotherapy for Children and Adolescents: Evidence-Based Treatments and Case Examples
Author: John Weisz
Publisher: Cambridge University Press, 2004
(For clinicians who want specifics about the implementation of evidence-based psychotherapies)
Paperback 540 pages

Depression

Clinical Practice of Cognitive Therapy for Children and Adolescents: Nuts and Bolts
Authors: Jessica McClure and Robert Friedberg
Publisher: Guilford Press, 2002
(For clinicians who want a concise and user-friendly summary of cognitive therapy techniques for youth)
Hardback 354 pages

Interpersonal Psychotherapy for Depressed Adolescents, Second Edition
Authors: Laura Mufson, Donna Moreau, Myrna Weissman, and Kristen Dorta
Publisher: Guilford Press, 2004
(For clinicians who want an example of a manualized evidence-based psychotherapy)
Hardback 315 pages

For Disruptive Disorders

Anger Control Training
Authors: Emma Williams and Rebecca Bellow
Publisher: Speechmark, 2007
Hardcover 186 pages

Multisystemic Therapy for Antisocial Behavior in Children and Adolescents, Second Edition
Authors : Scott Henggler, Sonja Schoenwald, Charles Bourdain, Melisa Rowland, and Phillipe Cunningham
Publisher: Guilford Press, 2009
Hardcover 324 pages

Parent Management Training: Treatment for Oppositional Aggressive and Antisocial Behavior in Children and Adolescents
Author: Alan Kazdin
Publisher: Oxford University Press, 2005
Hardcover 424 pages

Helping the Noncompliant Child Family-Based Treatment for Oppositional Behavior
Authors: Robert McMahon and Rex Forehand
Publisher: Guilford Press, 2005
Paperback 313 pages

Anxiety Disorders

Modular Cognitive–Behavioral Therapy for Childhood Anxiety Disorders (Guides to Individualized Evidence-Based Treatment)
Author: Bruce Chorpita
Publisher: Guilford Press, 2006
Paperback 335 pages

Phobic and Anxiety Disorders in Children and Adolescents: A Clinician's Guide to Effective Psychosocial and Pharmacological Interventions
Authors: Thomas Ollendick and John March
Publisher: Oxford University Press, 2004
Hardcover 592 pages

Child and Adolescent Therapy, Third Edition: Cognitive–Behavioral Procedures
Author: Philip Kendall
Publisher: Guilford Press, 2005
Hardback 528 pages

Childhood Anxiety Disorders: A Guide to Research and Treatment
Authors: Deborah Beidel and Samuel Turner
Publisher: Brunner-Routledge, 2005
Hardback 368 pages

Coping Cat Workbook, Second Edition
Editors: Philip Kendall and Kristina Hedtke
Publisher: Workbook Publishing, 2006
Spiral Bound 81 pages

Trauma
Treating Trauma and Traumatic Grief in Children and Adolescents
Authors: Judith Cohen, Anthony Mannarino, and Esther Deblinger
Publisher: Guilford Press, 2006
Hardcover 256 pages

Helping Abused and Traumatized Children: Integrating Directive and Nondirective Approaches
Authors: Eliana Gil and John Briere
Publisher: Guilford Press, 2006
Hardback 254 pages

Substance Use Disorders
Functional Family Therapy: An Evidence-Based Clinical Model for Working with Troubled Adolescents and Their Families
Author: Thomas Sexton
Publisher: Routledge, 2009
Paperback 320 pages

Adolescent Substance Abuse: Research and Clinical Advances
Authors: Howard Liddle and Cynthia Rowe
Publisher: Cambridge University Press, 2006
Hardback 528 pages

Adolescent Substance Abuse: Psychiatric Comorbidity and High Risk
Authors: Yifrah Kaminer and Oscar Bukstein
Publisher: Haworth Press, 2007
Hardback 532 pages

Multisystemic Therapy and Neighborhood Partnerships: Reducing Adolescent Violence and Substance Abuse
Authors: Cynthia Swenson, Scott Henggeler, Ida Taylor, Oliver Addison, and Patricia Chamberlin
Publisher: Guilford Press, 2009
Paperback 272 pages

Autism
Autism Spectrum Disorders in Infants and Toddlers: Diagnosis, Assessment and Treatment
Authors: Michael Powers, Katarzyna Chawarska, Ami Klin, and Fred Volkmar
Publisher: Guilford Press, 2008
Hardcover 348 pages

Applied Behavior Analysis, Second Edition
Authors: John Cooper, Timothy Heron, and William Heward
Publisher: Prentice Hall, 2007
Hardcover 800 pages

The TEACCH Approach to Autism Spectrum Disorders
Authors: Gary Mesibov, Victoria Shea, and Eric Schopler
Publisher: Springer Publications, 2004
Hardcover 211 pages

SUGGESTED WEBSITES

Cochrane Reviews: http://www.cochrane.org/reviews/
National Child Traumatic Stress Network: http://www.nctsnet.org
National Registry of Evidence-Based Programs and Practices: http://www.nrepp.samhsa.gov/
The Incredible Years: http://www.incredibleyears.com/
The Parent–Child Interaction Therapy: http://pcit.phhp.ufl.edu/
The Positive Parenting Program: http://www.triplep-america.com/
The Multidimensional Treatment Foster Care: http://www.mtfc.com/
The Multisystemic Therapy: http://www.mstservices.com/
The Collaborative Problems Solving: http://www.ccps.info/

REVIEW QUESTIONS

1. Research has shown that an evidence-based psychotherapy alone is a more efficacious treatment than medication alone in which of the following psychiatric disorders of childhood?
   a. Attention-deficit hyperactivity disorder (ADHD)
   b. Prepubertal-onset major depression
   c. Autism
   d. Obsessive–compulsive disorder
   e. Early-onset schizophrenia

2. Research has shown that a combination of evidence-based psychotherapy and medication is more efficacious than either treatment modality alone in which of the following disorders?
   a. Attention-deficit hyperactivity disorder (ADHD)
   b. Major depression
   c. Autism
   d. Anxiety disorders
   e. Obsessive–compulsive disorder

3. Family therapy is considered a "well-established" treatment for which of the following disorders of childhood?
   a. Attention-deficit hyperactivity disorder (ADHD)
   b. Anorexia nervosa
   c. Bipolar disorder
   d. Bulimia nervosa
   e. Autism

4. Which of the following agencies/institutions has what is considered the consensus rating system for evidence-based practice?
   a. American Academy of Child and Adolescent Psychiatry
   b. American Academy of Pediatrics
   c. The Cochrane Collaboration
   d. American Psychological Association
   e. None of the Above

5. Presently, which of the following is considered a "well-established" treatment for youth with a substance-use disorder?
   a. Brief Strategic Family Therapy
   b. Multisystemic Therapy
   c. Motivational Interviewing
   d. Functional Family Therapy
   e. Cognitive–Behavioral Therapy

Answers: 1-d, 2-b and d, 3-b, 4-e, 5-d

Community-Based Systems of Care

Introduction

The "system-of-care" model was articulated in 1986 by the Child and Adolescent Service System Program (CASSP) in response to reports that children and adolescents with serious emotional disturbance (SED) (9% to 13% of the child/adolescent population) were receiving fragmented, ineffective care largely in residential institutions far from their communities. The system-of-care model has now been widely accepted across the nation. Its core values are that services for children and adolescents with SED should be family-driven and youth-guided; coordinated and integrated across agencies and providers; culturally competent; and tailored to the needs of the individual child and family in the least restrictive environment possible. Federal funding for systems of care across the country have led to new community-based approaches supported by a growing evidence base, including care coordination, wraparound planning, and intensive home-based services. System-of-care values and approaches can be incorporated into office-based practice. The clinician caring for a child with SED should be prepared to actively collaborate with clinicians from different child-serving systems, and learn how to access community-based services. This chapter is intended to provide the primary care clinician or general psychiatrist with an understanding of how systems of care function for children and youth with significant mental health needs, so that they can more effectively interface with such systems; it also suggests some office-based practices that incorporate system-of-care strategies.

Systems of Care: A Paradigm Shift

From the 1960s through the 1980s several important reports on the state of children's mental health in the nation described shockingly inadequate services for children and adolescents with SED. These reports documented a disturbingly disorganized and fragmented "nonsystem" in which these children were sent to out-of-state residential facilities because services in their own communities were largely unavailable. When they returned from these centers there was minimal coordination with existing resources in their communities and whatever progress was made was difficult to sustain.

In response to these reports, the federal government established the CASSP under the auspices of the National Institutes of Mental Health. In 1986, Stroul and Friedman articulated CASSP's core values and guiding principles for a system-of-care for children and adolescents with SED. The CASSP principles have served as a template for subsequent system-of-care development all across the nation. A "system-of-care" was defined as a comprehensive spectrum of mental health and other services and supports organized into a coordinated network to meet the diverse and changing needs of children and adolescents with severe emotional disorders and their families. The major elements of the CASSP principles summarized in Table 27-1 include:

TABLE 27-1	Values and Principles of Systems of Care

Core values—systems of care are:
- Child-centered, family focused, and family driven;
- Community-based;
- Culturally competent and responsive.

Guiding principles—systems of care provide for:
- Service coordination or case management;
- Prevention and early identification and intervention;
- Smooth transitions among agencies, providers, and to the adult service system;
- Human rights protection and advocacy;
- Nondiscrimination in access to services;
- A comprehensive array of services;
- Individualized service planning;
- Services in the least restrictive environment;
- Family participation in ALL aspects of planning, service delivery, and evaluation.

From SAMHSA Mental Health Information Center. Available at: http://mentalhealth.samhsa.gov/publications/allpubs/ Ca-0029/default.asp.

(1) individualized care that recognizes strengths in the child, family, and community and is tailored to the individual needs and preferences of the child and family, (2) family inclusion at every level of the clinical process and system development, (3) collaboration and coordination between different child-serving agencies and integration of services across agencies, (4) provision of culturally competent services, and (5) serving youth in their communities, or the least restrictive setting that meets their clinical needs, utilizing natural supports in the community whenever possible.

There is sometimes ambiguity in usage of the term "system-of-care." Formal systems of care are *programs* organized around the CASSP principles. They have specific mechanisms and infrastructure such as blended funding from multiple agencies, to enable agencies, providers, families, and youth to collaborate more effectively. Formal systems-of-care facilitate and explicitly require that services are individualized, family-driven, youth-guided, and preferentially based in the child's community or in the least restrictive setting possible. System-of-care is also used to describe the *philosophy* defined by the CASSP values, which have reshaped practice in most child-serving systems. There is also a more generic use of system-of-care to describe the *existing child-serving systems*—child welfare, juvenile justice, developmental disabilities (DD), mental health, etc., in whatever state of organization, or lack of organization, they exist.

SAMHSA's Investment in Systems of Care

In 1992, the Center for Mental Health Services (CMHS), part of the Substance Abuse and Mental Health Services Administration (SAMHSA), made the largest investment ever in children's mental health services when they established The Comprehensive Community Services for Children and Youth and Their Families, which has recently been described by Stroul and colleagues. Through this initiative, SAMHSA has funded over 100 6-year system-of-care projects in diverse communities in all 50 states, Native American tribes, and U.S. territories. These programs provide a broad array of individualized, family-driven, and community-based services, and ensure the full involvement of families in the care of their children and development of local services. CMHS has defined the following specific performance measures for the grants: (1) increased interagency collaboration as measured by referrals from non-mental health agencies; (2) decreased utilization of inpatient or residential treatment by 20%; (3) improved child outcomes in areas such as school attendance and law-enforcement contacts; (4) decreased overall functional impairment of youth; (5) increased family satisfaction with services; (6) increased stability of living arrangements; and (7) decreased levels of family stress.

As reviewed by Mantueffel and colleagues, nationwide outcome data from this CMHS initiative indicate that system-of-care programs have reduced the number of hospital and out-of-home residential placements, improved school performance, improved youths' behavioral and emotional functioning, reduced violations of the law, and provided more services to children and families who need them. These outcomes have led to increasing congressional appropriations from an initial appropriation of $5 million to the current appropriation of over $100 million.

The primary target population of formal systems-of-care continues to be children and adolescents with SED, defined by SAMHSA as a mental or emotional disturbance listed in the Diagnostic and Statistical Manual of Mental Disorders (DSM), which must be associated with significant functional impairments interfering with major life domains such as home, school, and community. These children and adolescents are typically those with multiple psychiatric diagnoses, often comorbid with learning disorders (LD) and other DD. Objections have been raised to "SED" as stigmatizing and not conveying the psychiatric and neurodevelopmental complexity of this population. Another term that has been suggested is "emotional and behavioral disorders," now often used in educational settings. In this chapter, the two terms will be used interchangeably.

Children with SED served in systems of care often require the services of two or more child-serving agencies such as mental health, education, juvenile justice, child welfare, or DD, and, therefore, coordination among providers is important. However, according to SAMHSA, two thirds of these children do not receive any services. Therefore, basic access to care, especially in rural areas, needs to improve. Implicit in its public health orientation is that system-of-care methodology also has a place in preventive efforts for young at-risk children, and SAMHSA has followed suit by recently starting a grant program for children ages 0 to 8.

A primary goal of systems of care is to serve youth more effectively in their communities so they can maintain their relationships with families, schools, and neighbors. Community-based treatment and supports are provided to the youth and family, often in the home, to enable the youth to stay at home. These include an array of individualized services such as intensive home-based services, crisis shelter care, treatment foster care, mobile crisis services, skills building, and mentoring. The array of services is summarized in Table 27-2. The trend towards

---

TABLE 27-2 | **The Range of Community-Based Services that may be Included in a System of Care**

• Case management (service coordination)	• Legal services
• Community-based in-patient psychiatric care	• Protection and advocacy
• Counseling (individual, group, and youth)	• Psychiatric consultation
• Crisis residential care	• Recreation therapy
• Crisis outreach teams	• Residential treatment
• Day treatment	• Respite care
• Education/special education services	• Self-help or support groups
• Family support	• Small therapeutic group care
• Health services	• Therapeutic foster care
• Independent living supports	• Transportation
• Intensive family-based counseling (in the home)	• Tutoring
	• Vocational counseling

From SAMHSA Mental Health Information Center. Available at: http://mentalhealth.samhsa.gov/publications/allpubs/CA-0014/default.asp.

community-based services has received support from several sources, including the limited evidence showing effectiveness of hospital and residential treatment as described in the 1999 Report of the Surgeon General on Mental Health; advocacy from family organizations such as the Federation of Families for Children's Mental Health (FFCMH); and promising outcomes of home- and community-based interventions. Additionally, separating youth from their families to receive treatment carries the risk that the same problems in the home context will resurface after discharge. Most important, however, is that families have begun to demand more intensive services be provided in their communities so they can keep their children at home.

Family-Driven and Youth-Guided Care

The system-of-care model places the child or adolescent and family at the center of the clinical process and makes them full partners at all levels of system planning. Family advocacy organizations such as the FFCMH and National Association for the Mentally Ill (NAMI), strengthened by federal support, have made the concept of family-driven care the cornerstone of systems of care. As summarized in Table 27-3, family-driven care means that families have a primary decision-making role in the care of their own children as well as the policies and

---

TABLE 27-3   Definition of Family-Driven Care

Family-driven means families have a primary decision making role in the care of their own children as well as the policies and procedures governing care for all children in their community, state, tribe, territory, and nation. This includes:
- Choosing supports, services, and providers;
- Setting goals;
- Designing and implementing programs;
- Monitoring outcomes;
- Partnering in funding decisions; and
- Determining the effectiveness of all efforts to promote the mental health and well being of children and youth.

Guiding Principles of Family-Driven Care
- Families and youth are given accurate, understandable, and complete information necessary to set goals and to make choices for improved planning for children and families.

Families and youth, providers and administrators embrace the concept of sharing decision-making and
- Responsibility for outcomes with providers.
- Families and youth are organized to collectively use their knowledge and skills as a force for systems transformation.
- Families and family-run organizations engage in peer-support activities to reduce isolation, gather and disseminate accurate information, and strengthen the family voice.
- Families and family-run organizations provide direction for decisions that impact funding for services, treatments, and supports.
- Providers take the initiative to change practice from provider-driven to family-driven.
- Administrators allocate staff, training, support and resources to make family-driven practice work at the point where services and supports are delivered to youth and families.
- Community attitude change efforts focus on removing barriers and discrimination created by stigma.
- Communities embrace, value, and celebrate the diverse cultures of their children and families.
- Everyone who connects with children and families continually advances his/her own cultural and linguistic responsiveness as the population served changes.

From SAMHSA Mental Health Information Center. Available at: http://www.systemsofcare.samhsa.gov/headermenus/deffamilydriven.aspx.

procedures governing care for all children in their community, state, tribe, territory, and nation. When operationalized, family-driven care means that family members are present at any meeting in which decisions are made about their child; set the goals and desired outcomes for service planning; and constitute 50% or more of planning groups at the case and system levels. Family-driven care has significantly influenced national policy in adult mental health as well and was embraced by the President's New Freedom Commission on Mental Health in 2003; one of its six major goals is that *Mental Health Care is Consumer and Family-Driven.*

Family-driven care has been expanded to include youth-guided care, which means that youth provide meaningful guidance to mental health professionals based on their own experience as recipients of services. Youth-guided as defined by SAMHSA means that youth have the right to be empowered, educated, and given a decision-making role in the care of their own lives as well as the policies and procedures governing the care of all youth in the community, state, and nation. Youth voice is being developed by the national organization Youth M.O.V.E. (Motivating Others through Voices of Experience), which was organized with SAMHSA's support to improve services that support positive growth and development by uniting the voices of youth and young adults who have lived experience in various systems, including mental health, juvenile justice, education, and child welfare. Guidelines for family-driven and youth-guided care call for families and youth to be given complete information and included in all decision making about their care. Youth have become active as national speakers and educators of clinicians as to how to more effectively interact with them in clinical relationships. Youth leaders have helped to shape new local and federal initiatives to respond to the unique needs of young adults 16 to 21 years old who are in transition to adulthood and need a variety of age-appropriate social, educational, housing, and vocational supports.

Culturally Competent Care

The number of ethnically and culturally diverse children and youth in the United States is growing and is expected to rise to more than 50% by the year 2030. Children from diverse ethnic and cultural groups face many disadvantages, including language barriers, educational and health care disparities, and multiple forms of discrimination. Culture influences many aspects of family life, including parenting practices and normative expectations for development and adaptive behaviors. Culture is associated with differences in symptom expressions, understandings of mental illness and attitudes towards mental health services. The provision of culturally competent care is a key system-of-care value and was reiterated in the President's New Freedom Commission on Mental Health in 2003.

The cultural competence model has become widely accepted as the standard of care for culturally diverse youth and families. It involves using knowledge-based skills and attitudes about culture and cultural differences to develop effective, culturally appropriate prevention and treatment strategies. Such strategies include addressing the special mental health needs of diverse populations and disparities in their ability to access care. At the clinical level, cultural competence is essential to providing individualized, customized care that fits the needs of the child and family. It includes the recognition of the unique strengths and resources of the family's culture that could be protective and provide support to children (e.g., involvement of extended family or religious institutions), as well as recognition of cultural stressors, such as tensions that arise between the parental and children's generations due to differences in acculturation.

Culturally competent clinical practice begins with the mental health assessment and should include the family's history of migration, refugee trauma, cultural traditions, language, degree of acculturation, and current experience of being a member of a minority culture. It involves direct service practices such as explicit incorporation of the family's cultural values into treatment, use of culturally similar service providers (or at minimum language interpreters), and may entail adoption of specific cultural practices such as spiritual traditions, involvement of extended families, and cultural mediators. One clinical challenge is that few evidence-based practices have included ethnically diverse subjects and, therefore, modifications to existing evidence-based practices may have to be made. Organizations can incorporate cultural competence through offering culturally specific services and supports, translating printed material into diverse languages, hiring ethnically diverse staff, offering cultural competence training, and partnering with local businesses to cosponsor culturally diverse events.

The Interface of Children's Mental Health with Other Child-Serving Systems

Central to the systems-of-care approach is collaboration among the family, youth, and the providers of services and supports. When multiple providers from different agencies or systems are involved, direct communication is the only way to coordinate care and ensure that all efforts are aimed at the same goals. When it is not possible to meet with representatives from all systems, it becomes crucial for a clinician to learn about basic processes within other systems in order to make appropriate referrals and help parents advocate for necessary services. The following descriptions, summarized in Table 27-4, highlight features of the major child-serving systems relevant to clinical practice. Mental health and substance abuse services are discussed together although some states and localities organize and fund them separately.

Primary Health Care

Primary health care is the first system to be involved with a child, optimally starting with prenatal care and continuing with regular well-child visits. The primary care provider (PCP) has the capacity to develop a long-term relationship with the child and parents and is generally the first clinician to learn about a child's emotional, behavioral, or developmental difficulties. The PCP therefore constitutes an important pathway to early identification and treatment of these problems. As noted by Kelleher and colleagues in 2006, a significant percentage of mental health care is provided by PCPs in the United States and other countries, and there have been national efforts to enhance the role of the PCP in providing quality mental health screening and care through improving reimbursement, provision of training and appropriate consultation, and addressing barriers related to information sharing.

The medical home model for children with special health care needs, articulated by the American Academy of Pediatrics (AAP) in 2007 and endorsed by the U.S. Department of Health and Human Services, is one such initiative. Its premise is that the PCP, as a trusted person with whom the child and family have a continuous relationship, is well positioned to be the first point of contact and to provide preventive, acute, and chronic care that is coordinated and integrated with care from other providers. Another effort towards integration is the provision of easily accessible specialty mental health consultation to assist PCPs in providing mental health services. The Massachusetts Child Psychiatry Access Project (MCPAP) and the Washington State Partnership Access Line (PAL) that provide child psychiatric consultation to PCPs are two such examples; other programs have colocated child psychiatrists and other mental health specialists with primary health care providers.

Advocacy for integration of primary health care with care from other systems has been considerable for the early childhood population. These efforts have been strengthened by the National School Readiness Initiative, which provides funds for states to establish Early Childhood Advisory Councils (ECACs) to coordinate efforts of multiple child-serving agencies, as described below.

Early Childhood Services

Multiple systems are relevant to the health and welfare of young children. Among them are health care, child care, Early Intervention (EI), Head Start, Early Special Education, DD services, child welfare in cases of abuse or neglect, and adult mental health, addiction, and domestic

TABLE 27-4	Characteristics of Different Child-Serving Agencies
Primary care	• Separate funding streams, inadequate reimbursement pose barriers to integration with mental health services • Medical home model for children with special needs • Enhanced mental health services in primary care through mental health consultation
Early Childhood Services	• Relevant services include primary health care, child care, Early Intervention, Head Start, Early Special Education, Developmental Disabilities, Child Welfare in cases of abuse or neglect, parental mental health/addiction/domestic violence services • New SAMHSA system-of-care grants for children ages 0 to 8. • Prevention efforts and service integration promoted by state Early Childhood Advisory Councils • Use of alternative diagnostic system DC:0-3R as a way to improve access
Education	• Under Individuals with Disabilities Act (IDEA), child required to have Individualized Education Plan (IEP) • Section 504 of the Vocational Rehabilitation Act allows for individualized plan without full special education designation • Positive Behavioral Support model offers continuum of behavioral supports • School-based mental health services with continuum of supports in the school setting
Developmental Disabilities	• Serves youth with mental retardation and developmental disabilities that impact functioning • High prevalence of comorbidity between developmental and psychiatric disorders • Criteria must be met before age 18–21; eligibility criteria for specific services (e.g., intensive home-based supports) vary by state
Mental Health and Substance Abuse	• Continuum of care from outpatient to inpatient, with regional and community variations • Role of managed care Medicaid in controlling access • School-based mental health services and other integrated mental health models • Addictions often funded separately; underdiagnosed in youth population
Child Welfare	• Mandated reporting of abuse and neglect • Child welfare operates as legal guardian in cases of removal from parental custody • Adoption and Safe Families Act (AFSA) requires early permanency planning • High rates of mental disorders in child welfare population • Difficulty finding appropriate placements may contribute to longer residential placements
Juvenile Justice	• High rates of psychiatric disorders (50–70%) • Recent legislation requiring adult adjudication (punishment vs. rehabilitation) • Disproportionate representation of ethnic and cultural minorities. System-of-care interventions have reduced incarceration (MST, and wraparound) • Defining conduct disorder as a "behavioral" versus "mental health" disorder in some communities poses barrier to youth receiving needed mental health services

violence services. Many states have ECACs to coordinate efforts of these agencies. The intent is to not only support state efforts to implement requirements of the Improving Head Start for School Readiness Act of 2007, but to engage state-level leadership to maximize the councils' potential to drive effective policy decisions for children ages birth to five. ECACs include representatives from Head Start, EI, state educational agencies, child care, and local providers of health and mental health care. The intent is to identify barriers and opportunities for collaboration among the various early childhood programs.

There is a substantial body of research showing that children learn most rapidly in the early years. It is difficult to compensate for missing those opportunities due to developmental and environmental challenges. Children with developmental challenges often face disappointment, social isolation, stress, and frustration. Their difficulties may also affect the well-being of their siblings and families. For these reasons it is imperative that clinicians working with young children know resources available to address their social, emotional, or developmental difficulties and access those services without delay.

EI services were established in 1986 under the federal Program for Infants and Toddlers with Disabilities (Part C of IDEA). EI helps infants and toddlers from birth up to age three who have developmental delays or are at risk for such delays. Services are offered to children from birth up to age three who (1) are not developing typically for their age, (2) have a physical, emotional, or cognitive condition that may cause developmental delays, or (3) are at risk of developmental delays because of biological or environmental factors. Each state decides how EI services are organized and the specific eligibility criteria; in some states EI is housed in DD; others may have separate agencies paired with Early Special Education. When a referral is made, the EI agency must evaluate the child in five developmental areas: cognitive, communication, social/emotional, physical, and adaptive. After eligibility is established, a team develops an Individualized Family Service Plan (IFSP), which specifies the services to be offered. EI services available include speech/language, occupational, and physical therapy; behavior modification and counseling; and an array of family support services. Services are delivered in the most naturalistic setting possible. Children who turn three and are in need of continuing services may be referred to Early Special Education Services administered through the educational system. Head Start is an educational program for low-income children ages 3 to 5. 10% of Head Start slots are set aside for children with special needs, including those with emotional, behavioral, and developmental challenges. All children in foster care are eligible. Early Head Start was initiated in 1995 for children under age 3.

Despite recognition of a high prevalence of emotional and behavioral disorders among young children, mental health services for young children have been largely neglected. The likely reasons for this include lack of an early childhood-trained workforce, problems with applying diagnoses from the DSM-IV to young children, and general attitudes against diagnosing young children with mental disorders. Moreover, early childhood mental health requires a different skill set, including knowledge of early childhood development, how to assess young preverbal children, and how to assess and work with parent–infant dyads. Infant manifestations of mental health disorders may be different from those of older children and adolescents, and are not well-described by the childhood diagnoses in the DSM-IV. For example, a depressed infant may avert his or her gaze, fail to thrive, and be slow to achieve developmental milestones, as opposed to exhibiting sad, angry, or oppositional behavior more likely to be seen in the older child. The DC:0-3R (Diagnostic Classification of Mental Health and Developmental Disorders of Infancy and Early Childhood: Revised Edition) published in 2005 by ZERO TO THREE is more specific to young children and has been adopted by some states to address this need.

Given national data indicating that children with SED have had early referrals for special education and early involvement in child welfare, preventive interventions for SED should occur at a young age, before age 6. Responding to this need, SAMHSA system-of-care grants have been awarded to address high-risk children from ages 0 to 8. Clinicians should also consider how they might advocate for more services to young children with these early risk factors.

Education

The critical role of the educational system in every child's life as the context for a major part of his or her cognitive, social, and emotional development cannot be overemphasized. The school culture is unique in the system of care because, unlike other systems, it serves *all* children and is accountable to the society at large. Students with emotional and behavioral disorders have the highest risk of dropping out of school, which leads to other adverse outcomes such as unemployment, substance abuse, early pregnancy, and involvement with the criminal justice system. National data indicate that children with SED tend to be referred for special education before receiving any other services, making schools an ideal locus for prevention efforts. The Individuals with Disabilities Education Act (IDEA) Amendments of 1997 (PL 105–17) constitute the primary vehicle for ensuring that students with emotional and behavioral disorders receive assessments, services, and supports to enable them to be successful in school. Mental services provided in school settings have become widespread, as they have been shown to improve attendance, improve academic performance, and decrease behavioral problems. According to SAMHSA's web site, the majority of schools now provide a variety of mental health services such as prevention, mental health screening, behavior management, crisis intervention, mental health counseling, milieu-based programs such as intensive day treatment, medication management, and substance abuse services. The latter two services are available but are the least likely to be offered. School-based mental health services have been shown to reduce restrictive out-of-school and out-of-home placements.

A child's mental health problems more often than not manifest in school, making collaboration and information sharing between the mental health provider and teacher or school counselor of utmost importance. Information about the child's functioning in school is a necessary part of the mental health assessment; conversely, the mental health provider's clinical explanation for a child's challenging behaviors is often a key step in helping the school develop positive behavioral support strategies to augment the child's own adaptive capacities. Clinicians should become familiar with the steps involved in screening for special education services, and will usually be asked to provide supporting documentation.

The first level of intervention for a child with an emotional or behavioral disorder who requires "reasonable accommodations" is the development of a written plan under Section 504, led by a 504 coordinator; this level of intervention is not formal special education. If initial interventions are unsuccessful, or if the emotional/behavioral disabilities are more significant and require specialized instruction, the child will be more comprehensively evaluated for special education eligibility under IDEA and a Special Education Coordinator will form an Individualized Educational Plan (IEP) team to develop a detailed plan for intervention.

Developmental Disabilities

Children with DD, including intellectual disability, have higher rates of mental health conditions than the typically developing population, and are often in need of individualized services from multiple agencies. Departments of DD vary from state to state with regard to which conditions are covered and what services are offered. In many states, EI is part of DD and provides the eligibility criteria for children under 3. If EI is not part of DD, a child under 3 would require medical documentation of a functionally impairing disability to receive DD services. Conditions generally covered by DD services include mental retardation, cerebral palsy, epilepsy, autism, and other neurological conditions related to mental retardation or requiring similar services. Eligibility is based on intellectual testing and tests of adaptive functioning such as the Vineland Adaptive Behavior Scales or the Adaptive Behavior Assessment System (ABAS). The developmental disability usually must be present by age 18 to 21, depending on the state. DD services also vary from state to state and may include case management, in-home family support, intensive in-home supports, and 24-hour services in foster care or residential placement. Most states are increasingly emphasizing services that allow clients to stay in their homes and community.

Access to appropriate mental health services may be difficult for youth with co-occurring DD and mental disorders as many physicians and mental health clinicians feel ill-equipped to address this comorbidity. A useful resource to assist with more accurate diagnostic assessment is Fletcher et al.'s 2007 *Diagnostic Manual-Intellectual Disability (DM-ID): A Textbook of*

Diagnosis of Mental Disorders in Persons with Intellectual Disability. In addition, children and youth with DD benefit from specialized case management and individualized team-based service planning to facilitate access to appropriate behavioral health services, which often have to be customized to their needs.

Although LDs are generally not covered by DD, but are addressed within the educational system, they are briefly discussed here because of their relevance to the SED population. Prevalence of LDs in children with attention-deficit hyperactivity disorder, depression, conduct disorders, and other psychiatric conditions may range as high as 25%, compared with an estimated prevalence of 5% to 6% in the general school population. LDs and other DD such as autism spectrum disorders may be underdiagnosed in youth with SED, whose disruptive behavior often attracts more attention. This is problematic as LDs are often implicated in a child's disruptive behavior, and not addressing those problems contributes to the child's continued failure, lack of cooperation, and adverse outcomes. It is thus important for the clinician to investigate possible diagnoses that may gain the child access to developmental services that address his deficits in adaptive functioning.

Public Mental Health System and Substance Abuse Services

States vary widely with respect to how they organize public mental health and substance abuse services. States generally employ managed care strategies to assist with utilization of federal Medicaid funding through locally organized public mental health provider networks. PCPs generally practice separately from public mental health agencies; thus, when a child receives pharmacotherapy from his PCP and counseling from a separate agency, collaboration becomes imperative. However, barriers to coordination of care between the primary care and mental health sectors are common. Traditionally, mental health services have existed on a continuum including outpatient services, day treatment, residential treatment, acute hospital and long-term state hospital. More recently, and influenced by evolving systems of care, mental health services are provided in other settings such as Head Start programs and schools. Lengths of stay in long-term hospitals have decreased in favor of intensive services provided in less restrictive settings, and paraprofessionals serve as clinician "extenders" in community settings.

In a recent report on co-occurring substance abuse and mental disorders, SAMHSA confirmed high rates of co-occurring mental health and substance use problems in youth and adults. Youth receiving mental health services have shown rates of substance abuse disorders (SUDs) ranging from 50% to 80%. SUD is associated with psychosocial and academic deficits, as well as high rates of suicide attempts and greater lethality. SUDs are underidentified and undertreated in children's systems of care. Many mental health programs including residential treatment centers do not have SUD treatment, resulting in the SUDs not being addressed. Most mental health training programs do not offer adequate training in assessment and treatment of SUDs. Moreover, the two systems are often funded and located separately. Despite these problems, the prevailing view is that substance abuse and mental health treatment should be integrated, and that screening and assessment should occur within each system. Clinicians should access educational opportunities to improve their skills in assessment and integrated treatment of mental health disorder and SUD co-occurrence. SAMHSA has sponsored a program known as the Co-Occurring Center for Excellence which provides technical assistance, training, products, and resources in support of best practices for co-occurring disorders.

Child Welfare

It is estimated that as many as 75% of children involved in the child welfare system suffer from mental health disorders. The majority of these children are victims of neglect and/or abuse, and other environmental deprivations, putting them at high risk for attachment- and trauma-related disorders. Unfortunately, the child welfare system generally suffers from lack of resources and ineffective interventions. Too often children are moved from one foster home to another, which may not result in better care than the homes from which they were removed. Inadequate foster care resources often result in delayed discharge of children from mental health facilities. The scant availability of adult mental health and SUD services for low-income parents also contributes to children staying longer than needed in the child welfare system.

Child welfare agencies and family courts are trying new approaches to engage children's families so that children may not need to be removed from their parents' care. These include the use of parent partners to facilitate engagement in treatment; increasing adults' access to mental health, medical, and addictions services; use of evidence-based parent–child interaction therapies; and wraparound programs that address the needs of the entire family in a strengths-based, non-blaming manner. Child welfare agencies are now mandated under the Adoption and Safe Families Act to provide permanency planning for young children in a timely manner. Clinicians should be aware of state abuse and neglect reporting statutes as well as how to access family support services from the child welfare or mental health agency to intervene in the presence of risk factors for abuse or neglect.

Juvenile Justice

National data indicate that as many as 50% to 70% of youth involved with juvenile justice experience serious mental health disorders and associated functional impairment. In spite of the similarities of their populations, the juvenile justice and mental health systems have significant differences in philosophy and service orientation. National concerns about juvenile violence in the 1980s and 1990s led to more pressure towards incarceration and punishment; competing with this trend were federal mandates such as the IDEA and class action lawsuits whose settlements required that appropriate mental health services be offered to juvenile justice involved youth. There are still many barriers to juvenile offenders receiving the services they need. Ethnic minorities are disproportionately represented in the juvenile justice system, especially African-American and Latino youth. The unique needs of female offenders, who have higher reported rates of physical and sexual abuse than the general population, have been poorly addressed. The trend towards establishing mental health services within the juvenile justice system has led to increased funding, but with the unfortunate consequence of costly duplication and uneven quality of services. System-of-care strategies to prevent incarceration such as Henggeler's Multisystemic Therapy (MST), and wraparound have been successful and should be more widely available to this population. Ultimately, juvenile offenders have similar histories as youth with SED, but have had lower rates of mental health services utilization. Prevention strategies are urgently needed, and should target younger children with disruptive behaviors.

An Overview of Community-Based Interventions

A key aspect of the system-of-care movement has been the development and testing of specific intensive community-based interventions that offer alternatives to institution-based approaches for youth with significant mental health needs. Summarized in Table 27-5 and discussed below is a brief overview of some promising evidence-based interventions that have been used effectively in systems of care to achieve the system-of-care goals help kids "stay at home, in school, and out of trouble."

Wraparound

Formal systems of care (as defined in SAMHSA grants and implemented by a number of states) utilize wraparound, an evidence-based intervention. Wraparound is a definable *planning process* that results in a unique set of community services and natural supports that are individualized for a child and family to achieve a positive set of outcomes. Services and supports are "wrapped around" the child and family in their natural environments. Natural supports might include newly located family members who wish to become more involved with the youth; providing

TABLE 27-5	Overview of Some Intensive Community-Based Interventions		
Intervention	Essential Features	Who Provides Services	Where Services are Provided
Wraparound Planning Process	• Family-driven team with facilitator • Strengths-based/use of natural supports	• Any provider selected by team • Use of parent partners and natural supports	Community, home, or clinic
Multisystemic Therapy (MST)	• Ecological case formulation • 24/7 crisis availability • High fidelity to research model	• Clinical MST team (Mental health clinicians, psychiatrist)	Primarily home-based and community-based
Treatment Foster Care (Oregon MTFC model)	• Highly trained staff • Use of intensive behavior modification • Coordinated school/home plans • Family trained from outset	• Foster family and behavioral consultants	Foster home, school/community consultation
Intensive Case Management	• Intensive individualized services with assigned case manager	• Varies; some services by case manager	Usually home or community

support for the youth to develop an area of interest that may enhance his self-esteem; or providing a parent with a "parent partner" who can help her navigate the various child-serving systems. As originally defined by VanDenBerg and Grealish, wraparound planning process is child- and family-centered, builds on child and family strengths, is community-based, culturally relevant, flexible, and coordinated across agencies; it is outcome driven, and provides unconditional care. These components are shown in Table 27-6. Since its inception, wraparound has become well defined as an intervention with increasing attention given to maintaining fidelity to the model especially in relation to outcomes, as described by Bruns and colleagues.

TABLE 27-6	Essential Components of Wraparound

- Efforts are based in the community.
- Wraparound must be a team-driven process involving the family, child, natural supports, agencies, and community services working together to develop, implement, and evaluate the individualized plan.
- Families must be full and active partners at every level of the wraparound process.
- Services and supports must be individualized, built on strengths, and meet the needs of children and families across life domains to promote success, safety, and permanence in home, school, and community.
- The process must be culturally competent, building on unique values, preferences, and strengths of children and families, and their communities.
- Wraparound child and family teams must have flexible approaches and adequate flexible funding.
- Wraparound plans must include a balance of formal services and informal community and family supports.
- There must be an unconditional commitment to serve children and their families.
- The plans should be developed and implemented based on an interagency, community-based collaborative process.
- Outcomes must be determined and measured for the individual child, for the program, and for the system.

Winters and Metz note that the youth and family drive the wraparound team process by providing their vision of how they will know when things are better; selecting the team; identifying goals and desired outcomes of services to address specific needs; evaluating the effectiveness of services; and having a meaningful role in all decisions. The team views the family's expertise about itself as equally important to the professionals' expertise. No decisions are made about care plans without family participation. The team is facilitated by a specialist care coordinator trained in wraparound, and frequently there is also a paid "parent partner" who helps support family engagement in the planning process. The parent partner is a person who has experience raising a child with SED and often has a cultural background similar to the family.

There are some premises in wraparound that represent shifts from traditional ways of delivering services. The care coordinator and parent partner have a primary responsibility to facilitate a "no shame, no blame" atmosphere in the team meetings and model mutual respect. Importantly, the team begins with and maintains a focus on the youth and family's strengths and needs rather than on pathology. The team process facilitates interagency collaboration and all members contribute to identifying resources that promote better outcomes and resolving system barriers and conflicting agency mandates. If a plan is not successful in achieving its goals, the plan is understood as needing revision, not that the family should be ejected from services as having been uncooperative. Finally, rather than being driven by the priorities and limitations of categorical agencies (education, child welfare, juvenile justice, etc), the wraparound planning process must have access to flexible, noncategorical funding. Such funds can be spent for a broad array of home- and community-based supports such as home-based therapy, respite, and mentoring services. They may also be available to address individual needs important to treatment success (e.g., time-limited assistance with housing). Interventions designed to reinforce strengths of the child or youth and family may include nontraditional therapies such as specific skills training, mentored work experiences, or lessons to develop a youth's specific talents.

Wraparound is a team-based planning process, not a clinical treatment, and as such it must be informed by comprehensive clinical assessment and make use of evidence-based interventions. To be successful, interventions should be culturally relevant and able to promote sustained engagement of the child and family. Although not a clinical intervention per se, the wraparound process does offer a good deal of personal support and in so doing can promote increased self-esteem and adaptive functioning in the child and family.

Multisystemic Therapy

Multisystemic therapy (MST) was developed as an intensive home- and community-based family treatment model for youth at risk of out-of-home placement because of serious emotional and behavioral problems. It was developed for juvenile offenders, but has been successfully applied to youth in the child welfare system at risk for psychiatric hospitalization, and violent sex offenders. MST is an intensive intervention lasting 3 to 5 months; all services are provided by the MST team, which is in contrast to wraparound as a planning process only. MST interventions follow from a comprehensive assessment of the child and family using a social ecological model. MST has been carefully implemented in each new site to ensure adherence to the model. There have been nine randomized, controlled trials demonstrating its efficacy. One of the drawbacks to the full implementation of MST is the cost of full adherence to the model, and for that reason its wide implementation has been limited. This, however, is a universal issue in the transporting of well-researched treatment models to "real world" contexts.

Multidimensional Treatment Foster Care

Multidimensional Treatment Foster Care (MTFC) is a specific evidence-based treatment foster care model developed by the Oregon Social Learning Center as a home-based alternative to residential treatment for youths with mental health needs or antisocial behavior. MTFC includes close supervision of foster parents by experienced therapists who train them in behavior modification with consistent application of positive reinforcement and consequences. Two randomized controlled trials demonstrated superiority of MTFC to treatment as usual for juvenile justice-involved youth, and another study favored MTFC over treatment at a state psychiatric hospital. MTFC has also been applied successfully to troubled youth in the child welfare system and to address the needs of preschoolers with aggressive and oppositional behavior.

Intensive Case Management

Case management or care coordination is a frequent strategy used in systems of care to coordinate care and ensure access to an array of services that will meet a child and family's needs. Case management has generally been defined as including various functions including needs assessment, service planning and implementation, service coordination and monitoring, and advocacy. Although primary clinicians (including PCPs) often do some case management, children with SED are better served by formal case management in which a specialist case manager or care coordinator is assigned. The case manager either functions as a broker of services or, in more intensive models such as the Children and Youth Intensive Case Management model (CYICM) developed in New York, the case manager offers direct clinical support. There have been at least four randomized controlled trials of case management that have shown positive findings in relation to comparison groups. Variations in the intensity of case management across different models, however, make the findings difficult to assess.

Applications of Systems of Care for the Office-Based Clinician

As indicated in the 2007 American Academy of Child and Adolescent Psychiatry Practice Parameter on Child and Adolescent Mental Health Care in Systems of Care, many aspects of the system-of-care model can be applied by an individual practitioner. For example, psychiatric evaluations can assess factors in the child's wider "ecosystem," such as the contributions of the family's culture, community, and resources available to them in the system of care. This approach necessitates comprehensive gathering of information not only from the child and family, but from all the systems with which they are involved. Evaluation and treatment can be performed in a manner that is collaborative with families, emphasizes their strengths and needs, is driven by their goals, -considers use of community and natural supports, and incorporates the values of wraparound. In addition, by communicating directly with involved clinicians from other agencies, the practitioner can contribute to more coordinated, more integrated care. This may require exploration of funding mechanisms for such coordination. Table 27-7 summarizes factors underlying successful application of system-of-care principles to the office.

Conclusions

The system-of-care paradigm has brought about important reforms in children's mental health, especially for children and adolescents with high mental health needs. System-of-care approaches emphasize care that is individualized to the child and family's needs, well coordinated, driven by the strengths and goals of the family and youth, and is community-based whenever possible. Organized systems of care have developed strategies to coordinate and integrate mental health care with services provided by education, juvenile justice, child welfare, primary care, and DD. With this shift of emphasis towards providing care in the community some new treatment strategies have emerged that are accumulating a solid evidence base, such as MST, wraparound, and treatment foster care. The PCP, mental health clinician, and psychiatrist, each has an important role to play in the system of care and should actively collaborate with other service providers to coordinate care. The individual clinician should also integrate into his or her practice principles of family-driven, youth-guided, and culturally competent care; exploring community-based treatment options; and use of community and natural supports in addition to formal treatment options.

TABLE 27-7	Application of System-of-Care Principles to Office Practice

1. Clinical assessment and treatment approaches should be guided by an understanding of the ecological context of the child and family, incorporating information from all community systems with which they are involved, including formal services as well as natural supports.
2. The clinician should develop collaborative and strengths-based relationships with families, emphasizing partnerships at both the case planning and system planning level.
3. Mental health interventions should be actively coordinated with services by other providers, including primary care providers, and, whenever possible, integrated with interventions provided by other social agencies. This can occur at the case, program, and larger systems level.
4. Services should be culturally competent and should address the needs of underserved, culturally diverse, at-risk populations.
5. To achieve individualization of care for children with significant and complex mental health needs, clinicians should consider a wraparound planning process.
6. Treatment planning in systems of care should incorporate effective interventions supported by the available evidence base.
7. Child and adolescent psychiatrists' roles in systems of care should include, triage, provision of direct service (psychosocial therapies as well as pharmacotherapy), consultation to other service providers, quality improvement, program design, and evaluation and advocacy.
8. Pharmacotherapy should be performed by a physician or medical practitioner who is integrated into the interdisciplinary process and has completed a biopsychosocial assessment, including interviewing the child and his/her parent or caregiver and reviewing relevant ancillary data.
9. The clinician should be familiar with the organization and functioning of the system in which he/she is working in order to advocate effectively for adequacy of resources and practices to meet the needs of children and families served.
10. The clinician and the family share accountability for treatment success. The system of care through its component programs should be accountable for clinical outcomes and actively involved in quality improvement efforts.
11. Services should be delivered in the most normative and least restrictive setting that is clinically appropriate. Children should have access to a continuum of care with assignment of level or intensity of care determined by clinically informed decision-making.
12. Significant attention should be paid to transitions between levels of care, services, agencies, or systems to ensure that care is appropriate, emphasizing continuity of care.
13. Systems of care should incorporate prevention strategies in clinical practice and system design.

Adapted from 2007 AACAP Practice Parameter on Child and Adolescent Mental Health Care in Community Systems of Care.

CASE VIGNETTES

VIGNETTE 1: JOSE, A TODDLER AND CULTURALLY COMPETENT CARE

Jose, a 2.5-year old Latino boy is brought to see his PCP because he is oppositional and not following directions at home. Unfortunately, Jose's family (his single mother and two older children) just moved from a neighboring community and the family is new to this physician. It is not clear why Jose had not received regular health care before this visit. His mother speaks Spanish but her English is adequate. She provides limited information about Jose's history and appears to be anxious. On examination, Jose has significant speech delay, makes poor eye contact and is small for his age, although he is clean and seems well cared for. Jose's new PCP recognizes that Jose's mother is very stressed and schedules another longer visit with a Spanish language interpreter, and another staff member watches Jose while he speaks with the mother alone. He learns that Jose's mother recently left her violent alcoholic husband, and is anxious that he will find the family. The PCP expresses his support for her courage in doing the right thing for her family. He consults with the clinic social worker and makes a referral to a Latino specialty clinic that provides domestic violence and mental health services for Jose's mother. He makes an EI referral for Jose, who easily qualifies and he starts receiving speech therapy, behavioral support services, and nutritional counseling in the home. The Latino clinic offers case management and is able to get Jose's family some food assistance. The physician was periodically contacted by the EI specialist who gave him updates so that he could remain aware of Jose's progress. He scheduled a return visit 1 month later.

Discussion

Jose's PCP incorporated several system-of-care approaches. He showed cultural competence in scheduling extra time to talk to Jose's mother with a Spanish interpreter. He developed an ecological understanding of Jose's difficulties by talking with her in detail about the family situation. He identified the family's strengths and was nonblaming towards Jose's mother. He immediately referred Jose for EI services to address his developmental delay, and made a culturally appropriate referral for his mother.

VIGNETTE 2: AMANDA, A TEEN IN THE CHILD WELFARE SYSTEM

Amanda is a 14-year-old girl in foster care who is brought to a mental health counselor's office by her foster mother because she threatened to kill herself at school. The school wants her evaluated before returning. The counselor learns that Amanda has recently moved from another foster home in another county because the previous foster parent could not handle her rebellious behavior. She is on several medications, including a stimulant for ADHD and an antidepressant for depression. The foster mother wonders if the young lady might have bipolar disorder because she is so moody; she does not get along with peers at her new school, and often disrupts the class. Because Amanda is so new to her, the foster mother has little information about Amanda's history. The counselor meets alone with Amanda and is able to establish some rapport by asking Amanda about her interests. Eventually, she learns that Amanda was sexually abused by an older teenager in the previous foster home 3 months ago. She never told anyone about it but started using drugs, became more and more depressed, and started staying out on the streets late at night. She hates school and said she was suicidal to get out of attending. The therapist compliments Amanda on her forthrightness and ability to tell her story. She explains her dilemma that she does not want to act against Amanda's desire not to tell about the sexual abuse, but explains that she is legally required to report it. She tells Amanda she would like to see her again and will give her support while this incident is investigated. She contacts the school and explains that Amanda needs a higher level of services within the school and recommends screening for special education services based on an emotional and behavioral disorder. She offers to speak with the school counselor to explain her view of Amanda and offer recommendations. She schedules another meeting with Amanda and her foster mother to help them start communicating about what Amanda has experienced and what her needs are. She contacts the county care coordination unit and requests a care coordinator be assigned to Amanda's case for a period of time until a comprehensive service plan can be developed, including enhanced school services, assignment to a young adult peer mentor, a complete drug and alcohol evaluation, and a medication evaluation through the mental health center. She diagnoses Amanda with PTSD and recommends a course of individual therapy for her.

Discussion

Amanda's presentation demonstrates many of the problems in the child welfare system including instability of placements and exposure to abuse in foster care; lack of continuity of medical and mental health records; acting out and substance use in youth exposed to abuse and neglect; and barriers to youth receiving adequate services in the educational system. The mental health counselor was able to use youth-appropriate interviewing strategies, and had knowledge of county-based care coordination services that could help her develop a comprehensive, individualized plan of care in collaboration with Amanda and her foster mother.

REFERENCES

American Academy of Child and Adolescent Psychiatry. Practice parameter for child and adolescent mental health care in community systems of care. *J Am Acad Child Adolesc Psychiatry.* 2007;46(2):284–299

American Academy of Pediatrics Council on Children With Disabilities, Duby JC. Role of the medical home in family-centered early intervention services. *Pediatrics.* 2007;120:1153–1158.

Burns BJ, Goldman SK. Promising practices in wraparound for children with serious emotional disturbance and their families. *Systems of Care: Promising Practices in Children's Mental Health.* Washington DC: Center for Effective Collaboration and Practice, American Institute for Research. Vol. IV:77-100; 1998. Available at: http://mentalhealth.samhsa.gov/cmhs/ChildrensCampaign/practices.asp

Burns BJ, Hoagwood K. *Community Treatment for Youth: Evidence-Based Interventions forSevere Emotional and Behavioral Disorders.* New York: Oxford University Press; 2002.

Bruns EJ, Suter JC, Force MM, Burchard JD. Adherence to wraparound principles and association with outcomes. *J Child Family Studies.* 2005;14:521–534.

Bruns EJ, Suter JC, Leverentz-Brady MA. Relations between program and system variables and fidelity to the wraparound process for children and families. *Psychiatric Serv.* 2006; 57:1586–1593.

Fletcher R, Loschen E, Stavrakaki C, First, M., eds. *Diagnostic Manual—IntellectualDisability (DM-ID): A Textbook of Diagnosis of Mental Disorders in Persons with Intellectual Disability.* Kingston, NY: NADD Press; 2007.

Henggeler SW, Shoenwald SK, Borduis CM, Rowland MD, Cunningham PB. *Multisystemic Treatment ofAntisocial Behavior in Children and Adolescents.* New York: Guilford; 1998.

Kelleher KJ, Camp JV, Gardner WP. Management of pediatric mental disorders in primary care: where are we now and where are we going? *Curr Opin Ped.* 2006;18:649–653.

Knitzer J. *Unclaimed Children: The Failure of Public Responsibility to Children and Adolescents in Need of Mental Health Services.* Washington, DC: The Children's Defense Fund; 1982.

Manteuffel B, Stephens RL, Brashears F, et al.. Evaluation results and systems of care: a review. In Stroul BA and Blau GM, eds. *The System of Care Handbook: Transforming Mental Health Services for Children, Youth, and Families.* Baltimore, MD: Paul H. Brookes Publishing Co.; 2008; 25–70.

New Freedom Commission on Mental Health. Achieving the promise: transforming mental health care in America. Final Report. DHHS Pub. No. SMA-03-3832. Rockville, MD; 2003.

Pumariega, AJ, Winters NC, eds. *Handbook of Child and Adolescent Systems of Care: The NewCommunity Psychiatry.* San Francisco: Jossey-Bass; 2003.

Rowland MD, Halliday-Boykins CA, Schoenwald SK. *Multisystemic Therapy with youth exhibiting significant psychiatric impairment.* In: Epstein MH, Kutash K, Duchnowski AJ, eds. *Outcomes for Children with Emotional and Behavioral Disorders and Their Families.* Austin, TX: Pro-Ed; 2005; 401–420.

Stroul BA, Blau GM, Sondheimer DL. Systems of care: a strategy to transform children's mentalhealth. In Stroul BA and Blau GM, Eds. *The System of Care Handbook: Transforming Mental Health Services for Children, Youth, and Families.* Baltimore, MD: Paul H. Brookes Publishing Co.; 2008; 3–24.

Stroul B, Friedman R. *A System of Care for Children and Youth with Severe Emotional Disturbances* (rev ed.) 1986. Washington (DC): Georgetown University Child Development Center, National Technical Assistance Center for Children's Mental Health; 1986.

U.S. Department of Health and Human Services. Mental health: A Report of the Surgeon General. Rockville, MD: U.S. Department of Health and Human Services, Substance Abuse and Mental Health Services Administration, Center for Mental Health Services, National Institutes of Health, National Institute of Mental Health; 1999.

VanDenBerg JE, Grealish. Individualized services and supports through the wraparound process: philosophy and procedures. *J Child and Family Studies.* 5:7–21; 1996.

Winters NC, Metz PW. The wraparound approach in systems of care, *Psychiatr Clin N Am.* 2009;32:135–151.

ZERO TO THREE: Diagnostic Classification. *Diagnostic Classification of Mental Health and Developmental Disorders of Infancy and Early Childhood: Revised Edition.* Arlington, VA: ZERO TO THREE/National Center for Clinical Infant Programs; 2005.

RELEVANT WEBSITES

1. **Substance Abuse and Mental Health Administration (SAMHSA) Information on Systems of Care.**
   a. Information on Systems of Care. Available at: http://mentalhealth.samhsa.gov/child. Accessed 9/7/09.
   b. Values and Principles of Systems of Care. Available at: http://mentalhealth.samhsa.gov/publications/allpubs/Ca-0029/default.asp. Accessed 9/7/09.
   c. Range of Community-based Services in Systems of Care. Available at: http://mentalhealth.samhsa.gov/publications/allpubs/CA-0014/default.asp. Accessed 9/7/09.
   d. Information on Family-driven Care. Available at: http://www.systemsofcare.samhsa.gov/headermenus/deffamilydriven.aspx. Accessed 9/7/09.
2. **Federation of Families for Children's Mental Health.** The vision and mission of the Federation of Families for Children's Mental Health. Claiming Children 2001; summer. Available at: http://www.ffcmh.org. Accessed 9/7/08.
3. **Youth M.O.V.E.** (Motivating Others Through Voices of Experience). Available at: http://youthmove.us/. Accessed 11/4/09.
4. **Center for Mental Health Services Comprehensive Community Mental Health Services for Children and Their Families Program.** Available at: http://mentalhealth.samhsa.gov/cmhs/childrenscampaign/ccmhs.
5. **Information on Early Intervention and IDEA Part C:** National Early Childhood Technical Assistance Center. Available at: http://www.nectac.org/partc/partc.asp. Accessed 11/4/09.
6. **Links to Developmental Disability sites of the U.S. States.** Available at: http://www.ddrcco.com/states.
7. **SAMHSA Co-Occurring Center for Excellence (COCE).** Available at: http://coce.samhsa.gov/. Accessed 11/4/09.
8. **National Wraparound Initiative.** Available at: http://www.rtc.pdx.edu/nwi/

RECOMMENDED READINGS

1. Stroul BA, Blau GM. *The System of Care Handbook: Transforming Mental Health Services for Children, Youth, and Families.* Baltimore, MD: Paul H. Brookes Publishing Co.; 2008; 25–70 (most recent, comprehensive book on systems of care).
2. American Academy of Child and Adolescent Psychiatry. Practice parameter for child and adolescent mental health care in community systems of care. *J Am Acad Child Adolesc Psychiatry.* 2007;46(2):284–299.

REVIEW QUESTIONS

1. Which of the following is a CASSP Value?
   a. Services should be individualized
   b. Services should be culturally competent
   c. Families should be full partners in all aspects of treatment and system planning
   d. Services should be coordinated and integrated with services from other agencies
   e. All of the above

2. Which community-based intervention has the strongest evidence base for youths involved with juvenile justice?
   a. Treatment foster care
   b. Multisystemic Therapy
   c. Intensive case management
   d. Wraparound

3. Which would be the most appropriate referrals for a two year-old boy with motor delays?
   a. Head Start
   b. Medical evaluation
   c. Early Intervention evaluation
   d. Early Special Education

4. Which advocacy organization represents young adults who have been recipients of mental health services?
   a. NAMI
   b. Federation for Families
   c. Youth M.O.V.E.
   d. SAMHSA

5. Which of the following are not typically included in cultural competence approaches?
   a. Cultural assessment questionnaires
   b. Language interpreters
   c. Cultural mediators
   d. Traditional healing
   e. Culturally similar therapists

Answers: 1-e; 2-b; 3-b; c; 4-c; 5-a

INDEX

Page numbers followed by *f* and *t* indicate figures and tables, respectively.